"FATS" IN FACT

BY

LAURIE WRIGHT

WITH A MEMOIR FROM ERNIE ANDERSON

AND SPECIAL CONTRIBUTIONS BY
(in alphabetical order)

Morten Clausen Gene Deitch
Henry Francis Howard Rye
Courtney Williams/Nigel Haslewood

To Ron Jewson
a colleague sorely missed

ISBN 0 902391 14 3

Published by Storyville Publications and Co. Ltd
66 Fairview Drive, Chigwell, Essex IG7 6HS, England.

Binding by Petam Bookbinding Co. Ltd., Trinity Street, Enfield, Middx.

CONTENTS

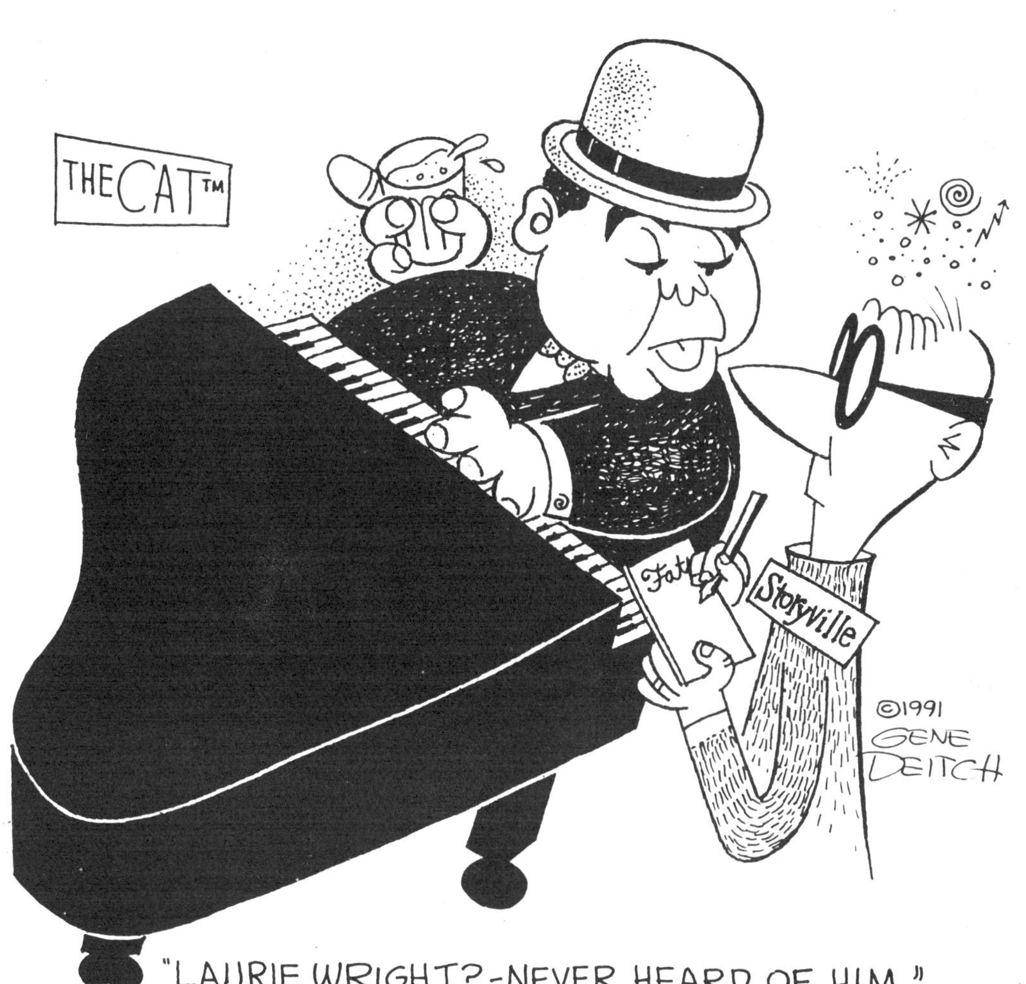

"LAURIE WRIGHT? -NEVER HEARD OF HIM."

FOREWORD

During his life, Thomas Wright "Fats" Waller spread oodles of Happiness and Joy. In radio interviews "Fats" was often asked for a definition of swing, jazz or whatever, and one reply he gave was, "You get that right tickin' rhythm man, and it's on!"

"Fats" was a Great Musician, a Great Composer and a Great Entertainer. I heard "Fats" the first time on a recording at the age of nine, and the inspiration he gave me was tremendous and will always be with me. Hearing him play and sing, with the side comments should lift anyone's spirits. He was a Master!

Laurie Wright, Ernie Anderson and all who contributed to this book have devoted much time and love in putting it all together.

My thanks to you.

Ralph Sutton

INTRODUCTION

This is a completely new study of the career and works of Thomas "Fats" Waller, and the reader might be excused for asking why yet another book on Fats when so many have already been published.

The answer is found quite simply in the title I have chosen (whichever way you care to interpret it), for all too often previous volumes have been more concerned with legend, myth and exaggeration than with what actually happened.

Although my interest in Waller's music goes right back to my first involvement with jazz, he was then but one of many figures whose music delighted me, and I first became involved in him from a publishing point of view when, at the time we were preparing the first edition of *Storyville* magazine, Bob Kumm wrote from New York. He asked if I would like to serialise his up-dated Waller discography. The answer was an unqualified "yes", and its forthcoming appearance was duly announced in our very first issue.

When Bob's manuscript arrived, I was somewhat disappointed to find that it was a xerox of Roy Cooke's revision of John R.T. Davies's original work, published in 1953 by the "Friends of Fats". In this, Bob had been entering microgroove catalogue numbers, but apart from noting the existence of the odd broadcast title, had done no new research.

Roy Rhodes fortunately had an almost complete collection of Waller recordings in some form or another and he volunteered to make these available. Together we sat and listened and made notes and our findings were serialised in *Storyville,* issues 2 to 12 using the same generic title as before.

It had been my intention to gather this material together with the notes and amendments which were already beginning to arrive from enthusiasts world-wide into a booklet to be published a year or so later and, in fact, I had almost completed the manuscript when a bombshell in the guise of a set of Victor recording sheets (courtesy of Roy Cooke) dropped into my hands. These revealed that much of what had been believed was inaccurate or incomplete. At the same time I had begun to acquire microfilm of the Negro Press in America and it soon became apparent that with all this new information, I should go right back to the beginning.

However, other more pressing matters occupied my attention, although for twenty-odd years I have been carefully gathering and filing information. Finally, in 1989 I began to assemble this mass of information into a chronological sequence. That done, I checked through previously published works and noted discrepancies where they occurred and sought to resolve them. In some cases this has not been possible and, as in my previous books, I have left the reader to assess the evidence and reach his or her own conclusion.

Also, as in previous books, I have attempted to provide a means of identifying which take may be held on a microgroove or other issue of the many alternative takes which exist. As far as possible beginnings and endings have been avoided (as these can easily be edited out) and where there are vocals these have usually provided a key. It has not always been easy and I have sought the help of a number of other enthusiasts in this respect and Roy Cooke, John R.T. Davies, Joyce and Doug Onslow and Louis Mazetier have all contributed and must be thanked. Special thanks are also due to my wife Peggy who has spent many, many hours listening with me and transcribing lyrics.

The book also contains a number of special features. Ernie Anderson responded most enthusiastically when I asked if he would write a short piece on the Carnegie Hall Concert which he promoted and promised "about 3,000 words" ... but it grew, and grew into the lengthy reminiscence you will find within. Henry Francis had written a piece on 'Stride Piano' for *Storyville* and had revised and re-written it with special reference to Waller for inclusion in the book when the project was first discussed. He too has updated his piece for inclusion here. The piano roll section has benefitted from the attentions of a number of specialist collectors as has the section devoted to Waller's compositions and copyrights. The visits to Europe have been enhanced by detailed research from Jo Beaton, Howard Rye, Alf Lavér and Morten Clausen as well as anecdotal material from those who saw and heard Fats and photographs and other visual material has come from many sources and is noted as appropriate.

At a very early stage I decided that I would not attempt to list microgroove, tape and CD issues as these are constantly being issued and deleted and, after consultation with Howard Rye he has agreed to compile these as a separate volume which can then be updated as required.

What you hold in your hands is the end result. It is not complete; no book of this nature ever is, and if you can add even one small fact, I shall be pleased to hear from you provided you give the source of your information.

Laurie Wright,
Chigwell, December 1991

ACKNOWLEDGEMENTS

The following have contributed information to the present volume, for which grateful thanks is due:

Abrams, Max
Airey, Les
Akeroyd, Ernest H.
Allen, Walter C.

Banfi, Mario
Barazetta, Giuseppe
Bastin, Bruce
Benford, Tommy (d)
Bennett, David
Besson, Pierre
Binyon, Larry (ts)
Blachman, Stanley L.
Boas, Günter H.
Burgis, Peter
Bushkin, Joe (p)

Cangardel, P-F
Carey, Dave
Carmichael, Hoagy (p)
Carr, Peter
Casey, Al (g)
Cheatham, A.A. 'Doc' (t)
Chisholm, George (tb)
Chivers, Eric
Clausen, Morten
Coldham, Reg
Coller, Derek
Collinson, John,
Cooke, Roy M.
Cowans, Herbie (d)
Crawford, Ken Jr.
Crump, Charlie
Cundall, Tom

Dalal, Jehangir B.
Davies, John R.T
Davis, Reg
Daylie, Holmes "Daddy-O"
Debroe, Georges
Delaunay, Charles
Dierckx, Léon
Dixon, Dave
Dobell, Doug
Douglas, J. Harold
Driggs, Frank
Duffy, Michael C.

Engstrøm & Sødrings Musikforlag

Fortier, Ray
Frankel, Mervyn
French, David
Freeman, Lawrence 'Bud' (ts)

Gaines, Lee
Gladen, Dave
Graf, Bob
Griffiths, David
Guerin, Daniel
Guiter, Jean-Paul

Hällström, Carl
Hardy, J.M.
Harris, Sheldon
Harvey, Kitty and Jack F.
Haslewood, Nigel
Heinz, John G.
Hilbert, Bob
Hofmann, Ralph
Holley, John
Holmes, D.V.
Howard, Darnell (reeds)
Howard, Earle (p)
Hunter, Alberta

Jackson, Franz (ts)
James, George (as)
Jennings, Ian
Jewson, Ron
Jouet, Jean

Kaminsky, Max (t)
Kennedy, Peter

Kirkeby, Ed.
Kuhoupt, Shirley
Kukla, Barbara
Kumm, Bob

Laird, Ross
Lasker, Steven
Lavér, Alf
Laverdure, Michel
Lipskin, Mike
Loudon, Don

Mackenzie, Harry
Macnic, Ray P.
Magnusson, Tor
Malham, Pat
Marquerie, Antonio,
Mazetier, Louis (p)
Minish, Geoffrey
Mitchell, Jack
Mitchell, Raymond F.
Morgenstern, Dan
Mueller, Klaus D.
Mundell, Hazel
Muscutt, Les, (g)
Dean-Myatt, Bill

Nevers, Daniel
Nicolaus, Dr. Peter
Nishijima, Tony

Onslow, Joyce & Doug

Panassié, Hugues
Parker, Henry (FW's cousin)
Parry-Jones, Mr. & Mrs. J.C.
Peak, Don
Peltier, Etienne
Pepper, Antony
Pernet, Robert
Pfau, Michel
Philippi, Hans
Pilkington, Art
Pozzi, Giovanni

Rains, Richard
Razaf, Andy
Rhodes, Roy E.
Richner, Hansjürg
Rust, Brian

Scherman, Bo
Shacter, Jim
Sherburn, Nevill
Simmen, Johnny
Skerritt, Freddie (ts)
Smith, Derek Hamilton
Smith, Harrison
Smith, John (g)
Snowden, Elmer, (bj)
Solgaard, Ib
Solsona, Pedro
Stevens, Norman
Stroud, Peter
Sugiyama, Yusaku
Sutcliffe, Mike
Suykerbuyk, Eugeen
Swinbanks, Eric

Taylor, Phil
Taylor, Eva
Temple, Henry M.
Thompson, Kay, C. (p)
Thornton, Theo
Traill, Sinclair
Turner, Alan

Utermahlen, G. Carroll

Vollmer, Al
Voran, Pierre
Vreede, Max E.

Wadley, Johnny
Walker, Edward S.
Waller, Maurice (Fats's son - p)
Wante, Steve
Warner, Tom
Webb, Ray
Whittle, John K.R.
Whyatt, Bert
Wilby, Ross
Wilkins, Dave (t)
Willé, Vernon
Williams, Bobby (t)
Williams, Courtney (t)
Williams, Franc (Francis) (t)
Wilmer, G.A.
Wilmer, Val
Wilson, John
Wondraschek, Ralph

The following books have been consulted with profit:

Albertson, Chris	*Bessie. A Biography of Bessie Smith.* Published by Barrie & Jenkins, London 1972.
Allen, Walter C.	*Hendersonia The Music of Fletcher Henderson and his Musicians* Published by the author as Jazz Monographs No. 4, N.J. 1973.
Basie, Count	*Good Morning Blues* An autobiography as told to Albert Murray. Published by William Heinemann Ltd., London 1986.
Biagioni, Egino	*Herb Flemming a jazz pioneer around the world* Published by Micrography, 1978.
Brown, Scott E. and Hilbert, Robert	*James P. Johnson A Case Of Mistaken Identity* Published by Scarecrow Press and the Institute of Jazz Studies, Rutgers University, Metuchen, N.J. 1986.
Bushell, Garvin	*Jazz From The Beginning* as told to Mark Tucker. University of Michigan (U.S.) and Bayou Press, Oxford (U.K.) 1988.
Chilton, John	*McKinney's Music: A bio-discography of McKinney's Cotton Pickers* Published by the author, London, 1978.
Chilton, John	*Who's Who Of Jazz*, Revised Edition, published by Macmillan, London, 1989
Clayton, Buck	*Buck Clayton's Jazz World* assisted by Nancy Miller Elliott. Published by Macmillan Press Ltd., London 1986.
Coleman, Bill	*Trumpet Story* English edition published by The Macmillan Press Ltd., London. 1990
Condon, Eddie	*We Called It Music* Jazz Book Club Edition, London, 1956.
Connor, D. Russell	*Benny Goodman, Listen To His Legacy:*Published by Scarecrow Press & Institute Of Jazz Studies, Rutgers University, Metuchen, N.J., 1988.
Cooke, R.M.	Revised Edition of *The Music Of Thomas "Fats" Waller* compiled by John R.T. Davies. Published by "Friends of Fats" 1953.
Dance, Stanley,	*The World Of Count Basie* Published by Charles Scribner's Sons, New York, 1980.
Dance, Stanley	*The World Of Earl Hines* Published by Charles Scribners Sons, New York, 1977.
Dial, Harry	*All This Jazz About Jazz* Published by Storyville Publications and Co. Ltd., Chigwell, 1984.
Dixon, R.M.W. & Godrich, J.	*Blues & Gospel Records 1902-1943* (3rd revised edition) Published by Storyville Publications and Co. Ltd., Chigwell, 1982.
Fox, Charles	*Kings Of Jazz, Fats Waller* Published by Cassell, London, 1960.
Kiner, Larry F.	*The Rudy Vallee Discography* Published by Greenwood Press, Westport, Connecticut, 1985.
Kirkeby, W.T. Ed.	*Ain't Misbehavin'* with Duncan P. Schiedt and Sinclair Traill. Published by Peter Davies, London, 1966.
Kukla, Barbara J.	*Swing City, Newark Nightlife 1925-1950.* Published by Temple University Press, 1991.
Lange, Horst H.	*Die Deutsche "78er" Discographie der Hot-Dance-und Jazz-Musik 1903-1958.* 2nd Edition. Published by Colloquium Verlag, Berlin 1978.

Lord, Tom — *Clarence Williams.* Published by Storyville Publications and Co, Ltd., Chigwell, 1976.

Magnusson, Tor — *Fats Waller with Gene Austin on the record* from *Journal of Jazz Studies, Vol. 4, No. 1,* New Brunswick, N.J., 1976.

Panassié, Hugues — *Cinq Mois A New York.* Published by Editions Corréa, Paris, 1947.

Rust, Brian — *Jazz Records 1897-1942, A-Z,* 2 volumes. 5th Revised edition: Published by Storyville Publications and Co. Ltd., Chigwell, 1983.

Rust, Brian — *The Victor Master Book Vol. 2.* Published by the author, 1969.

Schiffman, Jack — *Uptown: The Story of Harlem's Apollo Theatre* Published by Cowles Book Company, Inc. New York, 1971.

Sears, Richard S. — *V-Discs: A History and Discography.* Published by Greenwood Press, 1980.

Shaw, Arnold — *The Street That Never Slept.* Published by Coward, McCann & Geoghegan, Inc. New York, 1971.

Strateman, Dr. Klaus — *Negro Bands On Film. Volume 1: Big Bands 1928-1950.* Published by Uhle & Kleimann, 1981.

Sudhalter, Richard M., — *Bix Man & Legend* with Philip R. Evans and William Dean-Myatt. Published by Quartet, London, 1974.

Travis, Dempsey J. — *An Autobiography Of Black Jazz.* Published by Urban Research Institute, Inc., Chicago 1983.

Vreede, Max — *Paramount 12/13000 Series* Published by Storyville Publications and Co. Ltd., London E17, 1971.

Vreede, Max — *The Paramount Matrix Files.* Unpublished.

Waller, Maurice and Calabrese, Anthony — *Fats Waller* Published by Cassell Ltd., London, 1977.

Wells, Dicky — *The Night People* as told to Stanley Dance. Published by Robert Hale & Company, 1971.

Wiedemann, Erik — *Jazz i Denmark.* Published by Gyldendal, Copenhagen, 1982.

...as have numerous issues of the following magazines, periodicals and newspapers:

Aarhus Stiftstidende
Aftenbladet (Copenhagen)
Aftenposten (Oslo)
Baltimore Afro-American
The Billboard
Birmingham Gazette
Brighton Evening Argus
B.T. (Copenhagen)
Coda
Collectors Items
Dagbladet (Oslo)

Dagens Nyheter (Stockholm)
(Hull) Daily Mail
(Chicago) Defender
Downbeat
The Era
Evening Despatch (Edinburgh)
Glasgow Evening News
Göteborgs Handels-och Sjöfarts-Tidning
Hamilton Spectator
Helsingborgs Dagblad
Hot Notes
International Musician
Jazz
Jazz Information
Jazz Journal
Jyllandsposten
Lloyd's List
Lunds Dagblad
Matrix
Melody Maker
Nationaltidende (Copenhagen)
Music og Film (Copenhagen)
The Needle
New York Age
New York Amsterdam News
New York World-Telegram
Nottingham Journal
Orchestra World
Orkester Journalen
The Performer
Phonograph and Talking Machine Weeky
Pittsburgh Courier
Politiken (Copenhagen)
Radio Pictorial
Radio Times
Recorded Sound
Record Research
Social-Demokraten (Copenhagen)
Southern Daily Echo
The Stage
The Star (Sheffield)
Storyville
Svenska Dagbladet
Sydsvenska Dagbladet

Time
Tottenham and Edmonton Weekly Herald
Variety

Plus sleeve information to various LP issues as noted in the text.

Special thanks are due to the staffs of RCA, New York and RCA, Paris, and to Jeff Walden of the BBC Written Archives Centre, who gave every possible assistance in checking through all available extant material relating to Waller.
Thanks are also due to the staff of the Public Record Office.

Finally, my thanks must go to my wife, Peggy, for her constant support and encouragement in this and so many other things; for having assumed many of my own responsibilities during the final preparation period, for providing a second pair of ears in resolving some difficult points and transcribing lyrics and for her unfailing good humour when confronted with the chaos in our home brought about by literally hundreds of pieces of paper.

Notes To Users and Abbreviations

In the Bio-Discography an *Italic* face has been used as follows: In the linking text for tune titles, magazine, book and newspaper titles, musical shows and films and for direct quotes from whatever source these may come (and please note that these are always exactly as given including all mis-spellings, although occasionally 'sic' is used to emphasise this), as well as occasionally for emphasis. In the discography it is used to indicate uncertainty in the case of names, dates and instruments and, in the case of catalogue numbers, for dubbed issues. The term "Issued on LP" has been used as a blanket term to indicate issues of broadcast transcriptions and an initial issue on other than the originally intended 78 r.p.m. format and may take the form of a disc issued at any speed, a cassette or compact disc, and reference should be made to the separate volume compiled by Howard Rye.

Credits: All record credits are given exactly as on the copy of the original issue seen. Major variants on other issues are noted, but minor changes are not. Nor, to avoid constant repetition, are credits on foreign issues given. As a matter of interest German Electrola issues from the 'Rhythm' period usually use **Fats Waller und sein Orchester;** Italian HMV as **"Fats" Waller e la sua Orch. ritmica;** Spanish issues as **"Fats" Waller y su Ritmo** and so on. Also please note that the presentation of catalogue numbers also follows the copy first inspected. Where a record remained in catalogue for an extended period, frequent changes in typography and layout may have occurred; for example an HMV issue might be BD1234; B.D.1234; BD.1234, all with or without spaces between the prefix and the number! In the case of unissued takes, the information is as given in the company files where this has been available. To save space matrix letter prefixes are not given, as these often indicate nothing more than the size of the wax used.

Many Victor and occasionally other labels give a translation of the title in Spanish, this is not noted, nor are foreign language titles and band credits given.

Where known, the identity of the group and sometimes the actual title of the performance of the reverse of "single-sided" Waller issues is given, but this feature is by no means complete, and is not intended to be as with certain early sessions, even if the information is available, it would be too space consuming to carry out in full.

Alternative takes: The search for unissued versions of Waller performances has continued unabated and almost certainly others, presently unknown, will surface and be issued in future. As far as possible I have attempted to give a verbal description of differences which the listener may use to determine which take of a performance is held, despite the sometimes erroneous information given on reissue sleeves.

International Musician: A special note is required regarding entries in this monthly paper, the journal of the AFM. Listings are given of musicians who are working temporarily within the jurisdiction of a Local, but because of the layout adopted it is sometimes difficult to determine the beginning and ending of musicians in a group. Names are frequently garbled and although an educated guess may often be made, where there is doubt, the name will be shown as listed. Listings may refer to the month in which they are printed, but often refer back to a previous month. Information from Locals is presented in numerical order of the Local numbers, so these do not necessarily offer any chronology, but must be combined with other information where this is available.

The following abbreviations have been used:

Record labels (American unless otherwise noted)

AFCDJ	Association Francais des Collectioneurs de Disques de Jazz (French)
APS	Associated Program Service
ARC	American Record Company
ASR	Alberti Special Record (German) These numbers are derived almost entirely from Horst Lange's work
Ba	Banner
BB	BlueBird
Bm	Biltmore
Br	Brunswick
BRS	British Rhythm Society (American despite the name)
Bu	Buddy
Ce	Century
Ch	Champion
Ci	Circle
Cl	Clarion
Co	Columbia
Com	Commodore
De	Decca
Do	Domino
El	Electrola (German). Note that Horst Lange shows a number of Electrola test pressings which indicate at least an interest in issuing the item in Germany, but as these never made their way into a catalogue they are not listed.
Ge	Gennett
Ha	Harmony
Hg	Harmograph
HJCA	Hot Jazz Club of America
HMV	"His Master's Voice" and used for all issues other than Victor which bear the Dog and Gramophone trade mark. Certain English issues, notably those in the J.O. and J.F. series were intended for export, but were available to special order in the U.K. Although the vast majority of these were pressed at Hayes, Middlesex, some were also pressed in other countries, as were issues in the BD and B series; those known being duly noted. Certain French issues appeared on both the "La Voix De Son Maitre" label and on "Gramophone" using the K- 4-fig number. Also note that some issues in these series were also pressed in Belgium. Those pressed in France bear the legend "Made In France", those with no legend were pressed in Belgium.

Imp	Imperial
JC	Jazz Collector (English)
JSo	Jazz Society
LMS	Liberty Music Shop
Lon	London (English)
Me	Melotone
MW	Montgomery Ward
Od	Odeon
OK	OKeh
Or	Oriole
Pa	Parlophone
PA	Pathé Actuelle
Pe	Perfect
Pm	Paramount
Re	Regal
Ri	Ristic (English)
Rl	Royal (Canadian)
Ro	Romeo
RZ	Regal Zonophone
Sil	Silvertone
Sr	Sunrise
St	Sterling (Canadian)
Te	Tempo
UHCA	United Hot Clubs of America
V-D	V-Disc
Ve	Velvetone
Vi	Victor and RCA-Victor. Note that some issues appeared initially on the Victor label and later on RCA-Victor and possibly even RCA, without any change of catalogue number.
Vo	Vocalion

The following suffixes have been used to denote country of origin:

Au	Australia
Ar	Argentina
C	Canada
Ch	Chile
Cz	Czechoslovakia
E	England
Ei	Eire
Eu	General European distribution
Ex	Export (used on those HMV issues produced specifically for export)
F	France

Fi	Finland
G	Germany
H	Holland (The Netherlands)
In	India
It	Italy
J	Japan
N	Norway
SA	South Africa
Sc	General Scandinavian distribution
Sp	Spain
Sw	Switzerland
Tu	Turkey

Instrumental and other abbreviations used:

acc	accompanied by or accompaniment as appropriate.
as	alto saxophone
bb	brass bass (usually tuba or sousaphone)
bj	banjo
bar	baritone saxophone
bsn	bassoon
bsx	bass saxophone
c	cornet
cel	celeste
cl	clarinet
d	drums
g	guitar
k	kazoo
o	electric organ
p	piano
po	pipe or church organ
sb	string bass
sp	speech
ss	soprano saxophone
stg	steel or Hawaiian guitar
t	trumpet
tb	trombone
ts	tenor saxophone
vn	violin
v	vocal
vb	vibraphone
vc	violoncello

Miscellaneous

NSA National Sound Archive (formerly the British Institute of Recorded Sound)

PRO Public Record Office

UC Used to indicate a legend which appears entirely in upper case or capital lettering. i.e. FATS WALLER'S ORCHESTRA.

UC/lc Used to indicate a legend where only the first letter of each word is upper case. i.e. Fats Waller's Orchestra.

A NOTE FROM FATS

Although Fats Waller is one of the most written about and publicised figures in jazz, there is very little available written by Fats himself. The following was written by him (at least it bears his byline, although Ed Kirkeby may well have had a hand in it) for H.M.V. in 1939 and has previously appeared in 'Jazz Journal'. I am grateful to them both for permission to reproduce it here.

The life of a musician is certainly not a mess of chidlins, and the deeper you get into it, the tougher it gets. Here I am all set to get goin' on another eight week trip out of town when I'm asked to sub for a reviewer or sumthin'. It's such things as these that suggest some of my song titles to me, and in this instance it's *You Must Be Losing Your Mind.*

When I look back at the ground I've covered from way back in 1919 when I wrote my first professional song *Squeeze Me,* I guess I've been more used to being written about, than being on the writing end. Give me a piano to beat up and that's me; but as to this writing business, *I'm like a bear from the fair, I ain't nowhere.*

But there are a couple of things I'd like to say, and number one is: that I'm very glad to see that jazz, that much analyzed, classified, sublimated and much discussed type of music, has finally come back to its pappy *Melody.* Now that the jitterbugs are cooling off, and the Shag is no more, we're beginning to give the old masters a rest, and concocting some melodies of our own.

It is my contention, and always has been, that the thing that makes a tune click is the melody; and give the public four bars of that to dig their teeth into, and you have a killer-diller. And if you doubt this statement just take a look at the weekly Hit Parade.

Now I'm not a cat to preach without practising what I preach, and in all of the long line of hits I have had the fortune to write, there has always been a melodic line. Regardless of how sweet that line, how fast or slow, the good old left hand can always swing it out.

And it's melody that gives variety to the ear. That's what makes popular music endure. The fad of Boogie Woogie piano playing is burning itself out. Why? Because it's too monotonous—it all sounds the same.

I wrote a little tune in Chicago once, and called it the *Jitterbug Waltz.* My idea was to convey the picture of a jitterbug waltzing; thereby indicating a change in his techniques as of today compared with the past; that is, the

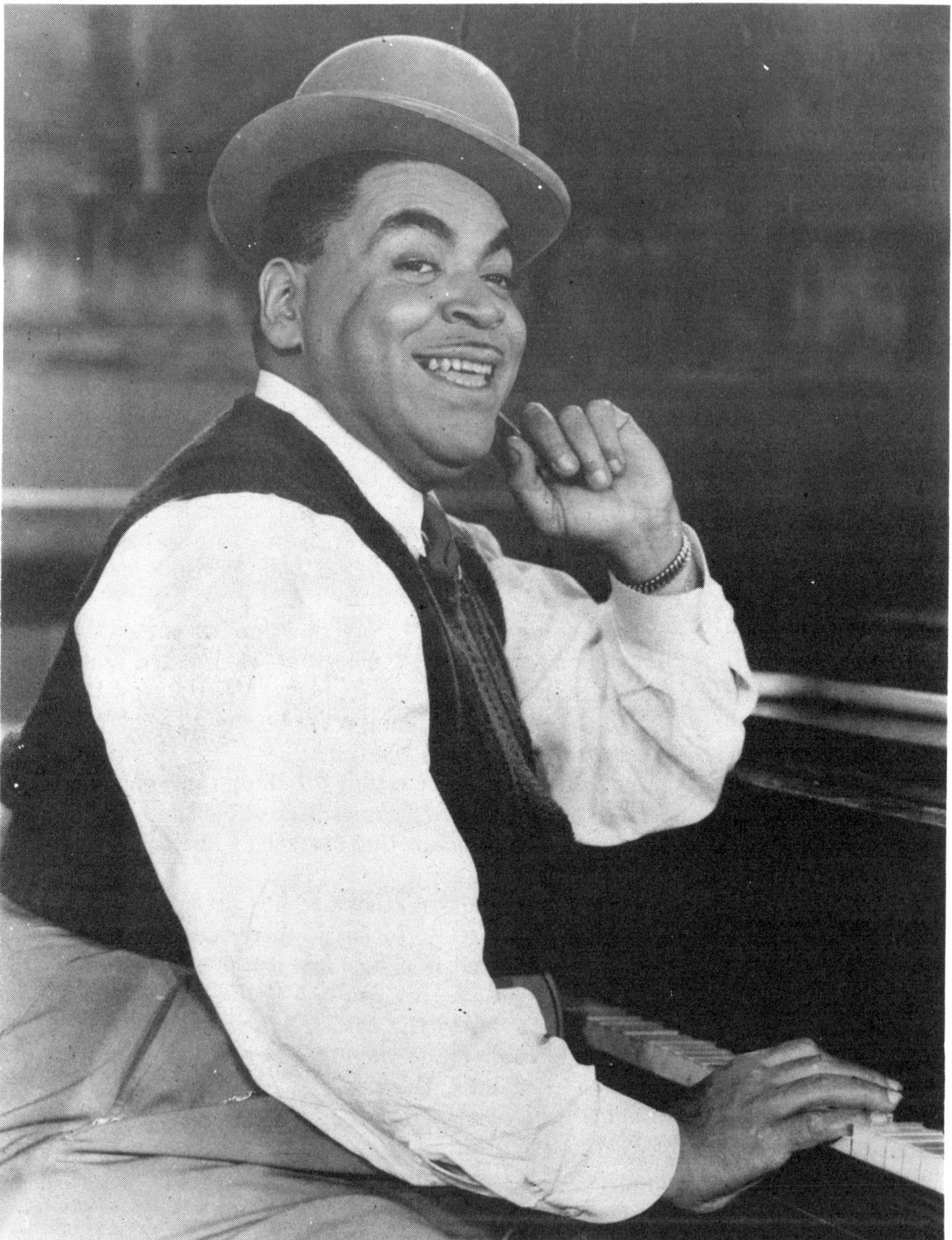

substitution of the romantic and exhilerating 3/4, for the wild and ludicrous hopping about he did in the 4/4 time. And that's what he has now come to enjoy and dance to—melody and rhythm instead of just plain spinebeat.

Ashton Stevens, music critic of the *Chicago-America* wrote: "The organ is the favourite instrument of Fat's heart; and the piano only of his stomach." Well, I really love the organ. I can get so much more colour from it than the piano that it really sends me. I have one at home, and a great many of my compositions originated there. Included is *We Need A Little Love, That's All,* my newest ballad. Ed. Kirkeby collaborated with me on this, and I remember that we stayed up until 11 o'clock the *next* morning finishing it up. That's the way songs are born. I will never forget how on a tour through the English provinces we were playing the Empire Theatre, in Sheffield. After theatre is our usual time for relaxation, and following dinner I roamed restlessly through the beautiful park there. At dawn the birds awakened, and out of their lively chirpings one short strain stood out. I went back to the hotel, and by 10 o'clock that morning with the aid of some delicious Amontillado Sherry, we had finished *Honey Hush.* You see, it's fifty per cent. inspiration and fifty per cent. perspiration.

Another thrill of my life was making the records in my organ album. I'll never forget sitting down at the console of that magnificent organ in the H.M.V. studio on the outskirts of London. It reminded me of that Wurlitzer Grand I played at the Lincoln Theatre in Harlem when I was a kid sixteen years old. I had myself a ball that afternoon, and the records really came easy.

Next to the grand organ there's nothing finer than a magnificent symphony orchestra. I get my kicks out of that kind of music as well as spontaneous jazz. Both kinds for different moods are solid senders, and each type has its place in this everyday world of ours.

THE EARLY YEARS

This first part of the book draws heavily on the accounts of Maurice Waller, in particular, and others and attempts to bring some order into the mass of written material. There are conflicting memories, and it is not always possible to resolve these.

*****

Thomas Wright Waller was one of eleven children, of whom six died in childhood, born to Adeline and Edward Waller at Waverly Place, in Greenwich Village, New York Cty and details of the siblings are by courtesy of Maurice Waller:

Charles A. b. September 1890 d as infant
Edward Lawrence b. 1892
William Robert b 1893
Alfred Winslow b. 1895 d. 1905
Ruth Adeline b. 1902 d. 1095
May Naomi b. 1903
Thomas Wright b. 21 May 1904
Esther b. 1906
Samuel b. 1907
Unnamed boy died in childbirth, 1909
Edith Salome 25 July 1910

*****

In the early 1900s, the Waller family, who were members of the Abyssinian Baptist Church, moved uptown to West Sixty-Third Street when their church moved to the same area. After trying several apartments, they eventually settled into 107 West 134th Street and it was this address that "Fats" gave as his birthplace in an interview with Dolores Calvin in 1942.

*****

It was apparently soon after moving into this apartment that Thomas, aged six, first came into contact with a piano; that owned by an upstairs neighbour. He was fascinated by the instrument and from then on, sought every opportunity to play on each and every piano he encountered. He also took his turn playing the harmonium in the street-corner missions run by his father who was a pastor in the church and in which the whole family were expected to participate.

William Robert was impressed by his younger brother's serious interest in the piano and although purchase of an instrument was beyond the modest income of the family, a step-brother of Adeline, was approached and the outcome was that a piano was installed in the Waller household. However, the cost of piano lessons too was almost too much for Adeline to find from her housekeeping, but eventually, Naomi and Thomas were sent to a Miss Perry, the local teacher. Her approach was the formal one of scales, scales and more scales and lots of practice, and both children quickly lost interest, Naomi before Thomas. Thomas had a wonderful ear and, on hearing and seeing a piece played was very quickly able to replicate it. Miss Perry, realising that Thomas was not prepared to practice his lessons soon advised Mrs Waller that she was wasting her money and formal training ceased for the time being.

At this time Thomas began to play the organ in his church as well as continue his informal musical education wherever he could find someone to show him a new tune. By the time he was old enough to attend school he had acquired a considerable repertoire.

By a fortunate accident of circumstance, the school he attended, Public School 89, had as its music teacher one of those unsung heroes of American music, a Miss Corlias, and through her hands there passed a number of musicians who became well-known on the jazz stage. Recognising the latent talent in the young Waller, she put him to studying string bass and violin as well as piano. The school orchestra was a well-drilled unit and initially Waller was considered too poorly equipped to participate, but was allowed to play the march music to which the boys entered for morning assembly. Eventually, he made the grade and was appointed pianist in the school orchestra and his father, sensing that perhaps if his son wouldn't follow in his own footsteps and become a preacher, he might become a classical pianist, bought tickets for a Paderewski recital at Carnegie Hall as a reward. It was an occasion which was to have an immediate and long-lasting effect on Thomas and, for the rest of his life he maintained a reverence for Carnegie Hall and was to perform there three times himself.

One of the celebrated musicians to pass through P.S.89 was Edgar Sampson, another was pianist Earle Howard and in a letter to me in January 1974, he spoke of his attendance there and gave what is probably the earliest first-hand account of a Waller performance:

My family first moved to Harlem in 1917 and September of that year found me attending P.S. 89 at 135th Street and Lenox Avenue. In assembly one morning, about a month after school started, the superintendent, Mr. Theobaldt, said as he called the morning exercise to order, "If you boys keep in order I have a surprise for you." So, at the end of the session, he called to his office and said, "send Thomas out here." Out from the office stepped a young kid about fourteen years old with a big grin on his fat face. After exchanging the morning greetings, Mr. T. said, "Thomas you have been absent without permission for several days so you must be punished. My punishment is that you must play the piano for the next fifteen minutes. With a smile the fat kid started playing and the assembly started rocking, and that was it.

Me, just two weeks out of the south, began asking questions. My seat-mate Gene Martin, being of a musical family, hipped me to what the cat's name was – "Fats" Waller, and added that he played every day after the news reel at the Lincoln Theater, which was right around the corner. When he came on his first tune was the popular saying that was in music 'Ya Dirty Mistreater' and the balcony would answer with a Charleston beat, "mop-mop". The Charleston hadn't been officially presented at that time. From that time on, until a few weeks before his death, Fats and I enjoyed a great friendship that meant that we would meet and ball every time we worked and met in the same town.

We lived in a part of Harlem that was only a block from the famous Lafayette Theater and three blocks from the Lincoln, and the Martin Smith Music School, where most of the kids attended, was four blocks away. Former students include Edgar Sampson, Johnny Russell, Proco, Dave Martin, etc. Fats and James P. were often in the neighbourhood and often we would meet to hear them get off. It was something for a kid to never forget. From then on, I was hooked on jazz music, so you can understand how I became jazz happy.

August of the year he died was the last time we met. He was working at a place called 'The Cave' in Philadelphia and he gave his usual farewell party for the staff at his hotel, and I was working in the neighbourhood.

*****

Adeline Waller and all her children had a something of a weight problem, and with the onset of diabetes, her health began to deteriorate to the point where she could no longer manage the stairs up to the family apartment, and new accomodation was sought in the locality. It was found at 134th Street and Lenox Avenue, right in the heart of Harlem. The children were encouraged to contribute to the family finances by after-school employment and Thomas's contribution was as a delivery boy for Eckert's Delicatessen. School holidays were also a time to seek more regular employment and, in the summer of 1918 father found Thomas and Naomi jobs with a jewel-box manufacturer. It didn't last though, as they soon discovered that Trinity Church in nearby lower Manhattan had a piano and a sympathetic sexton who allowed the two youngsters to play it in their lunch hour. The inevitable happened, and returns to afternoon work became later and later and, after threats and complaints to his father, Waller quit.

His new job was as a delivery boy for the Immermans, delivering bootleg liquor concealed about his ample person. This was far more amenable employment as it left him time to listen to music where he could and to practise, but it didn't please his family and led to many rows.

*****

It was possibly from this period that Willie 'The Lion' Smith first met Waller as he recounts in his book:

Whenever I would cut out from Leroy's, it was my custom to leave the piano in the custody of a trial horse. In this way I felt I could get my job back when it came time to return.

But there came one time when I really goofed and almost lost the job. That was when I left the stool in charge of a sixteren-year old fat boy, whose name I didn't even know at the time. He used to hang around wherever there was a piano on 135th Street. I was told they let him play the box at the Crescent dime movie down the street when the regular man was off. (This was long before this kid was bugging Maisie Mullins, the pianist-organist at the Lincoln Theater, to let him play the ten-thousand dollar Wurlitzer pipe organ.)

Yeah, man, I'll never forget how good old Fats, when he was still a stripling, would walk into Leroy's eating one of those caramel-covered apples on a stick. He was never without one.

*****

As Earle Howard says, Waller, by now known as "Fats" to his friends and schoolmates, but still as Thomas to his family, was playing the organ at the Lincoln Theatre. According to Maurice Waller this had come about in 1919, because on his way to the Immerman's every afternoon Fats passed the Lincoln and, curious about what went on in this "forbidden territory", bought a ticket to find out. The film impressed him little, but the ability of the pianist who accompanied the film fascinated him, and when the organist took over for the interlude and to play for the stage show, he was in heaven! It was to be the first of many visits which soon became a daily routine and it wasn't long before the pianist, Mazie Mullins, noticed the fat boy who was always in the front row and constantly stared at her. She asked his name and why he kept coming back. Fats told her and she invited him to sit in the pit to watch her better, beginning a fruitful

Right: Pianist/bandleader Earle Howard

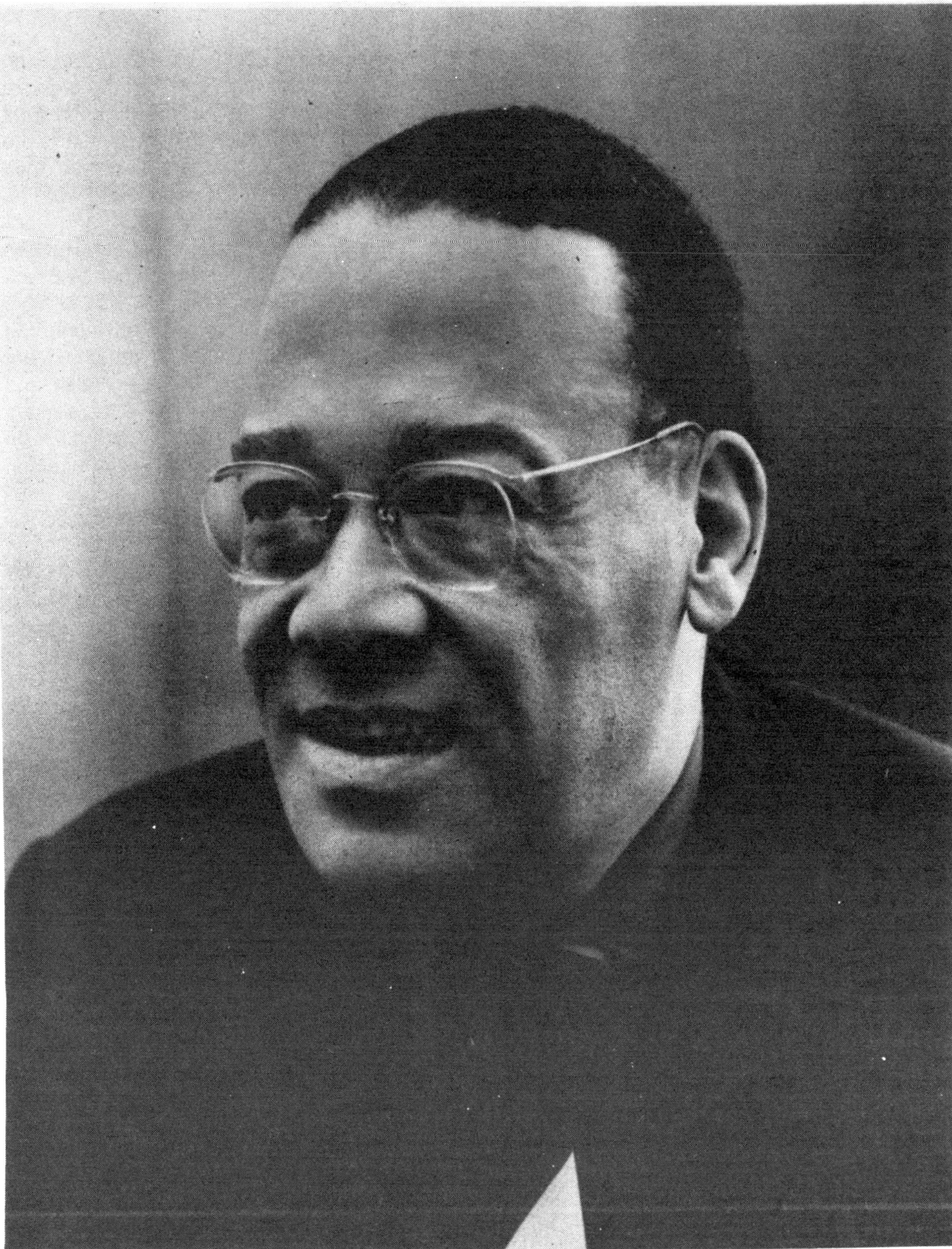

friendship for Waller.

Under her guidance and tuition it was not long before Fats was able to take over the piano stool whenever Mazie Mullins was in need of a break and soon after that he talked the organist (unnamed) into letting him play when he wanted a few moments off. When the organist went down with influenza and a replacement was urgently needed, Waller was able to persuade the theatre owner, Mrs Marie Downes to give him a try. He made out alright and was then engaged for ten days — his first paid job as a musician. His school friends soon found what he was doing and would pack the balcony to encourage him.

Among those who heard Waller during this ten-day period was local drummer Rueben Harris who needed a pianist for a job he had to play on a vacant lot on the corner of Brook Avenue and 165th Street. Would Fats be interested? Of course. It was a gig that was to have far-reaching results for among the people present that night was a young girl who caught the eye of the pianist. She lived just around the corner and Fats succeeded in attracting her attention for most of the evening, and thus began a courtship between Thomas Waller and Edith Hatchett that was doomed to failure. She too came from a middle-class and religious family and to the Waller family must have seemed the perfect choice to get their son back on the straight and narrow path. She might have stood a chance had fate not intervened again in the shape of the offer of a better paying job to the regular organist at the Lincoln (now recovered from his bout of influenza). He accepted, and Marie Downes immediately offered the job to Fats at $23 a week — a huge sum for that time.

Fats was presumably still at school, he was still only fifteen in 1919, and Maurice Waller talks of a year spent at De Witt Clinton High School. However, Sheldon Harris notes Waller touring with Bessie Brown in 1919 and when I queried this with him he pointed me to 'Walleresque' by Harrison Smith in *Record Research* of October 1955. In this Smith states, *In 1919, Waller teamed with George Williams & Bessie Brown and played the Putnam Theatre in Brooklyn, New York as well as other Toby Theatres. ... Fats was later destined to make his first recordings with Williams and Brown*

Williams & Brown's first known recordings were some time after those of Waller and were accompanied by Fletcher Henderson, named both in the files and on the labels, so that if Harrison Smith is correct, and although he is prone to exaggerate for his own self-aggrandisment, there is often a grain of truth in his claims, it would appear that on current knowledge any Waller accompaniments were unissued. I have not been able to confirm a date in 1919 for the Putnam Theater nor for the TOBA tour.

But whether he had left school permanently or not, Waller's life style led to constant battles with his father in which his mother did her best to intervene on hehalf of her son, often to the detriment of her own health. Eventually, after a serious row late in 1920 Fats became very concerned about his mother's obviously failing health; decided to become a reformed character and began to spend as much time at her bedside as he could, joining her in prayer. With all the temptations that surrounded him, it was a good resolution that was going to be difficult to keep, but in the event, he didn't have to try for too long. Adeline Waller suffered a massive stroke in the afternoon of Monday, 8 November 1920, and two days later she passed away. It was a blow from which Fats was never to recover fully for his mother had been the one who had always supported his ambition, even though at times it ran contrary to her own wishes and beliefs and for the rest of his life was likely to fall into a melancholic state at the

Right: An early shot of Fats Waller, date unknown

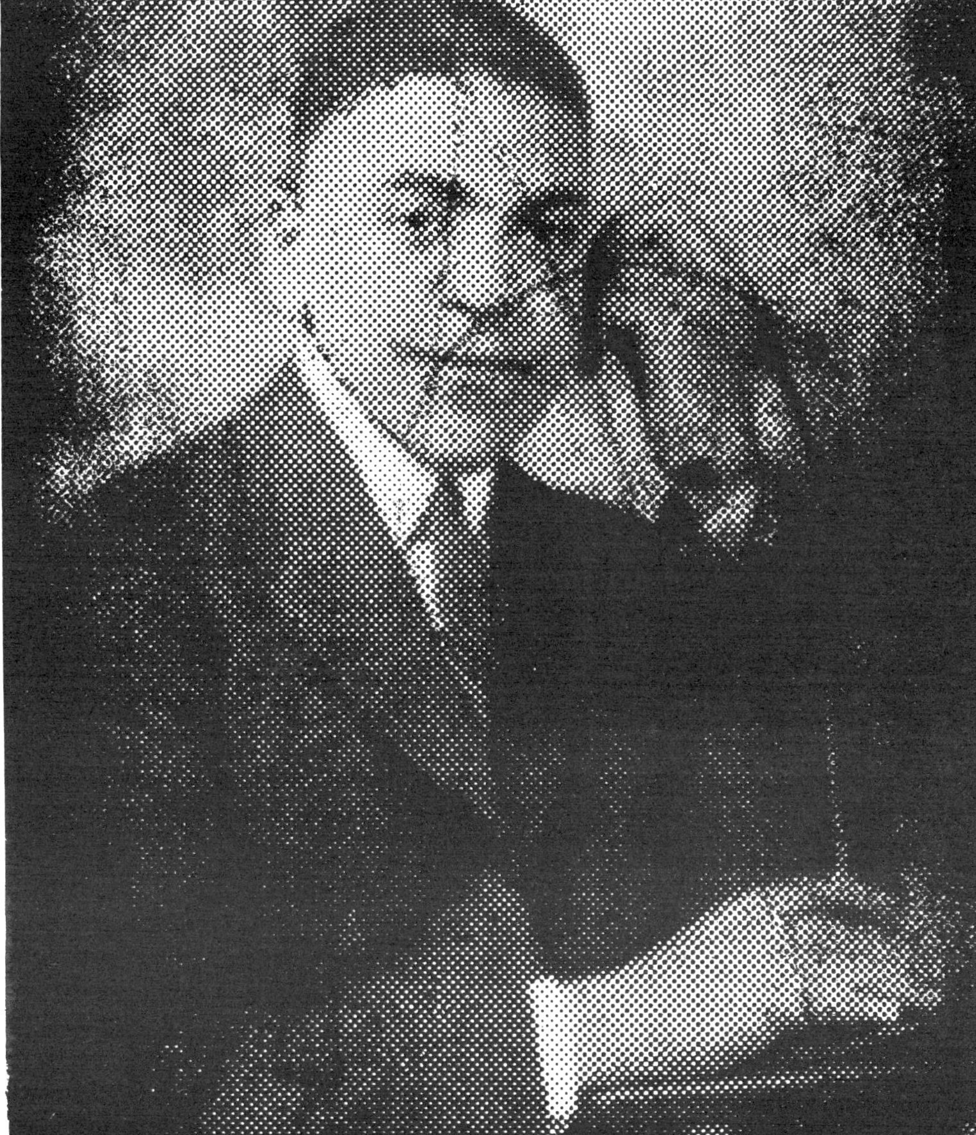

thought of her. Several musicians have recalled to me that he would feel impelled to play the spiritual *Sometimes I feel Like A Motherless Child,* but that the tears would come streaming down his face, and he was often so moved that he was unable to complete the number. It was almost as if playing it was a form of self-punishment for any unhappiness he had caused his mother.

*****

With his mother gone and the rows with his father a constant in his life, there was now nothing to keep Fats at home and after a particularly upsetting argument he left home and camped on the doorstep of his former classmate Wilson Brooks who, on returning home invited Fats to spend the night on the sofa. Next morning, a kindly Mrs Brooks decided to take the young man under her wing and arranged with Edward Waller that he should move in with them. Her own elder son was pianist Russell Books who had left home, so his room was vacant. It was a solution which satisfied both sides; Edward Waller was freed from the constant hassles of a wayward son and was able to satisfy his own conscience in that the Brook family was good and religious one and could be relied upon to keep an eye on Thomas; Thomas on the other hand, also freed from the daily arguements, moved into a more sympathetic musical environment — and a home which had a player piano and a collection of piano rolls.

*****

Russell Brooks had quite a reputation as a local pianist and was a friend of James P. Johnson and Willie 'The Lion' Smith. He'd more than a passing acquaintance with Fats and had heard him a number of times at the Lincoln and had advised the young pianist to broaden his scope by adding rags and shouts to his repertoire. He was fond of recounting how when playing a dance in a tent on Lenox and 140th Street, Fats had sneaked in and come over to the piano to watch him and said that he wanted to play as Russell had suggested, but lacked someone to show him. Not being a teacher himself, Russell then said he'd introduce the boy to James P. Johnson. Fats, all excited at the prospect, raced for the exit, caught himself up in the guy ropes and brought the whole tent down. From that moment the promise of an introduction was forgotten for a time.

Some time later Brooks returned home to visit his mother, and was surprised to find Fats sitting at the pianola teaching himself *Carolina Shout* from the piano roll, and he recalled his promise. There are two versions of how Brooks eventually brought Fats and James P. together. According to James P. Johnson himself, he first went to the Brooks home to hear Fats play a couple of things and then invited him to come to his sister's home where he was then living with his wife. The other version, related by Maurice Waller is that Russell Brooks took Waller to the Johnson home, where Johnson auditioned Fats, spent the afternoon teaching him, invited him to stay on for supper and then took him to Leroy's that night where Fats sat at the older man's side to absorb what was going on.

Under the tutelage of the older man, Waller quickly improved and James P. soon introduced him to the other stride piano players and to the rent party circuit where their skills were honed in competition with one another. It soon became apparent that the Waller talent was a very special one and, as the ideas and the compositions began to flow, Fats was introduced to others who could help him in furthering his career, first on piano rolls and later on record.

In the course of her own researches, Josephine Beaton has found a report from Local 310

Right: The photo of Fats used in the Q.R.S. advertising

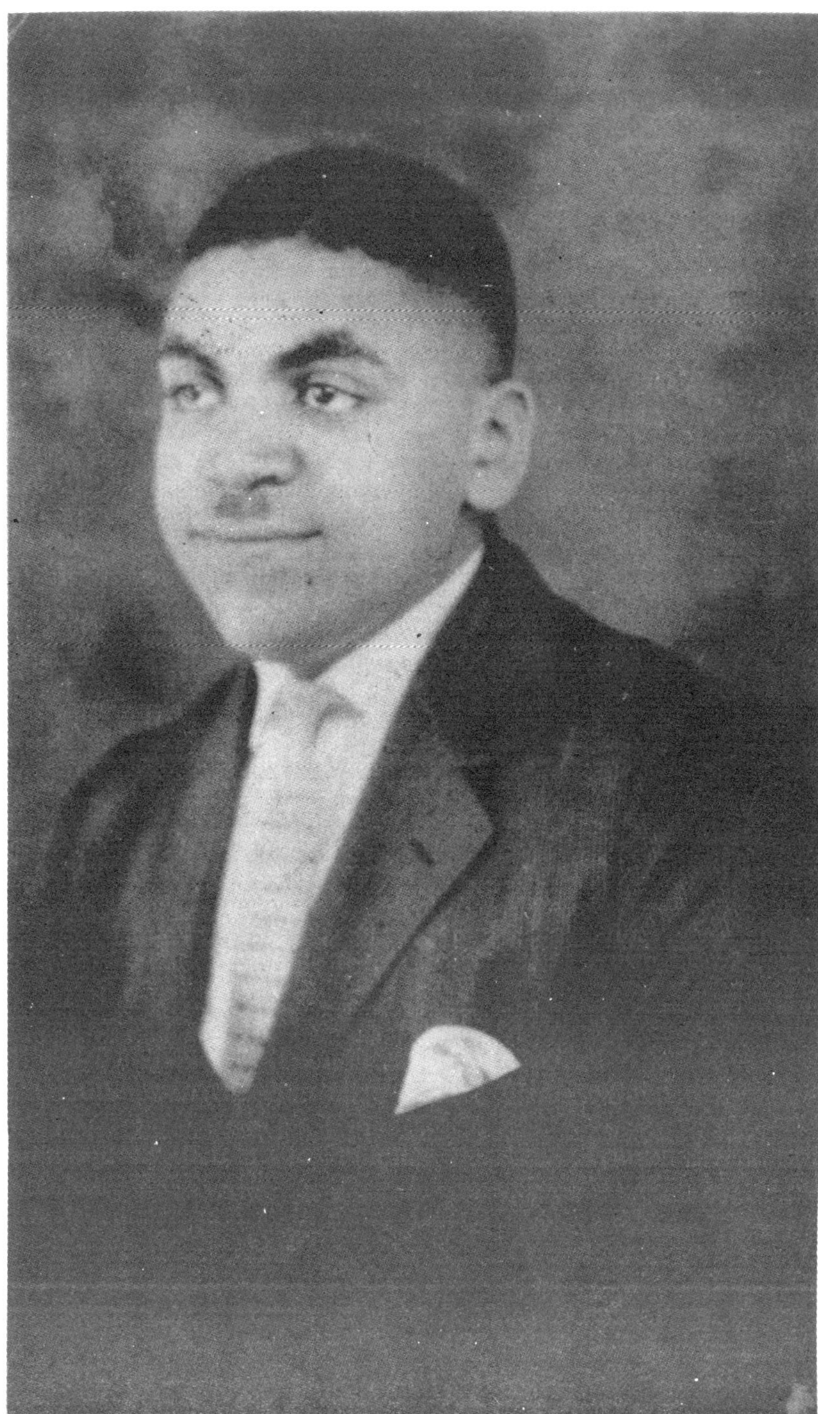

of New York in the *International Musician* of December 1920 that a Thos. Waller had been admitted to membership.

Sometime in 1921 Fats won a talent competition at the Regal Theater, New York playing *Carolina Shout.*

*****

Although I have been unable to find an exact date for the event, Fats continued to court Edith Hatchett and, according to available sources, married her when he was 17 years of age (i.e after May 1921) with the consent of his father as he was still a minor, and the newly married couple moved temporarily into the Hatchett family home on Brook Avenue in the Bronx before finding an apartment in Harlem. Married life made little difference to his life-style however and Edith, who soon became pregnant, wished for a quiet family life. It was not to be and conflicting interests soon led to friction between Waller and his wife and her family who were unable to come to terms with the life of a musician.

*****

Things took a decided turn for the worse when Willie 'The Lion' Smith fell out with the management at Leroy's and he and James P. Johnson engineered an invitation for Fats to replace him as resident pianist at Leroy's as accompanist and in a band which included Addington Major, c; Dope Andrews, tb; Ernest Elliott, cl; Leroy Parker, vn, and Tommy Benford, d. Waller quite naturally seized the opportunity and after a hastily organised afternoon session on the art of accompnying a singer and dancer put on by James P. and his wife who was both and had, in fact worked at Leroy's, Fats was taken down for the audition and approved.

*****

Thomas Waller Jr. was probably born in the Spring of 1922 — he was quoted as being 21 at the time of his father's death. Faced with increased financial obligations, and instead of seeking regular legitimate empbyment for which his wife and in-laws were agitating, Fats took a summer engagement in Asbury Park, New Jersey which, although it brought financial gain, eventually led to further family upsets as they were quite unable to see Waller's point of view or follow his reasoning. They felt he should be at home with his wife and son; he felt that the only way he could provide adequate support was to go where the pay was highest, even if it meant being separated.

Further details ot this summer engagement were given by Sonny Greer in an interview with Stanley Dance where he says that he had been working in the dining room of the Plaza Hotel on the boardwalk in Asbury Park, in a trio with Fats Waller and a violinist called (Ralph) 'Shrimp' Jones. At the end of the New Jersey engagement, Greer went to Washington where he met Duke Ellington for the first time, and Fats retumed to New York and followed Willie 'The Lion' Smith at the Capitol, a popular Harlem Club.

Maurice then refers to a short tour with a burlesque show, but since he gives no further information and in the light of other errors in chronology, it is almost certain that he is referring to the tour with 'Liza And Her Shuffling Sextet' as mentioned in the bio-discography which follows.

*****

A BIO-DISCOGRAPHY

Because no actual recording dates are known for any of the piano rolls which Waller made, these have been treated as a separate section and will be found at the end of the main listing.

According to a number of accounts, Fats Waller should have started his recording career a little earlier than he actually did. Clarence Williams had arranged for him to accompany Sara Martin for her OKeh recording of *Sugar Blues*, but Waller was already notoriously unreliable and failed to arrive at the studio at the appointed time and eventually Clarence himself played piano on the date.

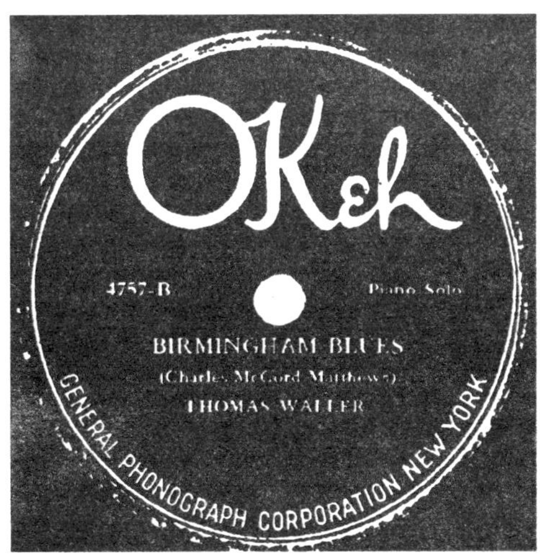

THOMAS WALLER
Piano solo

New York City, New York		c. Saturday, 21 October 1922
70948-a	Muscle Shoals Blues	OKeh rejected
70948-B	Muscle Shoals Blues	OKeh rejected
70948-C	Muscle Shoals Blues	OKeh rejected
70948-D	MUSCLE SHOALS BLUES (Geo. W. Thomas)	OK 4757-A, *Bm 1005, JSo AA-503*
70949-a	Birmingham Blues	OKeh rejected
70949-B	Birmingham Blues	OKeh rejected
70949-C	Birmingham Blues	OKeh rejected
70949-D	BIRMINGHAM BLUES (Charles McCord-Matthews)	OK 4757-B, *Bm 1005, JSo AA-503*

Although Maurice Waller states that the above were made in a single take of each title, the record proves otherwise and the somewhat high takes suggest that two sessions were involved. The original file cards no longer exist, but it seems possible that the issued takes were made at a re-make session about December 1922, possibly at the time of one of the Sara Martin sessions which follow. Fats himself said on several occasions that the Sara Martin sides were his first records, which supports this view and he may well have made only the first three takes of each title on his first visit to the OKeh studios and regarded that as an audition session, and this could also account for Maurice Waller's version (presumably related to him by his father) that a single take of each tune was cut.

OKeh 4757 was issued in February 1923.

Adjacent matrices: Those preceding are untraced.
S-709501/ are by the Rega Dance Orch.

*****

SARA MARTIN Contralto Solo Piano Accomp. by T. Waller
Sara Martin, v; acc: Thomas Waller, p

New York City, New York — c. Friday, 1 December 1922

S-71-068-a	'Tain't Nobody's Bus'ness If I Do	OKeh rejected
S-71-068-B	'Tain't Nobody's Bus'ness If I Do	OKeh rejected
S-71-068-C	'TAIN'T NOBODY'S BUS'NESS IF I DO (Porter Grainger-Everett Robbins)	OK 8043-B
S-71-069-a	You Got Ev'ry Thing A Sweet Mama Needs But Me	OKeh rejected
S-71-069-B	YOU GOT EV'RY THING A SWEET MAMA NEEDS BUT ME (Lemuel Fowler)	OK 8043-A

The original file cards for this session no longer survive, so it is not possible to state how many takes were made or what their disposition may have been.

Adjacent matrices are untraced.

*****

SARA MARTIN Contralto Solo Piano Accomp. By (or **by**) **Thomas Waller**
Sara Martin , v; acc: Thomas Waller, p.

New York City, New York — c. Thursday, 14 December 1922

S-71-105-a	Mama's Got The Blues	OKeh rejected
S-71-105-B	MAMA'S GOT THE BLUES (Clarence Williams Sara Martin)	OK 8045-B
S-71-106-a	Last Go Round Blues	OKeh rejected
S-71-106-B	LAST GO ROUND BLUES (Jimmy Cox)	OK 8045-A

As for the session above, the original file cards for this session no longer survive, so it is not possible to state how many takes were made or what their disposition may have been.

Adjacent matrices: S-71-103/4 are by J.J. Hochman's Jewish Orchestra.
S-71-1-7/8 are by Gus Goldstein & Co. (Jewish comedy songs).

*****

In *Blues Who's Who,* Sheldon Harris states that Fats toured with Sara Martin on the TOBA circuit in 1922-3, but this conflicts with the other evidence reported below and the date for this may have to be revised.

*****

A short article on Clarence Williams in the Baltimore *Afro-American* of 15 December 1922 covering his success as a song writer and publisher mentions that *Eva Taylor, Sarah Martin and Tom Waller and his band are on Mr. Williams staff for recording purposes.* This is the only reference I have been able to find of Waller fronting a band this early and conflicts with all the other available evidence and perhaps should not be taken literally.

*****

Around this time Fats was touring with 'Liza And Her Shuffling Sextet' and, in *Jazz From The Beginning,* Garvin Bushell recounts how Fats came to be hired and tells something of the act and conditions on the road at that time:

> *...Bert Adams was the piano player, and Clarence Robinson was the dancer and singer (he also produced a lot of the floor shows around New York). They got Seymour Irick on trumpet, Lew Henry on trombone, Mert Perry on drums, and myself. We didn't have any bass.*
>
> *Now, one night some fellow fought Bert Adams in the park and shot him. He got killed. So we had to revise the act, and got Fats Waller on piano. We put Katie Crippen into the act as the singer. One of the agents downtown thought up the name: Liza and Her Shuffling Sextet.*
>
> *At the time, Fats was just another good piano player. He hadn't composed anything then, and he was not seen opening his mouth. He drank as much, but he didn't sing. He was a big, happy, fat wrassler who could play a lot of piano. He used to come waddling down the street to the theater eating a big apple on a stick. Fats was a big baby. He never grew up.*
>
> *Clarence Robinson took over the act then, and I handled the business. ... I became part owner of the act with Clarence.*
>
> *Seymour Irick was an erratic Geechie. He had a good philosophy, and he was a pinchpenny. All he talked about was money. He kept himself clean and dressed well. But Mert Perry set the standard. He was a cocky little guy, like a little bantam rooster: immaculate and sharp, very sophisticated, very articulate. You'd think he was worth a half million or something when he talked with you, with his big cigar. So we all patterned ourselves after Mert. ...*
>
> *Our act usually opened with a fast instrumental number. Then out came the girl singer. Then the band did something special. After that, Clarence would come out and sing a song, and then maybe Katie would do another one, and join Clarence in one. Next Clarence would dance; he and Bert would do a duet together, like they had done in vaudeville (they'd been a big-time act on the Keith Circuit). To finish, we three horn players would put down our instruments, go out, and do a buck time step, then do "over the top" right along as a finale. We'd use something fast, like "Bandanna Days" or "Runnin' Wild." The pit band would pick it up, along with our drummer, and five of us would be doing the steps together in our tuxedos. It was a big finish. Many a time I sprained my ankle doing that "over the top." ...*
>
> *We were in Boston New Year's Eve of 1923, on the Poli time. Fats and I were sharing the front room in a brownstone in Back Bay. We'd been out of New York for three or four weeks. Everything was so old and depressing-looking in Boston in those days. This room had old furniture, old dark mahogany wood, dull yellow ceilings, and gaslights. There was also a bed and a piano. It was about quarter to midnight. Fats started noodling around on the piano, very soft. We were talking about being homesick for New York, wishing we*

were there. All of a sudden, at twelve o'clock the bells start ringing, people began shooting out the windows. And right then Fats came out with the theme to "Squeeze Me." He turned to me and said, "Hey Mackie, did you like that?"

I said, "Yeah, what is it?"

"I don't know."

"Does it have a middle part?" In those days, ninths were just becoming popular in bands, and you did it chromatically. Fats tried something, and said, "How's that?"

I said, "That closes it up. Put that on there." Then he put the whole thing together. He didn't have a title for it, but the next day, he said, "Hey Mackie, you know what I'm going to call that? 'Boy in the Boat.' Didn't have no hat, didn't have no coat." That was how he created it, right up there in that room.

On a trip down to Washington, D.C., a few of us went to hear a band in a little backstreet place. This group was headed by Elmer Snowden, the banjo player. There was a youngster playing piano named Duke Ellington, Toby Hardwick was on saxophone, Schiefe (Arthur Whetsol) on trumpet, and Sonny Greer on drums. After we heard the band, Clarence and I got in a terrific argument, and we decided to split up. So Clarence went to Snowden and said, "I've got a job for you." I kept the original band, with Fats on piano.

In the meantime, we had six and a half more weeks booked with the act on the Poli time. Clarence figured that he could take this new band and do the gigs, but I decided to beat him to the punch. Early Monday morning I went up to the Palace Theater office in New York. I said, "Clarence and I split up, and he's bringing in a strange band. I have the original one. Now, I could get a new dancer, or what do you want to do?" They got leery and canceled the whole six and a half weeks. So when Clarence arrived in New York with Snowden, Duke, and that bunch, they didn't have any work—I'd canceled all their jobs.

Towards the latter part of the act we had various dancers, and finally Bill Basie replaced Fats on piano. Then Seymour Irick was shot. He had a room in Johnny Hudgins's house, in the South Bronx, and a white girl shot and killed him. We couldn't get another good trumpet player.

The exact chronology of events is a little difficult to determine, especially as there are several versions extant of how (among other things) the Snowden band came to be in New York. Elmer Snowden gives a somewhat different account in a taped interview with Les Muscutt published in *Storyville 16:*

> *It was 1923 when I left* (Washington) *to go to New York, but Duke wasn't supposed to be my piano player. We were going in to play for a show ... the show had played Washington and had broken up in Washington, so the guy* (presumably Clarence Robinson) *was looking for a band to travel with the show because the band was quittin'. Now Fats Waller was in the band, so Fats came across to the place where we were working, and he assured us he wasn't quittin' ... he wasn't gonna leave him. ... we just got the group together and went on to New York. Just as we was leaving Duke came up and said, 'You got my drummer, what about me?' So I said, 'We don't need you Cutie, 'cause Fats is gonna play piano with us. That was a big deal you know, Fats Waller ... Anyway when we got to New York we couldn't find Fats ... we were there five days ... and we couldn't find the guy who told us to come to New York ... so we were stranded.*

This at least makes it clear that Fats was still with the group in Washington at the time of the split, but from Garvin Bushell's account it is not clear how long Fats had been with the group prior to the Boston date, nor when he left. In his own autobiography, Basie states that he replaced the piano player who had earlier replaced Fats. Thus it seems possible that the foregoing Sara Martin dates were made when Fats and the show were passing through (or perhaps playing in) New York. *Jazz Review* of April 1959 gives the show at the Lincoln Theatre, N.Y., but does not give a source for this nor a date, although Walter C. Allen thought c. October 1922, although on what grounds is not known. At this time the Lincoln Theatre featured a mixture of vaudeville and film, but except on special occasions their advertising did not note the artists concerned. Reviews in *The New York Age* were normally more concerned with what was on screen, and more often than not failed to even mention that there was anything happening on stage. However Bob Slater's 'Theatrical Jottings' column in the same paper does sometimes reveal who the headline act was and in the issue of 9 December 1922 it is noted that *Adams and Robinson with a jazz band are heading the bill at the Lincoln Theater, New York City.* I have assumed that this is the Adams and Robinson which concerns us and, as a matter of interest, they are first mentioned by Slater on 3 September 1921 through to the middle of December working theatres in the New York area. In December they added 'Saunders' (possibly Gertrude Saunders?) and then left on a tour of the West which lasted until April 1922, returning to New York and reverting to the 'Adams and Robinson' billing on 1 July 1922. Thereafter, they played the New York area and went no further afield than Massachusetts — they were reported in Springfield in the issue of 18 November, the last notice prior to that for the Lincoln Theatre. This latter is the first where a jazz band is mentioned and may be significant. It is also the final mention of Adams and Robinson, but there is no report of Katie Crippen up to this time or later.

Maurice Waller states that his father joined the show at the time it played the Lincoln Theatre, replacing the regular pianist who was sick, prior to heading out on tour. A search of the newspapers available to me has failed to uncover any report of the shooting of Bert Adams and hence a possible starting date for Fats with the group. The fact that Waller, a New York resident and *"just another good piano player"*, was recruited and that Adams was *"shot in the park"* without any identification of which park suggests Central Park and that the show was playing some other New York engagement which has not been traced.

A possible sequence of events is that Waller joined the show shortly before the Lincoln Theatre engagement in New York in December. The engagement probably ran for one week from Monday, 9 December and he thus made the Sara Martin records and the issued versions of his solos whilst there. The newspaper report was probably compiled from advance billing notices which would explain why the show is still shown under its original title. What is perhaps suprising is that although Adams and Robinson had been mentioned well over twenty times in the past year or so, the shooting incident failed to make the paper or, if it did, I have failed to find it. Then, up to Boston where they were playing at the end of December and into the New Year, followed by possibly other dates in New England.

The first reference to the new billing, which is not quite as Garvin Bushell recalled, in 'Theatrical Jottings' is in *The New York Age* of 5 May 1923 which states, *"Liza and "Shuffle Along" Six are at Commings Theatre, Fitchburg, Mass.* The following week was split between the Empire, Fall River and the Olympic, Lynn, Mass. Then in the issue of 19 May they are shown at Manchester, New Hampshire, but there is no entry for the week of 26 May or subsequently, but starting from 7 July there are references to the *"Shuffle Along" Four,* and these continue into February 1924 at which point 'Adams and Robinson' reappear and both groups are reported, so the shooting incident recalled by Garvin Bushell may not have been fatal as he thought. The show with Katie Crippen is known to have toured on the Keith and Poli vaudeville circuit, and the visit to Washington's Gayety Theatre, where it broke up must have been around May/June, because Snowden and company are believed to have made the trip to New York around 18 June. The Snowden band were advertised at Wonderland Park for 8 June, but were in New York prior to 27 July, when they made a test recording for Victor.

Katie Crippen, aged 34, died 25 November 1929 of cancer after an illness of several months according to an obituary in *The New York Age.* This also stated that she was a native of Philadelphia and was married to musician Lou Henry who is assumably the Lew Henry recalled by Garvin Bushell.

*****

Fats is reputed to have made his first broadcast some time in 1923 from the Fox Theatre in Newark, New Jersey, in company with Clarence Williams, but the exact date of this is not known.

*****

Alberta Hunter Acc. by Thomas Waller **Blues**

Alberta Hunter, v; acc. Thomas Waller, p.

New York City, New York c. July 1923

1455[1]	Stingaree Blues	Paramount unissued
1455[2]	Stingaree Blues (Clinton A. Kemp)	Pm 12049-A
1456[1]	You Can't Do What My Last Man Did (J.A. Johnson – Allie Moore)	Pm 12043-B
1456[2]	You Can't Do What My Last Man Did (J.A. Johnson and Allie Moore)	Pm 12049-B

1456: Beginning of second chorus

-1 "You can't do what my last man did
Toss (? boss) me around, treat me like a kid"

-2 "Daddy, you can't do what my last man did
I'd love you if you only could"

Recording date is estimated, but Paramount 12049 was first advertised in the Chicago *Defender* issue of 15 December 1923. Paramount 12043 is the subject of one of the biggest mix-ups in recording history with no fewer than five different backings to Alberta Hunter's *Mistreated Blues.* The first of these appears to have been Alberta Hunter with Eubie Blake in *I'm Going Away Just To Wear You Off My Mind,* (takes 1 and 2 were issued) and was advertised in this form in the *Defender* on 4 August 1923. Two versions appeared using 1456[1]; the first with labels showing 1456 is labelled **Alberta Hunter and Bubie Blake**, later versions showing 1469 on the label are labelled **Anna Jones Acc. by Thomas Waller**. The fifth version, using 1469[1] (see below) is correctly labelled as **Anna Jones Acc. by Thomas Waller**. These final versions were advertised in the *Defender* on 22 September 1923.

Adjacent matrices: 1453/4 and 1457/8 are by the Broadway Melody Makers.

*****

Alberta Hunter talked to Bob Kumm about this session in 1965:

On the first session that I worked with Fats we recorded into the old acoustical horns and the studio had sawdust on the floor. The recording was made on soft wax discs and the shavings would just fall on the floor while we were recording. Everything just came so naturally and we never had to do more than one or two takes. We didn't use any music of arrangements or anything like that. For instance, if we would start doing a number, we'd get some trick into it and just follow each other. I don't know how we did this, but it worked.

*****

Anna Jones Acc. by Thomas Waller **Blues**

Anna Jones, v; Acc. Thomas Waller, p.

New York City, New York c. July 1923

1468[1]	Sister Kate (I Wish I Could Shimmy Like My) (A.J. Piron)	Pm 12052-A, Hg 859
1468[2]	Sister Kate (I Wish I Could Shimmy Like My) (A.J. Piron)	Pm 12052-A (see note)
1469[1]	You Can't Do What My Last Man Did (J.A. Johnson – Allie Moore)	Pm 12043-B
1473[1]	Trixie Blues (Trixie Smith)	Pm 12052-B
1473[2]	Trixie Blues (Trixie Smith)	Pm 12052-B, Hg 859

1473: No original pressing has been available for study, so it has not been possible to provide a means of identifying take differences. All LP issues checked to date are aurally identical despite variations in playing time.

Paramount 12052 using 1468[2] has been seen advertised, but has not been located. The Harmograph issue likewise has not been inspected, but is reliably reported to use the -1/-2 take combination. The above may be the product of more than one session.

Adjacent matrices: 1466/7 are by the Metropolitan Dance Players.
1470/1 are by Frank Bessinger.
1472 and 1474/5/6 are untraced.

*****

Under the heading "New York News", the *Pittsburgh Courier* for 18 August 1923 lists a programme of "blues" to be broadcast on Saturday, 25 August. Among the artists scheduled to appear were Trixie Smith, accompanied by Thomas Walker (piano and QRS rolls). It seems almost certain that 'Walker' is a misprint for Waller.

*****

SARA MARTIN - CLARENCE WILLIAMS **Contralto-Baritone Duet with Piano Accomp.**

Sara Martin, Clarence Williams, v duet; Acc. Thomas Waller, p.

New York City, New York Thursday, 1 November 1923

S-71-984-a	I'm Cert'ny Gonna See 'Bout That	OKeh rejected
S-71-984-B	I'M CERT'NY GONNA SEE 'BOUT THAT (Tony Jackson)	OK 8108-B
S-71-985-a	Squabbling Blues	OKeh rejected
S-71-985-B	SQUABBLING BLUES (Sara Martin - Clarence Williams)	OK 8108-A

The original file cards for this session no longer exist, so it is not possible to state how many takes were made, nor what their disposition may have been, but probably there were no more than shown here.

OKeh 8108 was advertised in the Chicago *Defender* of 16 February 1924.
Adjacent matrices are untraced.

*****

Porter Grainger
Porter Grainger, v; acc. Fats Waller, p.
New York City, New York early 1924

31578 In Harlem's Araby (Trent-Waller) Ajax 17039-B

The reverse of Ajax is *Papa Don't Ask Mama Where She Was* (31571) by **Hazel Meyers and Her Sawin' Trio** without Waller.

Adjacent matrices: 31576/77 and 31579-80 are all untraced. The former are probably unissued takes by Hazel Meyers and Porter Grainger and the latter probably unissued takes by the Old Time Jubilee Singers, which group accounts for 31581/2.

*****

JAMAICA JAZZERS **Fox Trot**
Clarence Williams, Clarence Todd, k; Fats Waller, p; Justin Ring, percussion.
New York City, New York, c. Saturday, 10 May 1924

S-72-514-a You Don't Know My Mind Blues OKeh unissued
S-72-514-B YOU DON'T KNOW MY MIND BLUES OK 40117-A, OdG 312852, 03196
(Clarence Williams-Virginia Liston-Sam Gray)
S-72-515-A WEST INDIES BLUES OK 40117-B, OdG 312853, 03196
(Edgar Dowell-Spencer Williams-Clarence Williams)

The above personnel was given by Clarence Williams on being played the record by Bob Colton. File cards no longer exist for this session, so it is not possible to give details of number of takes made, nor of their disposition. It is likely that two takes were made of each side in line with normal OKeh practice at this time. OKeh 40117 was announced in the August 1924 *Phonograph & Talking Machine Weekly*. German Odeons 312852/3 are coupled.

Adjacent matrices: S-72-513/4 are by George McLennon's Jazz Devils, c. 9 May 1924.
S-72-516 is by Miller & Lyles, c. 12 May 1924.

*****

An advert in the *Pittsburgh Courier* of 29 March 1924 shows Thomas "Fats" Waller as the pianist with Eugene Aiken & Capitol Jazz Syncopators at New York's Capitol Palace Club.

*****

ETHEL WATERS Piano Accompaniment **Blues**
Ethel Waters, v; acc Thomas Waller, p
New York City, New York Friday, 1 August 1924

13452 Pleasure Mad Vocalion unissued
13453 PLEASURE MAD (Bechet) Vo B-14860, Sil 3014
13454 Back Bitin' Mama Vocalion unissued
13455 BACK-BITIN' MAMA (Waller) Vo A-14860, Sil 3014
13456-13458 are untraced
13459 Back Bitin' Mama Vocalion unissued

*****

HAZEL MEYERS Piano Accompaniment **Blue Ballad -1**
Blues -2

Hazel Meyers, v; acc. Thomas Waller, p.
New York City, New York Tuesday, 5 August 1924

13466	Maybe Someday	Vocalion unissued
13467	MAYBE SOMEDAY -1 (B. & J. SPIKES)	Vo B-14861, Sil 3012
13468	(I'm Gonna See You) When Your Troubles are Just Like Mine	Vocalion unissued
13469	(I'M GONNA SEE YOU) When Your Troubles Are Just Like Mine -2 (B. & J. SPIKES)	Vo A-14861, Sil 3012

Details of the above two sessions are from Steven Lasker who comments that the Aeolian files from this period are missing; the above details being from the inventory of parts. Only Vocalion 14861 of the various issues has yet been inspected and this is on brown wax. This was issued in October 1924. One copy of this issue has been reported as having composer credits and the title of 13469 U/C, but copies actually seen are as above.

Adjacent matrices: 13460-65 are untraced.
13470-73 are by the Florentine Serenaders.

*****

Little is known of Waller's movements or activites from this point until his next recording session below, a period of some eighteen months, although some of the time may have been spent in jail for failure to support his wife and child. Another possibilty that bears further investigation is the claim made in Waller's obituary notice in *The New York Age* that he had toured with Bessie Smith in 1925.

If we delve back a little further to allow for some error, Bessie's last tour in 1924 included a band led by Fred Longshaw, after which she played New York and made a number of recording sessions in that city in December/January. From June 1925 until the end of the year she had a band led by pianist Jimmy Jones. In between, she did go out on tour in February 1925 during which she was stabbed (reported in the Chicago *Defender* on 7 March and in other papers) and her accompanist on that tour was reported to be a pianist only. She was back in New York by May. At first sight this seems to be the only occasion when Waller might have toured with her, but it seems unlikely that given his later fame, no-one recalled him working with Bessie.

Certainly by the end of February he was working in Leroy Smith's Orchestra at Connie's Inn and was on hand for the week they played at Hurtig & Seamon's Theatre on 125th Street. This was reviewed by J.A. Jackson in the Baltimore *Afro-American* of 28 February 1925 and the part that concerns us reads:

> *An orchestra number was put on at this juncture, one that permitted the several musicians to demonstrate their individual abilities. "Fats" Waller, a rotund genial looking pianist creating grins the whole while with his eccentricities at that instrument.*

How long Waller had been at Connie's Inn is not known, nor is the length of his stay, but this dating would appear to invalidate any suggestion of being with Bessie Smith. Certainly, his place in the Leroy Smith band had been taken by Harry Brooks by October 1925 as noted in the Baltimore *Afro-American* of 24 October.

But pre-dating that, another firm reference to Waller is to be found in Jack Schiffman's book *Uptown: The Story of Harlem's Apollo Theatre* where he mentions that his father Frank and Leo Breecher had acquired the Lafayette Theatre on 132nd Street and Seventh Avenue and, after refurbishing it, re-opened in May 1925 with a show that featured a variety show, a chorus line of black girls and a small orchestra that included Thomas Waller on organ. Maurice Waller also makes reference to the Lafayette being purchased by *Ed Brecher and Frank Schiffman* who also owned the larger Lincoln, where they had installed a Robert Morton grand organ. Waller apparently doubled at both theatres for a time at a salary of $50 per week. Maurice places this as somewhat earlier, but it almost certainly refers to May 1925.

Maurice Waller says that Captain George Maines had appointed himself as a sort of unofficial manager to Waller in 1924 and had arranged for Fats to appear as a soloist over station WHN in New York. He also states that Waller shared a billing at the Kentucky Club, 203 W. 49th Street (the new name for the burned-out Hollywood Club) which opened in 1925, with Duke Ellington and his Washingtonians and singer-comedian Bert Lewis. Fats, in oriental costume and billed as "Ali Baba, the Egyptian Wonder" was Lewis's accompanist. The whole show was also booked into the New Amsterdam Theatre for one night each week and was there for nearly two months. Although Maurice implies that these events were in 1924, the Kentucky Club was not so named until re-opening after the fire which gutted the Hollywood Club in February 1925. In an interview with Stanley Dance, Sonny Greer also mentions Waller's appearance at the club with Bert Lewis, but gives no indication of the date. Note that Station WHN had a line into the Kentucky Club for regular broadcasts from there. I have not been able to trace the exact dates for these engagements, but the *Pittsburgh Courier* of 11 April 1925 reported Duke Ellington's Washingtonians in the Club Kentucky, saying it was formerly the Hollywood and *Billboard's* George Lottman waxed enthusiastically about the Ellington band and Waller in his coverage in the 5 December 1925 issue, but there is no indication how long Waller had been in residence.

*****

In his own book, Maurice Waller states that his father played the Sherman Hotel, Chicago in 1925, and this is repeated by Alyn Shipton in his study. However, I have been unable to find any confirmation of this.

*****

Mamie Harris **Vocal**

Rosa Henderson, v; acc. Fats Waller, p.

New York City, New York c. Tuesday 23 March 1926

106735	You Get Mad (Mike Jackson)	PA 7501-A, Pe 101
106736	What's The Matter Now? (S. Williams-C.Williams)	PA 7501-B, Pe 101B

The Perfect issue shows only a B side designation.

*****

Alta Browne & Bertha Powell **Negro Spritual Piano Acc., Thos. Waller**

Alta Browne, Bertha Powell, v; acc: Fats Waller, p.

Long Island City, New York Friday, 16 April 1926

X-71-A	Nobody Knows De Trouble I See	Ge 3318-B, Ch 15103
X-72-A	Couldn't Hear Nobody Pray	Ge 3308- , Ch 15103

Champion 15103 as **Caroline and May Floyd.** Stanley Blachman supplied details of Ge 3318,

issued in August 1926 and says that this is a "legitimate" performance of no jazz interest.
Adjacent matrices:

*****

Elkins Negro Ensemble
Vocal group acc. *Fats Waller,* p.
Long Island City, New York — Saturday 24 April 1926

X-98	Wheel In A Wheel (Ezekiel Saw De Wheel)	Ge 3318-A, Ch 15104

The above has not been seen or heard, but is reputedly a Fats Waller accompaniment. Even if it is, it is likely to be completely 'straight'.

The reverse of Ch 15104 is as **Southern Alabama Chorus**, and is by the same group, but unaccompanied.

Caroline Johnson "Fats' Waller at the Piano
Caroline Johnson, v; acc. "Fats" Waller, p.
Long Island City, New York — Saturday 24 April 1926

X-99-B	AIN'T GOT NOBODY TO GRIND MA COFFEE (Spencer Williams)	Ge 3307-A, Bu 8034- , Ch 15101
X-100	MAMA'S LOSIN' A MIGHTY GOOD CHANCE (Johnson-Allen)	Ge 3307-B, Bu 8033-B, Ch 15102

According to Harrison Smith, who says he organised this session, Caroline Johnson is a pseudonym for Alta Brown. Both Champion issues as **Flossie Porter**, and the reverses of these and both Buddy issues are by Alberta Jones. Bu 8033 is as the Gennett issue, and the label of that indicates a release date of July 1926. Some copies of Ge 3307-A include a hyphen between the two parts of Spencer Williams's name in the composer credit.

Adjacent matrices: X-96/7 are by Jack Kaufman on 21 April 1926.
X-101 is by Alberta Jones with piano by Carroll Boyd on 23 April 1926.

*****

A note in the *Pittsburgh Courier* of 10 July 1926 says: *At the Lincoln this week — Club Ciro's Creole Follies, a Leonard Harper presentation featuring Signor Thomas and Fats Waller...* In *The New York Age* of 17 July 1926 the advert for the Lincoln Theatre shows the revue to be in its second week and names the band as *Signor Fats Waller's Lincolnians.*

It was presumably during this spell on organ at the Lincoln theatre that Fats gave unofficial lessons to Count Basie as described by the latter in his autobiography. (pp69-71)

*****

During this period, Fats wrote tunes for *'Tan Town Topics'* and *'Junior Blackbirds',* both at the Lafayette theatre.

*****

In *Hendersonia,* Walter C. Allen relates how Waller had been recommended to Fletcher Henderson as a stand-in pianist and, knowing of his reputation, Henderson had waived his usual rule of no sitting-in with his band and permitted Waller to take over the piano chair. Waller fitted in so well that Henderson then frequently allowed him to repeat the exercise. One such occasion, and a presitigious one at that, is documented by a report in the November *Orchestra World* of a 'Battle of the Bands' at the Roseland Ballroom at Broadway and 31st Street on Wednesday, 13 October. The Henderson aggregation was pitched against the visiting Jean Goldkette Orchestra, and it seems to have been quite a night! Part of the report reads, ...*Thomas "Fats" Waller, the piano wizard relieved Fletcher once in a while, and the boys and girls stopped dancing to watch his fingers ramble...*

A friendship developed between Waller and Henderson and Fats began to write specifically for the Henderson Orchestra and sold both tunes and arrangements to Fletcher, some of which appeared with Henderson's name in place of Waller's according to certain claims. One story which gained credence and which probably has some basis in truth is that Fats wrote nine tunes in 1926/7 and, being short of ready cash, sold them to Henderson for the price of some hamburgers. The story was apparently originally told by Don Redman to John S. Wilson and has been repeated on a number of subsequent occasions. According to this, the nine tunes included *Top And Bottom* which was later recorded by Henderson as *Henderson Stomp*, *Thundermug Stomp* (which became *Hot Mustard*) and others which metamorphosed into *Variety Stomp*, *St. Louis Shuffle* and *Whiteman Stomp*. This latter, at least, seems unlikely in view of the report in *Variety* in March 1927. Henderson's recorded repertoire began to show signs of this association, and the first occasion when Waller actually participated in a Henderson recording date came soon after, as below.

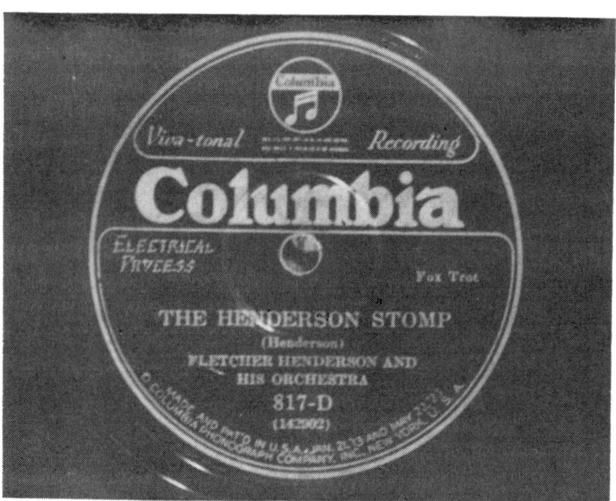

FLETCHER HENDERSON AND HIS ORCHESTRA **Fox Trot**

Russell Smith, t; Joe Smith, Tommy Ladnier, c; Benny Morton, tb; Buster Bailey, Don Redman, cl/as-2; Coleman Hawkins, cl/ts-2; Fats Waller, p-1/po-2; Charlie Dixon, bj; June Cole, bb; Kaiser Marshall, d.

New York City, New York — Wednesday, 3 November 1926

142902-1	The Henderson Stomp	Columbia rejected
142902-2	THE HENDERSON STOMP -1 (Henderson)	Co 817-D, CoE 4421, DB 5030, MC 5030, CoSd MC 5030, CoJ 132, Nipponophone 17150
142902-3	The Henderson Stomp	Columbia second choice
142904-1	The Chant	Columbia rejected
142904-2	THE CHANT -2 (Stitzel)	Co 817-D, CoJ 132, Nipponophone 17150
142904-3	The Chant	Columbia second choice

The first title was originally shown on the recording card as *Top And Bottom Stomp* and Walter

Allen suggests that this may have been one of the titles originally written by Waller. However, he also notes that the arrangements of both tunes are by Don Redman. The reverse of Columbia 4421 and all three of the Columbia 5030 numbers is *Tozol* by **Fletcher Henderson and His Orchestra** without Waller.

Adjacent matrices: 142899/90/91 are by The University Six.
142904 is by Art Gilham.

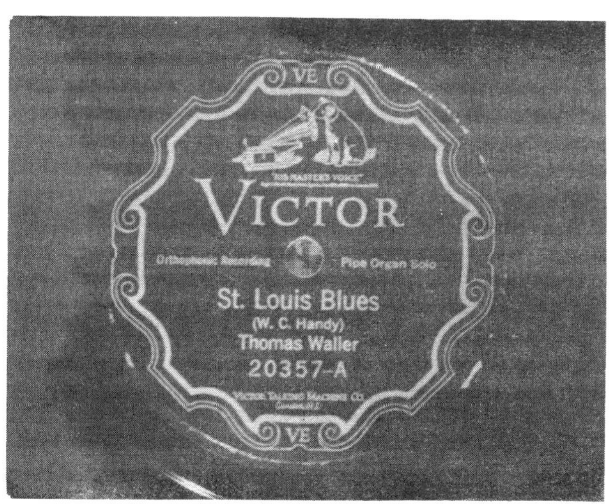

Thomas Waller **Pipe Organ Solo**

Thomas Waller, po.

Trinity Church Building, Camden, New Jersey — Wednesday, 17 November 1926
10:30 a.m. to 12:50 p.m. and 1:45 p.m. to 2:30 p.m.

36773-1	St. Louis Blues (W.C. Handy)	Vi 20357-A, HMV B8501, HMVF SG561
36773-2	St Louis Blues	Victor unissued 'Hold 30 days'
36773-3	St Louis Blues	Victor rejected, master destroyed
36774-1	The Church Organ Blues	Victor rejected, master destroyed
36774-2	The Church Organ Blues	Victor rejected, master destroyed
36774-3	The Church Organ Blues	Victor rejected, master destroyed
36774-4	Lenox Avenue Blues (T. Waller)	Vi 20357-B, HMV B8501, HMVF SG561

The Victor engineers did considerable experimenting when recording these sides and details of microphone placements are given on the recording sheets as well as the usual information on recordings levels, etc. A rather high level was employed and the results of this are evident on the issued sides where the modulation is such that grooves almost meet on loud passages. 36773-1 and 36774 -1 and -2 were recorded with a single microphone *57in from Shutters in line with Right Column.* All other takes were recorded using two microphones *29ft from Shutters in line with Right column.* This presumably refers to an internal column of the Church which was used by Victor because of its excellent acoustic qualities.

The recording sheet also gives Waller's address as 1006 Brook Avenue, Bronx and notes that no music was used for the first title. *The Church Organ Blues* may have been composed on the spot by Fats, for the recording sheet carries the note *Not Pub. Verbal Mr. Waller,* and when the record was issued the tune had been retitled.

*****

Six Hot Babies

Tom Morris, c; *Joe Nanton,* tb; *Bob Fuller,* cl; Nat Shilkret, p; *Thomas Waller,* po; *Bobby Leecan,* g; unknown d.

Trinity Church Building, Camden, New Jersey — Wednesday, 17 November 1926

36775-1	All God's Chillun Got Wings	Victor unissued
36775-2	All God's Chillun Got Wings	Victor unissued
36775-3	All God's Chillun Got Wings	Victor unissued
36775-4	All God's Chillun Got Wings	Victor unissued

No recording sheet was available for this session, which presumably followed straight on from that above. Details are from the Victor files via Brian Rust and Victor have advised that all four takes were subsequently destroyed.

Adjacent matrices: 36771/2 are by Gina Santelia on 16 November 1926.
36776/8 are by August Werner on 26 November 1926.

*****

It is interesting that Waller should have given his address to Victor as quoted above, as this was his wife's parents' home and in his book Maurice Waller has this to say:

By 1923 James P., Willie The Lion, Eva Taylor, Clarence Williams and Andy had replaced Edith and Thomas Jr. as Dad's family. Edith sought and won a divorce. The settlement was thirty-five dollars per week for child support and alimony. Dad agreed to pay, but from the very first installment the money came in late, and rarely was it the right amount.

Free from a marriage he no longer wanted, he found an apartment in Harlem...

And a few pages further on:

...Fats Waller and Anita Rutherford were married in 1926.

From the evidence of the recording sheet, it would appear that Maurice is a few years out in his dating, and his own birth-date of 10 September 1927 may have had something to do with this. I have been unable to find any evidence that Fats married Anita Rutherford in 1926 or at any other time, and the wording and content of the Waller will supports this view.

*****

Joe Sims and Clarence Williams **Vocal**

Joe Sims, Clarence Williams, v duet, acc. *Louis Metcalf,* c; Thomas 'Fats' Waller, p.

New York City, New York — c. January1927

2799[1]	What Do You Know About That (—)	Pm 12435-B
2799[2]	What Do You Know About That	Paramount unissued, test exists

2799: Patter following piano interlude:
-1 "Now you acting like you from the land of red beans and rice..."
-2 "Now you acting like you from down home..."

2800[1]	Shut Your Mouth	Paramount unissued, test exists
2800[2]	Shut Your Mouth (—)	Pm 12435-A

2800: Beginning of third vocal sequence:
-1 "There was some cheating done last night." "Shut your mouth."
-2 "There was some cheating done in the store last night." "Who was it?" "Shut your mouth."

The unissued takes appear on a two-sided Paramount test pressing. Recording date is

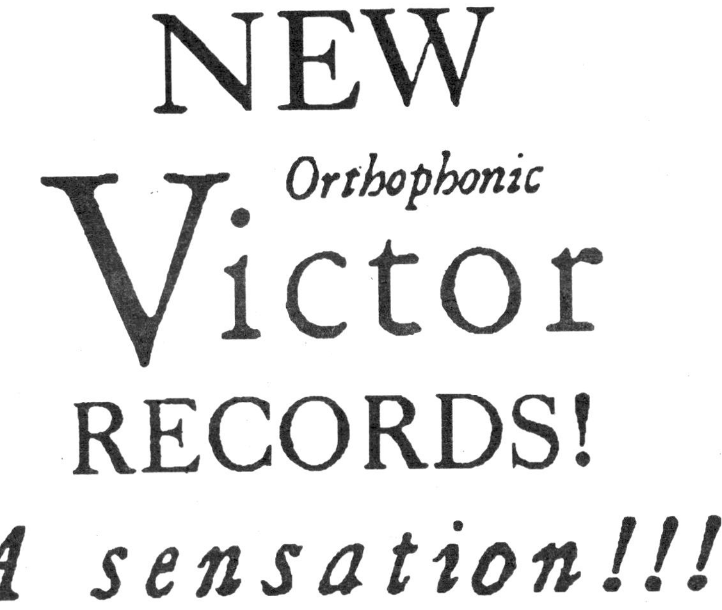

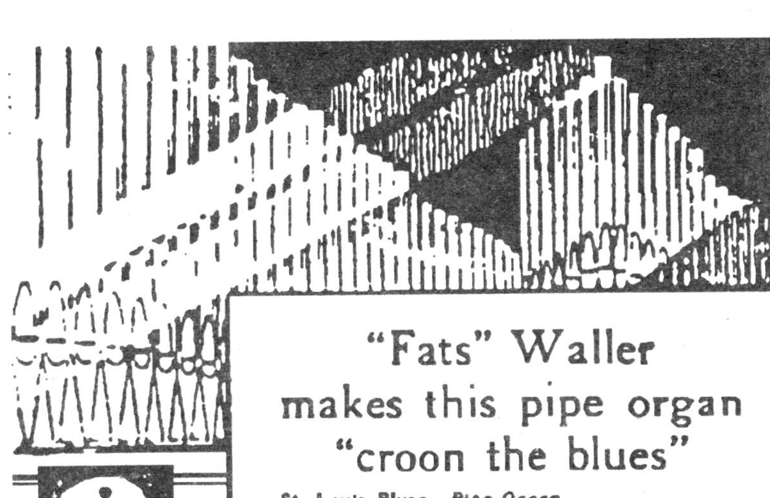

"Fats" Waller
makes this pipe organ
"croon the blues"
St. Louis Blues Pipe Organ
Lenox Avenue Blues Pipe Organ "Fats" WALLER
No. 20357. 10-inch. 75¢

Part of the Victor Display Advert in the Chicago *Defender* of 8 January 1927.

estimated, but Paramount 12435 was first advertised in the Chicago *Defender* issue of 12 February 1927.

Joe Sims was a vaudeville artist who had run his own company since at least 1924 and had appeared at many leading black theatres. Clarence Williams had presented a revue at the Lincoln Theatre in New York in the last week of September 1926 which included 'Sims and Crumbley' among others.

Adjacent matrices are untraced.

*****

Thomas Waller **Pipe Organ Solos**

Thomas Waller, po.

Trinity Church Building, Camden, New Jersey — Friday, 14 January 1927

10:00 a.m. to 12:15 p.m.

37357-1	Soothin' Syrup Stomp	Victor, hold and consult. Issued on LP?
37357-2	SOOTHIN' SYRUP—STOMP (Waller)	Vi 20470-A
37357-3	Soothin' Syrup Stomp	Victor, hold 30 days. Issued on LP?
37357: See note		
37358-1	Sloppy Water. Blues	Victor, hold and consult. Issued on LP
37358-2	Sloppy Water. Blues	Victor rejected, master destroyed
37358-3	SLOPPY WATER–Blues (T. Waller)	Vi 20492-B
37358	lead in to final chorus	-1 Four single notes followed by four answering chords and a right hand phrase -3 Four single notes followed by four answering chords and continuing with both hands
37359-1	Loveless Love. Blues Novelty	Victor, hold and consult.
37359-2	Loveless Love. Blues Novelty	Victor rejected, master destroyed
37359-3	LOVELESS LOVE-Blues Novelty (W.C. Handy)	Vi 20470-B, 23260-A

The recording sheet again notes that a single microphone, placed "7-ft from shutters in line with right column" was used.

I sought the help of pianist Louis Mazetier in attempting to notate the differences between the 'three' takes of *Soothin' Syrup Stomp* as differences appeared to be minimal and to defy verbal description. Louis's analysis confirmed my suspicion that takes -1 and -3 as presented on LP were identical, but since we have not had access to a test, it is not possible to state which is actually used, although John R.T Davies states that according to his files the tape version he holds comes from a test of take -3. Louis points out that Fats makes two slight mistakes in exactly the same places on 'takes' -1 and -3. They are on the 1st beat of the 8th bar of the third theme and on the 4th beat of the 3rd bar of the bridge passage of the repeated first theme which follows the third theme. The structure of the piece is as follows:

Takes -1 and -3 (as claimed on LP)	Take -2
Introduction	Introduction
1st theme, 32 bars with bridge	1st theme 32, bars with bridge
Transition	Transition
2nd theme, 16 bars	2nd theme, 16 bars
3rd theme, 16 bars in minor mood	3rd theme, 16 bars in minor mood
1st theme repeated softly	Modified 1st theme repeated
Riffs based on 1st theme	Riffs played softly, returning to the 1st theme melody for the final 8 bars.
Second series of (different) riffs, 16 bars.	Coda
Coda	

*****

Thomas Waller **Pipe Organ Solos**

Thomas Waller, po.

Trinity Church Building, Camden, New Jersey — Friday, 14 January 1927

1:30 p.m. to 4:15 p.m.

37360-1	Harlem Blues.	Victor rejected, master destroyed
37360-2	Harlem Blues.	Victor rejected, master destroyed
37360-3	Harlem Blues.	Victor rejected, master destroyed
37361-1	Messin' Around with The Blues.	Victor rejected, master destroyed
37361-2	Messin' Around with The Blues.	Victor, hold 30 days
37361-3	MESSIN' AROUND WITH THE BLUES (Phil Worde-Thomas Waller)	Vi 20655-A

37361: See note

37362-1	The Rusty Pail. Blues	Victor, hold 30 days. Issued on LP
37362-2	The Rusty Pail. Blues	Victor rejected, master destroyed
37362-3	THE RUSTY PAIL-Blues (T. Waller)	Vi 20492-A

37362 Opening -1 Three pairs of crisply struck chords plus a single chord leading into first phrase
-3 Two pairs of crisply struck chords followed by two groups of five and seven rapidly struck chords leading into first phrase

Second theme -1 The repeat of descending phrase by right hand/silent pause/longer descending phrase also by right hand
-3 Played right through by both hands

------1 I'd like to call you My Sweetheart. Fox Trot

The first title is shown as a W.C. Handy composition on the recording sheet, whilst the final title, without any serial number as above, bears the notation "Made as trial for Mr. Shilkret to hear. No Music." There is no disposition marking for it, and trials were normally not intended for issue. However, a letter from Hansjürg Richner in 1966 stated that he had been informed by RCA that the title bore the matrix 37363 and that the master was intact at the time he wrote to them in 1963. In the light of the extensive Waller reissue programmes since that date and search for unissued material, this seems highly suspect and it must now be assumed that unless a copy exists in Nat Shilkret's effects, it is lost to collectors.

Once again I sought the help of pianist Louis Mazetier in attempting to discover differences in the 'two takes' of *Messin' Around With The Blues,* and once again he confirms that LP issues available to us claiming to use take -2 are identical to the issued take -3. The timing and structure are identical, but the clinching factor is that Waller makes two minor errors in exactly the same place on both 'takes'.

Adjacent matrices: 37354/6 are by Geraldine Farrar on 13 January 1927.
37363/4 are by Lucy Levin on 17 January 1927.

*****

The New York Age for 22 January 1927 carries a short announcement to the effect that the Lincoln Theater installs music program: adds Wurlitzer organ and *engaged Thomas Fats' Waller to delight the patrons hourly with his renditions. Waller is now a record star for the Victor Phonograph Co.* The report went on to mention that Irving Pugsley and his Lincoln Theater Orchestra were also featured. The New York *Amsterdam News* of 19 January also showed Waller at the organ of the Lincoln Theater.

*****

Variety of 26 January also covered this as follows:

Tom (Fats) Waller, colored pipe organist, for some time employed by the Lafayette theatre (Harlem) is now organist at the Lincoln in the same uptown neighborhood.

Waller, regarded as the 'Jesse Crawford' of his race has recently been making solo records for both Brunswick and Victor machines. He is said to have no equal as a 'blue jazzist' on the pipe organ.

Needless to say, no trace has been found of Brunswick solos, and this is probably simply a case of misreporting.

*****

Thomas Waller **Pipe Organ Solos**

Thomas Waller, po.

Trinity Church Building, Camden, New Jersey Wednesday, 16 February 1927

9:30 a.m. to 12:00 a.m.

37819-1	Stompin the Bug. Stomp.	Victor, hold 30 days. Issued on LP
37819-2	STOMPIN' THE BUG (Phil Worde-Mercedes Gilbert)	Vi 20655-B
	37819: Bridge passage into last chorus	-1 based on descending phrase from Lenox Avenue Blues -2 Vamp
37820-1	Hog Maw. Stomp.	Victor, hold 30 days. Issued on LP
37820-2	HOG-MAW STOMP (Waller)	Vi 21525-B
	37820: Striking of metallic object in breaks in third theme	-1 two breaks in different rhythms -2 two breaks in same (Charleston) rhythm
37820-3	Hog Maw. Stomp.	Victor rejected, master destroyed
37821-1	Black Bottom is the latest fad Stomp	Victor, hold and consult
37821-2	Black Bottom is the latest fad Stomp	Victor rejected, master destroyed
37821-3	Black Bottom is the latest fad Stomp	Victor rejected, master destroyed
37822-1	Blue Black Bottom Stomp	Victor, hold and consult
37822-2	Blue Black Bottom Stomp	No designation given. Issued on LP

The recording sheet shows that the third title is a piano solo and, although there is no notation against it, the final title also proved to be a piano solo when it was issued on LP in August 1965. According to Mike Lipskin this derives from a contemporary test pressing, the master having been destroyed shortly after the recording session. It is possible that take -1 of this title was made on organ as the recording sheet implies and take -2 on piano.The composers of 37821 are shown as "Chas. Tyus & Effie Tyus', a vaudeville team in the Butterbeans and Susie style, and for 37822 'Mike Jackson and Thos Waller' are given.

Adjacent matrices: 37818 is an organ solo by Leroy Shield on 15 February 1927.
37823-6 are by Ezio Pinza on 17 February 1927.

*****

Waller's stint at the Lincoln appears to have been very short, for the following week (2 March) *Variety* reported that, *Waller closed last week at the Lincoln Theatre; now at Metropolitan (movie) theater, Chicago for eight weeks.* The Chicago *Defender* of 12 March also stated that *Thomas (Fatts) Waller, Race organist, is at the Metropolitan, Chicago picture house in the Race section, where he will be for eight weeks. Waller is signed by the Victor phonograph people to make records.*

****

It appears likely that the reason for Waller's sudden departure from New York and arrival in Chicago was as much to escape from his wife Edith, with whom relations had become strained, as in accepting work, but the "eight weeks" at the Metropolitan was cut very short, for on 19 March 1927, Dave Peyton in his 'Musical Bunch' column of the Chicago *Defender* says:

Fats Waller, famous organist, just in Chicago from New York City, will take the organ seat permanently in the Vendome theater this week. Mr. Waller is an artist on the instrument and exerts quite a lot of originality in portraying unique novelties. He will be an asset to the already wonderful musical organization of the Vendome theater.

However, Fats may not have begun work immediately as there is no mention of him in the Vendome advert of that week. The issue of 26 March 1927 carries the advert below and Dave Peyton says that *Fats Waller, the New York organist has made a big hit in Chicago. He is playing at the Vendome theater.* On the same page as the advert there is a review of the show by 'The Scribe' under the heading:

FATS WALLER STARS

I really enjoyed my visit to the Vendome theater this week. I was delighted with the organ playing of this man they call Fats Waller. Truly he is a genous (sic). *He is full of animation and pathos. Jazz playing is his strongest fort* (sic) *and he can play the classics too.*

He has definite control of the Vendome's master organ; he handles it as if it were a baby. Large and robust, he sits at the organ keyboard and pulls the modern novelties such as Jessie Crawford, Harold Yung, Joe Keates and many of the crack white organists pull. In the pit with the orchestra Mr. Waller played a jazz piano solo that made me think of Teddy Weatherford, who is now in China.

Music, music, music, and very good music is saturating the Vendome. Long lines are in evidence since the great Fats Waller has been there and they will be as long as he is there.

VENDOME THEATER
STATE STREET AT 32D STREET

ERSKINE TATE
AND HIS VENDOME SYNCOPATORS
STAGE SPECIALTIES
THOMAS WALLER
VICTOR RECORDING ARTIST, AT THE ORGAN
ON THE SCREEN
Thursday, Friday and Saturday, March 24, 25 and 26—
Ronald Colman in "The Winning of Barbara Worth."
Sunday, March 27—Bebe Daniels in "A Kiss in a Taxi."
Monday, Tuesday and Wednesday, March 28, 29 and 30—
Corinne Griffith in "The Lady in Ermine."
COME BEFORE 6:30 P. M. AND SEE THE ENTIRE EVENING PERFORMANCE AT MATINEE PRICES

Right: The Vendome Theater Advert from the Chicago *Defender* of 26 March 1927

Present day readers might well envy 'The Scribe' and patrons of the Vendome, for Tate's orchestra was a star-studded aggregation featuring Louis Armstrong (who was also leading his own group at the Sunset simultaneously), 'Flutes' Morton, 'Stump' Evans and Jimmy Bertrand among others, and the addition of Waller on piano for a feature number must have been the jam on already thickly-buttered bread. This was probably the first time that Waller and Armstrong had worked together, but it was not to last long.

Vendome Theater adverts in the paper show Fats still present the following week, but that of 9 April doesn't mention him by name. That same week, Dave Peyton comments that Louis Armstrong is to sever his connection with the Vendome and that his departure may affect business. The following two weeks, the advert restores Waller's name, but on 30 April the advert omits all mention of an organist and Dave Peyton reveals that:

> *Fats Waller, the organist of the Vendome theater, has been detained by the Chicago police. Facts concerning his sudden apprehension will be given out in our next issue. Domestic trouble is the reported cause.*

However, the following week Peyton offers only:

> *Fats Waller, who made a hit for a week or two at the Vendome theater, Chicago, is now in New York. Sorry to lose Fats as all Chicago was wild about his clever playing on the huge Vendome pipe organ. Come again, Fats.*

and the week after that he again laments Waller's absence from the organ at the Vendome.

The outcome of these various events was presumably a promise by Fats to pay alimony to his wife for he was soon back in the recording studio, but before passing to that, there are two brief announcements in New York-based papers which concern us.

*****

On 23 March 1927, *Variety* reported that, *Jack Robbins signs Milton Charles, Thomas Waller, Jo Trent to his music publishing house.* The report went on to say that Waller and Trent had written *Whiteman Stomp* in honour of Paul Whiteman.

*****

The *Billboard* for 16 April 1927 carries an announcement for, *Alligator Crawl by 'Fats' Waller; arr. by Frank L. Ventre (formerly with Charlie Dornberger orch); published by Triangle Music Co.*

*****

FLETCHER HENDERSON & HIS ORCHESTRA Fox Trot

Russell Smith, t; Tommy Ladnier, Joe Smith, c; Benny Morton, Jimmy Harrison, tb; Buster Bailey, cl/as; Don Redman, cl-1/as; Coleman Hawkins, cl-1/ts; Fletcher Henderson, Fats Waller, p; Charlie Dixon, bj; June Cole bb; Kaiser Marshall, d.

New York City, New York — Wednesday, 11 May 1927

144132-1	Whiteman Stomp	Columbia rejected
144132-2	WHITEMAN STOMP (Whiteman, Waller and Trent)	Co 1059-D, CoE 4561, *CoF BF 409, DF 3081, LF 227,* CoJ J 285
144132-3	Whiteman Stomp	Columbia second choice
144132-4	Whiteman Stomp	Columbia rejected
144133-1	I'm Coming Virginia *-1*	Columbia second choice
144133-2	I'm Coming Virginia *-1*	Columbia rejected
144133-3	I'M COMING VIRGINIA -1 (Heywood and Cook)	Co 1059-D, CoE 4561, *CoF BF 409, DF 3081, LF 227,* CoJ J 285

According to Walter Allen, both sides were arranged by Don Redman who confirmed that Waller was added for this date. Note that Whiteman's name has been added to the composer credit of the first title.

Adjacent matrices: 144122-31 are by Roy Harvey and Posey Rorer.
144134-6 are by the Dixie Stompers on the following day.

*****

REV. J.C. BURNETT assisted by Sisters Grainger and Jackson

Gospel Song Organ accomp.

Rev. J.C. Burnett, Ethel Grainger, Odette Jackson, sp/v; acc. Thomas Waller, po.
New York City, New York — Tuesday, 17 May 1927

144162-1	PREACH THE WORD (–)	Co 14317-D
144162-2	Preach The Word	Columbia second choice
144163-1	I'll Just Stand And Ring My Hands And Cry	Columbia second choice
144163-2	I'LL JUST STAND AND RING MY HANDS AND CRY (–)	Co 14242-D
144164-1	True Friendship	Columbia second choice
144164-2	TRUE FRIENDSHIP (–)	Co 14339-D, Cl 5148-C,Ve 7113-V
144165-1	The Christians' Trouble Is Ended	Columbia second choice
144165-2	THE CHRISTIANS' TROUBLE IS ENDED (–)	Co 14295-D

The organ playing on these sides is 'straight' and aurally, there is nothing to identify the presence of Fats, but his name is noted on the recording cards. The reverse of Velvet Tone and Clarion is by **Rev. J.M. Gates** and, despite the note in *Blues & Gospel Records 1902-1943* that these are as **Rev. Jackson And His Singers**, the copy of the Velvet Tone held here is as the heading. The reverses of all other issues are by **Rev. J.C. Burnett** without Waller.

Adjacent matrices: 144159/60/61 are from the same session without Waller.
144166/7 are by Fred Rich Orch. on 20 May 1927.

*****

Thomas Waller -1 — **Pipe Organ Solos -1**
Alberta Hunter Thomas Waller at Organ -2 — **Blues Singer with organ -2**
Alberta Hunter Thomas Waller at Organ -3 — **Singing with organ-3**

Thomas Waller, po -1 or Alberta Hunter, v; acc. Thomas Waller, po -2,-3.
Trinity Church Building, Camden, New Jersey — Friday, 20 May 1927
11:00 a.m. to 1:00 p.m.

38044-1	SUGAR – Fox Trot -1 (Maceo Pinchard)	Vi 21525-A, 23331-A, BB B-5093-B, MW M-4904-B, Sr S-3176-
38044-2	Sugar — Fox Trot -1	Victor, hold indefinitely
38045-1	Sugar. Fox-Trot -2	Victor rejected, master destroyed
38045-2	SUGAR -2 (Sidney Mitchell-Edna Alexander)	Vi 20771-B, *Bm 1020*
38045-3	Sugar. Fox-Trot -2	Victor rejected, master destroyed
38046-1	Beale Street Blues.	Victor rejected, master destroyed
38046-2	BEALE STREET BLUES -2 (W.C. Handy)	Vi 20771-A, *Bm 1020*
38047-1	BEALE STREET BLUES -1 (W.C. Handy)	Vi 20890-B
38048-1	I'm going to see My Ma. -3	Victor rejected, master destroyed
38048-2	I'M GOING TO SEE MY MA -3 (Clarence Todd)	Vi 21539-B
38049-1	I'M GOING TO SEE MY MA -1	Victor hold and consult

Note that the Victor copyright department got into a muddle over the composer credits for *Sugar*, giving a mis-spelled Maceo Pinkard (writer of the music) for the organ solo and the names of the lyricists for the vocal version! On the second Victor issue Pinkard's name is correctly spelled.

The reverse of Vi 21539 is *Police Done Tore My Playhouse Down* by **Elizabeth Smith** without Waller. Biltmore as *BEALE ST. BLUES.*

*****

Thomas Waller with Morris's Hot Babies **Organ with jazz band -1**
Thomas Waller with Morris' Hot Babies **Pipe Organ with orchestra -2**
Tom Morris, c; Charlie Irvis, tb; Thomas Waller p-1/po; *Eddie King,* d.
Trinity Church Building, Camden, New Jersey Friday, 20 May 1927
1:30 p.m. to 5:15 p.m.

38050-1 "Fats" Waller Stomp. Victor rejected, master destroyed
38050-2 "Fats" Waller Stomp. Victor, hold indefinitely. Issued on LP
38050-3 "FATS" WALLER STOMP -2 (T. Waller-C. Irvis) Vi 20890-A, *HMV B.10472, HMVSw HE3150*
38050 End of trombone solo -2 Cymbal crashes submerged in organ
-3 Two cymbal crashes in isolation
38051-1 SAVANNAH BLUES -1 (Thomas Morris) Vi 20776-A, HMV B5417
38051-2 Savannah Blues. -1 Victor, hold indefinitely. Issued on LP
38051: First and second choruses -1 Morris plays open lead
-2 Morris is muted and subordinate to the trombone
38052-1 Won't You take Me Home Fox-Trot Victor rejected, master destroyed
38052-2 Won't You take Me Home Fox-Trot Victor, hold indefinitely. Issued on LP
38052-3 WON'T YOU TAKE ME HOME-Fox Trot -1 Vi 20776-B, HMV B5417
(Thomas Morris-Phil Worde)
38052: Second cornet break -2 Played by cornet alone
-3 Played by cornet and organ

The recording sheet notes the instrumentation, but gives no names other than Waller's. Studio manager Eddie King loved to participate in recordings, much to the annoyance of most musicians, and could easily be responsible for the rudimentary drum-work audible here.

Adjacent matrices: 38040/3 are by Gilda Mignonette on 20 May 1927.
38053-60 are by Mikas Petrauskas on 26 May 1927.

*****

MAUDE MILLS Comedienne, Piano Acc. (Ba 6019, Re 8391))
MAY CRANE COMEDIENNE Novelty Accompaniment (Or 976)
MAY CRANE COMEDIENNE Piano Accompaniment (Or 949)
Maude Mills, v; acc. Thomas Waller, p.
New York City, New York c. early June 1927

7293 MY OLD DADDY'S GOT A BRAND-NEW WAY TO LOVE (Mike Jackson) Ba 6019-A, Do 3987-B, Re 8348, Or 949(b)
7294 ANYTHING THAT HAPPENS JUST PLEASES ME (Smith-Hunter) Ba 6019-B, Do 3987-A, Re 8348, Or 949(a)
7295-1 I'VE GOT THE JOOGIE BLUES (Edgar Dowell) Ba 6043-, Do 4022-, Re 8391-B
(1010-2) I'VE GOT THE JOOGIE BLUES (Edgar Dowell) Or 976(b)
7295: See note
Black Snake Blues Ba 6043-, Do 4006-A, Re 8371, Or 976(a)

Maude Mills, the sister of Florence, is recalled by many as a singer and dancer of lesser talent than her famous sister. She has a number of recordings to her credit and appeared frequently in cabaret and revue at locations like the Lafayette and Lincoln in the years 1923-1928. Don Redman recalled that she was a barmaid in Harlem in the 1950's, and she died 6 July 1959.

The piano accompaniment on the above is aurally Waller on the first three titles, but sounds unlike him on the fourth. It may be that Waller's name is given on the labels of one or more of the issues yet to be inspected. However, it is also worth noting that Carl Kendziora's Plaza listing in *Record Research* (see issue 111, July 1971) lists only matrix 7295 with blanks at 7293/4. The next nearest blank numbers are 7285 and 7305, which does support the view that Waller made only the first three titles.

Of the original issues, only those noted in the headings have been inspected. Oriole 949 bears controls 954-1/953-1 and Oriole 976 shows 1010-2/1009-2. 1009-2 is aurally identical to the performance on VJM VEP 34 which reputedly uses -1 on each side. Titles on both Orioles are U/C (Oriole 949b omits the hyphen) and composer credit for *Black Snake Blues* is (Spivey-Johnson). The matrix numbers on Banner 6019 appear in full on the labels as 17293/17294 respectively, but not in the wax. When such numbers do appear in the wax, the first digit is normally dropped. This issue shows only the controls 954-1 against 17293 and 953-1 against 17294, and in 1965 Hansjürg Richner reported that he owned Oriole 949 which also showed controls 954-1/953-1 respectively for the first two titles. He also said he had Regal 8391 showing 7295-1, which he suspected was the same as 1010-1 reported to him on Banner 6043. The only other known matrix is that on Regal 8391. Alternative versions of the first two titles are claimed to be in circulation on tape, but the source of these is not known and I have not been able to hear them. There is also an unconfirmed report that Regal 8348 shows matrix numbers 7294-1/7293-1 respectively and that these equate to controls 953-1/954-1. Only a rather battered copy of Oriole 976 was available for study and, although it appears to be slightly different to microgroove issues and is therefore listed as a separate item, it defied attempts to discover describable differences.

In a letter to John R.T. Davies in December 1970, Jeff Tarrer gave the side designations for the two Domino issues and voiced the opinion that the pianist on these (and several other records he listed) was "Mike Jackson rather than Waller, particularly when Jackson gets credit for composition on labels, not Waller." Unfortunately, his letter does not give the form in which the information is presented on the labels but does note that the reverse of Do 4006 is *Golden Brown Blues* by **Jones & Mills,** as is that of Re 8371. The reverse of Re 8391 is *Hard Headed Mama* by the same artists, but artist credits on Regal are not necessarily as on Domino. For a further discussion please see the "Non-Waller" section.

Adjacent matrices: 7292 is by Irving Kaufman.
7296 is by Colin O'More.

*****

The Chicago *Defender* of 25 June 1927 has a report of a charity concert given "on Monday night" (presumably 20 June) at the Alhambra Theater, New York, and among the long list of artists who were scheduled to appear was "Fat Waller" (sic). A full-page advert for Washington Belle Hair Victory (a hair dresser and straightener) also featured Fats Waller that week and included a photo of him at the organ console.

*****

A lengthy review of the show at the New York Lafayette Theater in the Chicago *Defender* of 9 July 1927 mentions that *Fats Waller wallers in jazz at the Robert Miller organ.* This presumably for the week commencing Monday, 4 July. The report goes on to mention a special show for "Friday Midnight", but it is not clear if this included Waller.

*****

The New York Age of 16 July 1927 carries a report of vocal star Mattie Wilkes's funeral which took place in the afternoon of Saturday, 9 July 1927 at St. James Presbyterian Church and notes that *Charles "Fats" Waller was at the organ.*

*****

Fats had apparently organised another group as the following advert from *The New York Age* of 13 August 1927 indicates. The following week there is no mention of Fats by name, only a 'snappy jazz band', so either this refers to the 'Harlem Serenaders' or Fats had gone on tour with the 'Brown Sugar' company or possibly had reverted to the organ alone.

LAFAYETTE

SEVENTH AVENUE AT 132nd STREET

One Week, Beginning Monday, August 15
Mrs. MARCUS GARVEY Presents

BROWN SUGAR

With SAM MANNING

Emmet Anthony George Cooper Jas. Liallard Fulton
Alexander, Anna Freeman, Lottie Brown
Margaret Johnson Ethel Tyler

16—BROWN SKIN BEAUTIES—16

Fats Waller and His Harlem Serenaders

ALSO A BIG PHOTOPLAY PROGRAM

*****

Waller's love life was again causing him problems as a short piece in *The New York Age* of 1 October 1927 indicates: *"Fats" Waller, who has been playing the organ at the Lafayette Theatre, was paid a visit by his wife one afternoon. She sat on the same stool with 'Fats' as he was playing. The management objected. Words. "Fats" quit there and then.*

*****

Eva Jessye's column in the Baltimore *Afro-American* of 5 November 1927 carries the note that *Benny Carter in cohoots* (sic) *with Thomas (Fats) Waller and Bud Allen has just completed a new fox-trot song entitled "Nobody Knows." Carter has also completed an orchestration for Fletcher Henderson's Roseland Orchestra and it will be recorded for Columbia.*

*****

Following a highly successful season in Europe, where she had charmed audiences in London and Paris, Florence Mills had returned triumphantly to New York in October. She was the darling of the black community and her sudden death on 1 November left everyone stunned and, in a genuine outpouring of grief, many of her contemporaries paid tribute to her on record. Fats was among them, both solo and in an accompanying role.

*****

Juanita Stinette Chappelle Soprano with grand organ accompaniment by Thomas Waller
Juanita Stinette Chappelle, v; acc. Thomas Waller, po.

Trinity Church Building, Camden, New Jersey — Monday, 14 November 1927

40077-1	Florence	Victor rejected, master destroyed
40077-2	FLORENCE (Chappie Chappelle)	Vi 21062-A
40077-3	FLORENCE	Victor, 'Hold Indefinitely'. Issued on LP?

Take -3 was originally marked as 'Hold Indefinitely' as shown above but, according to *Jazz Records,* then mastered and used. However, all copies inspected use take -2. Some LP issues claim to use take -3 but, the performances are 'straight', and no detectable differences have been noted.

Carroll C. Tate Tenor with violin and piano
Carroll, C. Tate, v; acc. Bert Howell, vn; Thomas Waller, p.

Trinity Church Building, Camden, New Jersey — Monday, 14 November 1927

40078-1	GONE BUT NOT FORGOTTEN — Florence Mills (Mandy Lee-Bob King)	Vi 21061-A
40078-2	GONE BUT NOT FORGOTTEN — Florence Mills	Victor, 'Hold Indefinitely'i
40079-1	You Live On In Memory	Victor, 'Hold Indefinitely'
40079-2	YOU LIVE ON IN MEMORY (Joe Trent)	Vi 21061-B

Dispositions for 40078 were originally, take -1 'M' and take -2 'HI', and although *Jazz Records* shows take -2 as the issued take, all copies inspected and reported to me use take -1. All four takes have since been destroyed. Note that despite the entry in *Jazz Records,* the performance credit is accurate and it is piano rather than pipe organ that Waller plays.

Bert Howell Tenor with grand organ accompaniment by Thomas Waller
Bert Howell, v; acc. Thomas Waller, po.

Trinity Church Building, Camden, New Jersey — Monday, 14 November 1927

40080-1	Bye-Bye Florence	Victor rejected, master destroyed
40080-2	BYE BYE FLORENCE (Mike Jackson)	Vi 21062-B

THOMAS WALLER
Thomas Waller, po.

Trinity Church Building, Camden, New Jersey — Monday, 14 November 1927
10:20 p.m. to 10:45 p.m.

40081-1	Memories of Florence Mills.	Victor, 'Master'
40081-2	Memories of Florence Mills.	Victor, hold and consult

Both takes are now believed to have been destroyed. Times for the sides in which Fats played as accompanist are not known, but it may be assumed that the entire session began in the early evening and was arranged at short notice.

Adjacent matrices: 40073/6 are by Cantor Savel Kwartin on 8 November 1927.
40082-4 are by Colin O'More on 16 November 1927.

*****

One must wonder which 'wife' it was that caused the fracas at the Lafayette Theatre reported in October, for the Chicago *Defender* of 10 December 1927 reported: *Thomas Waller, 23, of 107 West 133 St. sentenced to one to two years in prison, but sentence suspended pending his payment of $35 per week to Mrs Edith Waller, wife. Arrested while playing in Harlem theater.*

Variety of 21 December 1927 also reported: *Waller again promises to pay his wife Edith $35 per week alimony, in Brooklyn court; judge fines him $1,000 and brief jail sentence, suspended if he pays the above alimony.* Note that Waller's address has changed, but his wife and son were still living at the address quoted on the November 1926 Victor recording sheet and at the time of his jail sentence in 1928. The Brook Avenue address was in fact that of Edith's parents where the newly married couple had resided for a time after their marriage. The West 133rd Street address may have been the home they set up together and, after things became untenable, Edith returned to her parents with son Thomas.

*****

Thomas Waller Pipe-organ with Thomas Morris and his Hot Babies
Pipe Organ with orchestra and vocal refrain (Vi 21127-B)
Thomas Waller with Thomas Morris and His Hot Babies
Pipe Organ with orchestra (Vi 21358-B)
THOMAS WALLER Pipe-organ with Thomas Morris and His Hot Babies (Vi 21202-A,-B)
Thomas Waller Pipe-organ solo -2

Tom Morris, c-1; Jimmy Archey, tb-1; Thomas Waller, po/p-1/v-3; Bobby Leecan-g-1; *Eddie King*, d-1.

Trinity Church Building, Camden, New Jersey — Thursday, 1 December 1927
10:00 a.m. to 12:00 a.m. and 12:45 p.m. to 3:15 p.m.

40093-1	He's Gone Away. Fox-Trot -1	Victor, hold indefinitely
40093-2	HE'S GONE AWAY-Fox Trot -1 (Easton-Easton)	Vi 21202-B, *El EG 7892*
	40093: Piano solo -1 Waller plays 20-bar solo interrupted momentarily by Archey in 18th bar; -2 Waller plays 18-bar solo, then Morris and Archey enter together in eighteenth bar	
40094-1	I Ain't Got Nobody -2	Victor rejected (see note)
40094-2	I AIN'T GOT NOBODY (And Nobody Cares for Me) -2 (Roger Graham - Spencer Williams)	Vi 21127-A, 23331-B, BB B-5093-A, MW M-4904-A, Sr S-3176-
40095-1	The Digah's Stomp -2	*El EG 7892*
40095-2	THE DIGAH'S STOMP -2 (T. Waller)	Vi 21358-A
	40095: Break in trombone solo -1 Piano enters in second bar; -2 No piano in break, but guitar plays on second beat	
40096-1	RED HOT DAN-Fox Trot -1, -3 (S.Easton)	Vi 21127-B
40096-2	RED HOT DAN-Fox Trot -1, -3 (S.Easton)	Vi 21127-B, *HMV B.10472, HMVSw HE 3150*
	40096: Trumpet break in final chorus:1 -1 backed by guitar; -2 played solo	
40097-1	GEECHEE—Stomp -1 (R.A. Booker-C. Austin)	Vi 21358-B, *El EG 7882*
40097-2	GEECHEE—Stomp -1 (R.A. Booker-C. Austin)	Vi 21358-B
	40097: After intro: -1 One cymbal crash preceding organ solo; -2 Two cymbal crashes preceding organ solo	

40098-1 Please Take Me out of Jail. Fox-Trot. Victor, hold indefinitely. Issued on LP
40098-2 PLEASE TAKE ME OUT OF JAIL Vi 21202-A, *El EG 7882*
-Fox Trot (T. Morris–T. Waller)

40098: Break in piano solo -1 Left hand plays single notes
-2 Two fisted

Matrices 40094/5 were entered on a separate sheet which is no longer in the Victor files, so it is not possible to give details from it, but the likely dispositions were 'D' for 40091-1 and 'HI' for 40095-1. 40096-1 and 40097-1 were originally 'HI', but both were subsequently mastered and issued, the former being described on the recording sheet as 'Fox-Trot' and the latter as 'Stomp'.

Red Hot Dan is the first time that Waller's voice had been heard on record. A second voice, possibly that of Tom Morris is also heard on this. Despite previous listings, only the takes shown above were recorded and, as with the previous session with Thomas Morris and His Hot Babies, the instrumentation is noted, but no names other than Waller's are given. Eddie King may be the percussionist. Re-issues, from a somewhat later period when Waller was known to his public as "Fats", refer to him as such. *The Digah's Stomp* is an alternative title for *The Dream* or *The Digah's Dream*, by ragtime composer Jess Pickett. Note that previous listings and a number of LP issues are incorrect in assigning the takes of *Red Hot Dan* and the re-issues to take -1. Although these latter issues show matrix 40096-1A in the wax they are aurally take -2 as compared with an original Victor pressing.

Victor 21358 comes from a short period when the company began to show matrix numbers on the labels, and this issue shows (40095) and 40097) respectively.

Adjacent matrices: 40091/2 are by Ted Weems and his Orchestra on 25 November 1927.
40099 is a personal recording by Upper Darby High School Chorus with piano by David Haupt on 3 December 1927.

*****

JOHNNY THOMPSON Vocal Novelty accomp.

Andy Razaf, v; acc. Howard Nelson, vn; David Martin vc; Thomas Waller, p.

New York City, New York Tuesday, 17 January 1928

145533-1 BACK IN YOUR OWN BACK YARD Co 14285-D
(Jolson, Rose And Dreyer)
145533-2 Back In Your Own Back Yard Columbia rejected
145533-3 Back In Your Own Back Yard Columbia rejected
145534-1 Nobody Knows How Much I Love You Columbia rejected
145534-2 Nobody Knows How Much I Love You Columbia rejected
145534-3 NOBODY KNOWS (How Much I Love You) (Allen, Waller and Carter) Co 14285-D

The file cards for this session were originally made out in Andy Razaf's name which is then crossed out and 'Johnny Thompson' substituted. The accompanists are named on the cards. The record was listed in the April 1928 supplement.

Adjacent matrices: 145532 are by James Melton on 16 January 1928.
145535 is by Goodrich Silvertown Quartet on 17 January 1928.

*****

Paul Whiteman and his Orchestra

Paul Whiteman directing: 4 violins, 5 sax, 2 cornets, 2 trombones, 1 banjo, 1 piano, 1 tuba, 2 traps. Organist: Thomas "Fats" Waller.

Studio #1, Camden Church Building, Camden, New Jersey Thursday, 26 January 1928
9:30 to 11:35 a.m.

"After rehearsing 'Whispering', could not get arrangement to suit Mr. Whiteman. Date was called off."

The above information from the Victor files, is of an aborted session by Paul Whiteman's Orchestra which may have included Bix Beiderbecke as one of the two cornets. It is almost certainly this session that Fats recalled when he told Rochester in the 19 June 1941 interview that he had made records with Paul Whiteman, even though no recording actually took place, as the musicians would probably be unaware of whether waxes were cut or not. It may also be one of the occasions when he recalled working with Bix. Whiteman did make *Whispering* soon after, but without the organ, and without Fats.

*****

The Johnny Thompson Columbia date was the first occasion when the Waller and Razaf names had been linked. They were both members of the team which were working on the show 'Keep Shufflin'". This began its preview run at Gibson's Theater, Philadelphia for the week beginning Monday, 13 February 1928 according to an advert in the *Pittsburgh Courier* of 11 February 1928 reproduced opposite. Note the mis-spelling of 'Andy Raisof' and 'Henry Cramer'. A short publicity spiel on the same page retains these spellings and mentions *Twenty two novel and tuneful musical numbers...* The following week there is a much smaller boxed advert for the show, but no mention in the editorial columns. However, on 25 February there is a lengthy and enthusiastic review which mentions *the music by Jimmy Johnson, Fat Waller and Clarence Todd...* and further on, *Imagine Jimmie Johnson the man who wrote the "Charleston" and Fat Waller large and beaming, at the pianos. Jabbo Smith behind a bugle...*

Having completed a two-week preview run in Philadelphia, the show moved to New York and opened at Daly's 63rd Street Theater on Monday, 27 February, as an announcement in *Variety* of 7 March indicates. Basically, this duplicates earlier announcements, but says of the orchestra, *on white keys "Fats" Waller, on black keys Jimmy Johnson; behind bugle, Jabbo Smith.* — which is a direct quote from the programme for the show.

Back in New York, Fats was once again available for recording dates during the day but, despite earlier accounts, is not on the Shilkret Rhyth-Melodist sides made on Friday/Saturday 2 and 3 March 1928 as he would have been too busy at the theatre to have made the return journey to Camden, apart from other considerations.

See the non-Fats Waller section for details of these.

*****

PRIOR TO BROADWAY PRESENTATION

Con Conrad Inc., Takes Pleasure In Announcing to Philadelphia the Natural Entertainment Triumph of the Season

MILLER and LYLES

AMERICA'S FOREMOST COMEDIANS

IN

"KEEP SHUFFLIN"

THE NEW COLORED MUSICAL ACHIEVEMENT

WITH

90 OF THE WORLD'S MOST DAZZLING BEAUTIES **90**

THE PEPPIEST CAST OF PERFORMERS EVER ASSEMBLED

The Jubilee Glee Club, Lethia Hill, Clarence Robinson, Byron Jones, Jean Starr, Chris Jordon, Evelyn Keyes, Josephine Hall, John Vigal, Maud Russell

AND

Will Vodery's Symphonic Band

BRILLIANT MUSICAL SCORE BY

George Gershwin, Will Vodery, Jimmie Johnson, Cole Porter, Clarence Todd, Thomas Waller

Lyrics By

Ira Gershwin, Andy Raisof, Henry Cramer

COMING—LIMITED ENGAGEMENT

Gibson's Theater

BROAD AT LOMBARD STS., PHILADELPHIA

BEGINNING MONDAY, FEBRUARY 13th

For Reservations Phone Oregon 1077-1078 or Conway's Theatre Ticket Office, 217 S. Broad St. Phone Pennypacker 8900

DUNN'S ORIGINAL JAZZ HOUNDS **Fox Trot -1**
Blues Fox Trot -2

Johnny Dunn, c; *Herb Flemming*, tb; *Garvin Bushell*, cl-1/as; Herschell Brassfield, as; James P. Johnson, Fats Waller, p.

New York City, New York Monday, 26 March 1928

E-7232-W What's The Use Of Being Alone? -1 Vo 1176-A
— Bradford —
E-7233-W What's The Use Of Being Alone? Vocalion unissued
E-7234-W Original Bugle Blues Vocalion unissued
E-7235-W Original Bugle Blues -2 — Bradford — Vo 1176-B

The last three digits of the masters and the catalogue number with side designation are shown in the wax. The labels do not show side designations but, as is normal with Vocalion issues of this period, underline the catalogue number on the B side. A Vocalion sample pressing has also been seen which has plain white labels and stickers bearing information on the group, titles and matrix numbers. Although previously listed, no banjo is audible.

Adjacent matrices: E-7226-30-W are by Miami Marimba Band on 24 March 1928.
E-7236-9-W are transfers from C1784-7 by Rev D.C. Rice on 24 March 1928.

*****

Louisiana Sugar Babes **Orchestra-1**

Jabbo Smith, c; Garvin Bushell, cl-2/as-3/bsn-4; James P. Johnson, p; Fats Waller, po.

Studios 1 & 2, Church Building, Camden, New Jersey Tuesday, 27 March 1928
9.30 a.m. to 12.50 p.m. & 2.00 p.m. to 4.25 p.m.

42566-1 WILLOW TREE -1,-2,-3 Vi 21348-A
(Andy Razaf-Thomas Waller)
42566-2 Willow Tree – Slow drag. *-2,-3* Victor rejected
(A Musical Misery.
42566-3 Willow Tree – Slow drag. -2,-3 Victor rejected. Issued on LP
(A Musical Misery.

42566: Last eight bars of trumpet solo: -1 Jabbo plays the melody
-2 Jabbo improvises ascending arpeggios

42567-1 'SIPPI -1,-2,-4 (Conrad-Creamer-Johnson) Vi 21348-B
42567-2 'SIPPI -2,-4 (Conrad-Creamer-Johnson) BB B-10260-B

425677: Bridge into bassoon solo: -1 4 firmly struck organ chords
-2 legato organ phrase

42567-3 'Sippi – Slow Drag. *-2,-4* Victor rejected
42568-1 THOU SWELL -2,-3 (Hart-Rodgers) BB B-10260-A
42568-2 THOU SWELL -1,-2,-3, Vi 21346-B
(Lorenz Hart-Richard Rodgers)

42568: Organ break before alto sax solo: -1 one bar only
-2 two bars

42568-3 Thou Swell – Fox Trot. *-2,-3* Victor rejected
42569-1 PERSIAN RUG -1,-4 (Gus Kahn-Neil Morét) Vi 21346-A, HMVAu E.A.397
42569-2 Persian Rug – Fox Trot. *-4* Victor rejected

Although the recording sheet shows that studios 1 & 2 were used, it does not indicate which titles/takes were recorded in each, although from Garvin Bushell's recollections it appears that both were used simultaneously with Waller on the organ manual in one studio along with the other musicians and the organ pipes in the other – a very strange arrangement. The first two titles were from the show *Keep Shufflin'*, and this group was the pit band for the show, although Waller actually played piano in the theatre. Garvin Bushell also states that he doesn't recall playing the bassoon in the theatre but brought it to the studio on the insistance of James P. Johnson. The recording sheet shows that Nat Shilkret directed the first title, but no dispositions are noted for any title. For this reason previous listings have shown the second take of *Willow Tree* as issued on LP as either take -2 or take -3. However, when preparing their Jabbo Smith set, Retrieval Records discovered a Victor test which clearly showed take -3 in the wax. Note that the recording took place in a morning session and another in early afternoon, enabling the musicians to be back in New York in time for the evening performance. There was presumably no matinee on a Tuesday.

All three original issues bear the additional credit **Fox Trot** for each side and Victor 21346-B notes that 42658 comes from *A Connecticut Yankee*, whilst 21348 shows both sides from *Keep Shufflin'*.

The reverse of HMVAu E.A.397 is by **Hilo Hawaiian Orchestra**.

Adjacent matrices: 42563/5 are by Mary Lewis on 26 March 1928.
42570/1 are organ solos by Lawrence Munson on 28 March 1928.

*****

Garvin Bushell's recollections of the show and this recording date as chronicled in *Jazz From The Beginning* are worth quoting in full:

James P. Johnson wrote most of the music for Keep Shufflin' and Fats Waller contributed some numbers, too. Some of the comedy bits in the show were like "Shuffle Along". Two of the big songs were "Willow Tree" and "'Sippi." In the band we had tenor saxophonist Al Sears, who later went with Duke Ellington, also Jabbo Smith on trumpet. Allegretti was a dancer in the chorus, and Blanche Calloway was in the cast, too.

Jimmy conducted the pit orchestra, and Fats played piano. They had a two-piano thing where they played some of the same things they did down at Leroy's. The show could hardly go on after they got through.

Some Monday nights we'd have to send someone out to find James P. and Fats, since they'd have been out at parties since Friday night, playing piano, spending money, buying liquor. They'd just close the places up. Monday night they'd be ossified and you couldn't get them on. That was living in the fast lane, then.

In March I went down with James P., Fats, and Jabbo to record in Camden, New Jersey. Victor had bought this church there which had a great-sounding organ, and used it as a recording studio. The organ pipes were in one room and we were in another. Fats played organ on this date. The piano and the organ manual were together, but since the pipes were in the next room Fats had a real job, because the organ always sounded a fraction of a second late. It was quite a thing. And it was hard keeping time because we had no drums or bass. That morning, Fats didn't drink his fifth of gin until <u>after</u> we got through recording.

We did two songs from "Keep Shufflin'"—"Willow Tree" and "'Sippi"— also "Persian Rug" and "Thou Swell." I played some of the first jazz bassoon on those recordings. My sound was terrible then. I was fascinated by Adrian Rollini's style on bass sax, and my bassoon playing just came out that way, even though I wasn't trying to imitate him. On the record they called us the Louisiana Sugar Babes—I have no idea why, maybe Fats created the title. He always looked at the humorous side of things .

"Keep Shufflin'" started out at Daley's 63rd Street Theater, then moved down to the Eldridge Theater on 42nd Street. In the fall of 1928 we went out on the road, going to Michigan, Ohio, and as far west as St. Louis. In Chicago, Arnold Rothstein, the gangster who owned the show, was murdered in the barbershop of the Park Central Hotel. So the union closed the show, and everybody was stranded.

*****

The New York Age of 14 April 1928 has the following:

"Battle Axe" Kenny Is Host To Miller & Lyles

On Tuesday evening April 3 after the regular performance of Broadway's popular musical hit "Keep Shufflin'", Carl ("Battle Axe") Kenny, famous drummer, was host to the principals and musicians of the show at a banquet at the popular new Rose's dining room.

A chicken dinner served as only Rose can serve them was enjoyed by all present.

Those present were, Aubrey Lyles, Flournay Miller, principals and world famous comedians. Joe Jordan, conductor of the orchestra; Ossie Lyles, "Fats" Waller, James Johnson, pianists; Joe Lyman, Wesley Howard, violinists; Bert Hall, trombonist; Jabbo Smith, Brown, Ramsay, cornetists; Ruby (sic) *Jackson, Garvin Bushell, Herb Johnson, saxophonists; Marion Cumbo, cellist; Harry Hull, bass; and Battle Axe Kenny, drummer and host of the evening.*

*****

An advert in the New York *Amsterdam News* of 4 April 1928 announces a *Silver Jubilee Ball and Reception to Celebrate the 25-Year Anniversary of Flournay Miller and Aubrey Lyles Stars of "Keep Shufflin'" at Manhattan Casino on Saturday night April 14th.* Music was to be provided by *Jimmy Johnson's and Fat Waller's "Keep Shufflin'" Band plus Fletcher Henderson.* This was presumably also a late night affair commencing after the evening performance at the theatre.

*****

According to Scott Brown, in his collaboration with Bob Hilbert, *James P. Johnson A Case Of Mistaken Identity,* the show was at Daly's Theater for only a short period and then *moved downtown and opened at the Eltinge Theatre on 24nd St. West of Broadway on April 23.* This is assumably the 'Eldridge Theater' of Garvin Bushell's recollections above. These dates may be confirmed by reference to the 'Shows in New York And Comment' column in *Variety.* The show played 8 weeks at Daly's which is shown as having a seating capacity of 997 with an admission scale running up to $3.30 for the best seats. *Variety's* reason for the move to the slightly smaller Eltinge Theater (892 seats) was that business at Daly's had fallen below the break-even point and that in its last week there had grossed about $7,500. Despite its smaller size, the more central location of the Eltinge and a lower top price seat price of $2.75 ensured an average box office of around $9,000 to $10,000, but the arrival of the 'Blackbirds' show at the adjacent Liberty's Theater brought the show to an end in its 13th week as announced in *Variety* of 23 May 1928.

*****

Whilst he was conducting and playing in 'Keep Shufflin'', James P. Johnson had been

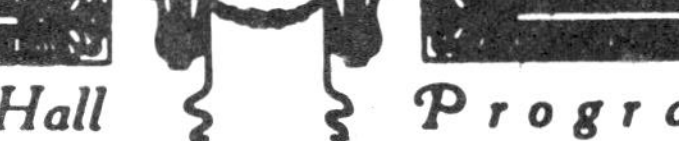

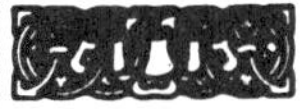

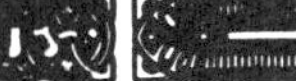

Carnegie Hall *Program*

CARNEGIE HALL

Friday Evening, April 27th, 1928.

W. C. Handy's Orchestra and Jubilee Singers

PROGRAM

PROLOGUE

a. "The Birth of Jazz"........Handy-Smith-Troy
b. "The Memphis Blues"..................Handy

SPIRITUALS—ARR. HANDY

1—a. "Steal Away To Jesus"
b. "Wheel In A Wheel"
c. "I've Heard of a City Called Heaven"
Orchestra and Chorus

BLUES

2—a. "Yellow Dog Blues"..................Handy
b. "St. Louis Blues"....................Handy
Solo-Messo Soprano Katherine Handy
c. "Beale Street Blues"..................Handy

PLANTATION SONGS

3—a. "Golden Slippers"..........James A. Bland
b. "Carry Me Back To Old Virginny"
James A. Bland
Tenor Solo—George E. Jackson
c. "My Old Virginia Home"..Rucker & Lofton
Tenor Solo—Russell Smith

SPIRITUALS—ARR. HANDY

4—a. "I'm Drinking From A Fountain"
b. "Give Me Jesus"
Orchestra and Chorus

WORK SONGS—ARR. HANDY

5—a. "Goin' To See My Sarah"
b. "Joe Jacobs"
Orchestra and Male Voices

PIANO SOLO

6—a. "Bamboula" ....Coleridge-Taylor
b. "Juba Dance" ....Nathaniel Dett
Sidney Brown

SPIRITUALS Arr. J. Rosamond Johnson

7—a. "Didn't My Lord Deliver Daniel"
b. "O Wasn't Dat A Wide River"
c. "Witness For My Lord"
J. Rosamond Johnson and Taylor Gordon

CHARACTER SONGS

8—a. "The Unbeliever",
Bert Williams-Smith-Bryan
b. "Wouldn't That Be A Dream"
Hogan-Jordan
Tom Fletcher
Accompanist, Bernardin Brown

Intermission

Part Two

9—Cake Walk.........Featuring Mme. Robinson
a. "Dark Town Is Out Tonight"
Will Marion Cook
b. "Exhortation" ....Will Marion Cook
Male Voices

NEGRO RHAPSODY

10—a. "Yamekraw"...........James P. Johnson
Orchestra
Piano—Thomas (Fats) Waller

SOPRANO SOLO

11—a. "Spring Had Come" (Hiawatha),
Coleridge Taylor
b. "Hear The Lamb A-Cryin'"..H. T. Burleigh
c. "Joshua Fit De Battle of Jericho",
Arr. Lawrence Brown
Minnie Brown
Accompanist—Andrades Lindsey

XYLOPHONE SOLO

12—"Maple Leaf Rag"..............Scott Joplin
W. C. Handy, Jr.

SOPRANO SOLO

13—"Africa" ....Ford Dabney
Josephine Hall

J. ROSAMOND JOHNSON

14—a. "African Drum Dance" No. 1,
J. Rosamond Johnson
Piano Solo
b. "Under The Bamboo Tree",
J. Rosamond Johnson
Baritone Solo

JAZZ FINALE

15—a. "Shimmy Like My Sister Kate",
Clarence Williams
Clarence Williams
b. "I Ain't Got Nobody"....Spencer Williams
Male Voices
c. "I'm Feelin' Devilish"......Maceo Pinkard
Orchestra
d. "St. Louis Blues"...................Handy
Organ Solo—Thomas (Fats) Waller
Orchestra and Chorus

STEINWAY PIANO USED

Management: Robert Clairmont

The programme for Handy's Carnegie Hall Concert was originally printed in single vertical column format, but to improve legibility it is here split into two.

composing a rhapsody which he called *Yamekraw* which he later expanded into a folk opera. Critics and friends alike were very impressed with this and W.C. Handy decided to feature it as a highlight in a Carnegie Hall concert he was scheduled to give on 27 April 1928 to celebrate the 25th anniversary of the publication of *Memphis Blues.* Handy wanted Johnson to take the solo piano role for this, but the owners of *'Keep Shufflin"* refused to grant him leave of absence for the evening. After considerable discussion, it was agreed that Waller could be spared for the evening and after auditioning for the sponsors of the Carnegie Hall function, during which he also played organ, it was agreed that not only would he take the solo part in *Yamekraw,* but would also contribute a set on organ. Anita is quoted by Maurice Waller in his book as saying:

> *"It was a Friday night, and the city was hit with a wild, spring storm. It rained all day and the streets were so windy you couldn't walk around. With all that bad weather you'd think that no one would go out and I was surprised to see that hall filled to capacity. Your father had recorded 'Beale Street Blues' the year before with Alberta Hunter, and W.C. Handy thought it would be the right selection for your father to play at Carnegie Hall."*

Maurice goes on to say that Fats first played *Beale Street Blues* as a solo, followed by a vocal version accompanying Katherine Handy, W.C's daughter.

A detailed review of the concert appeared in *The New York Age* of 5 May, and excerpts which concern us are *...The Program did not make known the identity of the pianist who was regularly used, but piano and organ specialties were played by Thomas Waller, whose first appearance was in rendering 'The Beale Street Blues'. Mr. Waller is familiarly known as "Fats" and his virtuosity as a jazz pianist quickly won favor with the large audience. ... A group of "blues" numbers included the "Yellow Dog Blues" "St. Louis Blues," (with the composer's daughter Katherine E. Handy, a mezzo soprano, singing the solo), and "The Beale Street Blues". The latter was repeated and then "Fats" Waller had to respond with a piano number as an encore. ... The most pretentious number of the evening was termed a Negro Rhapsody, "Yamekraw", written by James P. Johnson, and evidently, from the name, intended to typify life in the old Yamecraw section of Savannah, Ga. "Fats" Waller was again featured at the piano. ... The closing number was a jazz finale, including Clarence Williams' "Shimmy like my sister Kate," Pinkard's "I'm feeling devilish" and a grand climax was reached with another playing of "The St. Louis Blues," with "Fats" Waller at the organ, and the orchestra featuring a cornet cadenza.*

*****

JIMMY JOHNSON AND HIS ORCHESTRA **Fox Trot**

Cootie Williams, t; unknown, tb; Garvin Bushell, cl/as; unknown cl-1/ts; James P. Johnson, Fats Waller, p; Joe Watts, sb; Perry Bradford, sp-1.

New York City, New York — Monday, 18 June 1928

146539-1	Chicago Blues	Columbia second choice
146539-2	Chicago Blues	Columbia rejected
146539-3	CHICAGO BLUES (Biese, Altiere and Williams)	Co 14334-D
146540-1	MOURNFUL THO'TS -1 (Johnson)	Co 14334-D
146540-2	Mournful Tho'ts *-1*	Columbia rejected
146540-3	Mournful Tho'ts *-1*	Columbia second choice

Although an article in *Storyville 45*, p.90 reported that the bass was of the brass variety and added banjo and drums to the instrumentation as well as scat vocals, I do not hear any of these. There is a suggestion of banjo and some sort of percussion at the beginning of the first title, but I believe this is derived from the sound of the pianists and possibly someone (Bradford?) hitting something. It is unlikely that a banjoist and drummer would have been hired for this brief excursion. In 1989, John Heinz wrote to *Storyville* stating that he had played these sides to James P. Johnson before he suffered his stroke and that he had recalled Cootie Williams and Garvin Bushell, and Cootie himself recalled making them. Apparently, he was deputising for Jabbo Smith.

Adjacent matrices: 146538 is by Joe Davis (The Melody Man), piano acc. Rube Bloom on 19 June 1928.
146541/2 are by Paul Whiteman's Orchestra on 17(!) June 1928.

*****

Soon after the above date, Fats must have decided to leave 'Keep Shufflin", Maurice Waller says that Arnold Rothstein, who was the 'angel' behind the show, had fallen behind in his payments to Waller and that when an offer came to play piano and organ in the Grand Theatre in Philadelphia, Fats gladly accepted. Waller's departure date from the show is not known, but almost certainly would have been a Saturday as he would have worked a full week. 23 and 30 June 1928 were both Saturdays and an advert in *The New York Age* of 23 June for Hill's Social Club may give a clue for it shows that Waller was to be present at the Renaissance Casino to provide music along with Vernon Andrades (The strange reversal of dates may be explained by the fact that the cover date of a paper was not necessarily the actual publication date.) but a report of the event the following week says *Fats Waller gave no reason but did not show up...*

The *New York Amsterdam News* of 20 June reports Waller at the Alhambra for a benefit on 28 June.

He was also scheduled to appear at a benefit at the Lafayette on 5 July 1928 and was announced (as Fatts Waller) as one of the artists to appear for a one hour broadcast over New York station WABC on 6 July along with Will Vodery and Josephine Hall. It is not known if he honoured these engagements.

Fats may also have applied for work to the Regal in Chicago, for an announcement in *Variety* of 4 July 1928 says *James (Fats) Waller, colored organist, now permanently at Regal movie house, Chicago.* This obviously 'jumped the gun', for Fats actually went in a different direction.

By now Anita was pregnant with their second child and a steady income was required to support his family and keep up his alimony payments to Edith, which apparently had been maintained as long as the Wallers were in New York. However, it was a case of 'out of sight, out of mind' and it wasn't long before trouble loomed again. How long Fats stayed at the Grand is not known, but according to the report below, he was later at the Royal. After Waller's death, Charley McClane, who had signed Fats for the Royal recalled in *downbeat* of 1 February 1944 that the orginal contract called for Waller to play organ in the Royal Theater (a silent movie house operated by the Morris Wax circuit) for one month. He proved to be such a success that he stayed for "nine months", and that after his stint at the theatre, Waller would move on to the Sunset Grill where he played from midnight until 3:00 a.m. As is so often the case, the length of stay has become exaggerated in memory.

*****

The Baltimore *Afro-American* of 30 June 1928 datelined Philadelphia under the heading *FATS WALLER ONE OF TWELVE CHILDREN* goes on to say:

> *Out of a family of twelve brothers and sisters, Thomas 'Fats' Waller boasts of being the only one who went into the professional field for a career.*
>
> *Waller, who is filling a summer engagement at the Royal Theatre here, as organist is said to be one of the best in the country. He was born and reared in New York and began the study of music at the age of nine under a Mrs Alice Perry. When he was sixteen he took up organ under Edward V. Thomas and Carl Bohm, both white and the latter a German.*
>
> *Since going into music as a vocation, Waller has never been with but one show, and that was "Keep Shufflin' ". He has made several vaudeville tours and is well known in many of the night clubs in New York.*

*****

Fats was in matrimonial trouble again and the first news of this appeared in the Chicago *Defender* of 18 August 1928 in a report from New York:

> *"Fats" Waller, organist and composer and late of the Miller and Lyles show, was arrested and brought here from Philadelphia, where he had been playing under contract at the Grand theater, to answer charges of nonsupport brought against him by his wife. This is Waller's third appearance in court on the same charge. The case was tried before Judge Albert Cohen, who sentenced him to two years in prison and ordered him to pay $350 alimony. Attorneys Jaffe and Murray Becker appeared for Waller. Waller has one child.*

The Baltimore *Afro-American* of 15 September 1928 offered a slightly different version:

> *Failing six times to live up to his promise to support his wife and child, Fats Waller, Song-writer and pianist, was sentenced by Judge Cohn to serve from six months to three years in the New York Penitentiary. Waller, who has been in jail for the past thirty-one days, has been arrested on several occasions for the same offence. The last time being in the Royal Theatre in Philadelphia.*

Two weeks later, on 29 September, the same paper followed it up with:

> *Failing to pay his wife Mrs Waller the alimony allotted to her by the court has landed Fats Waller popular blues writer behind the bars to serve a term of from six months to three years in the County Penitentiary. Fats is charged with abandoning his wife and four year old son Thomas who live at 1006 Brooks Ave.*

This was also picked up and reported by *Variety* on 19 September.

From these reports it would appear that Fats was playing the Royal Theatre, Philadelphia in mid-August 1928 when he was arrested. He was presumably able to purge his contempt of the court and bring his alimony payments up to date for the *Afro-American* of 15 December 1928, datelined New York and under the heading *FATS WALLER FREED* reports *Fats Waller is back on Broadway after spending three months in the City Penitentiary for non-payment of alimony for his wife and child.*

Maurice Waller's account is somewhat different and he says that Fats and his wife and child (himself) had been in Philadelphia from June to October, during which time Waller had failed to make any alimony payments and that when they returned to Manhattan, Edith was waiting with an arrest warrant. He goes on to mention that Edward Waller had died while Fats was serving his time in prison and relates how Gene Austin came to the rescue and provided the bail money, convincing the judge that he needed Waller to make a record. However, he places this as after 4 November when Arnold Rothsetin was shot and then says that his father had been released prior to the birth of his brother Ronald, which took place on 26 October 1928. Also, there is no recording of Austin with Waller in October/November 1928 so his 'facts' do not tie up with each other.

In its edition of 24 November, the *Defender* reported that *'Keep Shufflin"* had closed following the murder of Rothstein, and two weeks after the above report, in its issue of 29 December, the *Afro-American* reported Fats back at the Lafayette Theatre.

*****

THOMAS WALLER PIANO SOLO -1

Fats Waller and His Buddies Hot Dance Orchestra -2

Charlie Gaines, t; Charlie Irvis, tb; Arville Harris, cl/as; Fats Waller, p/p solo-1; Eddie Condon, bj.

Liederkranz Hall, New York City, New York — Friday, 1 March 1929

3:10 p.m. to 3:30 p.m. and 4:55 p.m. to 5:20 p.m.

49759-1	HANDFUL OF KEYS -1 (T. Waller)	Vi V-38508-A, 27768-B, ViC 27768-B, HMV/Au B.4347, HMV B.4902, HMVIn N 4480, HMVSc X4480, HMVFr SG 543, ASR LB4347, LB4902
49759-2	Hand Full Of Keys -1	Victor rejected
49759-3	Hand Full Of Keys -1	Victor rejected
49760-1	The Minor Drag -2	Victor rejected
49760-2	THE MINOR DRAG-Fox Trot -2 (Thomas Waller)	Vi V-38050-A, 20-1583-B, *Vi/C20-1583-B,* BB B 10185-A, *RCA 420-0236,* HMV J.F.1, HMVSw HE2367, HMVAu E.A.3265, HMVFr K8196, HMVSc X.6252
49761-1	Harlem Fuss -2	Victor rejected
49761-2	HARLEM FUSS-Fox Trot -2 (Thomas Waller)	Vi V-38050-B, BB B 10185-B, HMVAu EA3713, HMVSw HE2367, HMVFr K8196, HMVSc X.6252
49762-1	Numb Fumblin' -1	Victor rejected
49762-2	NUMB FUMBLIN' -1 (T. Waller)	Vi V-38508-B, 25338-A, HMV/Au B.4347, HMV B4917, *HMVSw HE2381*, HMVSc X3944, X6292, ASR LB4347, LB4917

There is an amusing account of the above session in Eddie Condon's *We Called It Music* in which he relates how he had been engaged by the Victor company to get Fats to the studio on time and how he came to be playing banjo on it. He says that at the end of the session he was congratulated by one of the Victor executives on successfully achieving this and says that despite everything when the sides came out the titles had been reversed to actual content. Despite this, Dave Carey believes they are correctly labelled and points out that *The Minor Drag* is in a minor key and that *Harlem Fuss* could very well be descriptive of what is heard. Additional evidence in support of this theory comes from Jack Mitchell who says that the Australian HMV issue is one of those Victor derivative pressings that show some wax markings under the label either side of the centre boss. On one side is "BVE 49760 The ... " and "Fats ... Buddies" which suggests that the title inscribed at the time of recording is The Minor Drag. The reverse shows no trace of the title but, as Harlem Fuss is slightly shorter, it could well be accomodated in the area that has been machined smooth.

Amusingly, despite Condon's recollection, there is a cryptic note on the sheet saying "Date called for 1:45" so, despite all his efforts, the session was almost an hour and a half late in getting under way. The actual entries for the Buddies sides were made on a separate sheet which is no longer available. The sheet for the two solos notes Waller's address as 107 W 133 St. This look suspiciously like a misreading of 107 W 134 St., which was the Waller family home.

The Alberti Special Record issues have not been inspected, and may prove to be dubbed issues.

The reverse of HMV B4917 and HE2381 is *Call Of The Freaks* by **The Rhythm Kings**.

Adjacent matrices: 49757/8 are by Franklyn Baur on 28 February 1928.
49763/4 were not used.

*****

The Baltimore *Afro-American* of 18 May 1929 under the heading "Gets Radio Contract For Huge Orchestra" and datelined New York has:

> *Thomas "Fats" Waller, pianist and jazz organist, one of the guest artists on the Littman program Friday evening, has just signed a contract with station WABC to lead a twenty-six piece orchestra over that station during the Mason Mint Hour for a period of twenty-six weeks.*
>
> *This is the first time that a race orchestra has been engaged to feature the music of one of the big advertisers hours and is a tribute to Waller's ability as a pianist. His last appearance on Broadway was with "Rang Tang," when he was associated with Jimmy Johnson. Waller is a New York boy who has steadily climbed his way to the top, despite serious handicaps and obstacles.*

This is the only reference I have been able to trace referring to Waller taking an active part in *"Rang Tang"*. The show ran on Broadway in January/February 1928 at the Royal and Majestic Theatres and moved into the Lafayette for one week only ending on Sunday, 19 February 1928. For most of this period Waller was working on or with *"Keep Shufflin'"* so, although it is feasible that he took part in one or both of the Broadway presentations, he was certainly unavailable for the week at the Lafayette. It should be remembered that "shows" in those days were considerably different to what is found in London or on Broadway today. Generally they had a basic concept, a book of songs and a cast consisting of a number of principals and supporting acts. The actual content of a show might vary from performance to performance, partly according to audience reaction and partly to adjust to the availability of artists, so it is by no means inconceivable that Waller and Johnson did appear in *"Rang Tang"* at some time.

*****

Some time in the spring of 1929, Fats joined the staff of Joe Davis's music publishing empire and began to exploit his talent for writing and composing in a much more serious manner, and a whole string of fine compositions from him began to appear. With Harry Brooks and Andy Razaf, he worked on the score of a new show, *"Hot Chocolates"* and this opened at Connie's Inn in May 1929. It was so successful that Immerman decided to move it into a theatre and early in June it went into the Windsor Theatre in the Bronx for two weeks, then to the Hudson Theater, New York on 20 June 1929. It was staged by Leonard Harper and featured Baby Cox, Edith Wilson, Eddie Green, Billy Higgins and others. Two of the memorable numbers written for this show were *Ain't Misbehavin'* and *Sweet Savannah Sue*.

It is noteworthy that, with the settling into a more ordered existence, newspaper references to Waller became virtually non-existent! The only two I have been able to trace are in the Chicago *Defender* of 15 June and *The New York Age* of 19 July, both of which carried brief reports that Waller and Andy Razaf were writing the tunes for *"Hot Chocolates"*.

*****

Gene Austin Tenor with orchestra

Gene Austin, v; acc. Mike Mosiello, t; Andy Sanella, cl-1/as-2; Lou Raderman, Murray Kellner, Yascha Zayde, vn; Herb Borodkin, vc; Fats Waller, p; Carl Kress, g; Dick Cherwin, sb; Williams Dorn or Joe Green, d.

New York City, New York — Wednesday, 26 June 1929

53586-1	I've Got A Feeling I'm Falling *-1*	Victor unissued
53586-2	I've Got A Feeling I'm Falling *-1*	Victor unissued
53586-3	I'VE GOT A FEELING I'M FALLING -1 (Rose-Link-Waller)	Vi 22033-B, HMV B3117, HMVAu EA 593
53587-1	Maybe!-Who Knows? *-2*	Victor unissued
53587-2	Maybe!-Who Knows? *-2*	Victor unissued
53587-3	MAYBE!-WHO KNOWS? -2 (Tucker-Shuster-Etting)	Vi 22033-A, HMV B3117, HMVAu EA 593

The recording sheet for this session was not available for study.

Adjacent matrices: 53584/5 are by Bill Moore' Syncopators on 26 June.
53588/9 are by Gus Arnheim and his Orchestra on 27 June.

*****

Although *'Hot Chocolates'* was one of the more successful black shows it apparently followed the normal pattern in that it was subject to change, both of material and cast and, in this latter respect it has been extremely difficult to find exact datings for some important comings and goings. Waller had rehearsed the show before the opening at Connie's Inn, but there is no record of him actually participating initially. Louis Armstrong, who started as a featured soloist in the pit and later graduated to a main attraction, seems not to have come into the show until the tail end of the Bronx run. He is almost certainly the "unnamed member of the orchestra" who played *Ain't Misbehavin'* to the approval of the *New York Times* reviewer who covered the première at the Hudson. Fats himself certainly took part in at least part of the run of 219 apearances at the Hudson and for part of the time he, Edith Wilson and Louis Armstrong were billed as "A Thousand Pounds of Rhythm". The show itself seems to have been expanded from the original format before going into the Windsor Theatre, but adverse criticism led to it being pruned before the Broadway opening. During both theatre runs, the cast performed a shortened version back at Connie's Inn late at night and after closing at the Hudson and Connie's Inn it went on a brief road tour, but how many of the cast went on this and whether or not they included the principals is not known.

*****

Thomas Waller Piano Solo

Thomas Waller, p.

Studio #1, Trinity Church Building, Camden, New Jersey Friday, 2 August 1929
2:00 p.m. to 5:15 p.m.

49492-1	Ain't Misbehavin' From: "Hot Chocolates"	Victor unissued
49492-2	Ain't Misbehavin' From: "Hot Chocolates"	Victor unissued
49492-3	AIN'T MISBEHAVIN' (Razaf-Waller-Brooks)	Vi/C/Ar 22108-A, *Vi 20-1581-A*, ViC 22092-A, ViAr 68-0773-A, *RCA 420-0236*, HMV B3243, HMVAu EA 641
49493-1	Sweet Savannah Sue. From-"Hot Chocolates"	Victor unissued
49493-2	SWEET SAVANNAH SUE (Razaf-Waller-Brooks)	Vi/Ar 22108-B, BB B 10264-B, ViAr 68-0773-B, HMVAu EA 641
49494-1	I've got a Feeling I'm Falling.	Victor unissued. Issued on LP
49494-2	I'VE GOT A FEELING I'M FALLING (Rose-Link-Waller)	Vi/Ar/C 22092-B, ViC 22108-B, HMV B3243, HMVAu EA 622
49494-3	I've got a Feeling I'm Falling.	Victor unissued. Issued on LP

49494: End of verse -1 One 1-bar break
-2 Two 2-bar breaks
-3 No breaks

49495-1	Leave Me, or Love Me From: "Whoopee"	Victor unissued. Issued on LP
49495-2	Leave Me, or Love Me From: "Whoopee"	Victor unissued. Issued on LP?
49495-3	LOVE ME OR LEAVE ME (Gus Kahn- Walter Donaldson)	Vi/Ar 22092-A, BB B 10263-B

49495: End of verse: -1 No breaks
-3 Breaks

49496-1	GLADYSE (Thos. Waller)	Vi V-38554-B, HMV J.F.4, HMVSw HE2366
49496-2	Gladyse	Victor unissued. Issued on LP

49496: Fourteenth bar: -1 No break
-2 Half-bar break

49497-1	Valentine Stomp	Victor unissued. Issued on LP
49497-2	VALENTINE STOMP (Thos. Waller)	Vi V-38554-A, BB B 10263-A, HMV J.F.4, HMVSw HE2366

49497: Second half of bridge at end of first theme -1 Chords
-2 Single notes

The Victor clerical staff had at last acknowledged that Waller was known to all by his nickname and "(Fats)" is typed in above the recording sheet heading of "Thomas Waller (Piano Solos)". The composer credits for the last two tunes are also shown as "Fats Waller" and "Thomas Fats Waller" respectively. *Valentine Stomp* is named for Hazel Valentine, the madame of a popular brothel, The Daisy Chain, which was almost certainly unknown to the Victor staff.

Both sides of Victor 22108 bear the credit line **(From the Musical Comedy. "Connie's Hot Chocolates")**, and the A side of 22092 has **(From the Ziegfeld production, "Whoopee")**. Note the variations between what is found on the records and the recording sheet.

No dispositions are noted on the recording sheet and although this and the Victor ledger clearly give the recording date as "August 2nd", the test of 49494-3 equally clearly has "Aug 3-29" inscribed in the central area.

Matrix 49495-2 is reputed to appear on LP, but this has not been confirmed.

Adjacent matrices: 49488-91 are by Johnny Johnson Pennsylvanians on 2 August 1929. 49498/9 are piano duets by Hazel G. Kinscella and Myrtle C. Eaver on 9 August 1929.

*****

Thomas Waller Organ Solo -1

Thomas Waller, po.

Studio #1 Trinity Church Building, Camden, New Jersey — Thursday, 29 August 1929

9:00 to 11:05 (no indication of whether a.m. or p.m.)

56067-1 "Waiting At The End Of The Road" (Theme Song Of Hallelujah) — Victor unissued. Issued on LP

56067-2 "Waiting At The End Of The Road" (Theme Song Of Hallelujah) — Victor unissued. Issued on LP

56067: Opening of first chorus -1 First bar has sustained high note followed by single low note
-2 First bar has sustained high note followed by descending 4-note phrase

56068-1 "Baby-Oh Where Can You Be?" — Victor unissued. Issued on LP

56068-2 "Baby-Oh Where Can You Be?" — Victor unissued. Issued on LP

56068-3 "Baby-Oh Where Can You Be?" — Victor unissued. Issued on LP

56068: -1 Introduction followed by the chorus
-2 Introduction followed by the verse and then the chorus
-3 No introduction, piece begins with the verse from which the first notes appear to be missing

56069-1 "Tanglefoot" — Victor unissued. Issued on LP

56069-2 "Tanglefoot" — Victor unissued. Issued on LP

56069: End of first chorus -1 Extra bar
-2 No extra bar

56070-1 "Thats All" — Victor unissued. Issued on LP?

56070-2 THAT'S ALL -1 (Thos. Waller) — Vi 23260-B

Although the Victor files confirm that the above and the following session were made on the same day, the recording sheet for the piano solo session below is no longer available and it is thus not possible to say which of the two came first, especially as no indication is given as to whether the above is a morning or evening session. Camden matrix blocks were pre-assigned, which probably accounts for the wide divergence in matrix numbers. It is also likely that the piano solos were recorded in studio #2. Unusually, all four titles above are shown in double quotes, probably indicating a new clerk at work. Composer credits for the first two titles are to Irving Berlin; Thos. Waller & Sidney Easton for the third and Thos. Waller for the fourth.

Matrix 56070-1 is reputed to be issued on LP, but this is unconfirmed.

Adjacent matrices: These Waller recordings are the only ones listed for the 56000 block and Brian Rust suggests that the remainder of the block may have been allocated to Vitaphone soundtrack rcordings.

*****

"Fats" Waller and his Piano

Thomas Waller, p.

Trinity Church Building, Camden, New Jersey — Thursday, 29 August 1929

55375-1	WAITIN' AT THE END OF THE ROAD (Irving Berlin)	BB B 10264-A
55375-2	Waiting At The End Of The Road	Victor unissued. Issued on LP

55375: End of final chorus:
-1 4 left-hand vamp chords, which are repeated; followed by final phrase of melody and then by 3 left hand chords and a final right hand chord.
-2 melody is played through and piece ends with 3 single left hand notes.

55376-1	Baby, Oh! Where Can You Be?	Victor unissued. Issued on LP
55376-2	Baby, Oh! Where Can You Be?	Victor unissued. Issued on LP

55376: Middle eight of first chorus -1 First half in breaks, seiond half with rhythm
-2 Entirely in breaks

The recording sheet for this session was not available for study, but it seems probable that it took place in Studio #2, but whether before or after the previous session is not known.

Adjacent matrices: 55374 is by the Four Pals on 29 August.
55377 is a personal recording by Mr. Erdman on 3 September 1929.

*****

Thomas Waller Piano Solo

Thomas Waller, p.

44th Street Studio, New York City, New York — Wednesday, 11 September 1929
10:00 a.m. to 1:00 p.m.

56125-1	Goin' About.	Victor unissued. Issued on LP
56125-2	Goin' About.	Victor unissued. Issued on LP

56125: Repeat of first 16-bar theme -1 Is played at the same pitch as before
-2 Is played an octave higher

56126-1	MY FEELIN'S ARE HURT (Thomas Waller)	Vi V-38613-A
56126-2	My Feelin's Are Hurt	Victor hold and consult

Dispositions are shown only against the second title. Swiss HMV HE 3003 bearing the above pair of titles, and sometimes advertised as by Waller, was mis-pressed using masters which have nothing to do with him. Some copies of Victor V-38613-A show the composer credit as simply (Waller).

Adjacent matrices: 56123/4 are by Smith Ballew and his Orchestra on 6 September 1929.
56127/8 are by The High Hatters on 12 September 1929.

*****

THE LITTLE CHOCOLATE DANDIES — **Fox Trot -1**
Fox Trot with Vocal Refrain -2

Rex Stewart, c; Leonard Davis, t; J.C. Higginbotham, tb; Don Redman, cl-2/as/v-2; Benny Carter, as/v-2; Coleman Hawkins, ts; Fats Waller, p/cel-2; Bobby Johnson, bj; Cyrus St. Clair, bb; George Stafford, d; unknown, v-3.

New York City, New York — Wednesday, 18 September 1929

402965-A	That's How I Feel Today -3	OKeh second choice
402965-B	That's How I Feel Today -3	OKeh first choice
402965-C	THAT'S HOW I FEEL TODAY -1 (Redman)	OK 8728, PaE R.542

402966-A Six Or Seven Times -2 — OKeh rejected
402966-B Six Or Seven Times -2 — OKeh second choice
402966-C Six Or Seven Times -2 — OKeh rejected
402966-D SIX OR SEVEN TIMES -2 (Waller-Mills) — OK 8728, PaE R.542, R 2550, PaAu A 7483, PaSw PZ 11127, OdEx OR 2550

Note that a vocal version of the first title was originally selected for issue, but the choice was later changed in favour of the non-vocal take. Both tunes were arranged by Benny Carter.

Adjacent matrices: 402963/4 are by Frank Trumbauer Orch on 18 September 1929.
402967/70 are blank.

*****

THOMAS WALLER Piano Solo

Thomas Waller, p.

Liederkranz Hall, New York City, New York — Tuesday, 24 September 1929
10:00 a.m. to 11:45 a.m.

56710-1 Mashing Thirds — Victor unissued
56710-2 SMASHING THIRDS (T. Waller) — Vi V-38613-B, 25338-B, HMV B.4902, B8546, HMVFr SG 543, HMVSc X3944 ASR LB4902
56710-3 Mashing Thirds — Victor unissued

The title on the recording sheet is as given, but there is a note in manuscript "(Wiggle on the Third) — per Oberstein 8/29/30", but on issue it became the familiar *Smashing Thirds.* The sheet shows that Waller made only this one title, so that the adjacent matrices are more than usually interesting. Some copies of Victor V-38613-B show the composer credit as simply (Waller).

The Alberti Special Record issue has not been inspected and may prove to be a dubbing.

Adjacent matrices: 56707-9 are by P. Barchi on 20 September 1929.
56711/2 are by Helen Morgan on 24 September 1929. These are potential Waller items, but the issued takes come from a remake session and, unless tests exist from this first date we will never know.

*****

Fats Waller and His Buddies -Fox Trot — Vocal refrain by The Four Wanderers -1
Fats Waller and His Buddies -Fox Trot — Vocal Refrain by The Four Wanderers -2

Henry Allen, t; Jack Teagarden, tb/vb; Albert Nicholas, Otto Hardwick, as; Larry Binyon, ts; Fats Waller, p; Eddie Condon, bj; Al Morgan, sb; Gene Krupa, d; The Four Wanderers, v.

New York City, New York — Monday, 30 September 1929

56727-1 Lookin' Good But Feelin' Bad — Victor unissued
56727-2 LOOKIN' GOOD BUT FEELIN' BAD -1 (Santley-Waller) — Vi V-38086-A
56728-1 I NEED SOMEONE LIKE YOU -2 (Thomas Waller) — VI V-38086-B
56728-2 I Need Someone Like You — Victor unissued

The recording sheet for the above session was not available for study.

The Four Wanderers vocal group consist of Herman Hughes and Charles Clinkscales, tenors; Maceo Johnson, baritone, and Oliver Childs, bass. They had recorded previously with the Luis Russell band under Henry Allen's leadership. Henry Allen confirmed that Teagarden had played the vibes which "were standing in the corner."

Adjacent matrices: 56723-26 are by Bob McGimsey on 27 September 1929.
56729-31 are by Johnny Marvin on 30 September 1929.

*****

ED GREEN-BILLY HIGGINS AND COMPANY

Ed Green, Billy Higgins, J.E. Lightfoot, Billy Maxey, D. Campbell, J. Wilson, T. Hall, 'Jazzlips', A. Haston, sp; acc. Fats Waller, p.

Liederkranz Hal, New York City, New York — Monday, 14 October 1929
1:45 p.m. to 4:00 p.m.

56782-1	Big Business – Part 1	Victor unissued
56782-2	Big Business – Part 1	Victor unissued
56782-3	BIG BUSINESS – PART 1	Victor V-38552-A
56783-1	Big Business – Part 2	Victor unissued
56783-2	Big Business – Part 2	Victor unissued
56783-3	BIG BUSINESS – PART 2	Victor V-38552-B

The above is a sketch from the show *'Hot Chocolates'* by members of the cast with incidental piano by Waller. It is of little jazz interest.

Adjacent matrices: 56778-81 are by Frank Luther & Carson Robison on 14 October 1929.
56784 is a personal recording by Mabel Beck on 16 October 1929.

*****

An advert for the Alhambra Theater at 126th Street and Seventh Avenue, in *The New York Age* of 2 November 1929 shows a Benefit Show for Lincoln College Athletic Association to take place on "Sunday Midnite" (presumably 3 November). Elsewhere on the same page an editorial paragraph lists some of those scheduled to appear, and this list includes "Fats" Waller.

*****

McKinney's Cotton Pickers — **Fox Trot**
Slow Fox Trot Vocal refrain by Donald Redman -1

Joe Smith, Leonard Davis, Sidney De Paris, t; Claude Jones, tb; Don Redman, as/v-1; Benny Carter, as/cl-2; Coleman Hawkins, Ted McCord, ts; Leroy Tibbs, p-3; Fats Waller, p-4/cel-5; Dave Wilborn, bj; Billy Taylor, bb; Kaiser Marshall, d.

46th Street Studio, New York City, New York — Tuesday, 5 November 1929
1:45 p.m. to 5:00 p.m.

57064-1	Plain Dirt – Fox Trot *-3*	Victor unissued
57064-2	PLAIN DIRT -3 (C. Stanton)	Vi V-38097-B, *40-0115-A,* ViAr 62 0083, BB B-11590- , HMV B 4990, GrF K 6950
57065-1	GEE, AIN'T I GOOD TO YOU -1,-3 (Donald Redman)	Vi V-38097-A, ViAr J 5208, BB B 5205, BB B-10249-A, B 11590- , Sr S 3286, HMV B.4967, GrFr K6950, HMVSw JK 2155
57065-2	Gee, Ain't I Good To You – Slow Fox Trot -1, *-3*	Victor unissued

46th Street Studio, New York City, New York — Wednesday, 6 November 1929
1:45 p.m. to 5:30 p.m.

57066-1	I'd Love It – Fox Trot *-4,-5*	Victor unissued
57066-2	I'D LOVE IT -4,-5 (Redman-Hudson)	Vi/Ar V-38133-B, ViAr 62 0059, BB B-10706-A, HMV B.4967, HMVSw JK 2474
57067-1	THE WAY I FEEL TODAY -1,-2,*-3*,-4,-5 (Redman-Quicksell-Razaf)	Vi V-38102-B, ViAr 760-0001-B, BB B-10232-B, HMV B4901, B6204, HMVSw JK 2166
57067-2	The Way I Feel Today – Fox Trot -1, *-2,-3,-4,-5*	Victor unissued
57068-1	Miss Hannah - Fox Trot -1, *-3,-4,-5*	Victor unissued
57068-2	MISS HANNAH -1,*-3*,-4,-5 (Redman-Nesbit)	Vi V-38102-A, ViAr 760-0001-A, BB B-10232-A, HMV B4901, B6215, HMVSw JK 2166, El EG 2614

44th Street Studio, New York City, New York — Thursday, 7 November 1929
10:00 a.m. to 1:20 p.m.

57139-1	Peggy - Fox Trot *-4*	Victor unissued
57139-2	Peggy - Fox Trot *-4*	Victor unissued
57139-3	PEGGY -4 (Bismer-Buckley-Head)	Vi/Ar V-38133-A, ViAr 62 0059, BB B-10706-B
57140-1	Where Ever There's A Will. - Fox Trot -1,*-4*	Victor unissued
57140-2	WHEREVER THERE'S A WILL, BABY-1,-4 (D. Redman)	Vi 22736-B, BB B-10249-B, HMV B.D.135, HMVSw JK 2155
57140-3	Where Ever There's A Will. - Fox Trot -1,-4	Victor unissued. Issued on LP

57140: Redman sings: -2 Wherever there's a will… You know Rome wasn't built…
-3 Oh, wherever there's a will… Now, you know Rome wasn't built…

Note the change of recording studio for the final session. Arrangements for 57064 and 57139 are by John Nesbitt, the remainder are believed to be by Redman. The composer credit for 57139 represents the nicknames of Nesbitt, Wilborn and George Thomas.

These sessions are not by the regular McKinney group which was based at the Graystone Ballroom in Detroit and readers are referred to John Chilton's study, *McKinney's Music* for the full story leading to their appearance. For convenience, the entire group of sessions is given here, although it now seems likely that Waller is not on the first date. All three sessions were directed by Don Redman under the supervision of Mr. Watson, and Don commented in an interview with Hugues Panassié, published in the Irish magazine *Hot Notes* No. 12, that, "There were so many guys on those sessions." Hugues went on to say: *I also asked Don about the famous McKinney Cotton Pickers dates with Hawkins. He was positive that the piano on all sides but two was Fats Waller, not James P. Johnson. In the other two sides "It was a guy named Leroy Tibbs". As I wanted to be sure we listened together to 'Miss Hannah'. As for the sides in which Leroy Tibbs is on piano they are probably 'Plain Dirt' and 'Gee Baby Ain't I Good To You'. These sides were the first to be made and the pianist confines himself to background stuff.*

From Redman's remarks and aural study of the recordings, it appears possible that a slightly different personnel was assembled on each of the three days, although the recording sheets do give the same instrumentation of 3 cornets; trombone; 4 saxes; piano; banjo; tuba and trapman (drummer) for all three. Redman was clearly one of the saxes, although only the sheet for the third date actually states as much. In a letter to *Storyville* (issue 58), Les Airey reported that in a telephone call to Dave Wilborn the latter confirmed himself as the banjo player and also spoke approvingly of Tibbs as a "fine New York pianist". John Chilton points out that Bobby Stark claimed in the 1944 *The Needle* that he had recorded with McKinney's, but gave no further details, so he should be considered as a 'possible' here, but from there on it is mostly aural evidence. A manuscript note in the Victor files which was obviously used in the preparation of the booklet at the time of the re-issue of the Victor set refers to *I'd Love It/Plain Dirt* and was apparently approved by John Reed. A name that I can't read has been crossed out and Len Davis substituted; Prince Robinson is replaced by Joe Bettus (McCord's nickname); James P. Johnson by "Fats" Waller, and Cuba Austin by Kaiser Marshall. Other names are De Paris, Smith, Jones, Redman, Carter, Hawkins, Wilborn and Taylor. When the booklet appeared, these were the names given except that John Truehart was given on guitar in place of Wilborn despite the fact that it is banjo that is heard.

Reverses: Victor 22736 is by **Blanche Calloway and Her Joy Boys;** HMV B6204 is by **Irving Mills and his Modernists**; B6215 by **Jimmy Johnson and his Orchestra with Harry McDaniel**; B.D.135 by **Jimmie Lunceford and his Orch**.

Adjacent matrices: 57063 is a personal recording by Carolina de Keilhauer on 5 November 1929.
57069 is by Countess Olga Albani on 7 November 1929.
57138 is by Rudy Vallee on 6 November 1929.
57141 is by Rudy Vallee on 7 November 1929.

*****

Jimmie Johnson and His Orchestra **Vocal refrain by Keep Shufflin' Trio**

Joe 'King' Oliver, Davidson C. 'Dave' Nelson, t; James Archey, tb; two unknown, cl/as; *Charles H. Frazier,* cl-1/ts; James P. Johnson, Fats Waller, p; unknown, bj-2/g-3; Harry Hull, bb; unknown d. The 'Keep Shufflin' Trio', v, male trio, one of whom sounds like Waller

46th Street Studio, New York City, New York — Monday, 18 November 1929
10:00 a.m. to 1:15 p.m.

57701-1	You Don't Understand — Fox Trot *-3*	Victor unissued
57701-2	YOU DON'T UNDERSTAND — Fox Trot -3 (Jimmie Johnson)	Vi V-38099-B, HMVIt R 14398
57702-1	You've Got to be Modernistic — Fox Trot	Victor unissued
57702-2	YOU'VE GOT TO BE MODERNISTIC Fox Trot (Jimmie Johnson)	Vi V-38099-A, HMVIt R 14398

The instrumentation is confirmed by the Victor files which also state that Jimmie Johnson directed and that Mr. Watson was present. James P. Johnson himself gave the above personnel, with the exception of Frazier, to Walter Allen and also named Teddy Bunn on banjo/guitar. Walter Allen also interviewed James Archey who recalled a four-title session for Victor (he may have been thinking of four takes) under James P. Johnson's leadership and recalled *You've Got To Be Modernistic* as one of the tunes cut. He named both Waller and Johnson on pianos, Oliver, Nelson, himself, Teddy Bunn and recalled the bassist as Harry *Hall.* Although one of the voices in the vocal trio sounds like Bunn, and despite these recollections, Bunn himself stated in *Jazz Journal* November 1971, p.8, that he had *never* played banjo. Charles Delaunay once suggested Bernard Addison as the player here, but when I interviewed him he was evasive and the name is thus best left as 'unknown'. Charles Frazier had been recording with Oliver for Victor and, although he had no specific memory of this session, is probably the man present here.

Adjacent matrices: These numbers mark the beginning of a new matrix block allocated to the 46th Street studio. The previous block ended with 57092/57100 by Lionel Belasco Orch. on 15 November.
577003-8 are by Luke Jordan on 18 and 19 November.

*****

Gene Austin Tenor with orchestra

Gene Austin, v; Acc. unknown, c; tb; two cl; three vn; vc; Fats Waller, p; g; sb; d.

44th Street Studio, New York City, New York — Monday, 25 November 1929

4:00 p.m. to 5:05 p.m. Leonard Joy directing

57170-1	MY FATE IS IN YOUR HANDS (Andy Razaf-Thomas Waller)	Vi 22223-A, HMV/Au B3297

The recording sheet gives the instrumentation above, naming only Fats Waller among those present. A handwritten note also reveals that he was paid on 11 December – a different date to all the other musicians. It had been intended to make two takes of this title, but all the information for the second take is X'd out and at the bottom is typed: "Note on the above sel. we could only make one owing to fuse blowing in the switch box and Mr. Austin had to leave before electrician could make change."

Jazz Records offers a personnel for this recording which differs in several respects from the instrumentation on the recording sheet.

The reverse of both issues is by **Gene Austin** without Fats.

Adjacent matrices: 57169 is by Wellcome Lewis on 25 November 1929.
57171/2 are by Central American Marimba Band on 26 November 1929.

*****

Thomas "Fats" Waller Piano Solo

Thomas Waller, p.

New York City, New York — Wednesday, 4 December 1929

57190-1	My Fate Is In Your Hands	Victor unissued
57190-2	My Fate Is In Your Hands	Victor unissued
57190-3	My Fate Is In Your Hands	Victor unissued
57190-4	MY FATE IS IN YOUR HANDS (Andy Razaf- Thos. Waller)	Vi V-38568-A
57191-1	TURN ON THE HEAT (De Sylva-Brown-Henderson)	Vi V-38568-B
57191-2	Turn On The Heat	Victor unissued
57191-3	Turn On The Heat	Victor unissued

The recording sheet for this session was not available for study. Victor V-38568-B bears the additional credit **(From Fox Film "Sunny Side Up")**.

Adjacent matrices: 57188/9 are personal recordings by Josephine Bradlee on 3 December 1929
57192/6 are by Athenian Operetta on 5 December 1929.

*****

Fats Waller and His Buddies - Fox Trot **Vocal refrain by Orlando Roberson -1**

Henry Allen, Leonard Davis, t; Jack Teagarden, tb-2/vb-3; J.C. Higginbotham, tb; Albert Nicholas cl-4/as, Charlie Holmes, cl-5/as; Larry Binyon, ts; Fats Waller, p; Will Johnson, bj; Pops Foster, sb; Kaiser Marshall, d; Orlando Roberson, v -1.

Victor 44th Street Studio, New York City, New York Wednesday, 18 December 1929
10:00 a.m. to 1:30 p.m Mr. Watson directing

57926-1 LOOKIN' FOR ANOTHER
SWEETIE -1,-3 (Chick Smith-Sterling Grant)) Vi V-38110-A
57926-2 Lookin' for another Sweetie. -1,*-3* Victor rejected
57926-3 Lookin' for another Sweetie. -1,*-3* Victor rejected
57927-1 Ridin' but Walkin' -*-2,-3,-4,-5* Victor rejected
57927-2 Ridin' but Walkin' -*-2,-3,-4,-5* Victor rejected
57927-3 Ridin' But Walkin' -2,-3,-4,-5 (Waller) Vi V-38119-A, ViAr IAC-0135, HMV B.4971,
B.6390, HMVAu E.A.3265, HMVF SG-431
57928-1 Won't You Get Off It, Please -2 (Walller) Vi V-38119-B, ViAr IAC-0135, HMV B.4971,
B.6549, HMVAu EA-3713, HMVF SG 464
57928-2 Won't You Get Up Off It, Please *-2* Victor rejected
57929-1 When I'm Alone -1,*-3,-4,-5*
57929-2 WHEN I'M ALONE -1,-3,-4,-5 (Chick Smith) Vi V-38110-B

The recording sheet gives instrumentation and notes "Waller Dir. & Playing Piano." All four compositions are described as "Fox Trot", but no dispositions are noted.

The personnel quoted was supplied by Larry Binyon and agrees with the instrumentation in the Victor files and aurally with what is heard.

The reverse of HMV B.6390 is by **Bennie Moten** and that of B.6549 by **Paul Whiteman**.

Adjacent matrices: 57925 is by Fritz Kreisler on 17 December 1929.
57930/2 are by Fritz Kreisler on 18 December 1929.

*****

SEVEN GALLON JUG BAND **Fox Trot Vocal Refrain**

Ed Allen, c; unknown, cl; Frank Robinson, bsx/hca/v-1; *Willie 'The Lion' Smith,* p; Clarence Williams, j/v-1; Fats Waller, v-2

New York City, New York Friday, 3 January 1930

149638-1 For My Baby Columbia rejected
149638-2 For My Baby Columbia rejected
149638-3 For My Baby Columbia rejected
149639-1 What Makes Me Love You So? -1 Columbia rejected
149639-2 What Makes Me Love You So? -1 Columbia rejected
149639-3 What Makes Me Love You So? -1 Columbia rejected
149690-4 Wipe 'Em Off -1 Columbia second choice
149690-5 Wipe 'Em Off -1 Columbia rejected
149690-6 WIPE 'EM OFF -1,-2 (Williams and Johnson) Co 2087-D, CoD J880, PaE R.2329,
PaSw PZ11287, *OdG 028077*

When I played Columbia 2087-D to Maurice Waller I had not suspected that his father was present but, on hearing the second voice he immediately and excitedly shouted, "That's my dad!" He explained that his father often dropped into the recording studios, particularly when friends were recording and that in those days things were on a much more free and easy basis. Fats is certainly not the pianist and some authorities deny that it is his voice that is heard despite Maurice's conviction. The title is a remake from the session of 6 December 1929 by the same group and the reverse of the Columbia issues is *What If I Do* from that date. The reverse of the other three issues is by Bessie Smith.

Adjacent matrices: 149637 is by Musical Art Quartet on 2 January 1930.
149640/1 are by Art Gillham on 26 November 1929.
149689 is by Gene Autry on 5 December 1929.
149691 is by Seven Gallon Jug Band on 6 December 1929.

*****

Under the heading Thomas Waller, and datelined New York Feb. 21, the Chicago *Defender* of 22 February 1930 has: *Thomas Waller will be seen at Connie's Inn shortly, where an organ has been installed for the special performances to be given by Mr. Waller.*

*****

The *International Musician* of February 1930 has a report of what appears to be the Russell Wooding Orchestra from Local 9 of Boston which lists Russell Wooding, Bernard Parker, vn; Willie Hicks, t; Joe Marshall, d; Thomas Waller, p; Charles Green, tb, and Dallas Chambers, t.

*****

Thomas Waller - Bennie Paine **Piano duet**

Fats Waller, Bennie Paine, two p.

Liederkranz Hall, New York City, New York — Friday, 21 March 1930

3:00 to 5:10 p.m. Mr. Watson directing

59720-1	ST. LOUIS BLUES (W.C. Handy)	Victor 22371-A, ViAr 68-0830, ViJ JA-477-A HMV/Au B.8496, HMVAu EA770, HMVIt GW1341
59720-2	St. Louis Blues	Victor rejected, 'Destroy'
59720-3	St. Louis Blues	Victor 'Hold 30 days'
59721-1	AFTER YOU'VE GONE (Creamer and Layton)	Victor 22371-B, ViAr 68-0830, ViJ JA-477-B HMV/Au B.8496, HMVAu EA770, HMVIt GW1341
59721-2	After You've Gone	Victor rejected, 'Destroy'
59721-3	After You've Gone	Victor 'Hold 30 days'

This session is another example of the casual attitude that prevailed in the recording studios at that time, for Victor had planned a double sided release illustrating the 'old' and the 'modern swing' jazz piano styles featuring Jelly Roll Morton and Waller. Morton had failed to appear and, as Benny Paine was hanging around, an on-the-spot decision was made to record duets.

The Japanese Victor issue is on the usual 'curly' label; prints the Victor catalogue number and side designation, and uses a much reduced size label for the B side.

Adjacent matrices: 59719 is by Prof. Yau Hok Chau & Associates recorded on 21 March 1930.
59722 is by Metropolitan Opera House Chorus & Orch. recorded on 24 March 1930.

*****

During the Second Annual Fats Waller Memorial Week in 1945, Station WNEW Radio in New

York carried a series of tributes to Fats. The artists appearing on the show comprised a virtual 'who's who' of jazz at that time; James P. Johnson, Willie 'The Lion', Mildred Bailey, Red Norvo, Red McKenzie, Count Basie, Una Mae Carlisle and Tommy Dorsey, to name a few. In introducing Tommy Dorsey on the show, Ed Kirkeby asked him, "Say Tom, do you remember the Jackson Heights affair?" Tommy replied, "Yes indeed, Ed. That was the time the boys gave a little party for Hoagy Carmichael. Let's see, my brother Jimmy and I were there, and Bix Beiderbecke, Stan King, Joe Venuti and Eddie Lang and, of course, good old Fats — all 300 pounds of him! Man, oh man, what a clambake that one was!"

Bob Kumm sent a transcript of this programme to Hoagy Carmichael, with a request for any further information that he could supply, and he replied with the following:

> *...of course I saw Fats Waller many times in New York. But it is the same old story about musicians - when you see each other you shake hands and start talking about music or start a jam session. There is seldom a chance to become truly acquainted to the point where you can say something about the man, other than what everybody else might say - all superlatives. The party you mentioned was actually held (in 1930) on 31st Street at my apartment just off Park Avenue. It was supposed to have been a rehearsal for a recording session we were to make the following day for Victor. As usual, it turned into a jam session and my hoarded supply of liquor was totally consumed. Fats was not in on the recording date, but since everybody wanted to hear hin play and to play with him, my rehearsal went to pot. We were warned about our loudness by neighbors several times and finally 2 policeman closed us up around three A.M. We all left the apartment and boarded a trolly-car, with some of the boys still blowing on their instruments. We wound up the session on the trolly as dawn was breaking over Jackson Heights!*

Hoagy had recording dates with Victor on 21 May and 15 September in 1930, both of which featured Bix, Venuti and Lang, with Tommy Dorsey on the former and brother Jimmy on the latter, so either could be applicable, placing the "Jackson Heights Affair" on either Tuesday, 20 May 1930 (more likely) or Sunday, 14 September. It is possible that Fats was referring to this encounter as well as the aborted Paul Whiteman date of 1928 when he said in 1941 that he had worked with Bix.

*****

Waller and James P. Johnson had been collaborating again and produced the music for a short-lived revue at the Lafayette Theatre. Entitled *"Fireworks of 1930"*, it featured Geo. Dewey Washington, Mamie Smith and a cast of 40 with music provided by "Fats Waller's and Jimmie Johnson's Syncopators. Billed as a "Fourth Of July Special", the show opened on Saturday, 28 June 1930 and, despite claims made in other books, ran for one week only, being replaced by Bill 'Bojangles' Robinson the following Saturday. This was perfectly normal practice and Lafayette adverts in the black press showed what was featured that week with the following week's attraction boxed at the foot. The announcement of the show in the preceding week (reproduced here) mentioned the orchestra, but that of the week when the show was resident did not. However, *The New York Age* normally reviewed the shows in the principal black theatres and that for *'Fireworks Of 1930'* includes: *Mamie Smith, fascinating queen of the Blues, and a great jazz band under the leadership of Fats Waller and Jimmie Johnson, two of the finest song-writers and musicians in the country.* As usual, the advert itself states that the final performance would be at midnight on Friday. Occasionally, successful shows went on to appear at other venues, but I have been unable to trace any additional performances for this show.

Next Week—Beginning Saturday, June 28
Emory Hutchin's Glorious Holiday Revue

Fireworks of 1930

With GEO. DEWEY WASHINGTON
MAMIE SMITH — And 40 Others
MUSIC BY FATS WALLER'S AND JIMMIE JOHNSON'S SYNCOPATORS

Also the Dramatic Hit
"LADIES OF LEISURE"
With a Cast of Noted Talking Picture Stars

*****

A short paragraph in *The New York Age* of 23 August 1930 has: *Thomas (Fats) Waller, composer, pianist and organist is on a tour and is at the Regal in Chicago this week. He will also play in Detroit and will later go to Hollywood, where it is reported, he will compose for the talkies.*

*****

McKENZIE'S MOUND CITY BLUE BLOWERS

Red McKenzie, comb/v-2; Benny Goodman. cl-2; unknown, as/cl-1; Coleman Hawkins, Bud Freeman, ts-1; Fats Waller, p; Eddie Condon, bj; Josh Billings, suitcase.

New York City, New York — Thursday, 30 October 1930

10194-1	Girls Like You Were Meant For Boys Like Me	ARC rejected
10194-2	Girls Like You Were Meant For Boys Like Me	ARC rejected
10194-3	Girls Like You Were Meant For Boys Like Me -1	ARC rejected, issued on LP
10195-1	Arkansas Blues	ARC rejected
10195-2	Arkansas Blues	ARC rejected
10195-3	Arkansas Blues -2	ARC rejected, issued on LP

Despite the claims on LP sleeves, the issue of the second title is thought to be from take -3 as shown here. According to D. Russell Connor, Benny Goodman firmly identified himself on the second title, but not on the first. It still seems likely that he is responsible for the alto and clarinet work on that too.

Adjacent matrices: 10191-3 are blanks in the ARC ledgers.
10196-9 are by Elliott Jacoby's Orchestra, recorded on 31 October 1931.

*****

Fats Waller had again joined the revue at Connie's Inn where Fletcher Henderson was the resident band as a report in the Chicago *Defender* of 20 December 1930 indicates:

Thomas (Fats) Waller, who was the organist at the Regal Theater, Chicago, about a month ago, is now playing at Connie's Inn, New York, on an organ which was installed especially for him. Fats has been playing the radio and stage jumps. He was held in

Cleveland over WLW for more than three months. While in Chicago, at present the Mecca of all the big time bands, Fats made some arrangements for several North side units and was invited to dine with none other than Paul Whiteman. There's not a program featuring popular music going on the air that doesn't include one of the corpulent composer's numbers.

*****

Beginning 8 December 1930, Fats was the pianist on the Paramount-Publix show, 'Paramount On Parade', broadcast three time weekly over Columbia's New York Station WABC for 15 minutes from noon on Monday, Wednesday and Friday. Originally planned as a thirteen-week series, it proved so popular that from the fourth week it was expanded to a half hour show and then booked for a further thirteen weeks at the end of the initial run

*****

The advert for the Alhambra in *The New York Age* of 27 December 1930 announced Fats Waller and Alex Hill, Famous song-writers would appear in *'Hello 1931!'* The review of the show in the paper of the following week has:

Thomas Waller, whose name has been carried all around the world by his amazing succession of song hits — but "Fats" Waller to his friends in Harlem — is smiling his famous broad smile out of a gorgeous bower of roses at the Alhambra theatre this week in "Hello 1931". His pal, Alex Hill, looks out from the other side of the glowing rose garden and their song hits float out one after another, played as only the composers can play them. Each man has a piano cleverly concealed in the rich arbors of flowers.

Both the advert and the review stated that there would be a special Midnight show on New Year's Eve in addition to the usual programme. Virtually the same advert and much the same review appeared in the New York Amsterdam News of 31 December 1931 and from other evidence in this paper it may be deduced that *'Hello 1931!'* ran from Monday 29 December 1930 to Sunday 4 January 1931. Part of the advert from *The New York Age* is reproduced here.

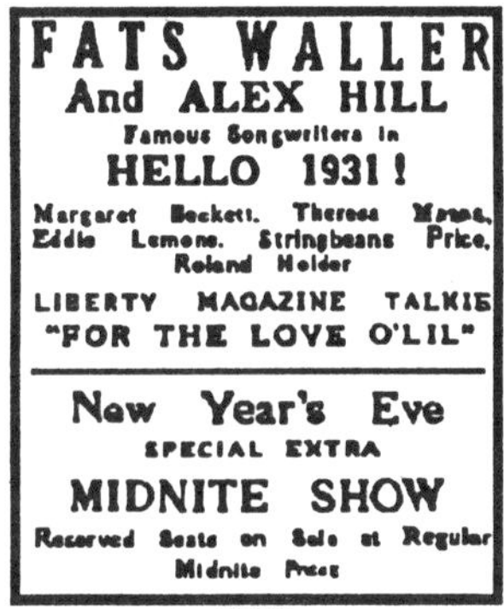
FATS WALLER
And ALEX HILL
Famous Songwriters in
HELLO 1931!
LIBERTY MAGAZINE TALKIE
"FOR THE LOVE O'LIL"
New Year's Eve
SPECIAL EXTRA
MIDNITE SHOW

*****

There was also a reference to Waller as a composer in *The Billboard* at this period. The issue of 31 January 1931 states that he was now free-lancing as a composer after completing a one-year contract with Santly Bros.

*****

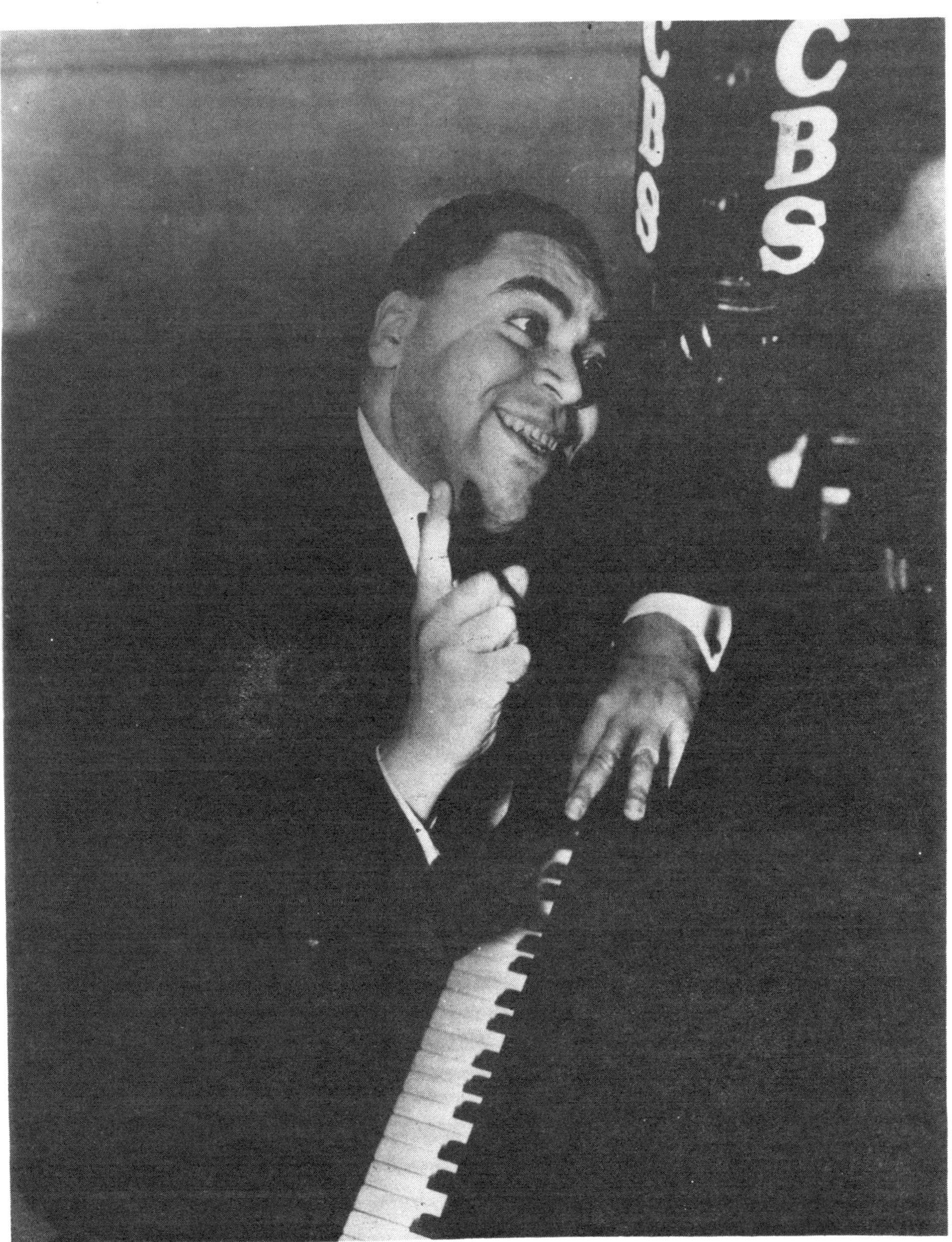

Above and overleaf: Two shots of Waller in the CBS Studios which may date from this period.

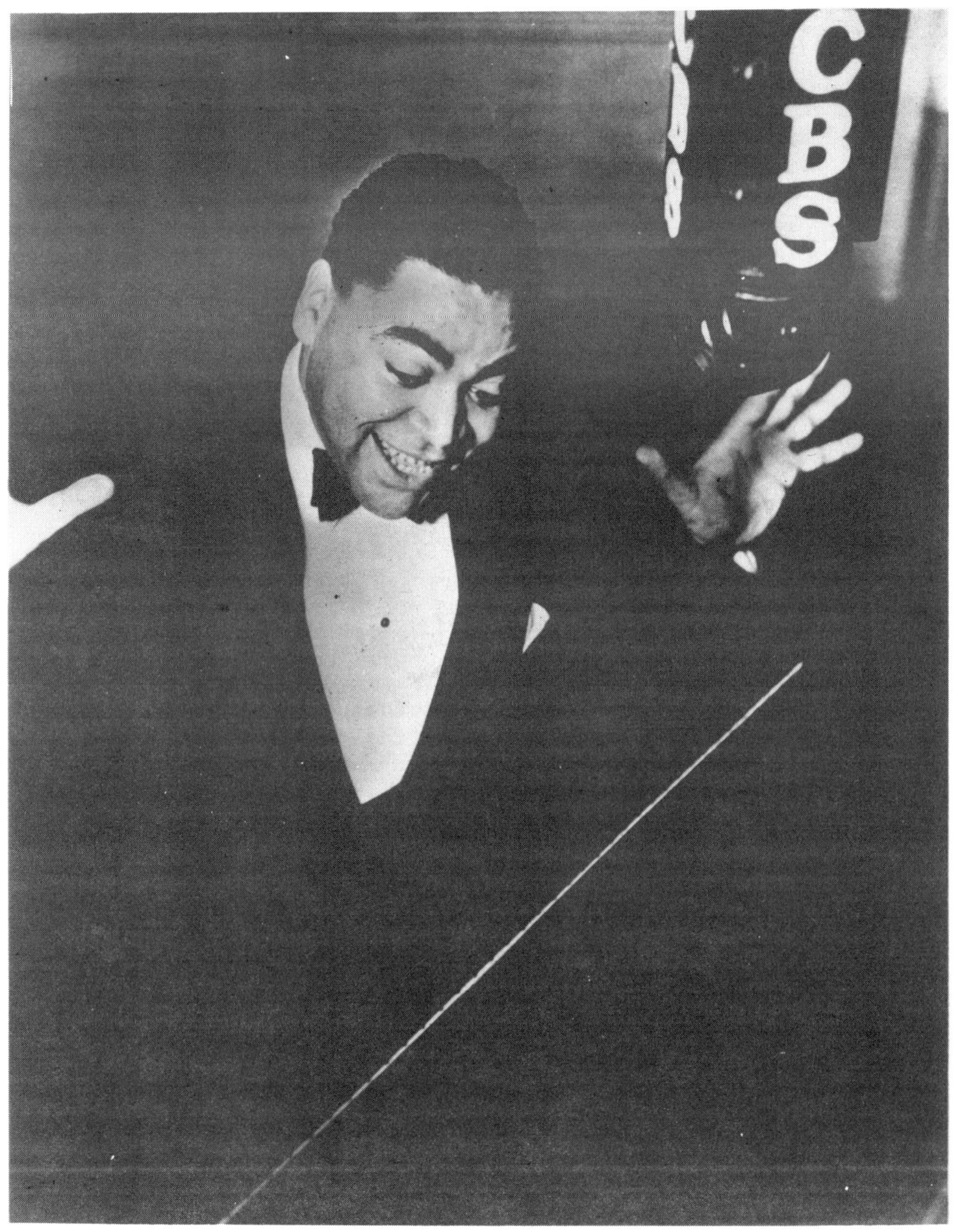
CBS

Ted Lewis AND HIS Band **Fox Trot Incidental singing by Ted Lewis** (1st title)
Fox Trot Incid. Sing. (2nd title).
Fox Trot Vocal Refrain (3rd & 4th titles)

Muggsy Spanier, c; Dave Klein, t; George Brunies, tb; Ted Lewis, cl-1/v-2/v interjections -3; Benny Goodman, cl; Hymie Wolfson, ts; Sam Shapiro, Sol Klein, vn-4; Fats Waller, p/v-5; Tony Gerardi, g; Harry Barth, bb-6/sb-7; John Lucas, d.

New York City, New York — Thursday, 5 March 1931

151395-1 Egyptian-Ella *-1,-2,-4,-6* — Columbia rejected
151395-2 EGYPTIAN-ELLA (Doyle) -1,-2,-4,-6 — Co 2428-D
151395-3 Egyptian-Ella *-1,-2,-4,-6* — Columbia 2nd choice, unissued
151395-4 Egyptian-Ella *-1,-2,-4,-6* — Columbia unissued, designation unknown
151396-1 I'M CRAZY 'BOUT MY BABY (And My Baby's Crazy 'Bout Me) (Waller and Hill)-4,-5,-6 — Co 2428-D

151396-2 I'm Crazy 'Bout My Baby *-4,-5,-6* — Columbia 2nd choice, unissued
151396-3 I'm Crazy 'Bout My Baby *-4,-5,-6* — Columbia rejected

New York City, New York — Friday, 6 March 1931

151397-1 Dallas Blues *-3,-4,-5,-7* — Columbia 2nd choice, unissued
151397-2 Dallas Blues *-3,-4,-5,-7* — Columbia rejected
151397-3 Dallas Blues -3,-4,-5,-7 (Wand and Garrett) — Co 2527-D, *35684, 38841*, CoE CB446, FB2820, CoAu DO2756, CoF DF765, CoG DW4053, CoEu DC136, CoJ J1255 *Ba 33412, Me M13379, Or 3132, Pe 16109, Ro 2506, BRS 1009*
151397-4 Dallas Blues *-3,-4,-5,-7* — Columbia unissued, designation unknown
151398-1 Royal Garden Blues -5,*-6* — Columbia rejected
151398-2 Royal Garden Blues -5,-6 (Williams) — Co 2527-D, *35684, 38841*, CoE CB446, FB2820, CoAu DO2756, CoF DF765, CoG DW4053, CoEu DC136, CoJ J1255 *OK 41579, BRS 1009*
151398-3 Royal Garden Blues -5,-6 — Columbia 2nd choice, unissued
151398-4 Royal Garden Blues -5,-6 — Columbia unissued, designation unknown

Matrix 151397-3 was dubbed to 17065-1 on 19 March 1935 and used on the ARC issues. Likewise, 151398-2 was dubbed to 17064-1 and used on OKeh 41579. Some of these issues may be as **TED LEWIS AND HIS ORCHESTRA.** BRS as **SPANIER-BRUNIES DIXIELANDERS.**

The piano on *Egyptian Ella* is unobtrusive and somewhat in the background, leading some authorites to conclude that it is not Waller on this title.

Adjacent matrices: 151394 is a violin solo by Efrem Zimbalist with piano recorded on 5 March 1931.
151399 is by Guy Lombardo and his Royal Canadians recorded on 5 March 1931.

*****

THOMAS "FATS" WALLER and His Hot Piano

Fats Waller, p/v.

New York City, New York — Friday, 13 March 1931

151417-1	I'm Crazy 'Bout My Baby (And My Baby's Crazy 'Bout Me)	Columbia rejected (H)
151417-2	I'm Crazy 'Bout My Baby (And My Baby's Crazy 'Bout Me)	Columbia 2nd choice
151417-3	I'M CRAZY 'BOUT MY BABY (And My Baby's Crazy 'bout Me) (Waller and Hill)	Co 14593-D, Vo 3016, PaE R1197, PaSw PZ11241, PaIt B71078, OdG 031817, OdF 279.476
151418-1	Draggin' My Heart Around	Columbia rejected (H)
151418-2	DRAGGIN' MY HEART AROUND (Hill)	Co 14593-D, Vo 3016, PaE R1197, PaSw PZ11241, PaIt B71078, OdG 031817, OdF 279.476
151418-3	Draggin' My Heart Around	Columbia 2nd choice

The Columbia files show (H) after the rejected takes as shown, the meaning of this is unclear, but is thought to indicate "Hold". Although Parlophone R1197 was pressed in England, it was also available to special order in Continental Europe.

Adjacent matrices: 151416 is by Art Gillham recorded on 12 March 1931.
151419 is by Kate Smith on 13 March 1931.

*****

Waller and Alex Hill had co-operated on a number of compositions by this time, and *The Billboard* of 14 March 1931 said they they, along with Bud Allen, were planning to form their own publishing company, but the plans seems to have come to nothing.

*****

The *'Paramount On Parade'* series over WABC finally ended in June 1931, and Waller was immediately engaged for a new series, *'Radio Roundup'* which began on 18 June 1931 and also featured the orchestra of Claude Hopkins. In addition to his radio work, Fats was also working in Otto Hardwick's band at the 'Hot Feet Club', situated at 142 West Houston Street in Greenwich Village. This was a late night spot, featuring bawdy entertainment and opening at 11.00 and running through the night as long as patrons were in the house. The band was quite a large aggregation and in *The World Of Duke Ellington* Stanley Dance states that it featured a five-man saxophone section (virtually unknown at that time) of Hardwick, Chu Berry, Wayman Carver, Garvin Bushell and Theodore McCord. No mention is made of the brass or rhythm other than Waller on piano. Because it was open after other places had closed, the club became a hang-out for musicians and much sitting-in and many battles of music took place. One such was against the full Ellington band which, by general consensus, was won by the resident band. Eventually the owner of the club was shot dead, the club closed and the band, minus Waller moved to other things.

*****

Another anecdote from Garvin Bushell appears to date from around this time. He relates how he'd been taking society gigs with Luckey Roberts and goes on to say:

> *Through Luckey I even made contact with the Vanderbilts. One particular afternoon W. K. Vanderbilt himself called me up.*

"Bushell, what're you doing?

"Nothin'."

Can you come out to the house?"

"Yeah, sure."

"Be sure and bring that fat one with you, the one that plays the organ."

I took along Fats Waller and Mert Perry. We hired a car and took it out to the Vanderbilt estate on Long Island. After you go through the gate it takes about six minutes to reach the house.

When we arrived, W. K. said, "I'm just lonesome and wanted to hear some music today." We played about two numbers and he said, "All right, come on, sit down here and let's talk." He wanted to know what we did, what made us tick. I'd been to Russia, and he wanted to know all about that. Then he said, "All right, play another tune." A little later, "Come on, let's drink." By that time a big dinner was ready.

W. K. loved Fats. He even had an organ in his house, and Fats played it. Vanderbilt said, "I'd give anything in the world if I was just free to do like you guys." I remember his exact words: "I don't know how to have fun."

So Fats stood up and said, "Mr. W. K., you give me some of your money and I'll show you how to have some fun!" That knocked him out.

The association with Fats and Mert Perry seems to confirm this approximate date as does the fact that Vanderbilt didn't know Waller's name. Had it been much later, after the commencement of the Rhythm series of recordings when Fats began to impinge upon white consciousness, he would certainly have known the identity of "the fat one who plays organ".

*****

Waller's writing activities for the Immerman's was paying dividends and when Fletcher Henderson left Connie's Inn in October 1931, Fats organised a band to take his place as reported in *The Billboard* of 10 October 1931. The report is datelined 'New York Oct. 3' and says, *'Fats' Waller, cowriter of 'My Fate Is In Your Hands' and other hits, has expanded his activities thru organizing a dance orchestra. He has placed his unit at Connie's Inn, replacing Fletcher Henderson's band.* Waller's presence there with a band is confirmed by *The New York Age* and *Variety*, but his stay ended on 15 November when Leroy Smith's Orchestra replaced him. No information has been found on the size or personnel of this Waller-led band, but it may be this group that Dicky Wells recalled in *The Night People*, or the band with Wells may have come from a slightly earlier period. His recollections of the acts that worked there, and of Jesse Crawford, may help to date his stay with Waller more accurately:

For a short period I played with Fats Waller at Connie's Inn. Frankie Newton was in that band, and Big Sidney, and Red Allen. They had this long organ in the corner, full size, for Fats to play. Jesse Crawford was the organist down at the Paramount Theatre then, and the talk of New York, but he used to live in the joint. We're supposed to finish at 4 o'clock, but Fats would put his derby on the piano after the second show and tell us to go home. They'd fill his derby up with money, and he'd be singing and composing songs, and we'd be on the street, or down the Hoofer's Club, or some place. That happened two or three times a week. The bosses were nice, treated us wonderful and paid us our money just the same. When Fats left there, Crawford would take him down to his house and Fats would stay there all night. Next night, same thing. All the people would gang around the piano and we'd quit about 2 o'clock. I got a kick out of playing wtih Fats, and the bosses were crazy about him.

One night, Frank Newton was playing a solo and Fats started to stride and overshadow him. So Frank stopped playing and asked Fats how much he wanted to cool it. Fats smiled and said, "Half a buck." Frank gave it to him and started blowing again—no hard feelings.

They had a great show at Connie's. Snake Hips Tucker and the Mills Brothers were there, and Louise Cook, a shake dancer, Bill Bailey, Jackie Mabley and Paul Myers.

*****

JACK TEAGARDEN & HIS ORCHESTRA

Charlie Teagarden, Sterling Bose, t; Jack Teagarden, tb/v; Pee Wee Russell, cl; Joe Catalyne, cl/ts; Max Farley, cl/ts; Adrian Rollini, bsx; Fats Waller, p/v-1; Nappy Lamare, g; Artie Bernstein, sb; Stan King, d.

New York City, New York — Wednesday, 14 October 1931

151839-1	YOU RASCAL YOU (Theard) -1	Co 2558-D, CoE CB424, CoAu DO667, CoG DW4079, *HJCA 611*
151839-2	You Rascal You	Columbia 2nd choice
151840-1	THAT'S WHAT I LIKE ABOUT YOU (Donaldson) -1	Co 2558-D, CoAu DO667, *HJCA 611*
151840-2	That's What I Like About You -1	Columbia 2nd choice
151841-1	CHANCES ARE	Columbia 2nd choice
151841-2	CHANCES ARE (Barris, Freed and Arnheim)	Ha 1403-H, Cl 5442-C, OK 41551, Ve 2502-V, CoEu DC-144
151842-1	I Got The Ritz From The One I Love	Columbia unissued, issued on LP

The reverse of CoE CB424 is by **The Knickerbockers** (Ben Selvin), of CoEu DC-144 by **The Dorsey Brothers**; that of CoG DW4075 is not known. Harmony/Clarion/Velvet Tone issues of matrix 151841 as **ROY CARROLL AND/& HIS SANDS POINT ORCH./ORCHESTRA** with vocal chorus attributed to **Dick Henry**, and a reverse by Jerry Fenwyck & His Orchestra. OKeh 41551 as **CLOVERDALE COUNTRY CLUB ORCHESTRA** with a reverse by a different band but using the same pseudonym.

It is not certain which of the two recorded takes of 151841 was actually used as none of the original issues inspected show this matrix, although it is almost certainly as given above. Dolf Rerink reported in *Storyville 63* that he owned a copy of CoEu DC-144 showing 151841-2, but it has not been possible to check this. A Columbia file card for 100589, which appears on the label and in the wax (both issues showing take -1) of Harmony 1403-H and Clarion 5442-C, bears the notation 'see 151841 and 405143' which presumably means that this master, at least was allocated an equivalent in these other series. Ray Batt confirms that his OK 41551 shows 405143-A in the wax, but in view of the dispositions noted on the orginal cards, this probably equates to take -2. What is certain is that all issues so far heard on 78 and LP are from the same take, which is probably take -2, the original 'first choice take'.

The original file card for the last title no longer exists, but is replaced by a 1939 card. HJCA 611 is a 12" issue with two titles per side, the reverse pair being by **Wingy Manone**.

Adjacent matrices: 151838 is by Ben Selvin and his Orchestra on 13 October 1931.
151843 is by Red McKenzie with Orchestra on 15 October 1931.

*****

Jack Teagarden and his orchestra -1
GENE AUSTIN AND HIS ORCHESTRA -2

Charlie Teagarden, *Sterling Bose*, t; Jack Teagarden, tb; *Matty Matlock*, cl; *Gil Rodin*, as; Eddie Miller, ts; Adrian Rollini, bsx; Fats Waller, p-1; *Fats Waller* or *Gil Bowers*, p-2; *Nappy Lamare*, g; *Ray Bauduc*, d; Gene Austin, v-2

New York City, New York — Tuesday, 10 November 1931

10976-1	China Boy -1	ARC unissued. Issued on LP
10977-1	Lies -2 (Springer-Barris)	Ba 32325-B, Or 2380-A, Pe 15542-B, Ro 1752-B, Me 91235-B, Do 51024, Rl 91235, St 91235, Ace 351024
10978-1	I'm Sorry Dear -2	ARC rejected
10978-2	I'm Sorry Dear -2	ARC rejected
10978-3	I'm Sorry Dear -2 (Weeks-Tobias-Scott)	Ba 32325-A, Or 2380-B, Pe 15542-A, Ro 1752-A, Me 91235-A, Do 51024, Rl 91235, St 91235, Ace 351024
10979-1	Tiger Rag -1	ARC unissued. Issued on LP

The file cards for the second and third title are made out as heading -2, and all issues are as this or as **GENE AUSTIN & HIS ORCH.** So little piano is heard on the vocal sides that it would be foolish to try and identify the artist and it could equally well be Waller or Bowers who was working with Teagarden at that time. It is also possible that both men are present on the first and last sides. Some authorities believe that the clarinet on this session is played by Pee Wee Russell.

Adjacent matrices: 10972-5 are by Frank Welling and John McGhee on 6 November 1931.
10980-83 are by The Arkansas Woodchopper on 6 November 1931.

*****

The New York Age of 20 February 1932 has: *Andy Razaff* (sic) *and "Fats" Waller on piano a few Sundays back on WMCA gave an appealing broadcast. Andy sang his own compositions. "My song of hate" reared its head prominently. "Fats" had a cute idea for "St. Louis Blues" as a solo.*

*****

Soon after this Waller may have gone to the West Coast as Buck Clayton recalled in his biography that, *Fats Waller came to the Cotton Club after Louie and was a success also ... Fats was funny, jolly, and one hell of a pianist and did very well in Los Angeles.*

The "Cotton Club" was that run by Frank Sebastian in Los Angeles where Louis Armstrong had been featured with Les Hite's Orchestra in the spring of 1932. It is presumably of this period that Buck is talking when he says that Fats came in after Louis, as Waller's movements from July 1932, when he was certainly in New York, are fairly well documented and since Clayton himself left the U.S. for Shanghai in 1934, his recollection has to be of some time prior to that.

Whether this is correct or not, Waller seems to have been back in New York around May, for John Hammond recalled being present at his 28th birthday party in the Waller home on 135th Street when Reginald Forsythe was among the other guests.

*****

JACK BLAND and His RHYTHMAKERS **Fox Trot Vocal Chorus Billy Banks** (Ba 32530)
Henry Allen, t; Jimmy Lord, cl; Pee Wee Russell, ts; Fats Waller, p/v-1; Eddie Condon, bj; Jack Bland, g; Pops Foster, sb; Zutty Singleton, d; Billy Banks, v; band vocal responses-1.

New York City, New York — Tuesday, 26 July 1932

12119-1 I'D DO ANYTHING FOR YOU — Ba 32530-A, Me M-12457, Pe 15651,
(Alex Hill-Bob Williams-Claude Hopkins) — BrFr A500316
12119-2 I WOULD DO ANYTHING FOR YOU — Ba 32530, Or 2534, UHCA 105,
(Alex Hill-Bob Williams-Claude Hopkins) — BrE 02508-B

12119: Lead into second vocal -1 trumpet with shake at end and very subdued tenor sax
-2 Straight note from trumpet and very prominent tenor sax

12120-1 MEAN OLD BED BUG BLUES -1 — Ba 32502, Me M-12457, Or 2554,
(???) — Pe 15669, UHCA 105, VoE 20-A, V.1021,
BrFr A500.315, ImpCz 6003, ImpG 18012
12120-2 MEAN OLD BED BUG BLUES -1 — Co 35882
-Jack Wood-

12120: Last line of second vocal chorus -1 "...chinch poison"
-2 "...bed bug pioison"

12121-1 Yellow Dog Blues — ARC rejected
12121-2 YELLOW DOG BLUES -Handy- — Co 35882
12121-3 YELLOW DOG BLUES — Ba 32502, Me M-12481, Or 2554,
Pe 15669, UHCA 107, VoE 20-B, V.1021,
BrFr A500.315, ImpCz 6003, ImpG 18012,
PaE R2810, PaAu A 7399,PaSw PZ11148,
Paln DPE.9

12121: Vocal chorus: -2 Sung throughout
-3 First half sung; second half scatted

12122-1 Yes Suh! -2 — ARC rejected, issued on LP
12122-2 YES, SUH! -2 (Razaf-Dowell) — Ba 32530-B, Me M-12481, Or 2534,
Pe 15651, UHCA 107, BrE 02078-A,
BrG A9940, *PaE R2810, PaAu A 7399,*
PaSw PZ11148, Paln DPE.9

12122: First line of vocal: "Does My Baby Call Me Honey?"
-1: 4th word emphasised and pitched higher, with last three words dipping in pitch.
-2: Whole phrase sung with even emphasis and at same pitch.

Title of 12119 on UHCA 105 becomes *I'D DO ANYTHING...*
Composer credit on Ba 32502 has not been seen. It is simply (Wood) on the English Vocalion issue. Variant band credits have been used for issues from this session as follows:
JACK BLAND AND HIS RHYTHMAKERS: All Perfect issues
CONDON AND BLAND'S RHYTHMAKERS: Me M12481
BILLY BANKS' CHICAGO RHYTHM KINGS: VoE 20, Imperial issues
CHICAGO RHYTHM KINGS: BrF issues
BILLY BANKS RHYTHMAKERS: VoE V.1021, UHCA issues (but **BANKS'**)
EDDIE CONDON AND HIS RHYTHMAKERS: BrE 02078, BrG A9940
THE RHYTHM MAKERS: PaE R2810, PaSw PZ 11148, Paln DPE.9

Reverses: BrE 02508 is by **Luis Russell & His Orch.**; 02078 is by **Alex Hill and his Hollywood Sepians**; BrF A500316 is under the same name but without Waller.

Adjacent matrices: 12117/8 are by Chick Bullock on 1 August 1932.
12123/4 are by Guy Lombardo on 27 July 1932.

*****

Shortly after this session, Fats set sail for Europe with Spencer Williams aboard the French liner *Ile de France* bound for Le Havre. He had apparently intended to visit England as well as France. The *Melody Maker* of August 1932 has *Fats Waller, the American Negro Singer-at-the-piano should be arriving in England early this month if negotiations went to plan.* (sic) The same paper for September has from John Hammond, datelined 9 August 32, *Fats Waller will be in London by the time this appears. His art can be as charming as that of any man's.* (sic) *We can only hope that he does not take it upon himself to play down to the public as he does to the music publishers on Broadway. Fats' best playing is too delightful to be missed by anybody.* However, the October issue, again from John Hammond, datelined 8 September 32. *Speaking of Fats, I am distressed to learn that he did not get to England after all because of some consular difficulty. It is really a shame, for he would have been greatly appreciated.*

Although some arrangements may have been made for Fats to play, not only in London, but elsewhere as well, none of these engagements took place as Fats had apparently become homesick and left Paris without warning to catch the boat from Le Havre back to New York and was back working again as indicated below.

*****

FATS WALLER/MONETTE MOORE

Monette Moore, v; Fats Waller, p

New York City, New York — Wednesday, 28 September 1932

TO-1210 A Shine On Your Shoes/ Louisiana Hayride — ARC "Test Only" recording, issued on LP

*****

Clyde Bernhardt joined Billy Fowler's Orchestra in September 1932 and, in his book, he recalls:

> *For a time Fowler backed Fats Waller at four different ballrooms in New York's Astor Hotel and on other jobs until Fats formed his own band. We be billed as Fats Waller and his band under the direction of Billy Fowler.*
>
> *Even though this was still Prohibition time, Fats never had to worry about drinks when we worked downtown. Always a big table in the bandroom lined up with all kinds of Canadian whiskey, scotch, gin, everything. Don't know where it cam from, but it was always there.*

This must have been in the period between Waller's return from his trip to France and his departure for Cincinnati in the autumn of 1932.

*****

Not long after the Columbia session above, and perhaps realising that his fortunes might take a turn for the better under the guidance of a white man in the then-prevailing atmosphere, Fats appointed Phil Ponce as a full-time manager and agent.

Station WLW in Cincinnati boasted one of the most powerful radio transmitters in the country at that time, with a coverage that extended far beyond the borders of the state of Ohio, and Ponce managed to get a booking for Fats which went over so well that he was able to persuade the station to build a show around his new charge. It was to be called 'Fats Waller's Rhythm Club', featuring Waller, a vocal group 'The Southern Suns' (four men and a girl who were all related) and a white studio house band and announced by Paul Stewart. The show went at 9.00 p.m. on Saturday nights and proved to be an immediate success. Later the vocal group spot was taken over by 'The King, The Jack And The Jesters' who, in later years changed their name and achieved international fame as 'The Inkspots'. Occasional guest artists were featured, and Fats himself introduced a very young Una Mae Carlisle for the Christmas week show of 1932. She proved to be such a success that her mother was persuaded to allow her to join the show on a permanent basis.

In addition to the WLW spots, Fats also broadcast over Station WSAI, which was then owned by WLW.

Anita and the two boys had joined Fats in a rented house in Cincinnati soon after the show had begun on a regular basis, but when the show became so popular that it went out on the road as a vaudeville attraction on the RKO circuit, they returned to New York.

In his account in *Ain't Misbehavin'*, Ed Kirkeby relates that the tour opened at Cincinnati Palace and mentions Indianapolis and Youngstown, Ohio as among the places played. The visit to Indianapolis is perhaps dated by a mention in the Chicago *Defender* of 25 February 1933, which says that *Fats Waller and Louis Armstrong featured jointly at Indianapolis last week, heard over the air from the Hoosier City in two fine broadcasts nightly. Fats is the Armstrong of the Ivories or is Louis the Fats of the cornet. Take your choice.* It was in Youngstown that the road show manager disappeared with the takings and the advance booking money, leaving the show stranded. A cousin of Una Mae's helped them get back to Cincinnati, where they resumed broadcasting and played an extended gig in a club. They also played a big country club (un-named) in Louisville and Ed Kirkeby relates another story highlighting Waller's continued irresponsible attitude. Also, according to Ed Kirkeby, Fats played the organ on the 'Moon River' programme during his time at WLW. This went out at 1.00 a.m. and featured romantic and classical music suitable for the hour and, because of the nature of the programme, few announcements were made and the organist was anonymous. According to other sources, playing the 'Moon River' programme was an unfulfilled Waller ambition. Fellow WLW artist Kay C. Thompson recalled the beginning of a friendship with Fats in the May 1951 *Jazz Journal: As I was concluding the final number on one of my regular stints, I chanced to look up, and there he was, making faces at me through the studio window. Since there was little else I could do at the moment, instinctively I made faces in return. Such, then, were the beginnings of our friendship.* She also recalls that, to her belief, it was Fats himself who conceived the title "Moon River" for the late night programme and that, although he invariably abided by the idea behind the show, his high spirits occasionally took over and *everything from Bach to Rimsky-Korsakov was rendered with resounding embellishements...*

The tour which Ed Kirkeby mentions was apparently only one of a number which the show undertook, usually accompanied by a band recruited for the occasion; Clarence Paige and his Band and Eddie Johnson and his Crackerjacks are two that have been mentioned in this connection, the latter by Eddie Johnson himself and also by Singleton Palmer who was in Johnson's group at the time. He explained: *You see what Fats did, I was in Cincinnati with Eddie Johnson, and some of the top musicians would pick up a whole band intact, and they would just go out under his name.*

Waller was certainly working with Clarence Paige and his Band in April 1933, as he fronted them for a dance at the Trianon Ballroom in Cincinnati on Sunday, 23 April as shown by the advertising shown here.

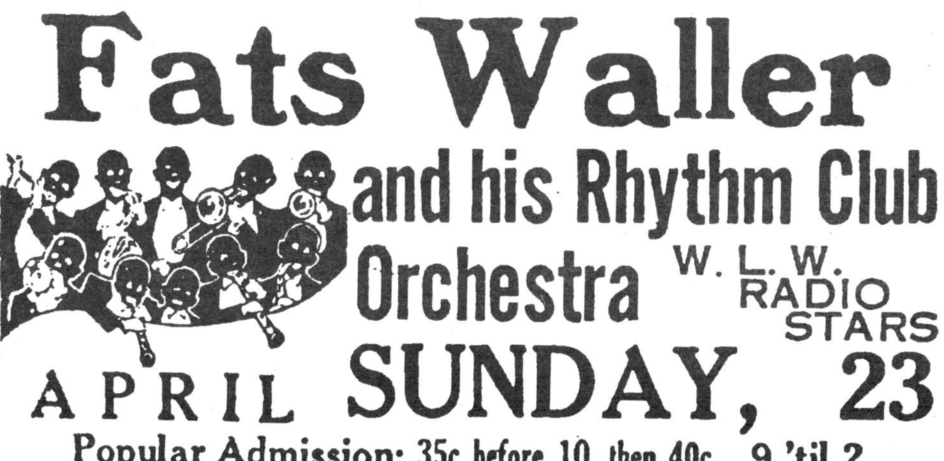
Fats Waller
and his Rhythm Club
Orchestra
W. L. W.
RADIO
STARS
APRIL SUNDAY, 23
Popular Admission: 35c before 10, then 40c 9 'til 2
TRIANON
PHONE RILEY 4839
BROADCASTING OVER W.F.B.M.

Apart from his regular tours, Waller also seems to have worked whatever gigs that came his way, probably in the early part of his stint at WLW. In *The World Of Count Basie,* Earle Warren recalls, *...I used to see and play shows with Fats Waller when I was at a club in Dayton, Ohio. He came out of Cincinnati, where he was on WLW, a radio station.*

Notes in the *Pittsburgh Courier,* which do not appear on a regular basis, show that 'The Rhythm Club' broadcasts over WLW had switched to a Saturday midnight transmission time by October 1933. These listings continued intermittently and showed the 'Rhythm Club' until the issue of 20 January 1934. In the next listing on 10 February it is absent and did not reappear, which may give a clue to the date when Waller quit the programme. In none of these is Waller mentioned by name. It is known that the WLW engagement came to an end early in 1934 when Waller had a misunderstanding with Phil Ponce and he returned to New York.

Back in New York, he played many of the Harlem clubs, usually on a casual basis, and also, as a result of his exposure over WLW, found himself in demand as a guest artist on radio shows. In March he appeared in the 'Saturday Revue'; in April in Morton Downey's 'House Party' and in 'Columbia Review'. It was not to be long before he had his own show again, but in the meantime, things were moving in another direction and Phil Ponce had secured a recording contract for Fats and a small band with Victor.

In 1960, the WLW library of some 9,000 historical programming material was donated to the Broadcasting Archives of Miami University, Oxford, Ohio. Bob Kumm asked the then director of the archive, Dr. Stephen Hathaway, if any of the Waller programmes were among them, but a search through the computerised listings proved negative.

*****

Before moving on to the formation of "Fats" Waller and His Rhythm, the following Waller broadcasts, all billed as "Fats Waller, Songs" over Station WABC of the CBS network are known from Lillian C. Irby's 'Ether Waves' notes in the *Pittsburgh Courier*:

Wednesday, 4 April 1934, 11:15 a.m.
Friday, 6 April 1934, 11:15 a.m.
Tuesday, 10 April 1934, 3:45 p.m.
Friday, 13 April 1934, 10:45 a.m.
Tuesday, 17 April 1934, 3:45 p.m.
Wednesday, 18 April 1934, 10:45 a.m.
Friday, 20 April 1934, 10:45 a.m.
Tuesday, 24 April 1934, 3:45 p.m.
Wednesday, 25 April 1934, 10:45 a.m.
Friday, 27 April 1934, 10:45 a.m.
Tuesday, 1 May 1934, 3:45 p.m.
Wednesday, 2 May 1934, 10:45 a.m.
Friday, 4 May 1934, 10:45 a.m.
Tuesday, 8 May 1934, 3:45 p.m.
Wednesday, 9 May 1934, 10:45 a.m.
Friday, 11 May 1934, 10:45 a.m.

*****

In his book *All This Jazz About Jazz* Harry Dial relates how he had come to New York and been engaged to play the show *'Emperor Jones'* at Small's Paradise beginning on 1 April 1934. It was there that he met Fats Waller, who came in several times a week and, as Harry relates it, Fats was impressed with his ability to play the show. Harry continues:

Fats Waller hadn't been working on a steady job for quite some time, but he had an income from ASCAP for the many hit songs he had written. Just at that time he got a contract with the Victor recording company to do one session each month for an extended time. He sent Bud Allen, a friend of his, to the Paradise one night to tell me to be at his house the next day for a rehearsal for that first session. He had Ben Whittet, sax and clarinet, Herman Autrey, trumpet, Al Casey, guitar, Billy Taylor, bass, himself, and myself.

Whittet didn't make more than two sessions because Oberstein said he didn't fit in the combination and he was right. 'Obie' was the recording manager.

We only had that one rehearsal at Fats's home. After that, all rehearsing was done in the studio and generally within our regular scheduled time. We didn't know what we were going to record until we reached the studio and Oberstein gave everybody a piano part. In just a few minutes of running over a tune we were ready to wax it — it was wax in those days, tapes hadn't been invented.

Al Casey recalled that Fats had taken him out on tour one summer while he was still at school, not to work, but as band-boy. This was presumably in 1933 via an introduction from the 'Southern Suns' who were his aunt and uncles. He said that his first professional job was when he he joined Waller for the first 'Rhythm' session when he was seventeen, although he was actually aged nineteen according to his accepted birth date.

*****

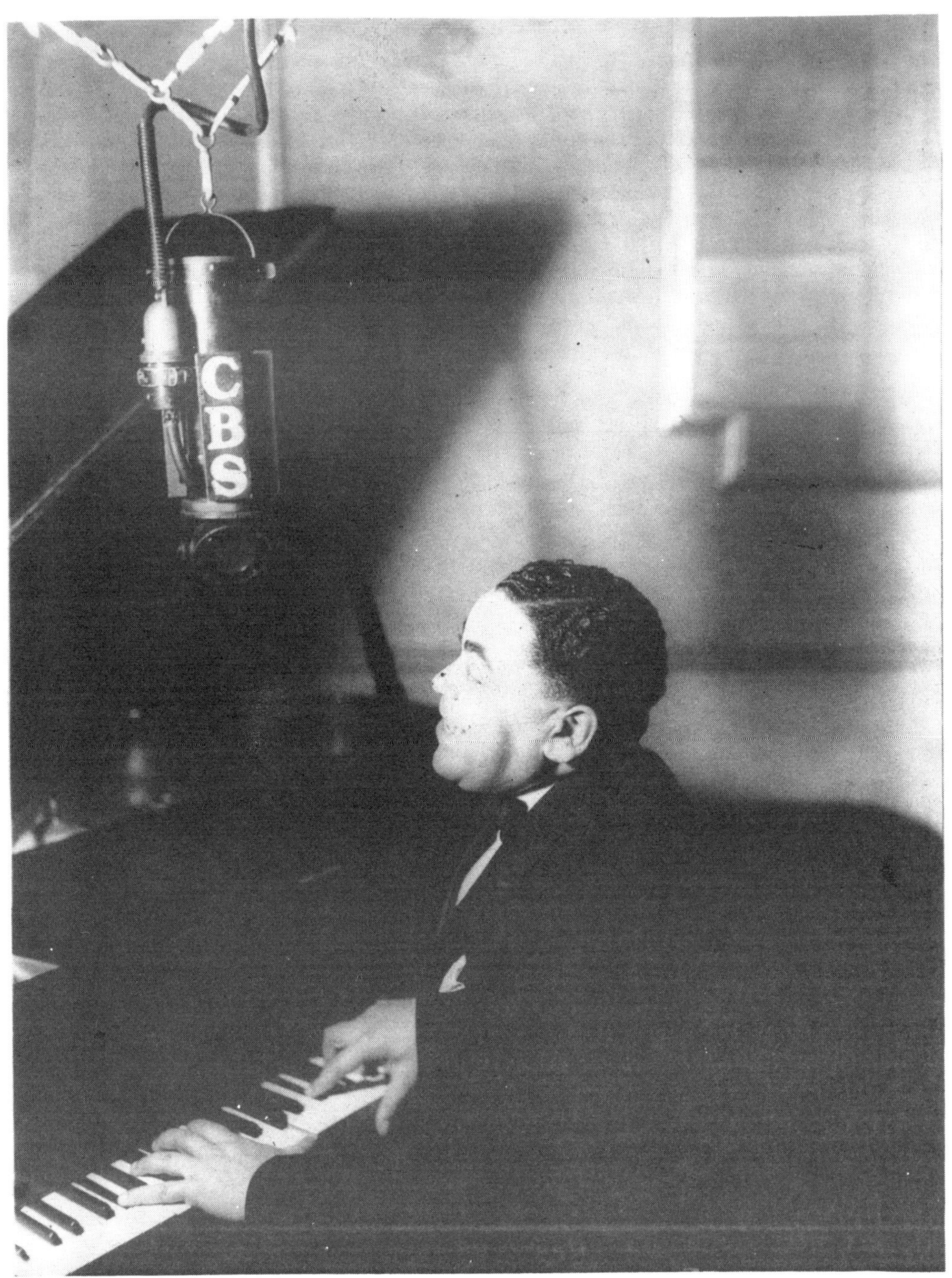

Another shot of Fats in the CBS Studios.

Thus was "Fats" Waller and his Rhythm born, and details of that first session are as follows. By this time, Victor were frequently using a twin-turntable recording system, with separate amplifiers connected to the microphones and each feeding a different turntable cutting head. Normally the amplifier settings were slightly different. This meant that if both resultant recordings were processed, musically identical but physically different discs would result. However, the virtually invariable disposition on the recording sheets for the alternative version, normally suffixed 'A', was "Hold". It seems pointless wasting space listing these out in full, so such recordings will be indicated by the use of an asterisk (*) after the matrix number, and if there is any variation from the standard disposition, it will be given in the notes to the session. Also, since Waller's recording sessions from this point on were very much self contained and pre-arranged affairs, there seems little point in detailing adjacent matrices as it is unlikely that he would have stayed on to sit-in with any other artist or group, and he seldom arrived early!

*****

"Fats" Waller and his Rhythm Fox Trot **Piano and vocal refrain by "Fats" Waller**

Herman Autrey, t; Ben Whitted, cl-1/as-2; Fats Waller, p/v; Albert Casey, g; Billy Taylor, sb; Harry Dial, d/vib-3

Studio No.2, New York City, New York — Wednesday, 16 May 1934

1:30 to 4:45 p.m. Eli Oberstein directing

82526-1*	A PORTER'S LOVE SONG TO A CHAMBERMAID -1,-3 (Andy Razaf-Jimmy Johnson)	Vi 24648-A, BB B10016-B, MW M7947, HMVAu EA2279
82527-1	I WISH I WERE TWINS -1 (De Lange-Loesser-Meyer)	Vi/China 24641-A, HMVJ.F.1, HMVAu EA1508, El EG3703
82527-2*	I WISH I WERE TWINS -1	Victor unissued, 'Hold', issued on LP
82527:	Interjection at end of third line of vocal:	-1 "Aw, you dog!" -2 "You dog!"
82528-1	ARMFUL O' SWEETNESS -1,-2 (Alexander Hill)	Vi/China 24641-B, BB B10149-, HMV J.F.7, HMVSw HE2358, RZAu G24194
82528-2	ARMFUL O' SWEETNESS -1,-2	Victor unissued, 'Hold'
82529-1	DO ME A FAVOR -1 (Jack Lawrence-Peter Tinturin)	Vi 24648-B, HMV J.F.7, HMVSw HE2358

The recording sheet notes that two microphones were used; one for Waller and one for the rest of the group. Some copies of Vi 24641 B omit the hyphen (thus). HMV J.F.7 uses the British spelling of FAVOUR. Note that Ben Whitted is the reedman recalled by Harry Dial as Ben Whittet; the confusion over the spelling arising because of the way the name was pronounced.

Rumours persist that matrix 82528-2 has been issued on LP, but at the time of writing, no copy using this is known to us.

The Chinese pressing of Vi 24641 shows the performance credit as **Piano & vocal ref. by Fats Waller**

*****

Published schedules for Station WABC show that Waller broadcast every Saturday evening at 8:45 p.m. from 19 May 1934. No indication is given of the nature of the programme, nor of its duration, but this is almost certainly a programme of organ music.

*****

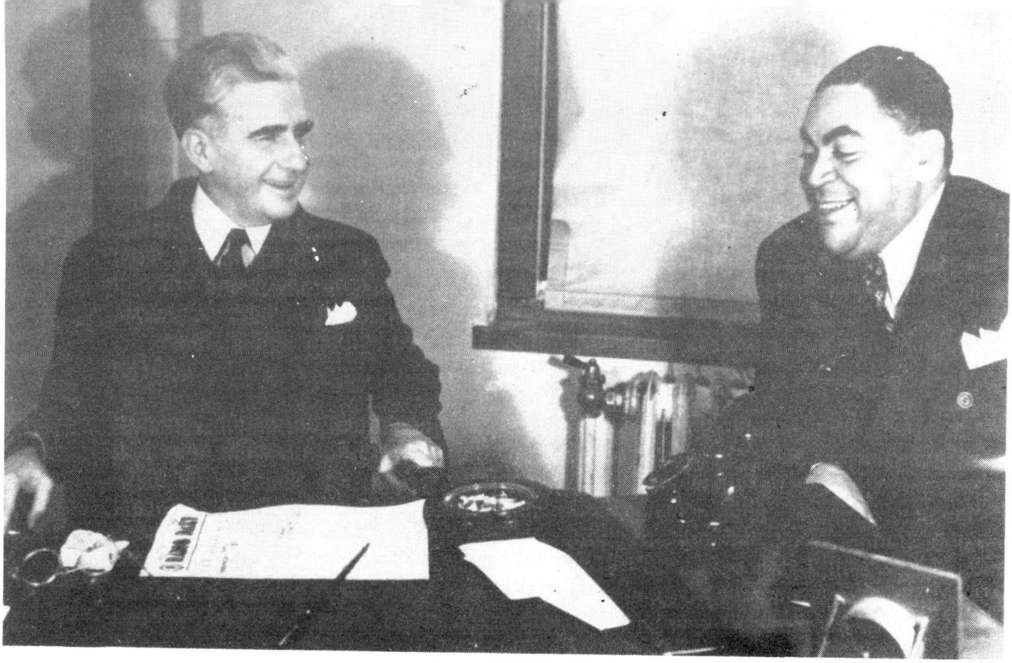

Two shots of a happy Fats Waller. Above: With Manager Phil Ponce in his office.
Below: Showing why he drove his managers to distraction.

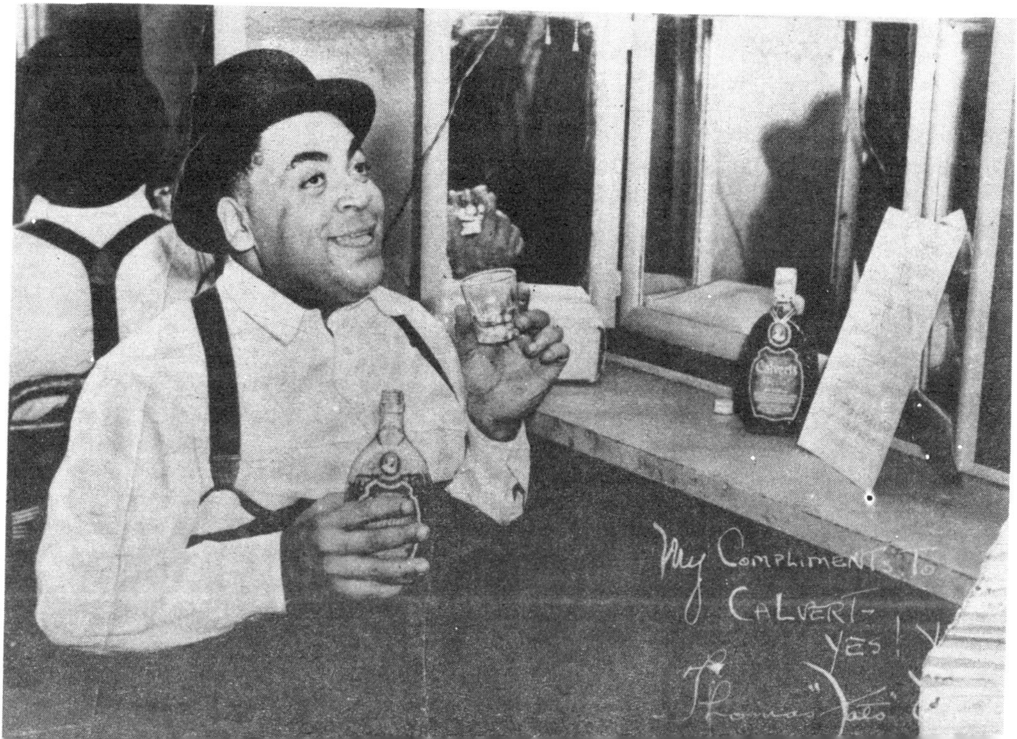

The Pittsburgh *Courier* had initiated a 'Defense Fund' to provide aid for the families of lynch victims and to fight civil rights cases on behalf of the National Association for the Advancement of Colored People (NAACP) and organised a benefit concert to take place at New York's Apollo Theatre from midnight on Saturday 26th May 1934. This was announced in the issue of 19 May and a big build-up followed the next week. This all showed Fats Waller with Bud Allen as appearing in a huge list of major artists. The issue of 2 June devoted much space to news items connected with the event and had two reviews showing that an all-star assembly, including *'Fats Waller & Andy Razaf, songs'* had been in attendance and "went over big". The second review said: *Fats Waller and Andy Razaf, famous song composers, next held the entire audience spellbound with their review of all the old well known songs written and featured by them. Fats played the piano with skill and precision beautiful to see, and Andy sang "Supposin'," "Ain't Misbehavin'," "Memories" and a dozen other old favorites.*

There is no mention of Bud Allen and the event was also covered by other black papers which also gave Waller and Razaf, and according to the *New York Age* reviewer, *they got going with a resume of their songs, well received..*

The New York *Amsterdam News*, noted that Fats Waller was scheduled to appear at a benefit concert for the Harlem branch of the Children's Aid Society at the Lafayette on Tuesday, 29 May 1934. It is not known whether or not he did so as there is no mention of him by name in the review of the concert the following week.

Also, on an unknown date in May, Fats was featured on the radio show 'Harlem Serenade', and commencing 4 June at 11:00 p.m. billed simply as "Fats Waller" he began broadcasting again over Station WABC on Monday evenings as well as Saturday evenings at 8:45 p.m. These two weekly broadcasts are listed until mid July. Then from mid July the following are known:

Monday, 16 July 1934, 11:00 p.m.	Fats Waller
Tuesday, 17 July 1934, 7:00 p.m.	Fats Waller's Rhythm Club
Friday, 20 July, 1934, 9:15 p.m.	Fats Waller's Rhythm Club
Saturday, 21 July 1934, 8:45 p.m.	Fats Waller
Monday, 30 July 1934, 11:00 p.m.	Fats Waller
Tuesday, 31 July 1934, 7:00 p.m.	Fats Waller's Rhythm Club
Friday, 3 August, 1934, 9:15 p.m.	Fats Waller's Rhythm Club
Monday, 6 August 1934, 11:00 p.m.	Fats Waller
Thursday, 9 August 1934, 9:45 p.m.	Fats Waller's Rhythm Club

*****

Harry Dial continues:

When I went to Fats's house to pick up my pay from that session he asked me if I knew a good clarinet player, which surprised me because I thought he knew everybody. I asked him if he knew Eugene Sedric and he said no. Well, Sedric had only been back in the country a few months; he had been in Europe with Sam Wooding for several years. His status of not being too well known by the local musicians was what I was trying to avoid by refusing to go to Europe with the Blackbirds. I told Fats he was a good clarinet and tenor man and he said to bring him on the next date, which I did, and he made an instant hit with Fats and Oberstein.

*****

"Fats" Waller and his Rhythm Fox Trot **Piano and vocal refrain by "Fats' Waller** or **Vocal refrain and piano by "Fats" Waller** (BB B-10078-B

Herman Autrey, t; Gene Sedric, ts; Fats Waller, p/v; Albert Casey, g; Billy Taylor, sb; Harry Dial, d/speech-1

Studio No.2, New York City, New York — Friday, 17 August 1934
12:00 to 3:30 and 4:30 to 5:30

83699-1	GEORGIA MAY (Andy Razaf-Paul Denniker)	Vi 24714-B, BB B-10078-B, HMV J.F.12, RZAu G24308
83699-2	GEORGIA MAY	Victor unissued, 'Hold'
84106-1	THEN I'LL BE TIRED OF YOU (E.Y. Harburg-Arthur Schwartz)	Vi 24708-A, HMV J.F.13
84106-2	THEN I'LL BE TIRED OF YOU	Victor unissued, 'Hold'
84107-1	DON'T LET IT BOTHER YOU -1 (Mack Gordon-Harry Revel)	Vi 24714-A, ViC 24738-B, HMV J.F.12, HMVIn N.4361, HMVSp AE4518
84107-2	DON'T LET IT BOTHER YOU	Victor unissued, 'Hold' then 'Process'
84108-1	HAVE A LITTLE DREAM ON ME (Rose-Murray-Baxter)	Vi 24708-B, HMV J.F.13
84108-2	HAVE A LITTLE DREAM ON ME	Victor unissued, 'Hold'
84108-3	HAVE A LITTLE DREAM ON ME	Victor unissued, 'Hold'

The recording sheet again notes that two mikes were used and, oddly, notes both sax and clarinet (as by separate people) in the instrumentation. A footnote after the third title says, *No:1 has a conversation between FATS WALLER & TRAPMAN, at beginning of Record, No.2 Starts with Band.* Vi 24714-A bears the additional note **(From RKO film "The Gay Divorcee")** (simplified on ViC 24738-B which shows all credits U/C-l/c), and Vi 24708-A has **(From "Second Casino de Paree Revue").** The disposition for 84107 was originally 'Hold', but this is x'd out and replaced by 'Process Both'.

The reverse of HMV N.4361 is by **Ramond Paige and His Orchestra** and that of HMVSp AE4518 by **Leo Reisman.**

*****

Following this record session Waller's broadcasts over Station WABC continued as follows:

Monday, 20 August 1934, 11:00 p.m. — Fats Waller
Thursday, 23 August 1934, 9:45 p.m. — Fats Waller's Rhythm Club

These broadcasts continued twice weekly at the same times and with the same billings until at least Friday, 13 September, at which point 'Ether Waves' disappeared from the *Pittsburgh Courier* for a short time.

*****

Ed Kirkeby relates how Fats and Willie 'The Lion' Smith attended a birthday party given for George Gershwin (his birthday was 26 September) by Sherman Fairchild in his Park Avenue apartment. Paul Whiteman was in charge of the music, and the two black pianists were present at his request. Among the guests was William Paley, head of CBS, and his young daughter, who drew her father's attention to Fats, who was at the piano as she came into the room. The girl was impressed by the Waller antics but Paley, with a shrewd eye for talent, gave Fats his telephone number with instructions to call him the following day. The result was that Fats Waller came to be the star of a sustaining programme over WABC. However, as so often with Kirkeby's statements, it is difficult to reconcile them with other known events, and Waller was assumably still based in Cincinnati in September 1933, and by September 1934

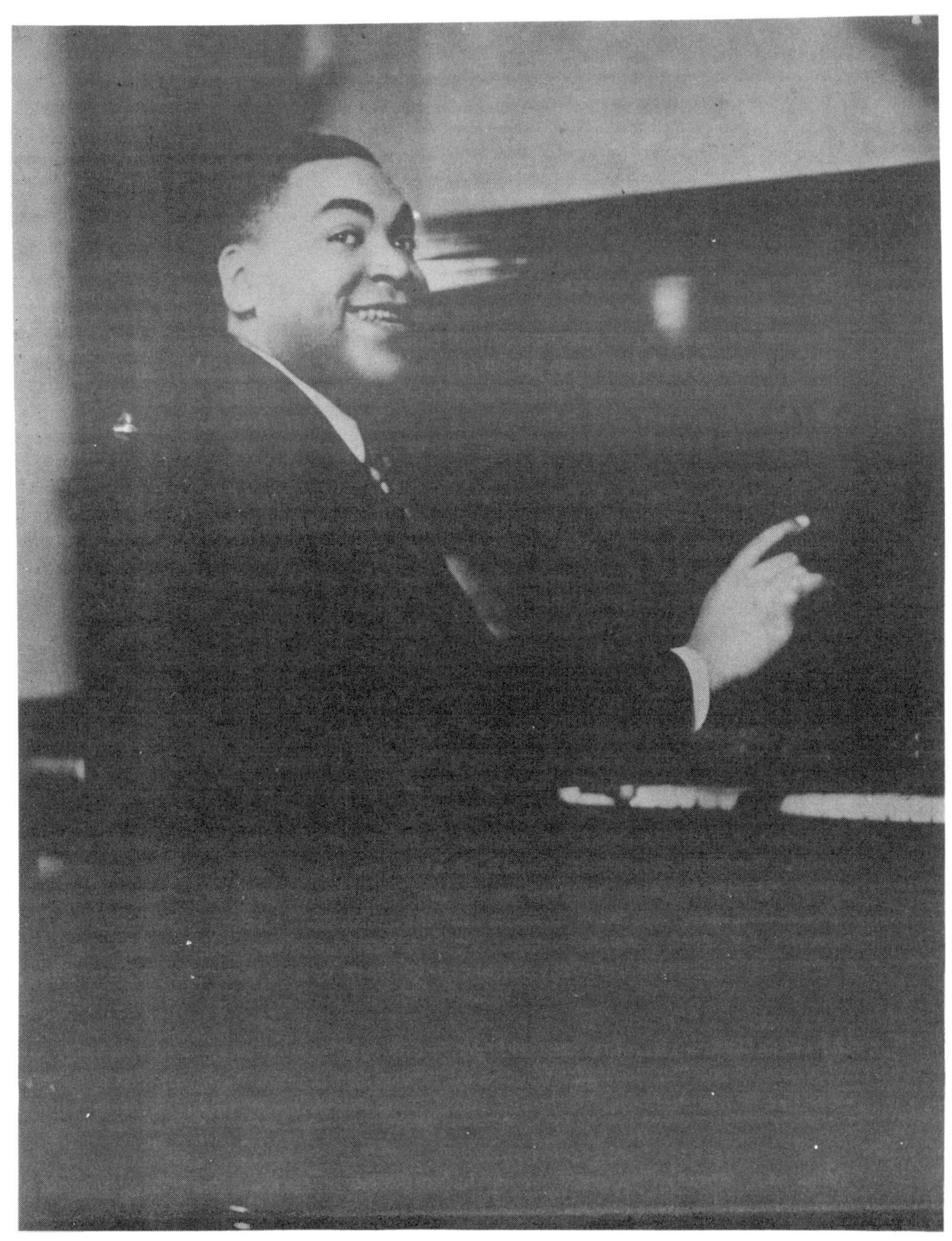

Fats at the piano at unknown date, but probably in the early '30s.

had been broadcasting regularly over WABC for several months.

An acetate is rumoured to survive of a broadcast from this period featuring Fats and Ethel Waters performing *Harlem On My Mind*, but no further details are available, nor has it been possible to ascertain when in Ethel Waters's busy schedule this broadcast might have taken place.

*****

Back to Harry Dial:

About the third session, Fats came up with Floyd O'Brien, trombone — he was good — and Milton Mezzrow, clarinet; those fellows were white, Fats was trying the integration move back then. However, Oberstein didn't like Mezzrow and said he was no improvement over Whittet and again he was right.

*****

"Fats" Waller and his Rhythm Fox Trot **Piano and vocal refrain by "Fats' Waller**
or **vocal refrain and piano by "Fats" Waller** (Vi 24737-A)
or **Vocal refrain and piano by "Fats" Waller** (Vi 24737-B)

Herman Autrey, t; Floyd O'Brien, tb; Mezz Mezzrow, cl-1/as-2; Fats Waller, p/sp-3/v-4; Albert Casey, g; Billy Taylor, sb; Harry Dial, d/vib-3

Studio No.2, New York City, New York — Friday, 28 September 1934

10:00 a.m. to 2:30 p.m. Ken Macomber directing

84417-1	SERENADE FOR A WEALTHY WIDOW -1,-3 (Reginald Foresythe)	Vi 24742-A, BB B10262-, HMV J.F.8, HMVF K7863, HMVIt GW1318, HMVSw HE2619
84417-2	SERENADE FOR A WEALTHY WIDOW *-1,-3*	Victor unissued, 'Hold'
84418-1*	HOW CAN YOU FACE ME? -1,-2,-4 (Andy Razaf-Thomas Waller)	Vi 24737-A, BB B10143-B, HMV J.F.14, HMVF K7863, HMVIt HN727, ASR L24737
84419-1	SWEETIE PIE -1,-4 (John Jacob Loeb)	Vi 24737-B, ViJ JA-404-B, BB B10262-, HMV J.F.8, HMVF K-7861, ASR L24737, HMVIt GW1318, HMVSw HE2619
84419-2	SWEETIE PIE *-1*,-4	Victor unissued, 'Hold'
84420-1	MANDY -1,-4 (Irving Berlin)	Vi/C 24738-A, HMV J.F.11, HMVSp GY281, HMVSc X4464, El EG7790
84420-2	MANDY *-1*,-4	Victor unissued, 'Hold'
84421-1	LET'S PRETEND THERE'S A MOON -2,-4 (Columbo-Hamilton-Stern)	Vi 24742-B, *HMV J.F.14,* HMVAu EA1510 HMVIn NE.219
84421-1	LET'S PRETEND THERE'S A MOON *-2,-4*	Victor unissued, 'Hold'
84422-1	YOU'RE NOT THE ONLY OYSTER IN THE STEW -1,-4 (Johnny Burke-Harold Spina)	Vi 24738-B, 20-2218-B, *20-2218-B,* ViJ JA-404-A, BB B10261-, HMV J.F.11, B.D.298, HMVF K-7861, K8526, HMVIt HN707, HMVSw HE2344, HMVSc X4464, HMVSp GY281
84422-2	YOU'RE NOT THE ONLY OYSTER IN THE STEW *-1,-4*	Victor unissued, 'Hold'

Waller's vocals include the usual interjections. Mezz Mezzrow is barely audible on matrix

84421-1. The J.F.14 issues of this title shows the matrix as 84421^{II}, but this is not take -2, merely E.M.I's method of indicating a dubbing at that time. Despite the note in *Jazz Records,* the recording sheet gives the takes made as above. Vi 24742-A omits the credit to Waller playing and singing, and the B side and the Indian HMV issue have the additional credit **(From Universal film "Wake Up and Dream")**. J.F. 11 of 84420-1 shows **(From Goldwyn film "Kid Millions" featuring Eddie Cantor).** *Jazz Records* shows Swiss HMV JK *and* HE 2344 for 84422-1, but a series of Swiss HMV catalogues held here show only the latter and enquiries among collectors indicate that the listing of JK 2344 is in error. HMVFr K-7863 omits the ? for matrix 84418-1.

The reverse of HMVIn NE.219 is a waltz by **Eddie Duchin and his Orchestra**.

*****

About this time, according to Ed Kirkeby, Fats played a stage show at the Academy of Music picture house on Fourteenth Street in Manhattan, sharing the bill with Charlie Turner's 15-piece Band, then resident at the Arcadia Ballroom. Both were well received and it apparently gave Phil Ponce the idea of putting Fats in front of the band and sending them out on tour, an idea which Turner is said to have found attractive. Fats's own feelings are not noted, but both Harry Dial's recollections and those of Ernie Anderson who knew Fats well, suggest that he did not warm to the idea, at least in the beginning.

*****

The *Pittsburgh Courier* of 6 October 1934 notes that: *Fats Waller and his Beale Street Boys are at the Palace Theatre, New York City.* In the same issue of the paper the 'Ether Waves' column re-appears for that one week and the following broadcasts over Station WABC are noted:

Thursday, 11 October 1934, 8:15 p.m.	Fats Waller's Rhythm Club
Friday, 12 October 1934. 11:00 p.m.	Fats Waller
Saturday, 13 October 1934, 8:15 p.m.	Fats Waller

*****

By this time Fats, who was notoriously uninterested in money and anything to do with organisation, had come to rely on Harry Dial to round up the musicians for the recording dates as they materialised. Harry was a dapper little man; a very fine drummer who was well aware of his own worth and ability, and of the lack of it in others which, by his own account, he was not slow to communicate. This did not exactly make him popular with his colleagues, and although he could always justify his words and actions to himself, it was all too easy to misinterpret something which happened as the following further extracts from his book make clear and also tell us something of what went on in the studio:

> *We did turn out some remarkably good records with no arrangements, nothing written at all, just those piano parts. When you listen to a tune like 'Serenade To A Wealthy Widow' you'll want to doubt that, but it is true.*
>
> *Fats was unbelievable in his ability to read music and interpret it so quickly. All those songs he sang on those records, except the originals and his compositions, he never saw or heard them before getting to the studio, yet, after playing a tune once or twice, he would perform as if he had been playing and singing it for at least a few weeks. Combined with his natural talent was extensive study and on several occasions Oberstein demonstrated Fats's ability to friends of his who would be visiting the studio by asking*

Fats to play something like 'Clair De Lune'. He said, "I don't want to hear 'Clair De Lune', but something in that vein." Almost without thinking, Fats would play a beautiful piece of music. That's how the 'Jitterbug Waltz' was born. On that occasion, Oberstein said, "Fats, I'd bet you could jazz a waltz." Not taking too much time to think, Fats began playing and what he played was later named the 'Jitterbug Waltz'. We all sat there flabbergasted and I think it is one of the most beautiful tunes ever written. Quite a few of the jazz groups play waltzes now but I don't think anyone did until after the 'Jitterbug Waltz' was done by Fats.

It's now August and we have come out of Small's and very shortly thereafter I was placed in the relief band at the Cotton Club by Wen Talbert. That was only a two-hour deal, ending not later than midnight, and soon after that I got a job at Jerry Preston's Log Cabin. It was an after-hour spot, so I went from the Cotton Club to 'the Cabin'. We sat around for a couple of hours or more doing nothing because we didn't have any business until after the regular places closed, which was at four o'clock. Located directly across the street from us was Dickey Wells's place, also an after-hour joint.

I went to work at the Log Cabin under Ralph Brown, a sax player I had known in Chicago. It was only a trio. Ralph quit a short time after I went there and left me in charge and during the period I was there I had such pianists as Bobby Henderson, Jelly Roll Morton, Charlie Prime — he was a great pianist, Willie 'The Lion' Smith, and Garnet Bradley. None of them stayed very long, they just considered themselves as helping me out. Fats would come by and 'sit in' as would other instrumentalists like Roy Eldridge, Vic Dickenson, Benny Carter, and a host of others. Billie Holiday was a frequent visitor, as was Bill Bailey, and so many other entertainers. On any given night, you could see a better show there than what you would pay for in the higher-priced places. Those performers and musicians would have a hell of a time just entertaining one another.

I stayed there until sometime in 1935, all the while still doing a record session once a month with Fats. Whenever Fats played organ on a session we were sent to Camden, New Jersey, where the company owned an old church that housed a mammoth great organ. For those sessions we were paid one hundred dollars.

On one of the record sessions that summer, Herman Autrey could not make the date because he was playing the Apollo Theatre with Charley Turner and Turner would not let him off to make the date. Since it was my job, as usual, to round up the players, I went to Fats's house — he didn't have a phone, and told him of the situation. I also suggested that if he would set the date back just one day Autrey could be there since they were finishing at the theatre on the same day as the recording. Fats told me to get a trumpet player and be in the studio at the appointed time. That night, I went to the Ubangi Club and engaged Coleman Johnson (Bill Coleman), *who was playing there with Teddy Hill. I would have gotten Joe Thomas, but he was out of town with Fletcher Henderson's band.*

Coleman made an instant hit with Fats and Oberstein, so much so that they wanted him to remain with the combo; he was a much better trumpet player than Autrey and fitted into the combo beautifully. Autrey never did know that I was ordered to get a trumpet player and always thought that I did it on my own, but if I had wanted to do that I could have done so on any date before that and it would have been Joe Thomas.

Bill Coleman's own recollections in *Trumpet Story* are somewhat different, and also a little muddled. He says it was Billy Taylor who contacted him to make a recording date with Waller and, although he gives the date correctly, he says it was made in Camden and he has clearly mixed recollections of his two dates with Fats in his mind.

*****

An enigmatic note is found in Marcus Wright's column in the *New York Age* of 3 November 1934. After making a number of comments about The Brittwood, which was a de-luxe supper bar and grill with entertainment provided, which had opened on 11 October to much acclaim, and then going on to other topics, he says: *Yes, it's true that Thomas (Fats) Waller can be seen nightly at the Brittwood.*

*****

"Fats" Waller and his Rhythm Fox Trot Vocal refrain and piano played by "Fats' Waller
Bill Coleman, t; Gene Sedric, cl-1/ ts-2; Fats Waller, p/v; Albert Casey, g; Billy Taylor, sb; Harry Dial, d/vb-3

Studio No.2, New York City, New York — Wednesday, 7 November 1934
1:00 to 5:15 p.m. Ken Macomber directing

84921-1*	HONEYSUCKLE ROSE -1 (Andy Razaf-Thomas Waller)	Vi/Ar 24826-A
84922-1	BELIEVE IT, BELOVED -1 (Whiting-Schwartz-Johnson)	Vi 24808-A, HMV B.D.134, J.F.15, HMVAu EA1509, HMVSp AE4484, HMVSc X.4430, X7475, El EG3703
84922-2	BELIEVE IT, BELOVED *-1*	Victor unissued, 'Hold'
84923-1*	DREAM MAN (Make Me Dream Some More) -1 (Joe Young-Milton Ager)	Vi 24801-A, BB B10261-, HMV B.D.117, HMVF K7454, K8526, HMVAu EA1457, HMVSw *HE2344,*
84924-1	I'M GROWING FONDER OF YOU-1,-3 (Young-Meyer-Wendling)	Vi 24801-B, HMV B.D.117, HMVAu E.A.1510
84924-2	I'M GROWING FONDER OF YOU-*1,-3*	Victor unissued, 'Hold' then 'Process'
84925-1	IF IT ISN'T LOVE -1,-2 (Val Burton-Will Jason)	Vi 24808-B, HMV J.F.15
84925-2	IF IT ISN'T LOVE *-1,-2*	Victor unissued, 'Hold'
84926-1	BREAKIN' THE ICE -1,-2 (McCarthy-Cavanaugh-Weldon)	Vi/Ar 24826-B, HMVAu E.A.1457
84926-2	BREAKIN' THE ICE *-1,-2*	Victor unissued, 'Hold'

Some copies of Victor 24826 omit the word **played** from the second part of the performance credit. Victor 24801-B bears the additional credit **(From RKO film "If This Isn't Love").** HMVSw HE2344 as by **Fats Waller And His Orchestra.** *Jazz Records* also shows HMVSw JK2344 for this title, but a Swiss HMV catalogue held here shows only the HE prefixed issue.

The original disposition for 84924-2 was 'Hold'. This is then X'd out and 'Process' written alongside it with 'Process Both' against take -1. As if to make sure that this instruction should not be missed, an additional 'NOTE:-PROCESS BOTH per Mr. Macomber' appears after the title. The recording sheet shows only clarinet in the instrumentation listed, but Sedric plays tenor sax as shown.

The reverse of HMV X.4430 is *Delta Serenade* by **Duke Ellington**.

*****

The Lafayette advert in the *New York Age* of 10 November 1934 is for a show *for one week only* headed by *Radio's Newest Sensation 'Fats' Waller* and commencing on Friday, 9 November with continuous performances from 10.00 a.m. to midnight and including a midnight show on Friday. As usual the stage presentation featuring Waller alternated throughout the day with a film. The show was reviewed in the same paper the following week as follows:

"Fats" Waller Massages The Piano At Lafayette

> *The biggest and best part of the Lafayette show this week is that champion ivory-tickler and piano massager, "Fats" Waller himself. He makes the piano actually talk to him whether at his own compositions or not, the big boy is not bad at crooning into the mike as well. The audience this week are enjoying every minute of him.*

From this it may be inferred that Waller was appearing as a solo act as the advert mentions only 'The Lafayette Orchestra' and the review refers to 'Kaiser Marshall's band' being fairly good at accompanying the acts, but not good enough for a stage presentation.

*****

"Fats" Waller Piano Solo

Fats Waller, p

Studio No.2, New York City, New York — Friday, 16 November 1934
1:30 to 4:00 p.m. Ken Macomber directing

86208-1	African Ripples	Victor unissued
86208-2*	AFRICAN RIPPLES (Thomas Waller)	Vi 24830-A, ViAr 68-0796, BB B10115-B, HMV J.F.41, B8546, HMVAu E.A.1458, HMVSw HE2289
86209-1*	CLOTHES LINE BALLET (Thomas "Fats" Waller)	Vi 25015-B, BB B10098-B, HMV J.F.35, HMVAu E.A.1254
86210-1*	ALLIGATOR CRAWL (Thomas "Fats" Waller)	Vi 24830-B, ViAr 68-0796, ViJ A1337, BB B10098-A, HMV J.F.41, B.8784, HMVAu E.A.1458, HMVSA 101, HMVF/Sw K8176, HMVEi IP370, HMVSp IW 89, AE 4581, HMVSc X.4490
86211-1	VIPER'S DRAG (Thomas "Fats" Waller)	Vi 25015-A, Vi/C 27768-A, BB B10133-, HMV B.8784, J.F.35, HMVAu E.A.1524, HMVF/Sw K8176, HMVEi IP370, HMVSp IW89, HMVIt HN2632, HMVSc X4480, HMVIn N4480, HMVSA 101

The reverse of HMV X.4490 is *Growlin* by **Charles Barnet & His Orchestra;** HMV AE 4581 is *After You've Gone* by **Trio Benny Goodman**. That of ViJ A1337 is not known.

*****

Harry Dial again supplies some background information on the personnel for the next session:

> *Turner had lost the job at the Arcadia Ballroom and things were really tough with him. I was visiting with Emmett Mathews one night and Charley's wife came by to borrow two dollars. I don't know why but it seems to be an unwritten law that once you establish yourself as a leader you must get your own job for nobody, but nobody, will give you even a gig, and there are very few exceptions in that case.*
>
> *When I was called to get the group together for the next record date, I was told that it*

would be in Camden, New Jersey, and, of course, an organ session. I always went to Billy Taylor's first because he only lived a few blocks from me, but this time I learned he had just joined Duke Ellington's band, so I rounded up the rest of the guys and went to Fats with the news about Taylor. All he said was, "Get a bass player and I'll see you at the station!"

On my way home, I thought about Turner and, although I knew he couldn't play, not to suit me anyway, I reasoned that Fats would be playing organ and the bass perhaps wouldn't matter too much anyway, and besides I could put a hundred dollars in Charley's pocket, which I knew he needed badly, so I hired him. As soon as we started to warm up, you could see the disappointed look on Oberstein's face, for the rhythm section of Waller, Taylor, Casey, and Dial was being hailed as the best in the business and Oberstein didn't like the idea of it being split up. However, we made the session and I think 'Obie' purposely played the bass down, or kept it from coming through as it might have.

*****

There is still considerable research to do on the movements of musicians and bands at this time. It is not clear from various recollections quite when Charlie Turner lost the job at the Arcadia Ballroom, nor what his personnel was. George James recalled that he was in the band at the Arcadia, so it seems likely that when Turner was discharged, he attempted to keep tabs on as many of his men as possible with a view to reforming and perhaps getting back in the Arcadia. James was not considered when the first Waller big band was formed, but was certainly in later versions of it, as will be seen.

*****

"Fats" Waller and his Rhythm Fox Trot **Piano and vocal refrain by "Fats' Waller"-3**
Organ and vocal refrain by "Fats' Waller"-4
Piano by "Fats" Waller -6
"Fats" Waller at the Piano -7

Bill Coleman, t; Gene Sedric, cl-1/ ts-2; Fats Waller, p-3/po-4/v-5; Albert Casey, g; Charles Turner, sb; Harry Dial, d

Camden Church Building, studio #2, Camden, New Jersey Saturday, 5 January 1935
10:15 a.m to 12:15 p.m. & 1:15 to 4:45 p.m. Eli Oberstein directing

87082-1	I'M A HUNDRED PERCENT FOR YOU -1,-3,-5 (Oakland-Parish-Mills)	Vi 24863-A
87082-2	I'M A HUNDRED PER CENT FOR YOU -*1*,-3,-5	Victor unissued, 'Hold'
87082-3	I'M A HUNDRED PER CENT FOR YOU -1,-3, -6 (Oakland-Parish-Mills)	Vi 24867-B, ViJ JA-491-B, HMV/H J.O.179, HMVF K7508, HMVSp IW96, AE4484
87083-1	BABY BROWN -1,-2,-3,-5 (Alex Hill)	Vi 24846-B, BB B-10109-B
87083-2	BABY BROWN -*1*,-*2*,-*3*,-5	Victor unissued, 'Hold'
87083-3	BABY BROWN -1,-2,-3,-7 (Alex Hill)	Vi 24867-A, ViJ JA-491-A, HMV J.F.45, HMVF K7508, SG464, HMVSw HE2361, HMVSp GY361, HMVSc X.4454
87084-1	NIGHT WIND -2,-4,-5 (Bob Rothberg-Dave Pollock)	Vi 24853-B, ViJ JA-489-B, HMVAu EA1482, HMVSp GY361
87084-2	NIGHT WIND -*2*,-4,-5	Victor unissued, 'Hold'

87085-1	BECAUSE OF ONCE UPON A TIME -2,-3,-5 (Young-Stride-Maltin)	Vi 24846-A, HMV B.D.134
87085-2	BECAUSE OF ONCE UPON A TIME -*2*,-3,-5	Victor unissued, 'Hold'
87086-1	I BELIEVE IN MIRACLES -2,-4,-5 (Lewis-Wendling-Meyer)	Vi 24853-A, ViJ JA-489-A, HMVAu EA1482, *HMVSw JK2796*
87086-2	I BELIEVE IN MIRACLES -*2*,-4,-5	Victor unissued, 'Hold'
87087-1	YOU FIT INTO THE PICTURE -1,-3,-5 (Bud Green-Jesse Greer)	Vi 24863-B, HMV B.D.5333, HMV/H J.O.179, HMVAu EA1509, El EG6369
87087-2	YOU FIT INTO THE PICTURE -*1*,-3,-5	Victor unissued, 'Hold'

Early pressings of the English issue of HMV J.O.179 are incorrectly labelled as using the vocal version of 87082. Although the recording sheet shows Waller playing organ for matrix 87087, the issued take has him playing piano. Victors 24863-A, 24867-B and HMV J.O.179 show 87082 as **(From the 25th Edition of the "Cotton Club Parade")**

The reverse of HMVSw JK2796 is *Mushmouth Shuffle* by **Jelly Roll Morton and his Red Hot Peppers,** and that of X.4454 is *Troubled* by **Frank Trumbauer and His Orchestra.** IW96 is not known.

*****

Bill Coleman gave a fine account of this session in his book, although mixing the dates for it and his first session with Waller. He says that the band took the train from New York to Philadelphia armed with two bottles of whisky which Fats passed around every time he wanted a drink. Two more bottles were bought by Fats for the short journey on to Camden. He continued:

> *The recording got off to a good start. Fats ad-libbed on all the singing numbers as though he had been playing and singing them all his life although the numbers were chosen by the recording company and not by himself, and he had not seen any of them before they were given to him in the studio. Before each number was recorded, Fats would run it down on the piano and then we would go over it a couple of times to set the solos and get the idea about what riff Sedric and I were going to play in certain spots. Then we'd rehearse once. With Fats, we fell into the groove from the start.*
>
> *Of course drinks were passed around between each number that was recorded and everybody stayed groovy. We recorded six numbers, but when Fats was playing the organ a reed broke on one of the pipes. It took an hour before someone found out which one it was that needed to be repaired. During that time we had a big meal, offered by the recording company, and more drinks.*
>
> *Finally we finished the session and took the train for New York. In Philadelphia, Fats bought two more bottles of whisky, which we drank before arriving at Pennsylvania Station in New York. I didn't feel drunk ...*

He then goes on to relate how he was unable to co-ordinate that night in his job with Teddy Hill and had to send in a substitute. He never again tried to match Waller in drinking. It is also interesting to note that the break in the recording was not just a simple case of stopping for lunch.

*****

Harry Dial again takes up the story:

> *Quite a few of the recordings we had made were turning out to be favourites on the juke-boxes and getting plenty of action from the discjockeys, so C.B.S. decided to book us on a tour. That knocked me out of joining Fats on his 'Saturday Night Rhythm Club' broadcast with Freddy Rich's band on C.B.S. I had already made the audition and had been accepted. The network booked the record combo on its first tour and Frank Daley's Meadow Brook was the first stop, then up through New England, lasting for several weeks, even though Eugene Sedric and Billy Taylor were not with the group. They were replaced by Emmett Mathews, who couldn't carry Gene's case as a tenor player, and Charley Turner on bass. They did weaken the combo but we were well received every place we played, mainly because of Fats.*
>
> *Sedric was not with us because he was working an exclusive Long Island spot with Broadway Jones and the pay was such that he wouldn't give up the job.*

This first tour probably took place early in 1935 and it seems that Waller found Mathews, whose speciality instrument was the soprano saxophone, to be unsuitable for recording purposes and, with Sedric presumably unavailable, Rudy Powell was brought into the recording band. Autrey returns in place of Coleman and Harry Dial also explains this by saying, *the only reason Coleman Johnson wasn't retained in the recording group was that he was having trouble with his wife and fled to Europe, where he has remained ever since.* In actual fact, although Bill Coleman may have been having trouble with his wife, it was to his home town that he went first and did not leave for Europe until later in the year. However, the tour was presumably of very short duration as there are several known dates in New York in the first couple of months of 1935.

*****

The Harlem Opera House advert in the *New York Age* of 12 January 1935 is for a revue featuring "Fats" Waller and Don Redman and His Orchestra with Harlan Lattimore (among others). Performances were for one week commencing Friday, 11 January, with the usual Saturday midnight show. Interestingly, the show for the following week was to feature Earl Hines (a great Waller fan) and Kathryn Perry, who was to feature with Fats at a later date.

The revue of this show in the following week's paper was as follows:

> *"Fats' Waller, Don Redmon* (sic) *Pleasing at Harlem Opera*
>
> *The good old Harlem Opera House continues its parade of big-time star attractions. Thomas "Fats" Waller, whose "hot" vocal and instrumental offerings comprise one of the most popular CBS radio programs and Don Redman and his orchestra ...*
>
> *"Fats" Waller, as big as ever, trots out some of his very best ivory-tickling, and when that boy does his stuff he does it well.*

*****

Waller, billed simply as "Fats Waller", broadcast over Station WABC at 4:14 p.m. on Monday 21 January 1935

*****

In a short note in the *Pittsburgh Courier* of 26 January 1935, Allan McMillan writing from New York says, *"Fats" Waller is always good. By the time you read this he'll have his own orchestra for Columbia.* The following broadcasts over WABC, but billed only as "Fats Waller" are listed, and in the light of the above and what follows, it may be assumed that these are by the newly formed orchestra.

Monday, 28 January at 4:15 p.m.
Monday, 4 February at 4:15 p.m.
Friday, 8 February at 5:45 p.m.
Monday, 11 February at 4:14 p.m.
Friday, 15 February at 5:45 p.m.
Monday, 18 February at 4:15 p.m.

*****

February 1935 was "Gala Anniversary Month" at New York's Apollo Theatre and featured one artist a week over a four-week period. Mrs. Louis Armstrong (Lill Hardin) opened the month, followed by Claude Hopkins and Louis Armstrong and, for the final week from Friday, 22 February to Thursday, 28 February in "Song Shop Revue", "Fats' Waller and his 14-piece Columbia recording band in what was claimed as their first appearance on stage. Among the supporting artists was 'Una Carlisle'. The advance write-up in the *New York Age* of 23 February 1935 makes interesting reading and includes:

> *...will offer to Harlem the first appeance on any theatre stage of "Fats" Waller and his orchestra of fourteen brilliant musicians who have become in short time the sensation of the Columbia Broadcasting System. The versatility of "Fats" Waller is familiar to Harlem, he composes, makes arrangements, sings, plays the piano and four other instruments, acts as Master of Ceremonies and if that isn't enough, personifies the wheeze that "Fats" Burns by burning up the microphone on his own sustaining programs over the WABC Columbia network.*
>
> *It is inevitable that this portly genial "Fats" Waller should seek a new outlet for his remarkable musical heritage obtained from his grandfather Adolph Waller who was one of the best known concert violinists of his day in Germany, and when he assmbled for the Columbia System an orchestra of fourteen men with himself at their head it was natural that "Fats" would turn to the 125th St. Apollo Theatre as a fitting background for his first appearance with his band.*

The review of the show in the following week's paper had:

> *"Fats" Waller, appearing on the stage for the first time with his own orchestra, presents a musical aggregation that is really good. His thrilling treble at the "grande" piano — a box just about twice the size of an ordinary music box — is augmented by the exceptional playing of Emmett Mathews, saxophonist and clarinetist, who receives a hand that brings him to the front of the stage. Aided by unusual delayed lighting effects, Waller presents "Tea For Two" in a new arrangement that is more than well received. He tops this effort in a really clean cut rendition of "Blue Moon" as an encore.*

From the above, it would seem that Fats had formed the big band immediately after appearting solo at the Harlem Opera House to have been broadcasting with it and become a 'sensation'.

*****

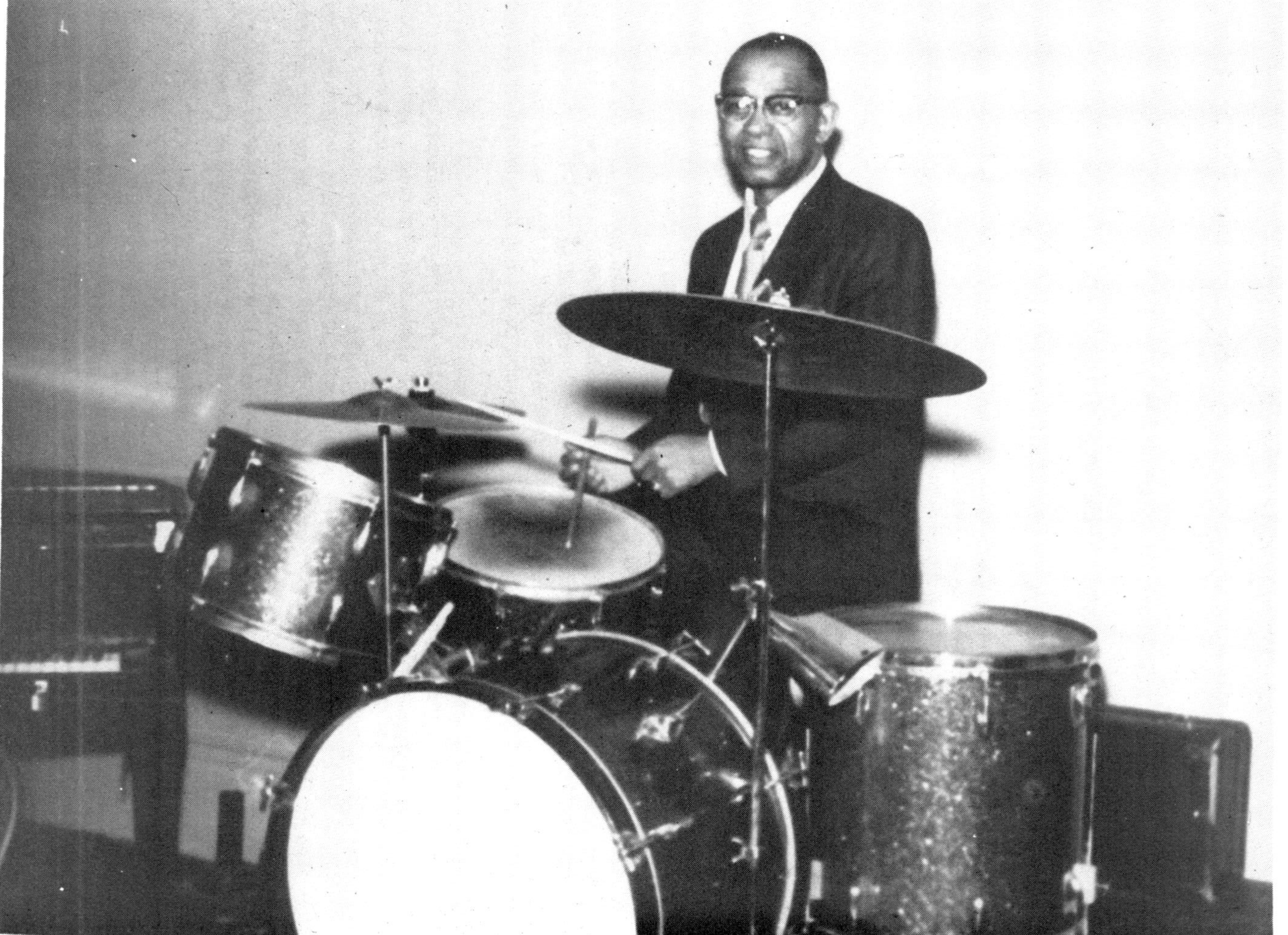

Harry Dial at his drum kit

"Fats" Waller and his Rhythm Fox Trot **Piano and vocal refrain by "Fats" Waller**
or **Vocal refrain and piano by "Fats" Waller**

Herman Autrey, t; Rudy Powell, cl-1/as-2; Fats Waller, p/v-3/cel-4; Albert Casey, g; Charles Turner, sb; Harry Dial, d.

Studio No.2 New York City, New York — Wednesday, 6 March 1935
Time not noted (see note) Eli Oberstein directing

88776-1 LOUISIANA FAIRY TALE -1,-3 — Vi 24898-A
(Parish-Gillespie-Coots)
88776-2 LOUISIANA FAIRY TALE -1,-3 — *HMVSw HE3083*
(Parish-Gillespie-Coots)
88776: Interjection in last chorus: -1: "Ah, ha. Oh latch, on latch on, yes."
-2: "Ah, mercy. Ah, you children, latch on latch on."
88777-1* I AIN'T GOT NOBODY (And Nobody Cares for Me) -1,-3 (Roger Graham-Spencer Williams) — Vi 24888-A
88778-1* I AIN'T GOT NOBODY (And Nobody Cares For Me) -1,-2 (Roger Graham-Spencer Williams — Vi 25026-A, HMV J.F.32, HMVSp AE4565, El EG3397
88779-1 WHOSE HONEY ARE YOU? -1,-3 (Haven Gillespie-J. Fred Coots) — Vi 24892-A, HMVAu EA1500
88779-2 WHOSE HONEY ARE YOU *-1*,-3 — Victor unissued, 'Hold'
88780-1* WHOSE HONEY ARE YOU? -1,-2,-4 (Haven Gillespie-J. Fred Coots) — Vi 25027-A, ViJ JA-508-A, HMV J.F.45, HMVF SG431, HMVSp GY362, HMVSw HE2361, El EG3398
88781-1 ROSETTA -1,-3,-4 (Earl Hines-Henri Woode) — Vi 24892-B
88781-2 ROSETTA *-1*,-3,*-4* — Victor unissued, 'Hold'
88782-1 ROSETTA -1,-4 (Earl Hines-Henri Woode) — Vi 25026-B, ViJ JA-537-B, A1241, BB B-10156-B, El EG3397
88782-2 ROSETTA *-1,-4* — Victor unissued, 'Hold'
88783-1* PARDON MY LOVE -1,-2,-3 (Milton Drake-Oscar Levant) — Vi 24889-A, HMV B.D.5278, HMVIt GW1103
88784-1 WHAT'S THE REASON (I'm Not Pleasin' You) -1,-3 (Poe-Grier-Tomlin-Hatch) — Vi 24889-B, 20-2643, ViJ JA-497-B, HMV B.D.156, HMVAu EA1500, HMVIt GW1103
88785-1 WHAT'S THE REASON (I'm Not Pleasin' You) -1,-4 (Poe-Grier-Tomlin-Hatch) — Vi 25027-B, HMV J.F.32, HMVSp AE4565, El EG3398
88786-1 CINDERS -1,-3,-4 (Lou Holzer-Harry Kogen) — Vi 24898-B
88787-1 (OH SUZANNAH) DUST OFF THAT OLD PIANNA -1,-3 (Caesar-Lerner-Marks) — Vi 24888-A, ViJ JA-497-A, HMV B.D.156, HMVAu EA1508, HMVSp IW 101, GY362

The available recording sheet covers only as far as matrix 88783-1A, at which point there is a note saying "Date Continued". Unfortunately, the sheet on which the remaining titles were entered is no longer available, so it is not possible to say how many takes were made or give their disposition (the ledger, which is not always reliable in this respect, shows only a single take of each). The times for the session, almost certainly a split one in view of the amount of material recorded, were presumably entered at the foot of the second sheet, and are thus not available.

Vi 24889-B and Vi 25027-B show the additional credit **(From M-G-M film "Times Square Lady")**, and HMV B.D.156 of this matrix omits the sub-title. Matrix 89787 shown on HMVAu EA1508 is in error. The performance credit on HMVSw HE3083 is **Vocal Refrain and Piano by "Fats" Waller**. Victors 25026, 25027 and Bluebird B-10156-B omit any performance credit.

The reverses of ViJ A-508 and HMV IW101 are not known.

*****

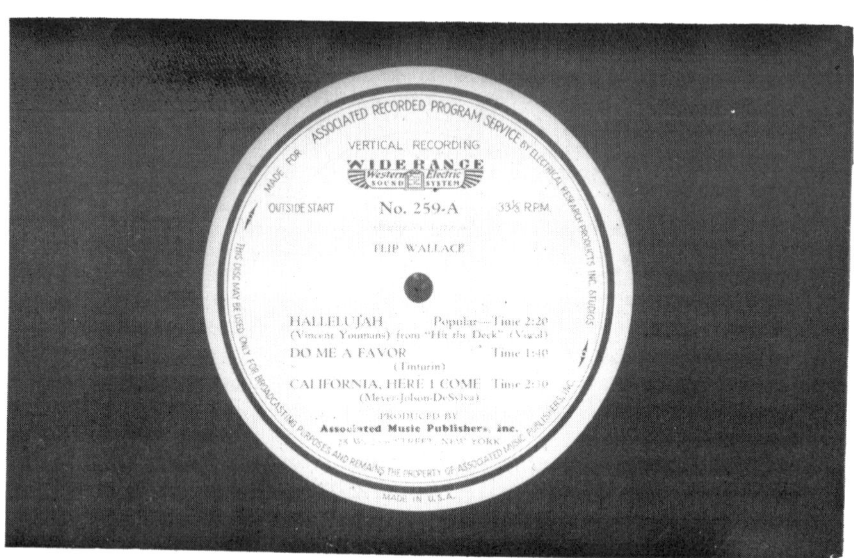

FLIP WALLACE

Fats Waller, p/v and/or comments-1; Rudy Powell, cl-2/as-3

Electrical Research Products Inc. Studio, Bronx, New York — Monday, 11 March 1935

Matrix	Title	Issue
A265-2	Baby Brown -1,-2 (ALEX HILL)	Associated unissued, test exists. Issued on LP (applies to all four titles)
	Viper's Drag (WALLER)	
	How Can You Face Me -1,-2 (WALLER)	
	Down Home Blues (WALLER)	
A266-2	Dinah -1,-3 (JOE YOUNG-HARRY AKST)	Associated No.182-A
	Handful Of Keys (FATS WALLER)	Associated No.182-A
	Solitude -1,-3 (DUKE ELLINGTON)	Associated No.182-A
A267-2	Crazy 'Bout My Baby -1 (WALLER)	Associated No.254-A
	Tea For Two -1 (YOUMANS — FROM "NO, NO NANNETTE")	Associated No.254-A
	Believe Me, Beloved -1 (J.C. JOHNSON)	Associated No.254-A
A268-2	Sweet Sue -1 (Victor Young)	Associated No.261-A
	Somebody Stole My Gal -1 (LEO WOOD)	Associated No.261-A
	Honeysuckle Rose (FATS WALLER)	Associated No.261-A

A269-2	Night Wind -1 (ROTHBERG-POLLOCK)	Associated No.253-B
	African Ripples (WALLER)	Associated No.253-B
	Because Of Once Upon A Time (STRIDE-MALTIN)	Associated No.253-B
A270-2	Where Were You On The Night Of June The Third? -1 (STEPT-TOBIAS)	Associated No.270-B
		Associated No.270-B
	Clothes Line Ballet (FATS WALLER)	Associated No.270-B
	Don't Let It Bother You -1 (GORDON-REVEL -FROM: "GAY DIVORCEE")	Associated No.270-B
A-271-2	"E" FLAT BLUES (WALLER)	Associated No.260-A
	ALLIGATOR CRAWL (WALLER)	Associated No.260-A
	ZONKY (WALLER)	Associated No.260-A
A-272-2	HALLELUJAH (VINCENT YOUMANS) FROM "HIT THE DECK"	Associated No.259-A
	DO ME A FAVOR -1 (TINTURIN)	Associated No.259-A
	CALIFORNIA, HERE I COME (MEYER-JOLSON-DESYLVA)	Associated No.259-A
A-273-2	I've Got A Feeling I'm Falling (WALLER-ROSE-LINK)	Associated No.263-A
	My Fate Is In Your Hands (WALLER-RAZAF)	Associated No.263-A
	AIN'T MISBEHAVIN' -1 (WALLER-RAZAF-BROOKS)	Associated No.263-A
A274-2	You're The Top (—)	Associated unissued, test exists. Issued on LP (applies to all three titles)
	Blue Turning Grey Over You (—)	
	Russian Fantasy (—)	

By now, Waller's popularity was such that he was invited by Associated Music Publishers, Inc., of 25 W. 45th Street, New York to produce a series of transcription discs intended as programme "fillers" for radio stations. Although *Jazz Records* states that these were made on 16" transcription discs, Ken Crawford Jr. wrote to me in 1966 as follows: "These were 12" 33⅓ rpm recordings, vertically cut, with one medley per side. All original issues were on the Associated Program Service label, under the name of 'Flip Wallace'. I know of no 78rpm issues under this pseudonym." The recordings were presumably in breach of Waller's contract with Victor, which may have been the reason for the pseudonym, although it is difficult to believe that anyone hearing them and owning a record by Fats Waller and his Rhythm would have been fooled for a moment. Be that as it may, when the material eventually achieved commercial release on microgroove, it was Victor and its overseas affiliates that issued it, so there may yet be something to discover about the circumstances of the original session. Ken Crawford Jr. then went on to give details of the three issues he then owned, two finished pressings and a test. Subsequently, Ken Crawford has completed a set of the original issues and also acquired a copy of the remaining selection in test form and details of these issues are by courtesy of him and Roy Cooke who also supplied photographic evidence. Ken also comments that all but master A-271-2 are presented as a continuous performance, but that issue has the titles separated by a scroll in the normal manner of LP issues. On *Blue Turning Grey Over You* in the final selection, Waller plays 16 bars of *How Can You Face Me* as a

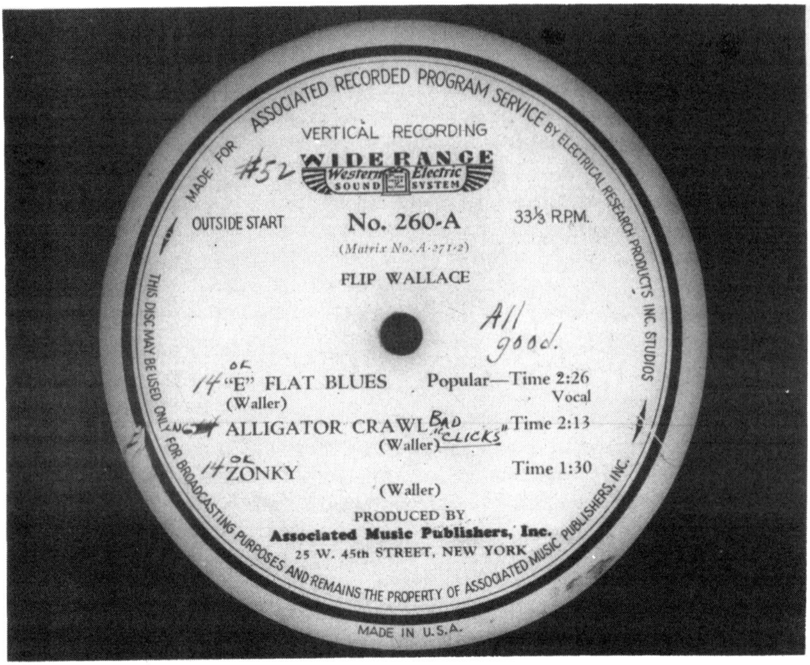

MADE FOR ASSOCIATED RECORDED PROGRAM SERVICE BY ELECTRICAL RESEARCH PRODUCTS INC. STUDIOS

VERTICAL RECORDING

WIDE RANGE Western Electric SOUND SYSTEM

#52

OUTSIDE START No. 260-A 33⅓ R.P.M.

(Matrix No. A-271-2)

FLIP WALLACE

All good.

14 OK "E" FLAT BLUES (Waller) Popular—Time 2:26 Vocal

NG ALLIGATOR CRAWL (Waller) BAD CLICKS Time 2:13

14 OK ZONKY (Waller) Time 1:30

PRODUCED BY
Associated Music Publishers, Inc.
25 W. 45th STREET, NEW YORK

THIS DISC MAY BE USED ONLY FOR BROADCASTING PURPOSES AND REMAINS THE PROPERTY OF ASSOCIATED MUSIC PUBLISHERS, INC.

MADE IN U.S.A.

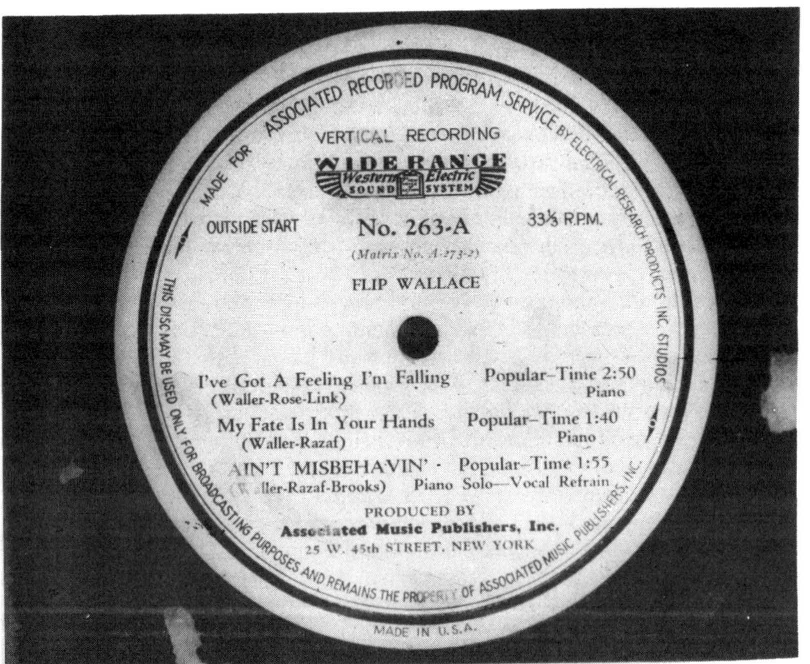

lead-in (probably in error as it was included in the first selection).

The label of No. 259-A incorrectly shows *Hallelujah* as '(Vocal)'.

Reverses: A-182-B is by **Green Bros. Novelty Band**; A-253-A by **Irene Beasley**; A-254-B by **Isham Jones Orchestra**; A-259-B, A-260-B, A-261-B, and A-263-B all by **Emil Coleman Orchestra**; and A-270-A by **Gertrude Nielsen with Johnny Green's Orchestra**

*****

In his 'Moon Over Harlem' column in the *New York Age* of 9 March 1935, Lou Layne says:

> *...When Fats leaves for the Coast next Monday to make a picture with Constance Bennett, he leaves his newly organized and grandiculous band in a sickle, for unless someone can be found to fill in for Emmett Mathews when he stands out front with his little baton, the orchestra stands in grave danger of going to the canines.*

Which is about as fine a piece of journalese as you'll find anywhere, but it does give a clue to the next event in the Waller story. 'Next Monday' would have been 11th March, but since Waller was certainly engaged in New York that day, and is listed broadcasting over WABC at 4:15 p.m. on 18th March, Layne presumably meant either the 18th and Waller left that evening, or he didn't actually leave on a Monday. Waller's name is absent from the broadcast schedules for the following week, and we do know that some time early in 1935, he went to Hollywood where he had been offered a short part in the RKO film *'Hooray For Love.'* The *Pittsburgh Courier* had run several pieces on the film and the role that black artists were to play in it and a piece from Bernice Patton, datelined California 28 February, noted that the film had started its schooting schedule 'yesterday'. It is almost certainly this film that Layne is referring to, and it was certainly completed prior to 14 June, as that is the date on which copyright was registered (No. L5661).

The following week, Layne reports that shooting of *'Hooray For Love'* has been held up for a while.

Fats's part in the film, which in the released prints ran for 72 minutes, was that of a removal man or bailiff evicting a young girl (Jeni Le Gon) from her Harlem apartment and stacking her possessions, which naturally include a piano, on the sidewalk. Spotting the piano, he goes to it, but the soundtrack is so badly synchronised with the action that the Waller sound is heard for several bars before he actually reaches the keyboard! The girl, understandably, looking upset at what has happened is comforted by the 'mayor' (Bill Robinson) who then indulges in some patter with Waller and Fats does his speciality of *I'm Living In A Great Big Way,* followed by a dance routine by Bojangles and Jeni Le Gon. The musical portions of this sequence have been issued on LP.

*****

Waller had presumably finished his part in the film by late March as a brief paragraph in the *Pittsburgh Courier* datelined Los Angeles, 28 March states, *"Fats" Waller, the star pianist and entertainer, who is in Los Angeles after his Columbia Broadcasting engagement, opened at the Sebastian Cotton Club here Tuesday night* (i.e. 26 March).

In his column in the *New York Age* of 6 April Lou Layne comments that while *Thomas "Fats" Waller may be enthralling audiences from Beverly Hills, Los Angeles and Boyle Heights at Sebastian's Cotton Club on the Coast, Harlem can hardly forget him...*

*****

The actual date of Waller's return to New York is unknown, but it seems likely to have been late April or early in May. A report in the *Pittsburgh Courier* of 11 May, datelined New York 9 May clearly has some inaccuracies. Under the heading *'Fats' Waller returns to Harlem* and sub-headed *Sensational Jazz Pianist and Outstanding Radio and Movie Star Plans to Start Tour In June With His Orchestra*, it states:

> *"Fats" Waller, Harlem's internationally known jazz pianist, composer and radio sensation is back in Harlem-town, after a seven-week sojourn in Hollywood.*
>
> *Waller and his famed orchestra went to the coast to be "shot" in "Hooray For Love" cinema hit, featuring Bill Robinson and Jeni LeGon.*
>
> *He returned to New York to be featured in a new movie, being made on Long Island, "The Broadcast of 1935". Jack Oakie, Burns and Allen and Jack Bennie are starred in the talkie.*
>
> *Waller will begin work on a series of new records for Victor this week and will play stage dates about the city until June 1. Then he prepares for a tour of the States, heading back towards Hollywood, where he and his band are scheduled to open at the Ambassador Hotel in Los Angeles in August.*
>
> *This engagement is reported to be the best ever made.*

It may be that Waller had returned earlier than the Courier reporter thought and that soon after he went out on tour briefly with his small group, for Harry Dial has this to say:

> *The first thing we heard upon returning to New York was that the band would be augmented for the next tour. Fats called the group together to discuss whom the new men would be. Since Al Casey had to leave town, Turner suggested that Fats use his band like Louis Armstrong was doing with Luis Russell's. Fats said no to that and added that the big band had to be built around the recording group, that R.C.A. and C.B.S. demanded it.*
>
> *We added two trumpets, a trombone, two saxes, and another piano. Turner was able to bring in Clarence Smith, Jimmy Smith (no relation), trumpet and guitar, Allen Jackson, sax, and Hank Duncan, piano, from his band, and I brought in Joe Thomas, Rudy Powell, and George Wilson, trumpet, sax, and trombone. I had said in the meeting that I would get Nat Story on trombone but when I reached him he had just joined the Mills Blue Rhythm Band. George Wilson used to come by and 'sit in' at Small's and I thought he was a very good trombonist, and he had asked me, if I ever had the opportunity, to try and get him a break with Fats. Fats liked him, so that was that.*
>
> *Immediately, Alex Hill was engaged to make arrangements for the band, and Rudy Powell also contributed in that capacity. I didn't consider the arrangements very hard but we were certainly having a hard time with some of them, primarily with Turner and the boys from his band. I remarked on several occasions that they should take their parts home and practice on them and try to take up less time in rehearsals. I never said those things in the presence of Fats. Since we had two pianos, he was coming to rehearsals late with the expectation that we would have ironed out any kinks in the arrangements before he arrived because they certainly did not present any problem to him. Several times he had arrangements passed in because he felt that the fellows were never going to play them.*
>
> *Finally, after about three weeks of rehearsals, we took to the road again, returning to a few of the towns made on the first tour, with Boston and some others added.*

It is possible that Harry has his chronology a little mixed up but, whatever the truth, before setting out on the tour and possibly while the big band was rehearsing, there was another record date to be fulfilled as noted in the Courier report above.

*****

"Fats" Waller and his Rhythm Fox Trot Vocal refrain and piano by "Fats" Waller-1
Herman Autrey, t; Rudy Powell, cl; Fats Waller, p/v; Albert Casey, g; Charles Turner, sb; Harry Dial, d.

Studio No.2 New York City, New York — Wednesday, 8 May 1935
2:00 to 6:00 p.m. Eli Oberstein directing

89760-1	LULU'S BACK IN TOWN (Al Dubin-Harry Warren)	Vi 25063-A, HMV J.F.47, HMVAu EA1563, HMVSp AE4571, HMVSw HE2631, ASR L25063
89760-2	LULU'S BACK IN TOWN	Victor unissued, 'Process'
89761-1	SWEET AND SLOW (Al Dubin-Harry Warren)	Vi 25063-B, HMV J.F.47, HMVAu EA1563, HMVSp AE4571, HMVSw HE2631, ASR L25063
89761-2	SWEET AND SLOW	Victor unissued, 'Hold'
89762-1	YOU'VE BEEN TAKING LESSONS IN LOVE (From Somebody New) (Winston Tharp-Grady Watts)	Vi 25044-B, *HMV B.10684, BRS 1013*
89762-2	YOU'VE BEEN TAKING LESSONS IN LOVE	Victor unissued, 'Hold'
89763-1	YOU'RE THE CUTEST ONE (Archie Berdahl)	Vi 25039-B, BB B-10129-B, HMVIt GW1214
89763-2	YOU'RE THE CUTEST ONE	Victor unissued, 'Hold'
89764-1	I'M GONNA SIT RIGHT DOWN AND WRITE MYSELF A LETTER (Joe Young-Fred E.Ahlert)	Vi 25044-A, 42-0037-A, 420-0234, ViC 25194-B, ViJ A1241, JA-537-A, HMV B.D.5031, *B.9935*, HMVF SG304, HMVIt GW1238, *HMVSw HE2362*, El EG3607, *Bm 1099, BRS 1013*
89764-2	I'M GONNA SIT RIGHT DOWN AND WRITE MYSELF A LETTER	Victor unissued, 'Hold'
89765-1	HATE TO TALK ABOUT MYSELF (Robin-Rainger-Whiting)	Vi 25039-A, HMVIt GW1214
89765-2	I HATE TO TALK ABOUT MYSELF	Victor unissued, 'Hold'

There is a note at the foot of the recording sheet that the orchestra was called for 1:00 p.m. but that recording didn't get under way until an hour later. Two microphones were used.

Vi 25063-A bears the additonal credit **(From Warner Bros. film "Broadway Gondolier")**. On Vi 25044-B 'Fox Trot' is abbreviated to **F.T.** Copies of Vi 25044 were imported into the U.K. by The Gramophone Co. and these bear a Victor 'Special' sticker over the top half of the original label. Biltmore 1099 as **FATS WALLER AND HIS ORCHESTRA**. Horst Lange quotes the Electrola issue number above for matrix 89764-1, whilst *Jazz Records* gives it as EG3602. It is not known which is correct.

Dave Dixon wrote about the cross couplings which occasionally appear on Canadian Victor, of which VicC 25194-B is an example. He says that the Canadian company would select what they considered to be the strongest sides from two U.S. issues and couple them. According to Dave, pre-war issues of ViC 25194 appear on the gold-on-black label and couple Vi 25044-A with Vi 25194-B. The situation is further complicated by the fact that the same catalogue number was retained for a late-war or post-war pressing on the pale yellow-on-black label which used dubbed masters of *Somebody Stole My Gal/Sugar Blues* (see sessions of 24 June and 2 August 1935).

*****

The *Pittsburgh Courier* of 25 May carries a photo of Waller congratulating Jimmie Lunceford backstage at the Palace Theater, New York after "Fats" had crowned Lunceford the "Syncopation King" on stage. The actual date for this is not known, but was in the first half of May.

*****

Some time after this recording date, possibly on the 1 June date mentioned above, the augmented band left on tour, the personnel comprising:
Herman Autrey, Joe Thomas, Clarence Smith, t; George Wilson, tb; Rudy Powell, as; Allen Jackson, ts; Gene Sedric, ts/cl; Fats Waller, Henry Duncan, p; James Smith, g; Charles Turner, sb; Harry Dial, d.

Again, Harry Dial has vivid memories of this tour:

On a couple of the engagements Fats was short with the pay-off; naturally, that irked everyone. Turner approached the men in the band who weren't with him previously and asked them if they wanted to return to the Arcadia Ballroom with him. When he spoke to me, I told him I would not work with Fats and be any part of a conspiracy against him. I said, "If the band breaks up, I'll work with the first guy who offers me a job, but this two-faced business, I'll have no part of it." I imagined that he thought that I told Fats what he was attempting to do, but I never opened my mouth.

Charley and his clique began to work against me and got so strong with it that Herman Autrey said to me on intermission time at the Colonades Hall in Washington, D.C., "Nigger, we're gonna get you outa this band!" I felt he was still harbouring the thought that I purposely knocked him out of the Camden record date.

The band came to New York to play the Apollo Theatre. During the rehearsal of the show, the clique blames everything that goes wrong on the drummer, trying to make me look bad. I fluffed off everything because I knew that Fats was aware of my ability. We opened on Friday, as scheduled, and the grumbling about me continued. After each show, Turner and Autrey repaired to Fats's dressing room and to make sure that enough whiskey was on hand they carried some with them, and they finally succeeded in talking Fats into letting me go and hiring Slick Jones, Turner's drummer. What I don't think Fats knew was that Turner was trying to get men in the band who would co-operate with him in the event he could go back to the Arcadia Ballroom.

That Sunday, on my way home for dinner after the second show, I met Luis Russell on the street and he said to me, "Harry, I hear you are coming out of Fats's band and, if it's true, you can come with me. I have the new Cotton Club contract," (it had moved down town), "and Paul Barbarin," (his drummer), "has gone back to New Orleans to live." I told him I knew the clique was trying to get me out but I had not received a notice or any word from Fats. I said I would speak to Fats about it when I got back to the theatre. Luis said, "I will have to know tomorrow because I start show rehearsals on Tuesday."

On returning to the theatre, I went to Fats's dressing room and told him about the conversation I had had with Luis Russell. I said, "If this is true, tell me now; I have a job waiting for me." Fats told me, "Don't let it bother you," the title of a song we had recorded, so I contacted Russell on Monday and told him I was remaining with Fats, but on Tuesday, when I came back from dinner, my instruments were down in the basement and Slick Jones was ready to go to work.

That actually broke my heart for two reasons. First, I had remained loyal to Fats as well as to the fellows; I said nothing to him about the poor ability of some of the other players, as some of them may have thought. I wouldn't insult Fats's intelligence by telling him who could or could not play, and he certainly knew my ability. Second, by him lying to me, I lost out on the Cotton Club job by just one day. When I went back to Russell he had engaged Walter Conyers. It was doubly painful because had I not taken it upon myself to engage Turner for that record date, in all probability he wouldn't have been there in the first place!

I had to go to Fats's house the following Thursday night to collect my salary and I went with a pistol in my pocket. After I had been paid, I called Turner and Fats every dirty name I could think of — Autrey had left — and if they had gotten out of their seats I would have shot them; they must have sensed it, for they didn't move and said very little. I told Fats that a couple more slips with the money and his band would be sittin' up in the Arcadia!

I must say this about Fats and money. It meant practically nothing to him. The couple of times he paid us off short I figured he had been out balling a lot of down-an'-outers and went overboard.

Although Harry was deeply distressed by what had happened, he does allow that Fats had little or no regard for money other than for his immediate needs. Also it is apparent that, with the friction that developed within the band, Fats would have taken the easy option and got rid of the 'odd man out'. In his book, Harry goes on to relate another occasion when Fats's cavalier attitude to money left Alex Hill and himself gasping and also says that when Eli Oberstein heard about his dismissal, he offered Harry a job as a studio musician which would have meant working with Fats and, for this reason Harry declined.

Although Harry Dial's memories are normally accurate, his story at this point contains a number of inconsistencies and it would appear that he has brought together memories, incidents and personalities that are actually unrelated. There was no engagement at the Apollo after the week in February and Waller did not return to the Apollo as an artist until the beginning of 1936, although he was seen there in *'Hooray For Love'*, which was the featured film for the week beginning 30 August, when Louis Armstrong headed the stage presentation. Indeed, there is no mention at all of Fats Waller that I have been able to trace in the *New York Age* for the months of April-July; the next being the note in the 10 August issue. Although Slick Jones may have replaced Harry on drums, it was Arnold Boling who took his place in the recording group when they travelled to Camden for the next date, and although Harry Dial thought that Charlie Turner had lost the job at the Arcadia and did not return there, other evidence points to the fact that Turner had some sort of loose arrangement with the management there and was in and out of the place over the next year or so at least.

*****

Details of the route followed by the orchestra for the above tour, which was booked by the Southland Orchestra Service, are sparse, and the only confirmed date is that at the Municipal Auditorium, Macon Georgia on Monday, 17 June, after which they headed north for New York and a recording date for Victor by the 'Rhythm'.

*****

Meanwhile, *'Hooray For Love'* was previewed at Hollywood's Hillstreet Theater on 6 June and reports indicate that the finished prints had edited out much that had been filmed by LeGon, Robinson and Waller to the dismay of those who had been associated with the production.

*****

"Fats" Waller and his Rhythm Fox Trot Vocal refrain and piano by "Fats" Waller -1
Herman Autrey, t; Rudy Powell, cl-2/as-3; Fats Waller, p/v; James Smith, g; Charles Turner, sb; Arnold Boling, d.

Camden, Studio #2, Camden, New Jersey — Monday, 24 June 1935
10:00 a.m. to 5:00 p.m. Mr. Kikeby (sic) directing. Waller arrived at 10:45

88989-1*	DINAH -1,-2 (Lewis-Young-Akst)	Vi 25471-A, 29988-, ViJ JA-869-A, HMV J.F.46, B.D.5040, HMVF SG383, HMVIt HN2996, HMVSw H.E.2356, HMVSp AE4555, HMVSc X8004, HMVAu EA2083, El EG3683
88990-1*	TAKE IT EASY -2,-3 (Jimmy McHugh-Dorothy Fields)	Vi 25078-B, HMV B.D.5199, El EG 3643
88991-1*	YOU'RE THE PICTURE (I'm The The Frame) -2 (Bob Rothberg-Jack Golden)	Vi 25075-B, *HMV B.10830, HMVSw HE3083, HMVFi TG224*
88992-1*	MY VERY GOOD FRIEND-THE MILKMAN -2 (Johnny Burke-Harold Spina)	Vi 25075-A, *HMV B.D.1218,* B.D.5376, HMVIt HN2584, ASR LB5376
88992-2	MY VERY GOOD FRIEND THE MILKMAN	Victor unissued, 'Hold'
88993-1*	BLUE BECAUSE OF YOU -2 (Carpenter-Dunlap-Wilson)	BB B-10322-B
88994-1*	THERE'S GOING TO BE THE DEVIL TO PAY -2 (Billy Hueston-Bob Emmerich)	Vi 25078-A
88995-1*	12TH STREET RAG -2 (Sumner-Bowman)	Vi 25087-A, ViAr 68-1358, ViJ JA-585-A, A1114, HMV B.D.262, HMVF K7601, SG.174, HMVIt GW1236, GW1900, HMVSp GY886, HMVSc X8004
88995-2	12th STREET RAG *-2*	Victor unissued, 'Hold'
88996-1*	THERE'LL BE SOME CHANGES MADE -2 (Billy Higgins-W. Benton Overstreet)	BB B10322-A, Vi 20-2216-A, *Vi 20-2216-A*
88996-2	THERE'LL BE SOME CHANGES MADE *-2*	Victor unissued, 'Hold'
88997-1*	SOMEBODY STOLE MY GAL -2 (Leo Woods)	Vi/C 25194-A, *ViC 25194-A,* ViJ JA-691-A, HMV J.F.46, HMVAu E.A.1630, *Bm 1099*

88998-1 SWEET SUE -2,-3 (Will J. Harris-Victor Young) Vi 25087-B, ViAr 68-1358, ViJ JA-585-B, A1114, HMV B.D.298, HMVSp AE4555

88998-2* SWEET SUE -2,-3 Victor unissued, 'Process', issued on LP

88998: First vocal: -1 "without you dear, I don't know what I'd do, ha-ha"
-2 "without you dear, I don't what I'd do, you sweet thing."
Final comment: -1 "Yes, Yes, Yes"
-2 "One more beat, o-n-e m-o-r-e beat"

1935-1 Somebody Stole My Gal Test made for Raymond R. Sooy

This was, by Ed Kirkeby's own account, his very first session as an A&R man for Victor and the first time he had met Fats Waller. This would account for the mis-spelling of his name on the recording sheet, as the studio clerk would not have known him. Kirkeby says that when he arrived, things were in full swing, but the sheet reveals that Waller was 45 minutes late arriving and it seems doubtful that Kirkeby would have been late for his very first assignment, so his statement is probably a bit of journalistic licence. Al Casey recalls that when asked to record *12th Street Rag,* Fats was very reluctant to tackle it, saying that it was not the right sort of material for the band. However, Kirkeby insisted, and it came out sounding as if it had been written for them.

Vi 25075-A and BB B-10332-A show "Fox Trot" abbreviated to **F.T.** American pressings of Vi 25194 couple *Somebody Stole My Gal/Sugar Blues* whilst some Canadian versions (see note after 8 May 1935 session) couple the first with *I'm Gonna Sit Right Down And Write Myself A Letter,* and show the titles UC/lc. Several Victors from this period appear on the normal 'curly-edge' label *and* on the 'Swing Classic' label and these latter show a personnel on the label which names the drummer as *Scrippie Boling*. BM 1099 as **FATS WALLER AND HIS ORCH**. Oddly, all the waxes for this session, except 88998-2/2A are prefixed BS, whilst these latter have BVE.

*****

Waller was apparently planning to be around New York for a while after this recording session, because a small advert from Lebon in the *Pittsburgh Courier* of 15 June indicated that he was available for bookings in the Tri-State District at the end of June/beginning of July, but thereafter it became almost a set pattern that short tours were interspersed with recording dates back in New York. Many of these tours, which sometimes lasted no more than a few days, featured return engagements, and there were no doubt changes of personnel in the group, so it has proved virtually impossible to plot them from the recollections of band members or those of Ed Kirkeby which, for this period were based mainly on what others had told him, as he was not to become Waller's manager until some time later when Phil Ponce's declining health and the problems of dealing with the unpredictable Waller brought about his retirement from the post.

*****

The film *'Hooray For Love'* was screened at the Roxy Theatre, 50th Street and Seventh Avenue on Friday, 12 July with a personal appearance by Bill Robinson. This is the first announcement I have been able to find in the black press and no mention is made of Waller's participation in the film.

*****

However, a second tour, mentioned some weeks earlier in the *Pittsburgh Courier,* had been planned well in advance and, under the auspices of the LeBon Social Club, Waller and the orchestra were at the Labor Lyceum in Pittsburgh on Friday, June 28 at the same time as *'Hooray For Love'* was being featured at the Stanley Theater in the city, and the *Pittsburgh Courier* of 29 June has a report datelined Columbus, Ohio that:

> *"Fats" Waller, greatest radio pianist in the country, with his sensational recording and radio orchestra, is heading into Ohio and West Virginia.*
>
> *According to authoritative information, Waller will play a four-day engagement in West Virginia and Ohio about the middle of July.*
>
> *In addition to playing here, he is tentatively scheduled to appear in Charleston, Bluefield and Beckley, W. Va.*

The only other reference is a very brief one indeed by 'Tattler' in the *Pittsburgh Courier* of 27 July which says, *Fats Waller in town for a few hours ... last week ... En-route*

*****

"Fats" Waller and his Rhythm Fox Trot **Vocal refrain and piano by "Fats" Waller**

Herman Autrey, t; Rudy Powell, cl; Fats Waller, p/v; James Smith, g; Charles Turner, sb; Arnold Boling, d/*vb*-1.

Studio 2, New York City, New York — Friday, 2 August 1935

11:00 a.m. to 3:00 p.m. W.T. Kirkeby directing

92915-1*	TRUCKIN' (From 26th Edition "Cotton Club Parade") (Ted Koehler-Rube Bloom)	Vi 25116-A, HMV B.D.262, HMVF K7601, SG.174, HMVIt GW1236, HMVSp GY886
92916-1*	SUGAR BLUES (Lucy Fletcher-Clarence Williams)	Vi 25194-B, *ViC 25194-B,* ViJ JA-691-B, HMVAu E.A.1630
92917-1*	JUST AS LONG AS THE WORLD GOES 'ROUND AND 'ROUND (And I Go around with you) (Harry Woods)	*HMVSw HE3018, HMV/H J.O.291, HMVF SG492*
92918-1	GEORGIA ROCKIN' CHAIR (Fred Fisher)	Vi 25175-A, ViJ A1261, BB/C B-10288-A, HMVAu EA1608, HMVSp AE4606
92918-2	GEORGIA ROCKIN' CHAIR	Victor unissued, 'Hold'
92919-1	BROTHER, SEEK AND YE SHALL FIND -1 (Frank Crum-Robert G. Stewart)	Vi 25175-B, ViJ A1261, HMVAu EA1608
92919-2	BROTHER SEEK AND YE SHALL FIND	Victor unissued, 'Hold'
92920-1	THE GIRL I LEFT BEHIND ME (Leslie-Rose Meyer)	Vi 25116-B, HMV B.10439, HMVAu E.A.1605, HMVIt HN3171, HMVFi TG156
92920-2	THE GIRL I LEFT BEHIND ME	Victor unissued, 'Hold'

A note on the recording sheet gives, *(Date Called 9:30)(Fats Waller Arrived 11:00)*, and in all cases Fox Trot is abbreviated to FT. Vibes are heard on 92919, presumably played by Boling, but possibly by Waller himself.

HMVJO291 omits the first word of the title (as on the recording sheet).

*****

Soon after the above date, the band were off on tour again, and several locations have been found. An advert in the Baltimore *Afro-American* shows them due to appear at the Rainbow Ballroom, Hyannis, Massachusetts where they were billed to play for dancing from 9 to 3 on Thursday, 8 August. The same advert also says their next appearance would be in a tent at Boston on 12 August. Under the heading *Fats Waller Starts Tour,* and datelined Norwalk,

Conn. the *New York Age* of 10 August 1935 has, *Fats Waller and his orchestra will begin their New England tour by opening at Roton Point here next Sunday.* This is presumably 11 August and between the two engagements above.

*****

The personnel of the touring band was given in *Jazz Hot No.5* for September-October 1935 as follows, and this almost certainly relates to a period at least a month prior to that date, possibly the New England tour mentioned above. This same personnel also appears in *Swing Music* for November-December 1935, but it is not known whether this was just picked up from the French paper, or is the result of a separate report. The original extract is:

> *The personnel of Fats Waller's Band is now Rudy Powell, Emmet Mathews, George James, Freddie Skerritt, saxes, Herman Autry, C.E. Smith, Eddie Anderson, trumpets, Fred Robinson, George Wilson, trombones, Hank Duncan & Fats, piano, Charlie Turner, bass, Arnold Bolden, drums.*

Note that no mention is made of guitarist James Smith.

*****

"Fats" Waller and his Rhythm Fox Trot Vocal refrain and piano by "Fats" Waller -1
Vocal refrain by "Fats" Waller & Herman Autrey -2

Herman Autrey, t/v-2; Rudy Powell, cl/as-3; Fats Waller, p/v/cel-4; James Smith, g; Charles Turner, sb; Arnold Boling, d.

Studio 2, New York City, New York Tuesday, 20 August 1935
12:00 a.m. to 4:00 p.m. & 4:30 to 6:30 p.m. W.T. Kirkeby directing

92992-1 YOU'RE SO DARN CHARMING Vi/C 25120-A, ViJ JA-605-A
(Johnny Burke-Harold Spina)

92992-2 YOU'RE SO DARN CHARMING Victor unissued, 'Hold,' then 'Process'
Issued on LP

92992: 2nd line of vocal: -1 "It seems you do everything, baby, so perfectly ... yes"
-2 "It seems you do everything so perfectly ... yes"

92993-1* WOE! IS ME -1 Vi 25140-B, HMV B.D.5031,
(Cavanaugh-Sanford-Emmerich) HMVAu EA1590, *HMVSw HE2362,*
HMVIt GW1238, El EG3602

92994-1* RHYTHM AND ROMANCE Vi 25131-A, HMV B.D.5199,
(Whiting-Schwartz-Johnson) HMVAu EA1587

92995-1* LOAFIN' TIME -2,-3 Vi 25140-A, HMVAu EA1590
(Arthur Altman-Milton Ager)

92996-1* (Do you intend to put an end to) A Vi 25131-B, HMVAu EA1587
SWEET BEGINNING LIKE THIS -1,-4
(Joe Young-Fred E. Ahlert)

92997-1* GOT A BRAN' NEW SUIT Vi 25123-B, ViJ JA-623-B, HMV B.D.5012,
(Howard Dietz-Arthur Schwartz) HMVEx/H J.O.196, HMVSw HE2896,
HMVIn N14065, El EG3702

92998-1* I'M ON A SEE-SAW Vi/C 25120-B, ViJ JA-605-B, HMV/H J.O.291,
(Desmond Carter-Vivian Ellis) HMVF SG492, HMVSw HE3018,
HMVAu E.A.1605, El EG3702

94100-1* THIEF IN THE NIGHT Vi 25123-A, ViJ JA-623-A
(Howard Dietz-Arthur Schwartz)

The original disposition for matrix 92992-2 was 'Hold', but this is crossed out and 'Process' written against both takes -1 and -2. The Canadian issue of Vi 25120 is on the "round" label and legends are UC/lc. Victor 25123 (both sides) and HMV J.O.196 bear the additional credit **(From musical production "At Home Abroad")** and HMV B.D.5012 bears the additonal sub-title **("Follow The Sun")**. HMV E.A.1605 bears the additional sub-title **("From "Jill Darling"]**, and J.O.291 has **(Introduced in the London production "Jack and Jill")**.This latter is also noted on the recording sheet. In his book *Fascinating Rhythm* Peter Cliffe states that the show was originally called *'Jack And Jill'* for its Glasgow try-out, but renamed *'Jill Darling'* by the time it reached London's West End.

Matrix 92999 was not used and, at this point, the Victor matrix system jumped straight to 94100.

*****

Probably during the late summer of 1935, Fats and Anita journeyed to Hollywood where he had been offered a part in the 20th Century Fox production 'King Of Burlesque'. Dressed in white tie and tails, he plays and sings *I've Got My Fingers Crossed* accompanied by an unknown group which is reputedly that of Les Hite's band, possibly augmented for the occasion, and certainly featuring trumpeter Teddy Buckner miming with a trombone on screen. This film merits further investigation as, in 1966 Bob Kumm noted that Fats is heard on the soundtrack playing piano accompaniment to the tune *I'm Shootin' High.* A letter to the Music Librarian of 20th Century Fox brought the additional information that Fats also recorded *Too Good To Be True* and *Oh! Susanna, Dust Off That Old Pianna,* but these were apparently not used in the film as released which ran for 90 minutes. No further information has been found.

Whilst in Hollywood, Fats appeared as guest star at Sebastian's Cotton Club where the Hite band was resident.

*****

The following were recorded for use in the film 'King Of Burlesque'. Only the first title was used in the film as issued, so it is not possible to state whether the remaining titles were by Fats Waller alone or with the accompanying band.

Fats Waller, p/v; acc. unidentified orchestra, featuring Teddy Bucker, t.-1

20th Century Fox Studio, Hollywood, California. 1935

I've Got My Fingers Crossed -1	Issued on LP
Oh, Susannah, Dust Off That Old Pianna	Not used
Shooting High	Reported used in the film
Too Good To Be True	Not used

Details of the unissued material by courtesy of 20th Century Fox. Information on the recording date has not been found, and all that can be said is that it took place prior to 3 January 1936, when copyright was registered under No. L6373.

*****

A small mystery is raised by Walter Allen in *Hendersonia* (p.322) when attempting to establish the personnel of the Henderson orchestra in the 1935 period. Herman Autrey was a member of this and in an interview with Walt, said that the reason he had joined Henderson was that Fats Waller, his regular employer, was absent in Europe and that he was thus out of work. As Walt points out, Waller's only known trips to Europe were 1932, 1938 and 1939 and it seems likely that Autrey (the interview was in 1971) was either confusing his employment with Henderson with that he was forced to seek whilst Waller was in Hollywood or, on the later occasions when

Fats was away.

*****

I interviewed saxophonist George James at length about his career and, talking of his time with Fats Waller during the period 1935-1938, he had this to say:

After the Bearcats, I guess my next regular job was with Charlie Turner over at the Arcadia Ballroom — we were called Charlie Turner's Arcadians. That was the band that Fats Waller took over when he went out on tour. He'd only had a little band himself before that, but they needed a big band to fit the image and took over Charlie's band, and put in some of the guys, like Herman Autrey, Gene Sedric and Al Casey out of Fats's own band. The reed section was me playing lead alto, clarinet and baritone; Gene Mikell, 3rd alto; Al Washington, 2nd tenor; Gene Sedric, 4th tenor, and Emmett Mathews, 5th baritone and soprano. We were touring with Fats for the best part of a year — right to the West Coast and back again. I remember that we were in Dallas at the same time that Paul Whiteman was playing The Fairgrounds there, and Paul decided that he was going to come over and join us one night — play with us. Now Paul Whiteman at that time had a girl pianist ...I think her name was Margo, and when the band came in and she sat down on the piano bench with Fats they almost had a riot. A white girl just didn't do that at that time I guess. A white girl probably wouldn't do it even now in Dallas whether it was Fats or not. Anyway, they finally got the place calmed down and it was alright for her to play the piano as long as she sat on the bench by herself. But the funny thing was that the guys in Paul's band were so upset by the attitude of the police, they wanted to fight, but we dissuaded them because it would only have made more problems for us in the end. We told them they'd only make it bad for us if they started another riot and to forget about it ...but they were really mad.

While we were in Dallas we played a Graduation Prom. — this was up on the Roof Garden of the Dallas Hotel. We were all in white uniforms and Fats was dressed in white tails. Somebody made a disparaging remark about Fats and his white tails, and our drummer, Slick Jones, took offence at this, and we almost had another riot on our hands. But we kept telling him to cool it, "We are on the Roof Garden you know," we told him, "and it's a long way down!" Oh yes, we had some incidents down there, it was quite nerve-racking.

One reference to this tour is given in the *Pittsburgh Courier* of 28 September which says: *Fats Waller, famous radio and recording star, will invade Chattanooga, October 2nd where he is to play an engagement at the Grand Theatre.*

*****

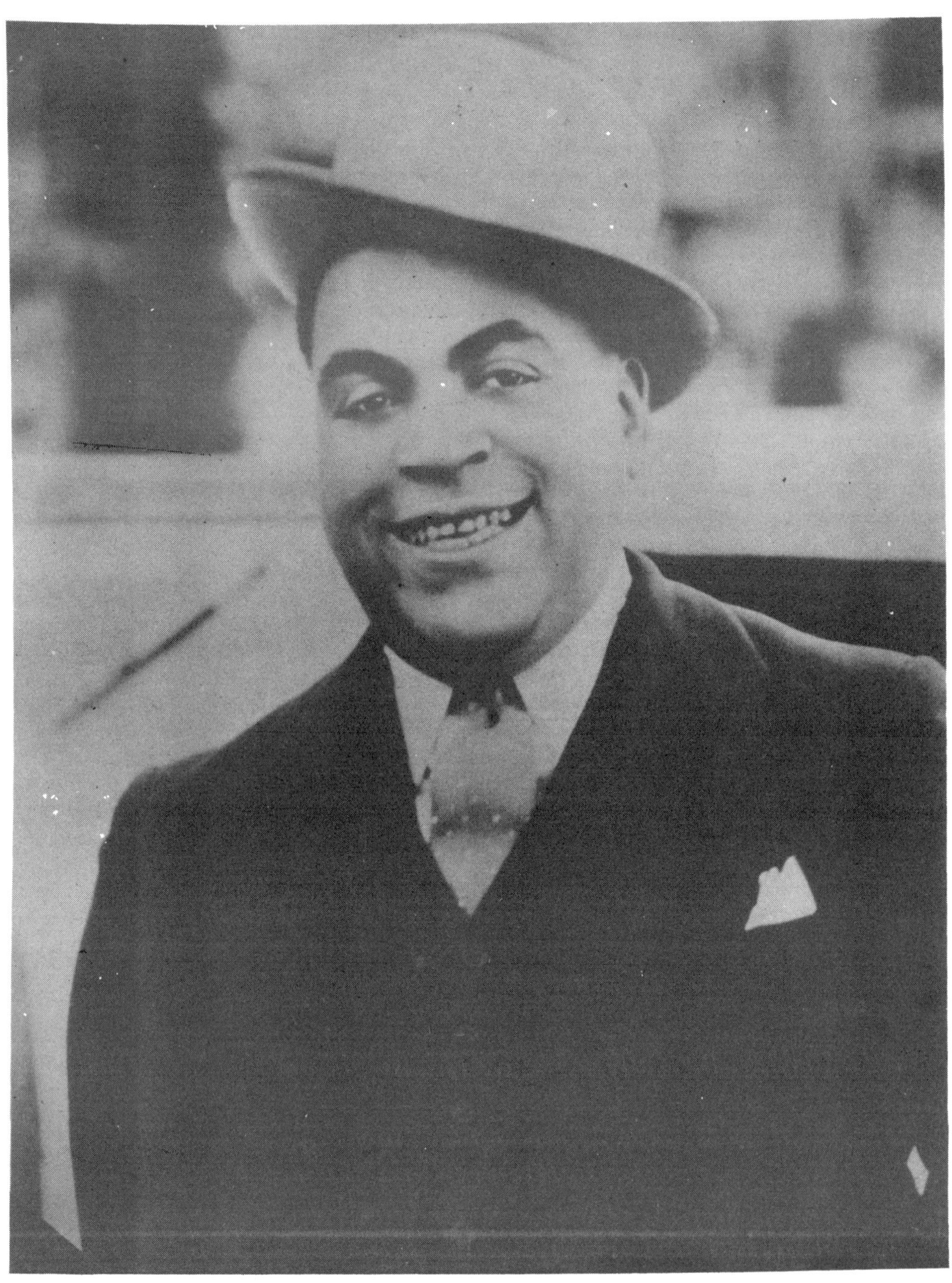

Fats snapped somewhere in the midwest sometime in the 1930's.

"Fats" Waller and his Rhythm Fox Trot **Vocal refrain and piano by "Fats" Waller**

Herman Autrey, t; Rudy Powell, cl-1/as-2; Fats Waller, p/v/cel-3; James Smith, g; Charles Turner, sb; Arnold Boling, d.

Studio 2, New York City, New York — Friday, 29 November 1935

2:30 to 6:30 p.m. W.T. Kirkeby directing.

98172-1*	WHEN SOMEBODY THINKS YOU'RE WONDERFUL -1,-2 (Harry Woods)	Vi 25222-B, HMV B.D.5040, HMVF SG383, HMVSw HE2356, HMVIt HN2996, El EG3683
98172-2	WHEN SOMEBODY THINKS YOU'RE WONDERFUL *-1,-2*	Victor unissued, 'Hold'
98173-1*	I'VE GOT MY FINGERS CROSSED -1,-2 (Ted Koehler-Jimmy McHugh)	Vi/China 25211-A, HMV B.D.5052, HMVEi IM122, HMVAu EA1637, HMVIn NE.286
98174-1*	SPREADIN' RHYTHM AROUND -1,-2 (Ted Koehler-Jimmy McHugh)	Vi/China 25211-B, ViJ DC14, HMVAu EA1637, HMVIn NE.286
98175-1*	A LITTLE BIT INDEPENDENT -2,-3 (Edgar Leslie-Joe Burke)	Vi 25196-A, HMV B.D.5012, HMVAu, EA1631, El EG3702
98176-1*	YOU STAYED AWAY TOO LONG -2 (Whiting-Schwartz-Johnson)	Vi 25222-A, 20-2216-B, *20-2216-B*,
98177-1**	SWEET THING -2 (Young-Baer-Ahlert)	Vi 25196-B, HMVSp AE4606, HMVAU EA1631

Later pressings of HMV BD. 5040 (sic) on the maroon and silver label are retitled as *When Someone...* Both sides of Vi 25211 bear the additional credit **(Feat. in 20th Century-Fox film "King of Burlesque")**, shortened on the Chinese pressing and Indian HMV. The recording sheet abbreviates Fox Trot to FT and has *Note:- Date called for 1:30. Held up by Audivision Recording started at 2:30.* Matrix 98177-1A has a figure 2 typed to the left of the 1A which is then x'd out. Apparently two simultaneous recordings were made of this; the second bearing 98177-2A, but there is the academic possibility that this might be a genuine second take.

It is interesting to note that although 98172 was selected as the 'B' side of the original issue, it went on to become one of Waller's greatest hits.

*****

"Fats" Waller and his Rhythm Foxtrot

Herman Autrey, *C.E. Smith, Eddie Anderson,* t; *Fred Robinson* or *George Wilson,* tb; Rudy Powell, George James, as; Emmett Mathews, ss-1/ts; Gene Sedric, ts; Freddie Skerritt, bar -2; Fats Waller, p/v/3/vib4; Henry Duncan, p; James Smith, g; Charles Turner, sb; Allen 'Yank' Porter, d/vib 5; Band vocal -6.

Studio 2, New York City, New York — Wednesday, 4 December 1935

10:00 a.m. to 1:30 p.m. W.T. Kirkeby directing

98196-1*	FAT AND GREASY -1,-2,-3,-4,-5,-6	Victor unissued, issued on LP
98196-2	FAT AND GREASY -1,-2,-3,-4,-5,-6	Victor unissued, 'Hold', issued on LP

98196: First line of second vocal: -1 "He's got big fat liver lips."
-2 "Ah, he's got a big pair of liver lips."

98197-1*	Functionizin' from Harlem Living Room Suite (Fats Waller, opus 1—3 Gins)	*HMVSw HE 2902, HMVF SG315*
98198-1*	I got Rhythm (Fast) (—) -1,-3	*HMVSw HE 2902, HMVF SG315*
98198-2	I GOT RHYTHM *-1,-3*	Victor unissued, 'Hold'

This was the first recording by Waller's touring band and the Victor clerical staff were clearly

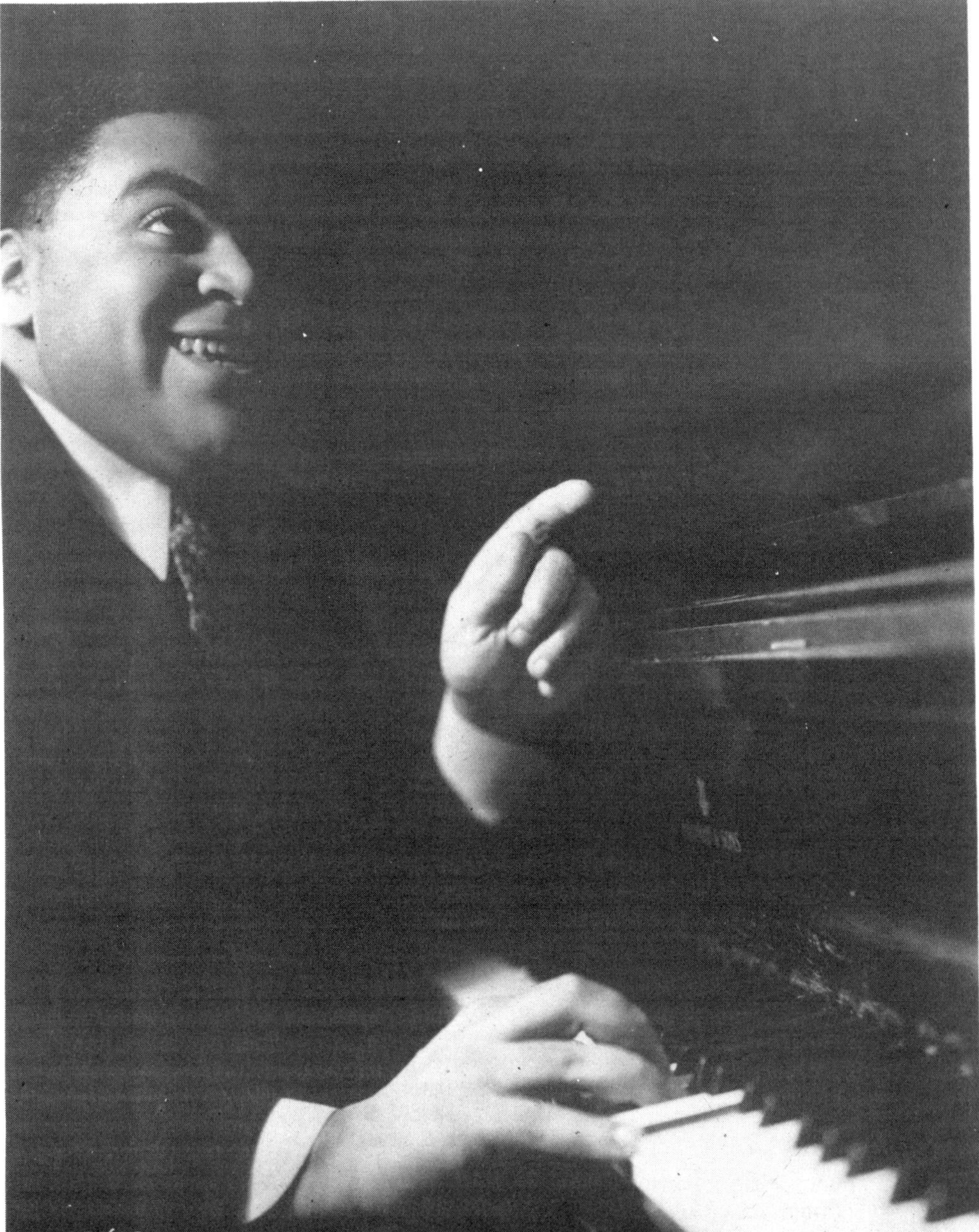

unsure as to how to show them as the recording sheet simply has **FATS WALLER AND** typed in and *his Rhythm* added later in manuscript, which is how the last two sides were issued when they appeared in Europe, despite previous reports to the contrary. The instrumentation given; *5 Saxes - 3 Trumpets - Trombone - Guitar - Str. Bass - 2 pianos - & Trapman,* agrees fairly closely with that quoted in *Jazz Hot* and *Swing Music* and it seems much more likely that the personnel is drawn from that rather than as previously given which is based almost entirely on aural recognition and therefore suspect. Arnold Boling, the band's regular drummer, was beginning to have health problems, which led to a series of temporary and then permanent replacements being used when he was unable to play. However, the report in Ed Kirkeby's book that he died in the late '30s appears to be in error as Johnny Simmen wrote to me in September 1966 that both Doc Cheatham and Herbie Cowans had met and spoken with Boling as recently as that August, but both stated that he had long given up playing. None of the sides achieved release with the United States until the advent of the microgroove.

The recording sheet shows the composer credit for the first title as *Charles Johnson & Porter Grainger*; has a note *NO Vocal (Fats Directing)* against the second. This is also shown as *-Opus 1-3 Gins (From:- Harlem Living Room Suite).*

Fats wrote his *'Harlem Living Room Suite'* in 1935 and it comprised *Functionizin', Corn Whiskey Cocktail* and *Scrimmage.* Only the first of these was published (by Mills Music, New York — the recording sheet shows *Millson's Mus.*) and this item, arranged by Alex Hill, is the only one of the three parts to have been recorded as far as present knowledge allows. *I Got Rhythm* (described as *Fast FT* on the recording sheet), arranged by Don Donaldson, is a shortened version of the routine used by the Waller big band to close their theatre shows.

The *Victor Master Book, Vol.2* notes that no trombone was used on the first title, although there is nothing on the recording sheet to indicate so.

98198-1 on HMVSw HE 2902 has the additional credit **Vocal by "Fats" Waller.**

*****

Following the release of *I Got Rhythm* on the Victor 'Vintage' series, Bob Kumm contacted Hank Duncan for his recollections of the piece:

> *Oh, we used that as the closing of the bill on our theatre tours,* Hank Duncan recalled, *I'd be at the keyboard for the opening of the show, where we'd usually begin with two or three fast instrumentals, Then Fats would come out and do one or two of his currently popular numbers, before settling into the groove for some of the 'standard items' from his repertoire.*

Duncan's use of the words 'standard items' caused him to chuckle, and he continued:

> *Fats himself probably never considered anything to be standard, he was always improvisin' on the lyric to nearly everything he sang, with an almost endless variety of verbal 'illuminations'. The guys in the band were never distracted by Fats's unpredictability, instead he was a constant source of inspiration to everyone who worked with him. I think that it might have been at the Grand Theatre in Philadelphia where we first expanded the 'I Got Rhythm' arrangement to include the piano cutting contest ... the number just sort of grew into a freewheeling bit of improvisation, with a lot of solo spots for the guys in the band and the two piano thing with Fats and I as the finale. It eventually ran for nine or ten minutes, and frequently inspired the audience to respond with a standing ovation, I think that the standing ovations were the primary factor in Fats's decision to use*

the number to close the show.

*****

A tape is in circulation among collectors (source unknown) which is believed to date from around this time as follows:

Fats Waller, p
Unknown location — probably late 1935 or early 1936

Here 'Tis
Humpty Dumpty

*****

Before leaving 1935, it should be noted that *Who's Who Of Jazz* shows trombonist Snub Mosley with Waller in 1935. When I interviewed him, he made no mention of having worked with Fats this early and placed his stay with Waller as coming after his period in the Luis Russell band, fronted by Louis Armstrong, and a short period with Fletcher Henderson when Chu Berry was in the band which seems to place it as in the autumn of 1937. This information is also repeated in *The World Of Count Basie,* and the appropriate quotation will be found at the approximately correct chronological point.

*****

The Apollo Theatre advert in the *New York Age* for 4 January 1936 shows 'Fats' Waller, described as 'Composer, Humorist, Musician and All-Around Star' heading the stage presentation with Charlie Turner's Arcadians and Emmett Mathews and a supporting cast for the week commencing Friday, 3 January.

The revue of the show in the paper of the following week includes:

> *..."Fats" Waller is the central attraction and Turner's Arcadians with Emmett Mathews ... Six shows were given Sunday, unprecedented in the history of the Apollo. ... In his dressing room, "Fats" confides he is on the water wagon, a New Year's resolution, but six months ago he started confining his libations to sherry.*

*****

"Fats" Waller and his Rhythm -Fox Trot — Vocal refrain and piano by "Fats" Waller

Herman Autrey, t; Gene Sedric, cl-1/ts-2; Fats Waller, p/v/cel-3/vb-4; James Smith, g; Charles Turner, sb; Yank Porter, d.

Studio 2, New York City, New York — Saturday, 1 February 1936
12:00 a.m. to 6:30 p.m. Mr. Kirkeby directing

98894-1	THE PANIC IS ON -1,-3 (G. & B. Clarke-W. Tharp)	Vi 25266-A
98894-2	THE PANIC IS ON *-1,-3*	Victor unissued, 'Hold'
98895-1*	SUGAR ROSE -1,-3 (Phil Ponce-"Fats" Waller)	Vi 25266-B, HMV B.D.5062, B.9885, HMVEx J.O.133, HMVEi IM133, HMVSw HE2813, HMVIn N14052, HMVIt GW1282, HN2763, El EG7622
98896-1*	OOOH! LOOK-A THERE, AIN'T SHE PRETTY? -1,-3 (Clarence Todd-Carmen Lombardo)	Vi 25255-B, 20-2218-A, HMVAu EA1722
98896-2	Oooh! LOOKA-THERE, AIN'T SHE PRETTY *-1,-3*	Victor unissued, 'Hold'
98897-1*	MOON ROSE -1,-2 (Fred Rose-Fred Fisher)	Vi 25281-A, HMVAu EA1704

98898-1*	WEST WIND -1,-2 (Ager-Newman-Mencher)	Vi/Ar 25253-A, HMV B.D.5052, HMVEi IM122, HMVAu EA1677, El EG3680
99034-1*	THAT NEVER-TO-BE FORGOTTEN NIGHT -2 (Charlie Tobias-Sammy Fain)	Vi 25255-A, HMV B.D.5062, HMVEi IM133, HMVAu EA1722, HMVIt GW1282
99035-1*	SING AN OLD FASHIONED SONG (To A Young Sophisticated Lady) -2 (Joe Young-Fred E. Ahlert)	Vi/Ar 25253-B, HMV B.D.5135, HMVAu EA 1677
99036-1*	GARBO GREEN -1 (Fred Fisher)	Vi 25281-B, HMVAu EA1704

98894-2 is originally typed as -1A, the 1 then has a 2 typed over it with a 2 added to the right. There is a discrepancy over the matrix for *That Never-To-Be-Forgotten Night.* The recording sheet (as shown here) gives it as 99034-1 and -1A; the *Victor Master Book, Vol 2,* and *Jazz Records* show it as 98899-1, which is entirely logical, as this would mark the end of a matrix block. This latter number also appears on the label of the HMV B.D. issue and is also stamped in the wax. Horst Lange gives the Electrola issue number shown above for matrix 98898-1, but *Jazz Records* shows it as EG 3660, but this latter is almost certainly incorrect.

The recording sheet notes after the session times *(Started recording At 2:00 P.M.)* but offers no explanation for the delay.

HMV B.D.5135 omits the sub-title.

*****

Fats Waller

Fats Waller, p/v.

Radio Broadcast, Station WHIS Bluefield, W. Virginia — Sunday, 2 February 1936

I'm Crazy 'Bout My Baby	Issued on LP
Truckin'	Issued on LP

Station WHIS in Bluefield, W. Virginia, is now a centre for 'Country and Western' music, but in 1936 appears to have included other styles in its transmissions. Waller would hardly have travelled this considerable distance between the termination of his record session the previous evening for a single broadcast and, given his normal life style as recounted by Ernie Anderson elsewhere in this volume, it seems more likely that this broadcast was from a pre-recorded acetate than a 'live' transmission. If this is so, then the disc would have almost certainly been used in transmissions from other stations around this time. Alternatively, the broadcast has been incorrectly dated, and possibly took place during the tour noted below.

Waller and his orchestra were booked to play in West Virginia in the first week of February according to a report in the *Pittsburgh Courier* of 18 January. After the usual blurbs, the report went on to say that Waller was recently returned from the Pacific Coast where he'd taken a role in 'King Of Burlesque' and that he'd been booked by George Morton of Beckley, West Virginia to play four dates: *Parkersburg on the fifth; Logan on the sixth; Welch the 7th and Charleston the eighth.* In the same paper the following week this was further enlarged and somewhat changed and the engagements were now given as Market Auditorium, Wheeling, 5 February; the Armory, Logan on 6 February; Bluefield on 7 February and in the Armory, Charleston on 8 February. The orchestra was noted to be 14 pieces.

The week after that, in the issue of 1 February, there was a much longer piece, parts of which are interesting:

... will leave Broadway on Wednesday of next week ... Waller, who croons, has

composed five national musical hits, plays the violin with dexterity and can play the piano upside down, is a comedian of the first rank. He has made Q-R-S roles (sic) *... played in leading nite clubs of America, England, Paris and Austria, including the Kit Kat Club of London and Moulin Rouge in Paris ... he studied under Godowsky of Vienna and Carl Bohn of New York ... Fats is to specialize in "Trucking" ... The trumpet section of his band is to pantomime "The Music Goes Round And Round" while Fats is to direct the comical section of this sensational musical hit, ... is to play "How Jazz Was Born", "I Got A Feeling I'm Falling", "My Fate Is In Your Hands" and "Honeysuckle Rose" and "I'm Gonna Sit Right Down And Write Myself A Letter' ...*

The report goes on to say that Waller travels with his own amplifying equipment, then a relatively new arrangement, and confirms the dates given the previous week except that the Bluefield engagement is now shown to be in the City Auditorium. Performances were to start at 9:30 p.m. except for that at Charleston which was to start about an hour earlier, and continue until 1:00 a.m. Note that much of this 'Press Release' — for it was clearly that, was still in use at the time of Waller's next visit to Europe.

The *Pittsburgh Courier* of 11 January had reported that Waller was to play St. Louis on Valentine nite (sic) (14 February), and the issue of 8 February said he was booked into the Forest Club, Detroit on 17 February (said to be his second visit to the city).

*****

In 1936 a controversy arose over the amounts of royalties collected by ASCAP for 'serious' music as opposed to 'popular' music, and the estate of John Philip Sousa took the matter to Congress. The *New York World-Telegram* sought the opinion of a 'popular' composer and, in an article published on 6 March quoted Fats Waller at length. As background, it mentioned that: *Recently he has been playing one-night stands, but his "acid condition" forced him to return to Harlem three weeks ago. Tonight he is leaving for Washington, where he will play in a theatre ...* From this report it may be that Waller's tour after the 1 February Victor date above, was cut short and he developed home sickness earlier than usual — "acid-condition" being one of his standard excuses for getting back home in a hurry. It would also seem that he played a Washington theatre around the beginning of March, but it is not known whether the engagements listed above were honoured before his 'acid condition' sent him hurrying back to Harlem.

*****

The *International Musician* of March 1936 has a report from Local 9, Boston listing Thomas Waller. Because of the layout used, it is not clear whether he was appearing as a 'single' or fronting the band which follows, the names for which are given (all sic) as: Philip Ferguson (Baron Lee); A.S. Harris; Trenton Harris; Reuben Reeves; Frederick Pedro; E.R. Reynolds; Herbert Cowans; Wendell Scoggins; Nesor Acevdo; Herbert Thomas; Leo Mosley (all 802); Henry Thompson (496); Scoville Brown (208); Gerald Reeves (208); Milton Fletcher (627). Either way, this may have been a 'one-off' engagement, for the same issue of the paper also gives the personnel of a recognisable Waller band from Local 308, Binghampton, New York. Apart from Waller himself, the others are named as: Herman Autrey; Al Washington; George James; Emmett Mathews; Edward S. Powell; James S. Smith; Clarence E. Smith; Eduard Orrell Anderson; Henry J. Duncan; Alan H. Porter; Fred L. Robinson (all 802). The same band minus James S. Smith, but adding Eugene P. Sedric, Eugene Fields and Charles M. Turner (all 802) are also listed by Local 471, Pittsburgh. The April issue of the paper then shows these same 14 musicians listed by Sub 2 St. Louis Local and Indianapolis, Local 3. Note that both combinations of names here produce a rather unusual line-up. 'Edward S. Powell' is almost certainly Rudy Powell and his name seems to have caused considerable problems in the paper, with something like half a dozen variant spellings over the next six months. Likewise, Eduard Orrell Anderson (4 variants noted) is amost certainly Edward 'Andy' Anderson.

*****

Rather surprisingly, following the coverage given to the filming of *'Hooray For Love'*, the *New York Age* made no mention of Waller and his second film, and the first mention of *'King Of Burlesque'* is in an advert for the Roosevelt Theatre on Seventh Avenue at 145th Street where it was screened from 28 February until 2 March. Later, when Waller's impact in the film had become more apparent, he began to receive top billing over the principals as in the advert for the Regal Theatre of 28 March 1936 in Chicago shown here. Victor too seized upon the potential offered by this exposure of Fats, took one of the film's publicity shots (shown on page 116); added a facsimile Waller signature and the words "Exclusive Victor Recording Artist" at the foot, and distributed it widely.

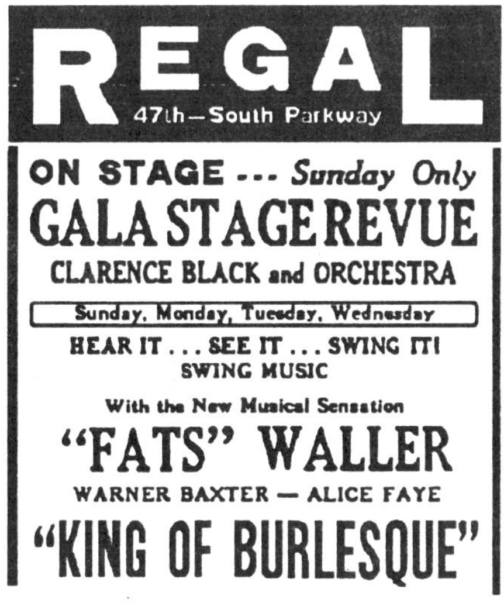

*****

A 'filler' in the *Pittsburgh Courier* of 21 March 1936 has, *Strange as it seems, the good Mr "Fats" Waller, eloquent master of swing music, once shared an organ loft in Belgium with a gifted disciple of the late Cesar Franck, well known composer of serious works.*

*****

Datelined New York City, 2 April, the *Pittsburgh Courier* of 4 April has a report of an engagement on Broadway for Waller and news of forthcoming events:

> *Broadway has been sizzling during the past week with some super torrid syncopation and modern swing music as done by "Fats" Waller and Miss Maud Russell, who topped the bill at Loew's State theatre ... Miss Russell ... was forced to take three and four curtain calls*

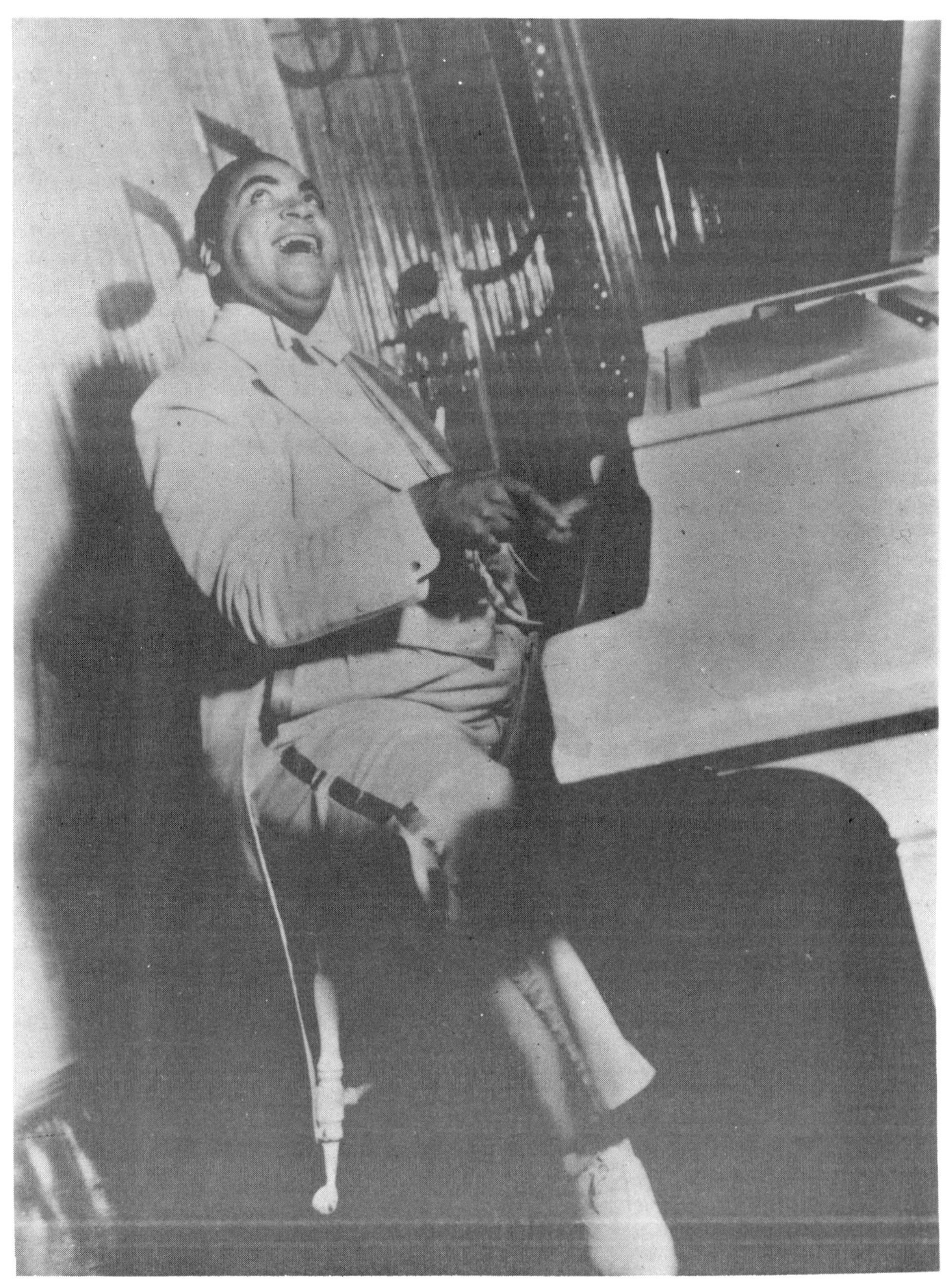

Two publicity shots for 'King Of Burlesque'

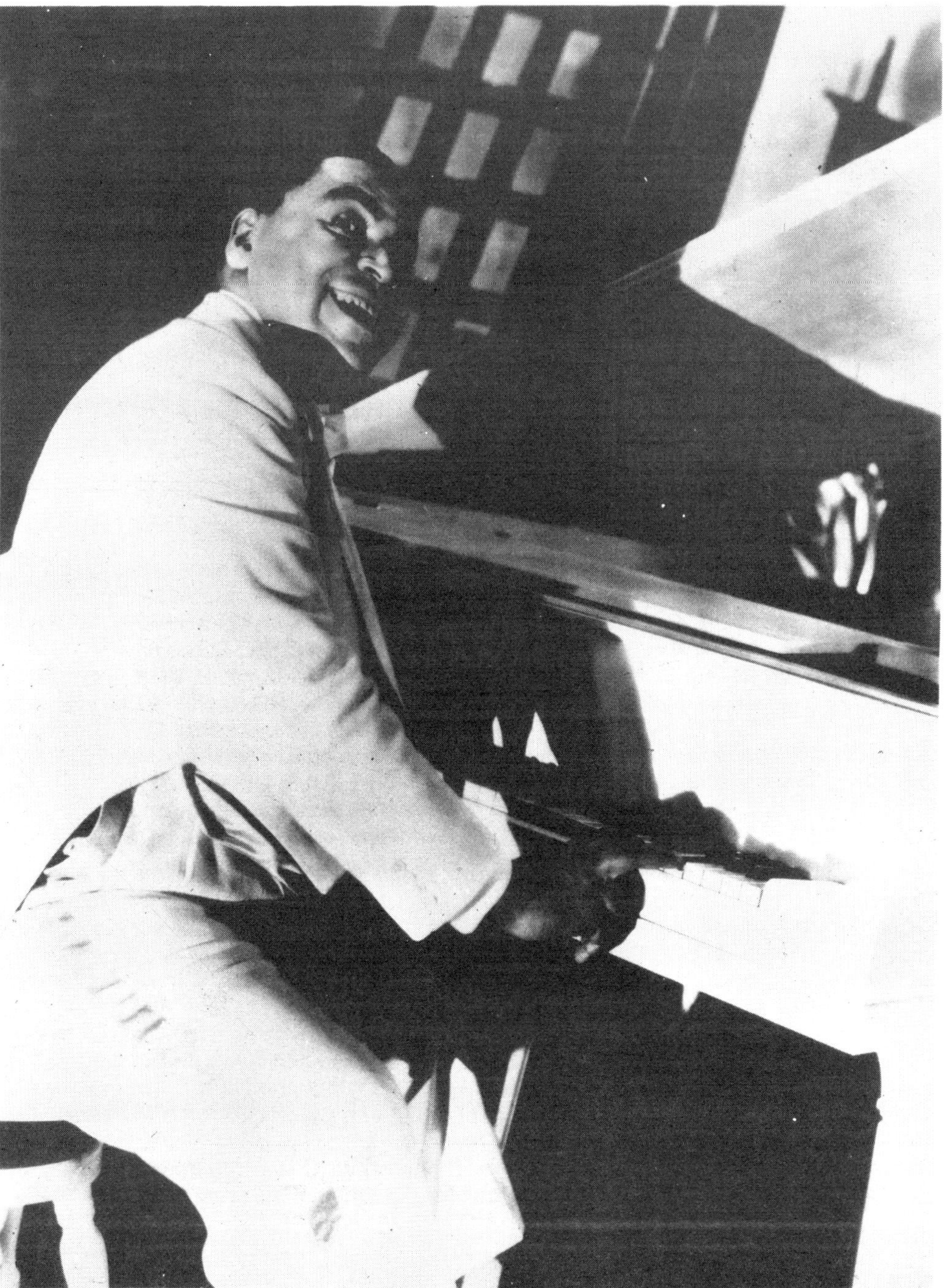

... stopped the show with a "Fats" Waller arrangement of ... "Give A Little Bit — Take A Little Bit". ... Waller featuring "Sugar Rose" ... Following a series of dance dates beginning this Sunday night (ie. 5 April) *which are slated to last about 10 days, Sir Waller, Miss Russell and the orchestra, will resume their delux theatre presentation at the Fox Detroit, on April 17.*

The dance dates were presumably in the New York area and the following recording session was made before leaving on tour again.

*****

"Fats" Waller and his Rhythm -Fox Trot **Vocal refrain and piano by "Fats" Waller**

Herman Autrey, t; Gene Sedric, cl-1/ts-2; Fats Waller, p/v/cel-3; Al Casey, g; Charles Turner, sb; Yank Porter, d, Elizabeth Handy, v-4.

Studio 2, New York City, New York — Wednesday, 8 April 1936

1:30 to 5:15 p.m. E. Kirkeby directing

Matrix	Title	Issues
101189-1*	ALL MY LIFE -1 (Sidney Mitchell-Sam H. Stept)	Vi 25296-A, HMV B.D.5077, HMVEi IM144, HMVAu EA1726, HMVSp GY487
101190-1*	CHRISTOPHER COLUMBUS (A Rhythm Cocktail) -2 (Andy Razaf-Leon Berry)	Vi 25295-B, ViJ JA-1086-B, HMVAu E.A.1744, El EG3682
101190-2	CHRISTOPHER COLUMBUS (A Rhythm Cocktail) -2	Victor unissued, 'Hold'
101191-1*	"CROSS PATCH" -1 (Tot Seymour-Vee Lawnhurst)	Vi 25315-A, HMV B.D.5098, AX4029, HMVAu EA1729, El EG3690
101192-1*	IT'S NO FUN -1 (Newman-Mencher-Ager)	Vi 25296-B, ViJ JA-749-A, HMV B.D.5087, HMVAu EA 1726, El EG3718
101193-1*	CABIN IN THE SKY -2,-3 (Edgar Leslie-Joe Burke)	Vi 25315-B, ViJ JA-749-B, HMV B.D.5077, HMVEi IM144, HMVSp GY897 (see note), HMVAu EA1729, El EG3690
101194-1*	US ON A BUS -1 (Todd Seymour-Vee Lawnhurst)	Vi 25295-A, ViJ JA-1086-A, HMVEx JO.123, HMVAu E.A.1744, El EG3682
101195-1	STAY -2,-4	Victor test recording, issued on LP
101195-2	STAY -2,-4	Victor test recording, unissued

Unusually, the recording sheet gives the names of the participants and, despite *Jazz Records*, the Trapman (Victor's normal term for a drummer) is shown as Allen H. Porter. The matrix number for the final title is that quoted by Victor (it does not appear on the recording sheet), but the test of take -1 actually bears the number T-24081, indicating that it was a test recording not intended for issue. The date typed at the head of the recording sheet is April 7, 1936, but this is altered manually to read April 8.

HMV AX4029 is listed in deference to *Jazz Records*, although nothing is known of it by anyone connected with this project, nor are any other issues bearing this prefix. The Spanish issue of 101193 has been variously given as GY497, GY487 and GY897. Only the last of these has been inspected. 101189 on HMV B.D.5077 bears the additional credit **(From the Film: "Laughing Irish Eyes")**. Vi 25295-A bears the additional credit **(From the musical production "Summer Wives")**, and this is shortened to **(From "Summer Wives")** on E.A.1744. Vi 25296-A has **(From the Republic film "Laughing Irish Eyes")**.

*****

The Waller stage show was presumably on tour between these two recording dates, but the only indication of this is the mention of the Detroit date on 17 April noted earlier. Waller may have returned to Detroit very soon after that for a note in the *Pittsburgh Courier* of 9 May, datelined Detroit, May 7 says, *Fats Waller will be honoured at the Celebrity Dance at the Black Cat the yawning* (sic) *of the 12th.*

*****

Two further reports from the *International Musicians* should be considered at this point. Both are in the June 1936 issue as 'for May' (i.e. probably late April dates) and are from Local 269, Harrisburg and Local 550, Cleveland. Fats Waller is noted for the first only, but otherwise the same 13 musicians are given: Charles M. Turner; Herman Autrey; Al Washington; George James; Emmett Mathews; Everett (Rudy?) Powell; Clarence E. Smith; Edward Anderson; Henry J. Duncan; Allen H. Porter; Fred L. Robinson; Eugene P. Sedric; Eugene Fields.

Also in the same issue (but probably relating to early May engagements) are reports from Local 40, Baltimore and Local 471, Pittsburgh. These too list the same musicians noted above with Waller present on the first, but absent on the second. Additionally, George Wilson is added for both dates and Paul Girland (a name unknown to me, but he may have been a guitarist) for the first.

*****

Fats Waller and his Rhythm

Herman Autrey, t; Gene Sedric, cl-1/ts-2; Fats Waller, p/v; Al Casey, g; Charles Turner, sb; Yank Porter, d.

Broadcast, 'Magic Key of Radio' from RCA studios, New York City, New York

Sunday, 24 May 1936

I'm Gonna Sit Right Down And Write Myself A Letter -1	Issued on LP
Christopher Columbus -2	Issued on LP

Waller's vocals on the above include spoken comments and interjections.

*****

The Apollo advert in the *New York Age* of 30 May 1936 shows "Fats" Waller with Turner's Arcadians with Emmett Mathews for the week beginning Friday, 5 June. However, the date in the advert is in error and should read 29 May. The advance editorial announcement in the same issue makes this clear and also mentions that: *Last Sunday he was the star of NBC's International broadcast — the ace hour of radio broadcasting. Some of the world's most famous stars appeared on the same program and it was the general consensus that Fats Waller dominated all.* The paper's radio reviewer thought similarly and said: *Fats Waller and Turner's Arcadians really put on their act during that Philly Theatre show. (WIP 10:30 p.m.)* The same words are used for both Saturday and Sunday — obviously a typesetting error.

The review by Joe Bostic the following week under his heading 'Seeing The Show' makes one wonder whether he did, for, after eulogising Waller and ending: *...doing his bit, which is quite a lot, in the best Waller tradition.* He continues, *Next in line comes the rousing rhythms and high scoring individual performers in Turner's Arcadians. Reading from left to right of course is ace rhythmaster and songster Emmett Mathews who all but broke up the Monday dinner show; then Hank Duncan who must have been born with a golden clarinet in his mouth; and last Al Washington, a piano playing fool from way back. ...* And so it goes on!

*****

Fats Waller and his Rhythm

Unknown personnel, possibly drawn from Waller's big band and certainly including Gene Sedric, cl-1/ts-2; Fats Waller, p/v/p solo-3

Broadcast, 'The Fleischmann Hour', NBC Studios, New York City, New York
Station WEAF 8:00 p.m. Thursday, 4 June 1936

I've Got My Fingers Crossed -1	Issued on LP
Honeysuckle Rose -3	Issued on LP
Chistopher Columbus -1,-2	Issued on LP

The 'Fleischmann Hour', hosted by Rudy Vallee, was broadcast every Thursday over almost ten years, and it became so closely associated with him that it is usually known incorrectly to enthusiasts as the 'Rudy Vallee Show'. Almost everyone who was anyone in the various aspects of show business appeared on it at some time. Waller's appearance, which was on the final day of his week at the Apollo, seems to have been a riotous occasion from the fragments that have survived and his 'vocals' include the usual spoken ad libs and encouragements.

The broadcast was noted in the *New York Age* which commented that Waller would *continue to play dance engagements until the first of August when he would take a much needed rest.* This was repeated almost word for word in the *Pittsburgh Courier.*

Waller had apparently also broadcast on the Wednesday evening over Station WMCA at 11:00 p.m. in the 'Amateur Night In Harlem' program. The same paper's radio reviewer said that, *Fats Waller after a dismal performance on the amateur show the previous night* ... and went on to praise him highly for his perfomance on the Rudy Vallee show.

*****

"Fats" Waller and his Rhythm -Fox Trot **Vocal refrain and piano by "Fats" Waller**

Herman Autrey, t; Gene Sedric, cl-1/ts-2; Fats Waller, p/v/cel-3; Al Casey, g; Charles Turner, sb; Yank Porter, d, band vocal -4.

Studio No.2, New York City, New York Friday, 5 June 1936
2:00 to 7:00 p.m. L. Joy directing

101667-1	IT'S A SIN TO TELL A LIE -1 (Billy Mayhew)	Vi 25342-A, *20-1595-B*, *42-0037-B*, ViJ A1230, JA-769-A, HMV B.D.5087, HMVEx J.O.205, HMVSc X7475, HMVAu E.A.1773, El EG3718, *V-D 359B*
101667-2*	IT'S A SIN TO TELL A LIE *-1*	Victor unissued, 'Hold'
101668-1	THE MORE I KNOW YOU (The More I Love You) -2 (Benny Davis-J.Fred Coots)	Vi 25348-B, ViJ JA-851-B, HMV B.D.5159
101668-2*	THE MORE I KNOW YOU (The More I Love You) *-2*	Victor unissued, 'Hold'
101669-1**	YOU'RE NOT THE KIND -2,-3 (Will Hudson-Irving Mills)	Vi 25353-A, ViJ JA-785-A, HMV B.D.5115, HMVSc AL2307, HMVAu EA1779, El EG3767
101670-1	WHY DO I LIE TO MYSELF ABOUT YOU? -1 (Benny Davis-J. Fred Coots)	Vi 25353-B, ViJ JA-785-B, HMV B.D.5150, HMVIt GW1390, *HMVSw HE2360*, HMVAu EA1779,
101670-2*	WHY DO I LIE TO MYSELF ABOUT YOU? *-1*	Victor unissued, 'Hold'

101671-1 LET'S SING AGAIN -1,-4 (Gus Kahn-Jimmy McHugh) — Vi 25348-A, ViJ JA-851-A, HMV B.D.5098, HMVIt GW1345
101671-2* LET'S SING AGAIN *-1,-4* — Victor unissued, 'Process'
101672-1 BIG CHIEF DE SOTA -2 (Andy Razaf-Fernando Arbelo) — Vi 25342-B, ViJ A1230, JA-769-B, HMVAu E.A.1773
101672-2* BIG CHIEF DE SOTA *-2* — Victor unissued, 'Hold'

Once again the recording sheet helpfully names the personnel and also (and most unusually) has a note *Date called for 2:00 (Orchestra were here 1:00) to 7:00P.M.* — one of the few occasions when Fats was not just on time, but actually early for an engagement! For matrix 10169 -1, -1A and -2A are given, but in the absence of a matrix 10169-2, the take -2A presumably indicates that three turntables were in use for this title.

Vi 25348-A and the B.D. issue bear the additional credit **(From the RKO Radio film "Let's Sing Again")**. Reverse of Italian HMV GW 1345 is *Nobody Sweetheart* by **Trio Benny Goodman.**

*****

"Fats" Waller and his Rhythm -Fox Trot **Vocal refrain and piano by "Fats" Waller**

Herman Autrey, t; Gene Sedric, cl-1/ts-2; Fats Waller, p/v; Al Casey, g; Charles Turner, sb; Yank Porter, d.

Studio No. 3, New York City, New York — Monday, 8 June 1936
9:30 a.m. to 1:45 p.m. L. Joy directing

102016-1* BLACK RASPBERRY JAM -1,-2 (Thomas Waller) — Vi 25359-A, ViJ JA-801-A, HMV B.D.5376, ASR LB5376
102016-2 BLACK RASPBERRY JAM -1,-2 — Victor unissued, 'Process', issued on LP

102016: Intro: -1 "I've got mine, mine's black raspberry. Look out here 'tis."
-2 "I've got my jam. Look out, here 'tis, I'm throwing it at you."
Coda: -1 "Take your finger out of my jam."
-2 "Diga, Diga, jam."

102017-1* BACH UP TO ME -2 (Thomas Waller) — Vi 25536-B, HMV B.D.5225, HMVIt GW1597, *HMVSw HE2368*
102017-2 (BACH) UP TO ME *-2* — Victor unissued, 'Hold'
102018-1* FRACTIOUS FINGERING -1 (Thomas Waller) — Vi 25656-B, 25652-B, HMVSc X6014
102019-1* PASWONKY -2 (Thomas Waller) — Vi 25359-B, ViJ JA-801-B, HMV/In B.D.5354, HMVF SG92, K8227, HMVSw HE2345, El EG6383
102020-1* LOUNGING AT THE WALDORF -1 (Thomas Waller) — Vi 25430-B, HMVF SG92, K8227
102021-1* LATCH ON -2 (Thomas Waller) — Vi 25471-B, ViJ JA-869-B

Once again the personnel is given on the recording sheet, but note the change of studio. This session is unique in that all six titles are Waller compositions. Waller's vocal contributions are more in the nature of ad lib commentaries than vocals in the accepted sense and the recording sheet bears a number of handwritten comments such as "just jabbered a few phrases" after the first title and "They all have gibberish" at the bottom. This has provided headaches to the issuing companies around the world in that some have decided a title is 'vocal', whilst others are quite happy to label the same item as 'non-vocal'.

Matrix 012018 quoted on HMVSc X6014 is in error. *Jazz Records* also shows 102019-1 as issued on HMVSw JK2345, but a Swiss HMV catalogue held here shows only the HE prefixed issue. Vi 25652 bears a different performance credit: **"Fats" Waller at the piano**, and The reverse of this issue is *The Big Apple* by **Tommy Dorsey & his Clambake Seven**. Although Waller's voice is heard on Vi 25536-B, the performance credit is simply **Piano by "Fats" Waller**.

*****

Between this session and the next, the big band obviously went out on tour. The only firm engagement traced is that given in the Chicago *Defender* of 4 July 1936 which has a report of the Fats Waller Orchestra at the 8th Regiment Armory, 'last week' with a personnel of *Charles Turner, Henry E. Duncan, E. Fields, Allen Porter, Al Washington, E. Sedric, George James, E. Mathews, Ed Powell, Ed Anderson, C.E. Smith, H Autrey, George Wilson, Fred Robinson and Thomas Waller.*

From Chicago they must have headed south for the *Pittsburgh Courier* of 18 July has an interesting report datelined Little Rock, Ark. July 16:

> *Paying a ten per cent federal tax, a two per cent State tax, and a three per cent tax to the white musicians' union was all right, but paying another $98 to the union for an "unseen orchestra" was too much. So 300 white persons who had gathered at Cinderella garden in Fair Park Wednesday night* (15 July) *did not hear Fats Waller and his celebrated orchestra.*
>
> *According to James Bryant, manager of the piano star, a union representative at the last minute demanded that Bryant pay for a "stand-in" orchestra at $7 a man for every man in Fats' band of 14 musicians. This stand-in orchestra, of course, does not play and serves merely to salve union members. Bryant declared he had never before been required to pay for a stand-in band on a one night stand and the deal was off. He and Fats Waller and his orchestra pack up their instruments and march away as the 300 whites arrive wondering why there was no dance.*

Another possible engagement was in Kansas City for, in his autobiography, Count Basie recalls that at some unspecified time before he left the Reno Club (i.e. before the end of 1936) Fats Waller came in one night and was crazy about the Basie band, and returned every night while he was in town to hear them. It may have been from a little earlier, but either way Basie errs in recalling that Kirkeby was Waller's personal manager at the time, as Kirkeby didn't take over until Ponce retired somewhar later. However, it would appear from Basie's account that it was with the big band rather than the rhythm that Fats was on tour.

Additional clues are provided by four reports in the August 1936 *International Musician*. They are from Sub Local 2, St. Louis; Local 38, Richmond, Virginia; Local 71, Memphis, and Local 627, Kansas City. The names quoted in the *Defender* report of 4 July (above) are confirmed except that Emmett Mathews is present only in the Richmond report where Eugene Fields is absent. Note that the *Defender* lists 'Ed Powell', but that the reports here list him as Everett, except for that from Memphis where he becomes 'Rudolph', hence the supposition that all these reports refer to the same man.

*****

"Fats" Waller and his Rhythm -Fox Trot **Vocal refrain and piano by "Fats" Waller**
Herman Autrey, t; Gene Sedric, cl-1/ts-2; Fats Waller, p/v; Al Casey, g; Charles Turner, sb; Slick Jones, d.

Studio No 2, New York City, New York — Saturday, 1 August 1936
9:45 a.m. to 1:45 p.m. L. Joy directing

102400-1	I'M CRAZY 'BOUT MY BABY (And My Baby's Crazy 'Bout Me) -1 (Alexander Hill-Thomas Waller)	Vi 25374-B, HMV B.D.5120, HMVIt GW1343
102400-2	I'M CRAZY 'BOUT MY BABY (And My Baby's Crazy 'Bout Me) *-1*	Victor unissued, 'Hold'
102401-1*	I JUST MADE UP WITH THAT OLD GIRL OF MINE -1 (Little-Pease-McConnell)	Vi 25394-B, HMV B.D.5159
102401-1	I JUST MADE UP WITH THAT OLD GIRL OF MINE -1	Victor unissued, 'Process'
102402-1*	UNTIL THE REAL THING COMES ALONG -2 (CAHN-CHAPLIN-FREEMAN)	Vi 25374-A, *20-2640-A*, ViJ JA-791-A, HMV B.D.5115, HMVSc AL2307, El EG3767
102402-2	(IT WILL HAVE TO DO) UNTIL THE REAL THING COMES ALONG *-2*	Victor unissued, 'Process'
102403-1*	THERE GOES MY ATTRACTION -1,-2 (Neiburg-Levinson-Bunch)	Vi 25388-B, HMV B.D.5120, HMVF K-7779, HMVIt GW1343, ASR LB5120
102403-2	THERE GOES MY ATTRACTION *-1,-2*	Victor unissued, 'Hold'
102404-1*	THE CURSE OF AN ACHING HEART -1 (Henry Fink-Al. Piantadosi)	Vi 25394-A, HMV B.D.5116, HMVAu EA1791, ASR LB5116
102404-2	THE CURSE OF AN ACHING HEART -1	Victor unissued, 'Hold', issued on LP

102404: Last line of patter prior to vocal proper -1 "I got to tell you something. Yeah! Here 'tis..."
-2 "I got to tell you this. Look here, here 'tis..."

102405-1*	BYE BYE, BABY -2 (Walter Hirsch-Lou Handman)	Vi 25388-A, HMV B.D.5116, HMVAu EA1791, HMVF K-7779, ASR LB5116

The title for 102402 is shown on the recording sheet all three times as for -2. The sub-title for 102400-1 is omitted on HMV B.D.5120. Band credit on HMVF K-7779 is to **FATS WALLER et son Orchestre avec Refrain vocal**. Matrix 102400-1 is also rumoured to appear on Japanese Victor JA791. However, this issue is not included on the check list of Japanese issues sent by Yusaku Sugiyama, and is thus not shown above.

*****

Fats Waller and his Rhythm
Herman Autrey, t; Gene Sedric, cl-1/ts-2; Fats Waller, p/v; Al Casey, g; Charles Turner, sb; Arnold Boling, d.

Broadcast, 'Magic Key of Radio' from RCA studios, New York City, New York
Sunday, 9 August 1936

It's A Sin To Tell A Lie -1	Issued on LP
Until The Real Thing Comes Along -2	Issued on LP
I'm Crazy 'Bout My Baby -2	Issued on LP

This is 'Scrippie' Boling's last recorded appearance with Fats Waller and his Rhythm. His declining health deteriorated to the point where he had to hand over to 'Slick' Jones on a permanent basis. As usual, on such occasions, Waller's vocals are a mixture of spoken comment and singing. Audience applause is heard after each selection, but this does not necessarily mean the performance was before a live audience.

*****

Two further reports in the September *International Musician* of September 1936 suggest that the big band was on the road again in the last half of August. These come from Local 3, Indianapolis and Local 23, San Antonio. Names listed are: Fats Waller; Charles Turner; Herman Autrey; Al Washington; George James; Edw. (Rudy?) Powell; Clarence Smith; Edward Anderson; Henry Duncan; Allen Porter; Fred Robinson; Eugene Sedric and George Wilson. Paul Girlando (slight variation in spelling) reappears in Indianapolis, but is replaced by Eugene Fields in San Antonio.

*****

"Fats" Waller and his Rhythm -Fox Trot **Vocal refrain and piano by "Fats" Waller**
Herman Autrey, t; Gene Sedric, cl-1/ts-2; Fats Waller, p/v; Al Casey, g; Charles Turner, sb; Slick Jones, d.

Studio No 2, New York City, New York — Wednesday, 9 September 1936
1:30 to 5:00 p.m. L. Joy directing

0339-1*	S'POSIN' -1,-2 (Andy Razaf-Paul Denniker)	Vi 25415-B, 20-2220-A, BB B-10156-A, HMV B.D.5135
0340-1	COPPER COLORED GAL -1 (Benny Davis-J. Fred Coots)	Vi 25409-A, ViJ JA-823-A, HMV B.D.5133
0340-21A	COPPER COLORED GAL -1	Victor unissued, "Hold" (see note)
0341-1	I'M AT THE MERCY OF LOVE -1 (Benny Davis-J. Fred Coots)	Vi 25409-B, ViJ JA-823-B, HMV B.D.5133 ASR LB5120
0341-2	I'M AT THE MERCY OF LOVE *-1*	Victor unissued, 'Hold'
0342-1*	FLOATIN' DOWN TO COTTON TOWN -1,-2 (Jack Frost-F. Henri Klickmann)	Vi 25415-A
0343-1	LA-DE-DE LA-DE-DA -1,-2 (Sam Lewis-Peter De Rose)	Vi 25430-A, HMV B.D.5150, HMVAu EA1850, HMVIt GW1390, *HMVSw HE2360*
0343-2	LA-DE-DE LA-DE-DA *-1,-2*	Victor unissued, 'Hold'
0344-1	YOU DON'T LOVE RIGHT	(See note)
0344-2	YOU DON'T LOVE RIGHT	Victor unissued, 'Hold'

The recording sheet again names the personnel, spelling Autrey as 'Autery', and notes that titles recorded on matrices 0340, 0341 and possibly 0344 are *From the 27th. edition of "COTTON CLUB PARADE — 1936"*. This final title is x'd out, but sufficient is visible beneath the xing to read the title, that it has a vocal by Fats and enough to suggest that it is as shown above; and that the first take was originally selected for issue with the second take designated "Hold". Despite all this, there are no serial numbers entered for the waxes used. The second 'take' of 0340 has the figure 1 directly below that of the first take, which is how these figures normally appear, with the 'A' following and the '2' preceeding it, so it may be that it was originally intended as a simultaneous turntable version of the first take, but changed to become a genuine second recording. 0342 has steamboat and water effects.

Both sides of Vi 25409 bear the additional credit (From the 27th edition of "Cotton Club Parade-1936').

*****

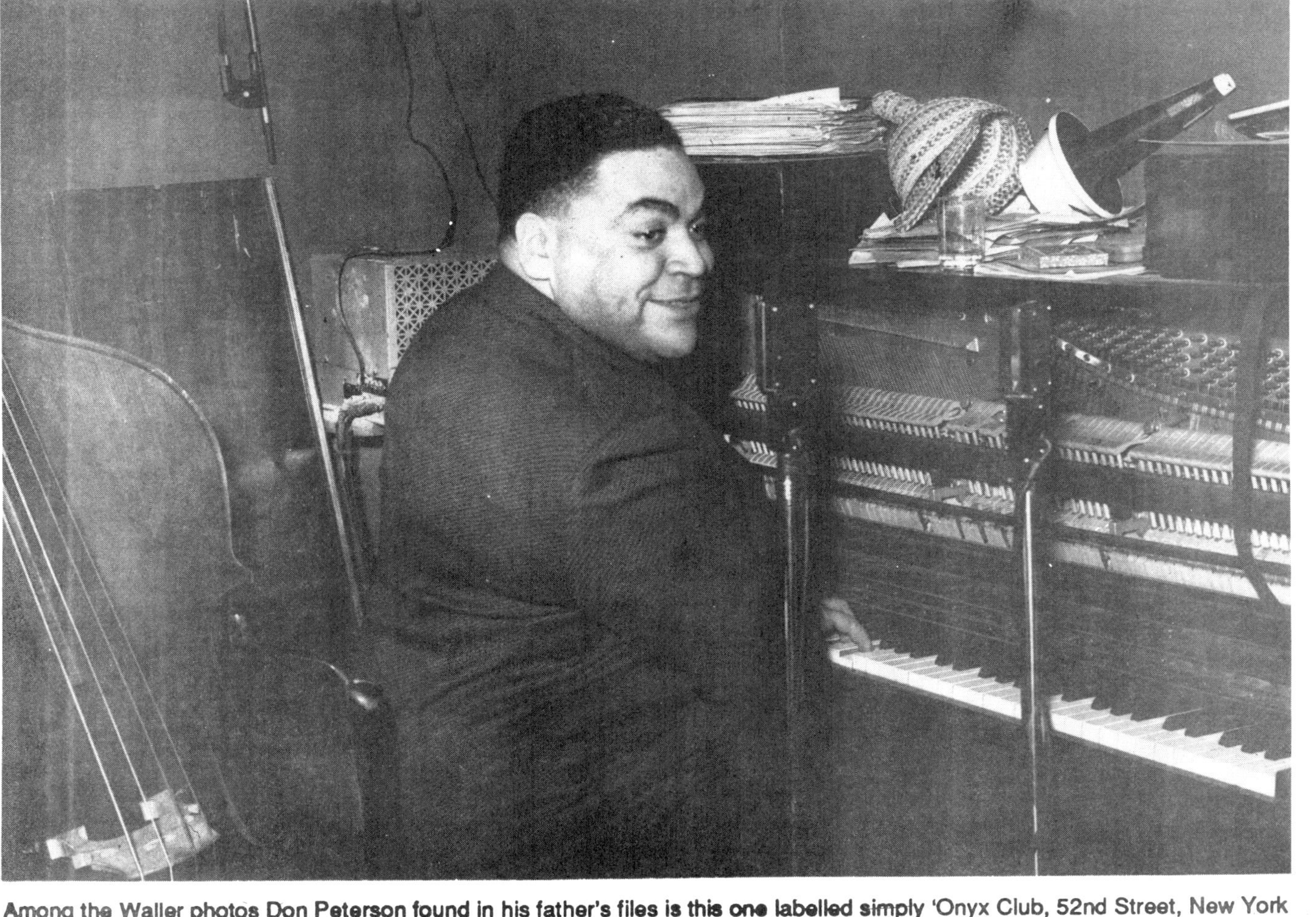

Among the Waller photos Don Peterson found in his father's files is this one labelled simply 'Onyx Club, 52nd Street, New York City, 1936'. It is not known if this was an engagement or simply an occasion when Fats dropped in and was persuaded to play.

The next reference to Waller is found in Billy Rowe's 'Harlem Note Book' column of the *Pittsburgh Courier.* He features short, snappy comments which are often valuable to researchers and to save space, future extracts will give his name and date only. On 19 September he commented: *The lovely Lovey Lane was the center of attraction at the Lincoln in the Quaker City with Fats Waller last wk.* Lovey Lane was a beautiful exotic dancer who performed in the briefest of costumes.

*****

The Royal Theatre, Baltimore was refurbished during the summer and opened on Friday, 25 September with a gala performance by Fats Waller. From the available report it is not clear whether it was a one night stand or an engagement for the week. The latter seems more likely.

*****

Waller played another week at the Apollo Theatre commencing Friday, 2 October 1936 and it is perhaps interesting that the advertising for this gave Emmett Mathews greater prominence than Turner's Arcadians. The personnel on this engagement was almost certainly that which toured Canada in the autumn of 1936. A report in the *International Musician* for November from Local 406, Montreal, gives the following personnel: C.E. Smith, Herman Autrey, Ed Anderson, Fred Robinson, George Wilson, Emmett Mathews, Eugene Sedric, Rudy Powell, George James, Al Washington, Fats Waller, Henry Duncan, Al Casey, Chas. Turner, Elmore (Wilmore 'Slick'?) Jones.

The issue for December has a reports from Local 149, Toronto, and Local 9, Boston, (which lists 'Rudy Ponce'!) giving an identical personnel except for Sedric who is omitted in Toronto. Because of the delay which often took place between the event and publishing the personnel in the *International Musician,* and the lack of definite details on appearances in Canada, it is not possible to state whether they took place before or after the next engagements and the session in Chicago.

The Waller show played the Fox Theatre, Detroit for a week commencing Friday, 20 November. A report in the *Pittsburgh Courier* of 21 November noted that Myra Johnson, 'The Manhattan Madcap' was a featured artist with the show and that she had *been with Fats all season and is now a regular feature with the band whether they play theatres or dances.*

At the end of the Detroit engagement, the show travelled to Youngstown, Ohio for a 'Post Turkey Day Dance' for the city's Progressive Club held in the Central Auditorium on Friday, 27 November from 9:00 p.m. to 1:00 a.m. A reception and dawn party were promised for Fats and his orchestra with a variety of foods and drinks on hand.

Following that, the group proceeded to Chicago for a record session; the first by the 'Rhythm' away from New York.

*****

"Fats" Waller and his Rhythm -Fox Trot **Vocal refrain and piano by "Fats" Waller -3**
Herman Autrey, t; Gene Sedric, cl-1/ts-2; Fats Waller, p/v-3; Al Casey, g; Charles Turner, sb; Slick Jones, d.

Chicago Studio C, Chicago, Illinois Sunday, 29 November 1936
12:00 a.m. to 4:00 p.m.

01801-1* HALLELUJAH! THINGS LOOK ROSY NOW -2,-3 (West-Flatow-Magine) Vi 25478-B, ViJ A1144, HMV B.D.5178

01802-1* HALLELUJAH! THINGS LOOK ROSY NOW -2 (West-Flatow-Magine) Vi 25489-A, HMVF K8228, HMVSc X4817, El EG3895

01803-1* 'TAIN'T GOOD (Like A Nickel Made Of Wood) -1,-2,-3 (Whiting-Bernier-Haid) — Vi 25478-A, HMV B.D.5178, HMVAu EA1850, El EG3880
01804-1* 'TAIN'T GOOD (Like A Nickel Made Of Wood) -1,-2 (Whiting Bernier-Haid) — Vi 25489-B, HMVF K8228, El EG3895
01805-1* SWINGIN' THEM JINGLE BELLS -1,-2,-3 (John Hancock) — Vi 25483-B, *Vi/Ar20-1602-A,* ViJ A1144, BB B10016-A, HMV B.D.1229†, HMVF SG65†, HMV/H J.O.81, HMVIt HN2426, HN2599†, HMVSw HE2672†, HMVAu EA2302
01806-1* SWINGIN' THEM JINGLE BELLS -1,-2 (John Hancock) — Vi 25490-B, ViJ JA-953-B, MW M7949, El EG3893

01807-1* A THOUSAND DREAMS OF YOU -2,-3 (Paul Webster-Louis Alter) — Vi 25483-A, ViJ JA-953-A, HMV B.D.5184, HMVAu EA1868, *HMVSw HE2359*
01808-1* A THOUSAND DREAMS OF YOU -2 (Paul Webster-Louis Alter) — Vi 25490-A, El EG3893
01809-1* A RHYME FOR LOVE -1,-3 (Leo Robin-Ralph Rainger) — Vi 25491-A, HMVAu EA1856, HMVIn NE329
01810-1* I ADORE YOU -1,-2,-3 (Leo Robin-Ralph Rainger) — Vi 25491-B, HMVAu EA1856, HMVIn NE329

The recording sheet notes the instrumentation and has the note *(Same Names as on Lawst* (sic) *Recording).*

Issues of 01805-1 marked † are as simply ***JINGLE BELLS.*** 01807 is originally typed on the recording sheet as *A THOUSAND DRAMS OF YOU* which would no doubt have pleased and amused Fats! Vi 25483-A and 25490-A bear the additional credit **(From the Walter Wanger film "You Only Live Once")**, other issues shorten this to **(From the Film "You only live once")**, and Vi 25491 (both sides) has **(From the Paramount film "College Holiday")**. Victor 25490 omits any performance credit.

*****

"Fats" Waller and his Rhythm -Fox Trot — **Vocal refrain and piano by "Fats" Waller**
Herman Autrey, t; Gene Sedric, cl-1/ts-2; Fats Waller, p/v; Al Casey, g; Charles Turner, sb; Slick Jones, d.

Studio No 2, New York City, New York — Thursday, 24 December 1936
10:00 a.m. to 1:00 p.m.

03840-1* HAVIN' A BALL -1,-2 (Andy Razaf-James P. Johnson) — Vi 25515-B, ViJ A1246, BB B-10100-B
03841-1* I'M SORRY I MADE YOU CRY -1,-2 (N.J. Clesi) — Vi 25515-A, ViJ A1246
03842-1* WHO'S AFRAID OF LOVE? -1 (Sidney D. Mitchell-Lew Pollack) — Vi 25499-A, HMVAu EA1851, HMVIn NE332, El EG4010
03843-1* PLEASE KEEP ME IN YOUR DREAMS -1 (Tot Seymour-Vee Lawnhurst) — Vi 25498-A, ViJ JA-888-A, HMV B.D.5184, HMVIn NE333, *HMVSw HE2359*
03844-1* ONE IN A MILLION -2 (Sidney D. Mitchell-Lew Pollack) — Vi 25499-B, HMVAu EA1851, HMVIn NE332
03845-1* NERO -2 (Razaf-Denniker-Davis) — Vi 25498-B, ViJ JA-888-B, HMVAu EA1868

The recording sheet notes the use of one ribbon microphone and one unidirectional one and also lists the personnel but not the session director. Victor 25499 bears the additional credit **(From the 20th Century-Fox film "One In A Million")** on both sides and BlueBird B-10100-B shows **(From the musical comedy "Policy Kings")**. On Victor 25498-A "Fox Trot" is abbreviated to **F.T.**

The reverse of HMVIn NE333 is by **Guy Lombardo.**

*****

Fats Waller and his Rhythm

Herman Autrey, t; Gene Sedric, ts; Fats Waller, p/v; Al Casey, g; Charles Turner, sb; Slick Jones, d.

Broadcast, 'Magic Key of Radio' from RCA studios, New York City, New York

Sunday, 3 January 1937

Hallelujah! Things Look Rosy Now	Issued on LP
A Thousand Dreams Of You	Issued on LP

*****

The *Pittsburgh Courier* of 16 January, in a report dated 14 January, noted Fats Waller and his band at Loew's State Thetre, New York and gave Myra Johnson, Emmett Mathews and Al Washington among those featured.

In the *Defender* of 16 January and datelined "New York City, January 15, Alan MacMillan wrote a glowing review of Waller's week at Loew's State Theater, which was probably from 8-14 January:

> *...Most amazing variety performance of the past week was that of Fats Waller at Loew's State theater. Last Sunday night we went to hear him, but were forced to stand in line for almost an hour. Backstage, the femme admirers swamped the corridor leading to his dressing room, seeking autographs. When we finally got inside and were seated the stage show was on. Every act was a click, gaining thunderous applause, but when Fats came on to close the bill there was a full three-minute ovation. And Maestro Waller really went to town and we'd like to cast a personal nomination for Myra Johnson, the talented hotcha girl who was given a chance to make good on the main stem by Fats Waller...*
>
> *Another great coast-to-coast broadcast was that of the Joe Cook show, during which time the clever comedian presented Babe Ruth, John McCormick, Johnny Weissmuller and Fats Waller. The program was aired from New York City at 9.30 throughout the NBC network and this was one of the most expensive Shell programs that Joe Cook has presented so far.*

The following week, Billy Rowe commented that the Broadway critics had disliked Waller's 'double talk', saying it wasn't suitable for a family audience, but that it was OK for Milton Berle to do likewise. He went on to note that despite the adverse criticism, Waller had been chief guest star on WABC's Saturday night swing music programme and scored his usual success.

*****

While Waller was playing Loew's, Dee Lloyd, billed as 'The Female Fats Waller' played the Apollo Theatre for the second week of January 1937 and the next week, beginning Friday 15 January, was followed by the real thing. For the first time the advertising was for 'Fats' Waller and his band with no mention of Turner's Arcadians or Emmett Mathews, although the *New York Age* editorial comments mentioned them in the advance announcement and review of the show which was couched in the usual glowing terms. The issue dated Saturday, 23 also devoted an editorial paragraph (unfortunately mutilated on the copy held here) which stated that Waller had been a guest on the CBS *'Swing Program' last Saturday.* It seems he was appearing in a solo capacity, and *played 'Hallelujah!', 'Things Look Rosy' and 'St. Louis Blues'.* The station received 327 telegrams of congratulation on Waller's performance from listeners. The date of this broadcast is assumably Saturday, 16 January, and the same broadcast as that mentioned by Billy Rowe above, and would have taken place whilst the film was being screened at the theatre. The *Pittsburgh Courier* reported Waller's success at the Apollo and noted him as fronting Turner's Arcadians.

*****

At this point mention should be made of a report in the *International Musician* of February 1937. It is a long entry from Local 136, Charleston, West Virginia and probably covers events for several months and, given the names involved and the knowledge of Waller's movements over the preceding weeks, suggests an engagement in the summer of 1936. The names are: Fats Waller; Charles Turner; Herman Autrey; Al Washington; George James; Emmett Mathews; Everard (Rudy?) Powell; Clarence Smith; Edward Anderson; Henry Duncan; Allen Porter; Fred Robinson; Eugene Sedric and Eugene Fields.

*****

Walter Allen provided two scraps of information (source not noted) that showed Fats Waller and His Rhythm playing at the Aragon Ballroom, Boston on Friday, 5 February 1937 and at the Recreation Ballroom, Lawrence, Massachusetts on the following day.

*****

In a report datelined Rome, N.Y. Feb. 15, the *Pittsburgh Courier* of 27 February has:

> *Thomas "Fats" Waller ... escaped with only minor injuriesa and a slight shake-up when his shiny sedan was involved in a collision with a truck-trailer a few miles west of here last Thursday (11 February). ... was travelling east on Route 5 between the cities of Syracuse and Utica when the accident occurred. According to State Trooper C.F. Sloane, who investigated the accident, the musicians attempted to pass the trailer on the three-strip road just as a west-bound machine ... approached. Waller stated later that he was temporarily blinded by the the driving snow beating against his windshield, and in trying to avoid hitting the oncoming car crashed into the trailer. ... Waller was able to continue on his way.*

*****

"Fats" Waller and his Rhythm -Fox Trot **Vocal refrain and piano by "Fats" Waller**

Herman Autrey, t; Gene Sedric, cl-1/ts-2; Fats Waller, p/v/cel-3; Al Casey, g; Charles Turner, sb; Slick Jones, d.

Studio No 3, New York City, New York — Monday, 22 February 1937
9:30 a.m. to 3:45 p.m.

04949-1*	YOU'RE LAUGHING AT ME *-1,-3*	Victor unissued 'Process'
04949-2*	YOU'RE LAUGHING AT ME -1,-3 (Irving Berlin)	Vi 25530-A, HMV B.D.5215, HMVIn NE342 El EG4010
04950-1*	I CAN'T BREAK THE HABIT OF YOU -1,-2 (Razaf-Beal-Causer)	Vi 25530-B, HMVAu EA1933
04951-1*	DID ANYONE EVER TELL YOU? -1 (Harold Adamson-Jimmy McHugh)	Vi 25537-B
04951-2*	DID ANYONE EVER TELL YOU? -1	Victor unissued, 'Process'. Issued on LP

04951: End of guitar chorus before vocal:
-1 Waller runs his right hand up the keyboard in a glissando
-2 Waller plays with both hand

04952-1 WHEN LOVE IS YOUNG -2 Vi 25537-A
(Harold Adamson-Jimmy McHugh)
04952-2a2* WHEN LOVE IS YOUNG -2 Victor unissued, 'Hold'.
04953-1* THE MEANEST THING YOU EVER DID WAS KISS ME -1 VI 25536-A, 20-2219-A, HMV B.D.5431, HMVAU EA1933, EL EG6676
(Lewis-Newman-Mencher)
04953-2 THE MEANEST THING YOU EVER DID WAS KISS ME *-1* Victor unissued, 'Hold'

Victor 25530-A bears the additional credit **(From the 20th Century-Fox film "On The Avenue")**, and both sides of Victor 25537 have **(From the Universal Film "When Love Is Young')**.

The reverse of HMVIn NE342 is by **Richard Himber**.

*****

"Fats" Waller and his Rhythm -Fox Trot **Vocal refrain and piano by "Fats" Waller**
Herman Autrey, t; Gene Sedric, cl-1/ts-2; Fats Waller, p/v; Al Casey, g; Charles Turner, sb; Slick Jones, d.

Studio No 3, New York City, New York Thursday, 18 March 1937

06413-1* CRYIN' MOOD -2 (Andy Razaf-Chick Webb) Vi 25551-B, HMV B.D.5278, HMVAu EA1939
06414-1* WHERE IS THE SUN? -1 Vi 25550-A, ViJ JA-1016-A, HMV B.D.5212, HMVEi IM292, HMVFr K7936
(John Redmond-Lee David)
06415-1* YOU'VE BEEN READING MY MAIL -1 (Joseph Meyer-Bob Rothberg) Vi 25554-B, ViJ A945-B, HMV B.10191, HMVEx J.O.274, HMVAu EA1960, HMVFr SG357, HMVSw HE2997, HMVIt HN3128, HMVIn N.14080, El EG7719
06416-1* TO A SWEET PRETTY THING -1 Vi 25551-A, HMVAu EA1939
(Joe Young-Fred E. Ahlert)
06417-1* OLD PLANTATION -1 Vi 25550-B, ViJ JA-1016-B, HMV B.D.5212, HMVEi IM292, HMVFr K7936
(John Redmond-Lee David)
06418-1* SPRING CLEANING -2 Vi 25554-A, ViJ A945-A
(Samuels-Whitcup-Powell)

A small mystery is posed by matrix 06418 on the recording sheet. Originally it is shown as *YOU HIT THE NAIL ON THE HEAD* written by Marty - - - and Milton Ager with vocal by Fats, and the usual -1 marked "A" (indicating selected for issue) and -1a marked "Hold". However, no wax numbers are shown for these and presumably the title was not actually recorded. The whole entry is X'd out and the same matrices used for the following title as indicated above which, on the recording sheet, has the sub title *(Getting Ready For Love).* This final title has "vacuum cleaner sound effects". Both sides of Victor 25550 and HMV B.D.5212 bear the additional credit **(From the "Cotton Club Revue 1937")**.

*****

When Count Basie first played the Apollo in New York for the week 19-25 March 1937, he recalls that Fats Waller came in one night to check the band out and rescued him from an awkward situation:

He was sitting over in a box seat enjoying the show, and I was just about to start the next number, somebody in the audience hollered out.

"Jam session. Jam session".

And that got me. I didn't know what to do. I was scared to death up there, because right away everybody was asking for a jam session. I just stood there holding up my hand. Then I finally got nerve enough to introduce Fats and ask him to come up on the stage

So he jumped over the railing and came on and called a couple of other guys up there. We introduced them, and everybody was still hollering, clapping and stompin, and when they kept on, old Fats held up his hands and stretched his big eyes at them. "Hey, wait a minute. You said you wanted a jam session, didn't you?"

And they said yes.

And he said, "Well, get quiet so you can hear it."

Then he sat down at the piano, and he and those guys tore it up in there, and that was the only thing that saved me. Old Fats. That's the kind of man he was. He could take charge of the situation.

*****

JAM SESSION AT VICTOR -Fox Trot

Bunny Berigan, t; Tommy Dorsey, tb; Fats Waller, p; Dick McDonough, g; George Wettling, d.

New York City, New York — Wednesday, 31 March 1937

06581-1	HONEYSUCKLE ROSE (–)	Vi/Ar 25559-A, ViAr 68-0864, ViJ A1245, HMV/Au B.8580, *HMVIt GW1473*, HMVSw JK2296, HMVFr K7921, El EG7551
06852-1	BLUES (–)	Vi/Ar 25559-B, ViAr 68-0864, ViJ A1245, HMV/Au B.8580, *HMVIt GW1473*, HMVSw JK2296, HMVFr K7921, El EG7551

The recording sheet for this session was not available for study. Victor 25559 appears as a "Swing Classic" in both "Curly" and "Round" label versions and late pressings of the latter use a dubbed master of 06581-1. All issues inspected show the personnel on the label and the English and Italian HMV (Disco Gramofono) issues show a composer credit of (Garret & Wand) for 06582 but, oddly, none for 06581. This credit is absent on the Australian pressing of B.8580. Horst Lange notes that some pressings of the Electrola issue show *Blues* as *Dallas Blues.*

*****

"Fats" Waller and his Rhythm -Fox Trot — **Vocal refrain and piano by "Fats" Waller or Piano by "Fats" Waller -4**

Herman Autrey, t; Gene Sedric, cl-1/ts-2; Fats Waller, p/v-3; Al Casey, g; Charles Turner, sb; Slick Jones, d/vb-4.

Studio No 2, New York City, New York — Friday, 9 April 1937

E. Oberstein directing

07745-1*	YOU SHOWED ME THE WAY -2,-3 (Fitzgerald-McRae-Webb-Green)	Vi 25579-A
07746-1*	YOU SHOWED ME THE WAY -2,-4 (Fitzgerald-McRae-Webb-Green)	Vi 25565-A, ViJ A1062-A, El EG4005
07747-1*	BOO-HOO -1,-2,-4 (Heyman-Lombardo-Loeb)	Vi 25563-A, HMV B.D.5229, HMVAu EA1938, HMVSp GY394

07748-1*	THE LOVE BUG WILL BITE YOU (If You Don't Watch Out) -1,-2,-4 (Pinky Tomlin	Vi 25563-B, HMV B.D.5229, HMVSc X4863, HMVAu EA1938, HMVSp GY394
07749-1*	SAN ANTON' -1,-3 (Andy Razaf-Paul Denniker)	Vi 25579-B
07750-1*	SAN ANTON' -1,-4 (Andy Razaf-Paul Denniker)	Vi 25565-B, ViJ A1062-B, BB B-10109-A, HMV B.D.5215, HMVCz X4918
07751-1*	I'VE GOT A NEW LEASE ON LOVE -1,-3, -4 (Joe Young-Fred E. Ahlert)	Vi/China 25580-B, *HMV B.10684,*
07752-1*	I'VE GOT A NEW LEASE ON LOVE -1 (Joe Young-Fred E. Ahlert)	Vi 25571-B, HMVFr SG.95, K-8262, El EG4005
07753-1*	SWEET HEARTACHE -2,-3,-4 (Ned Washington-Sam H. Stept)	Vi/China 25580-A, HMV B.D.5225, HMVIt GW1597, *HMVSw HE2368*
07754-1*	SWEET HEARTACHE -2 (Ned Washington-Sam H. Stept)	Vi 25571-A, HMVFr SG.95, K-8262, HMVCz X4918
07755-1	HONEYSUCKLE ROSE -1,-2 (Razaf-Waller-Immerman)	Vi 36206-A, *25779-B* (see note), ViJ JB185, NB6004, HMV C.2937, HMVAu EB114, HMVSw FKX121, HMVFr L1041, HMVIt S10610, ASR LC2937

The final title is a 12" recording and bears no performance credit. It was edited to fit a 10" issue, given the dub matrix number 17697 and issued in this form on Victor 25779 with performance credit -4.

The recording sheet shows only as far as matrix 07754-1a, and then has a note at the foot "Date continued on page 2" which is unfortunately missing from the files. Thus, it is not possible to give the session times.

Victor 25571 is, I believe, the only finished Victor pressing I have ever seen where the matrix number is visible beneath the labels and the -A side of this and the -A side of Victor 25580 (both issues) bear the additional credit **(From the Republic film "The Hit Parade")** with a shortened version on HMV B.D.5225 and on HMVFr SG.95 and HMVFr K-8262.

*****

Waller was presumably on a brief tour after the above date as the *Pittsburgh Courier* of 24 April had a paragraph datelined Charleston, W.Va., April 22 to the effect that promoter George E. Morton had booked the Fats Waller and Jimmy Raschel orchestras for a 'Battle Of Music' in the Armory on Saturday night (i.e. 24 April).

*****

Clarence Williams' Swing Band

Ed Allen, c; Buster Bailey, cl/as-2; Russell Procope, as/cl-3; Cecil Scott, ts/cl-3; Clarence Williams, p/sp-5; unknown, sb; Floyd Casey, d; William Cooley, v-1; Fats Waller, sp-6 unidentified voices-4.

New York — c. Thursday, 29 April 1937

MS 07862-1	Feel De Spirit -1	Lang-Worth Program 268
	Old Time Religion -1,-4	
	Lord Deliver Daniel -5	
	Sweet Kisses -2,-6	

MS 07863-1 Go Down Moses -1 Lang-Worth Program 270
Do You Call Dat Religion? -1,-5
Jericho -1,-2,-3,-4
Lazy Swing -2,-3,-4

Howard Rye drew my attention to Waller's presence on *Sweet Kisses.* He had recognised Waller's voice when attempting to discover the origin of the soundtrack to 'Soundie' 7M5 by the Mitchell Brothers and Evelyn Keyes which bears the same title as the tune. Waller is heard encouraging Buster Bailey at the beginning of the clarinet solo but, unless he is one of the unidentified voices on *Old Time Religion,* there is no other evidence of his presence. It may be presumed that he just drifted into the studio where his old friend was working and, finding no gin, just drifted out again after contributing to the general atmosphere. These recordings play at 33¹/₃ r.p.m and although it seems likely that all the sides listed were made at the same time, this is not necessarily so. The date given is probably a transfer date and is estimated from nearby Victor matrices; the actual recording date may have been the same, but probably a few days earlier. Reverses and adjacent matrices are unknown.

*****

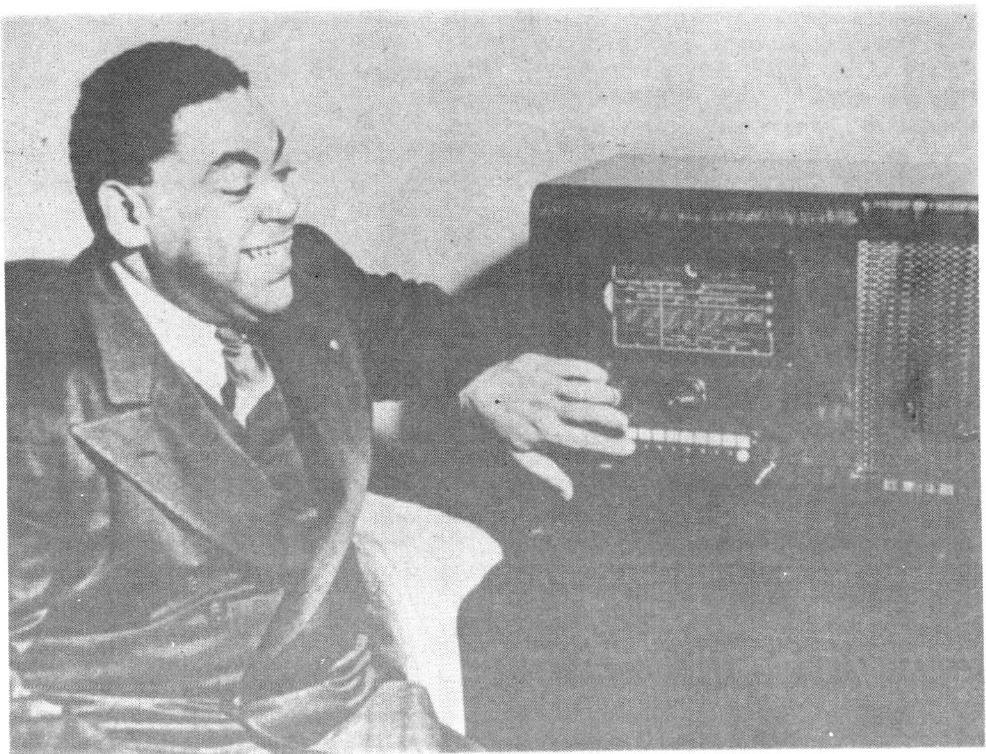

Another shot of Fats used as publicity by RCA Victor. It also exists cut so that the left hand and the radio are omitted.

The *International Musician* for April 1937 has a report from Local 40, Baltimore, Md. listing Thomas (Fats) Waller, Charles Turner, Henry C. Duncan, Al Casey, W. Jones, Fred Robinson, George Wilson, Edward Anderson, Herman Autrey, Clarence Smith, Emmett Mathews, A. Washington, Eugene Sedric, Eugene Mikell and George James. As usual it is not possible to date the engagement, but it is worth noting that the Waller band were in Charleston W. Virginia (as noted on page 132) in April, and it may have been this personnel.

*****

In its issue of 1 May 1937 and a report datelined Detroit, April 29 the *Pittsburgh Courier* notes that Fats Waller and his Orchestra have been booked in to the ballroom at Eastwood Amusement Park which is claimed to be the largest permanent ballroom in the world with a capacity of 8,000 dancers. Although no dates are given for Waller's engagement, the implication is that it is for the following week.

The following week the same paper carries a boxed advert for **Fats Waller and His Famous Orchestra** playing a dance on "Tuesday nite (sic), May 11 in Textile Hall, Greenville, S.C. from 9:30 p.m".

Waller was still in the Carolinas the following week according to a report from Durham, N.C. datelined May 27 which said that he had played a dance in the city 'last week' and that the local sheriff had served a writ of attachment for $1,300 brought by promoters Logan and Hill in respect of bookings they had made for Waller the previous autumn. It was claimed that Waller had 'walked out' to take more lucrative engagements elsewhere. The dance continued while Waller and his manager Edward Melchor conferred with the plaintiffs and settlement was agreed in the sum of $500.

In the *Pittsburgh Courier* of 15 May on page 12, there is a paragraph under the heading 'To Book Fats' which is unfortunately illegible in the copy held here, but from what I am able to decipher seems to indicate that the Waller organisation was to be booked by Moss and that something had been arranged commencing May 24.

*****

Another scrap of information from Walter C. Allen which fails to note the source show Fats Waller and His Rhythm opening the season at Nuttings on the Charles, Waltham, Massachusetts opposite Mal Hallett.

*****

In the *New York Age* of 21 May 1937 (oddly, the entire paper is dated Saturday, 21 May when it should have been 22 May!), Fats Waller was announced as the headline act at the Apollo along with Myra Johnson and Emmett Mathews and the editorial paragraph covering this stated that this engagement marked the end of a nationwide tour by the band. The engagement was from 21-27 May. If this information on a tour is correct, then Waller would have been away until very shortly before the Apollo opening date and 23 May can be ruled out for the private recordings which follow as he would have been fully engaged at the theatre. Thus, 30 May is the likely date. It is possibly of note that a benefit show took place at the Apollo from midnight on 30 May and neither Waller nor any of his known guests are among those scheduled to appear or listed in the review the following week.

In the paper of the following week, Waller is panned for the first time:

The show at the Apollo ... is one of the best in spite of the fact that the animated corpulent and clumsily clowning Fats Waller is supposed to be the featured performer. ... Tim Moore

... really stopped the show. ... The handsome and lively Emmett Mathews ... an appealing voice and baby! Can he toot a horn! ... He's invariably there when Waller barges in, which is our reason for going. Well, Mathews made the mountainous musician look like a molehill ... he won over the entire house ... the way His Corpulency cut up on the boards this week while Emmett is going through his act, that Waller is determined not to let this happen again. And so our piano-playing friend makes himself vastly unnecessary, cavorting heavily about and spoiling the slight impression he did make — when he was taking his pubic (sic) *piano practise.*

Did the reporter catch Waller on a bad night ... or had Waller upset him and we have a bad case of sour grapes?

*****

In March 1962, John R.T. Davies received from Maurice Waller via Bill Krasilowsky, the attorney acting for the Waller Estate, a parcel containing a number of private recordings on glass-based acetates and studio recordings. Many of these had failed to make the transatlantic journey, but after three years of intermittent work on repair and restoration, sufficient music had been reassembled to enable a double LP to appear as issue 22/23 on the Ristic label. Dates no more accurate than a month and year can be assigned to most of this material, and it will be inserted at the appropriate points with as much information as is available. The first group appear to come from around May 1937 as follows:

Home recordings, in the Waller Home probably Sunday, 30 May 1937

The Gathering	In which the voices of Fats, Willie 'The Lion' Smith, Eubie Blake, James P. Johnson and Andy Razaf are heard. Piano introduction by Willie'The Lion'.
Medley: Baltimore Buzz/Old Fashioned Love	Fats Waller, p.
Im Crazy 'Bout My Baby	Fats Waller, p/v.
Liza	James P. Johnson, p.
Until The Real Thing Comes Along	Naomi Waller, v; Fats Waller, p.
I'm Coming Virginia	Naomi Waller, v; Fats Waller, p.
Lost Love	Andy Razaf, v; Fats Waller p.
(A second, almost identical, version of this last title was not used in the Ristic set)	
Blues Is Bad No. 1	Gene Sedric, ts; Fats Waller, p.
Saxophone Doodle	Gene Sedric, ts.
Blues Is Bad No. 2	Gene Sedric, ts; Fats Waller, p.

Bob Kumm played these recordings to Eubie Blake who recalled that, for the first time in a number of years, the itineraries of himself and the other three pianists coincided and they were in New York at the same time. They had assembled at Waller's house one Sunday afternoon for a party to celebrate Fats's thirty-third birthday [Friday, 21 May] and had continued until late in the evening.

"We spent much of the day telling stories and recalling the early days. While there was much discussion of the early stride cutting contests, surprisingly, no challenge was given and no attempts to outdo each other at the piano were made. I guess we'd all matured somewhat by that time and were just glad to be able to get together for a private party and

> *enjoy each other's company and companionshp. After all, it had been a long time since all of us were able to socialise like that, what with the hectic pace that we had been maintaining in travelling about the country during the 'thirties. This was a sort of grand reunion, and there was much happy conversation and plenty of good food. The day passed all too quickly, and the party broke up at a rather 'respectable' hour, with everyone able to navigate themselves home in a sober, or at least near-sober state."*

Willie 'The Lion' Smith's piano introduction on *The Gathering* was identified aurally by Mike Lipskin. He also identified the female voice in the second group as that of Lillian Wright (Mrs. James P. Johnson). However, in a letter to me dated 21 April 1971 Henry Parker, Waller's 'cousin', wrote as follows:

> *...Waller made quite a few records of his own at his home in N.Y.C. He had a record player and record maker combined. Some of these records have come to light, but not all of them ... some were sent to London a few years back ... it's known to no-one but Waller, his sister Naomi and myself that the voice of the lady singing on them is his sister. She sang 'I'm Coming Virginia' and 'Until The Real Thing Comes Along' ... this was not known when the records were shipped over.*

Henry Parker amplified this information in a later letter dated 18 September 1971 in which he says that Naomi visited him in June and, on being played the recordings, recalled that they were all made on the same day. He goes on:

> *..."I'm Coming Virginia" was one of her best favourites; her mother came from Virginia. She told me all about the day they were at his home making the records. James P. Johnson, Andy Razaf, Willie 'The Lion' Smith, Eubie Blake and many more were there.*

As a family member Henry should know, and he supplied the photos of himself with her and others of the family which are found in this book. Although Henry Parker always called himself Waller's cousin and was extremely active in promoting the memory of Fats and was very clearly a member of the Waller clan, I have been unable to clarify the exact relationship and Henry never responded to my enquiries along these lines.

*****

During Waller's week at the Apollo, photographer Charles Peterson took a superb series of photographs, mostly in the street behind the theatre between shows. Two of the series are shown here with more in the 'Waller Scrapbook' section. Peterson had himself been a musician, being the guitarist in Rudy Vallee's Connecticut Yankees when that band was a top attraction in the country. Later he took up photography and focussed his attention on the great jazz players of the day. In the shot opposite, taken in Waller's dressing room, Peterson stands between Fats and Eddie Condon who had brought along his new protégé from Providence, Rhode Island, Bobby Hackett, to play for Fats. Peterson had set his camera, stepped into the shot and got Buster Shepherd to trip the shutter. Overleaf Fats is talking with Anita who sits at the wheel of his big green Lincoln car. The choice of make was not lost on the black community, and Fats told Ernie Anderson, "Lincoln freed the slaves, and not only that, when Raymond Massey played Lincoln he got so carried away that he went up to the Cotton Club and freed all those chorus girls!"

*****

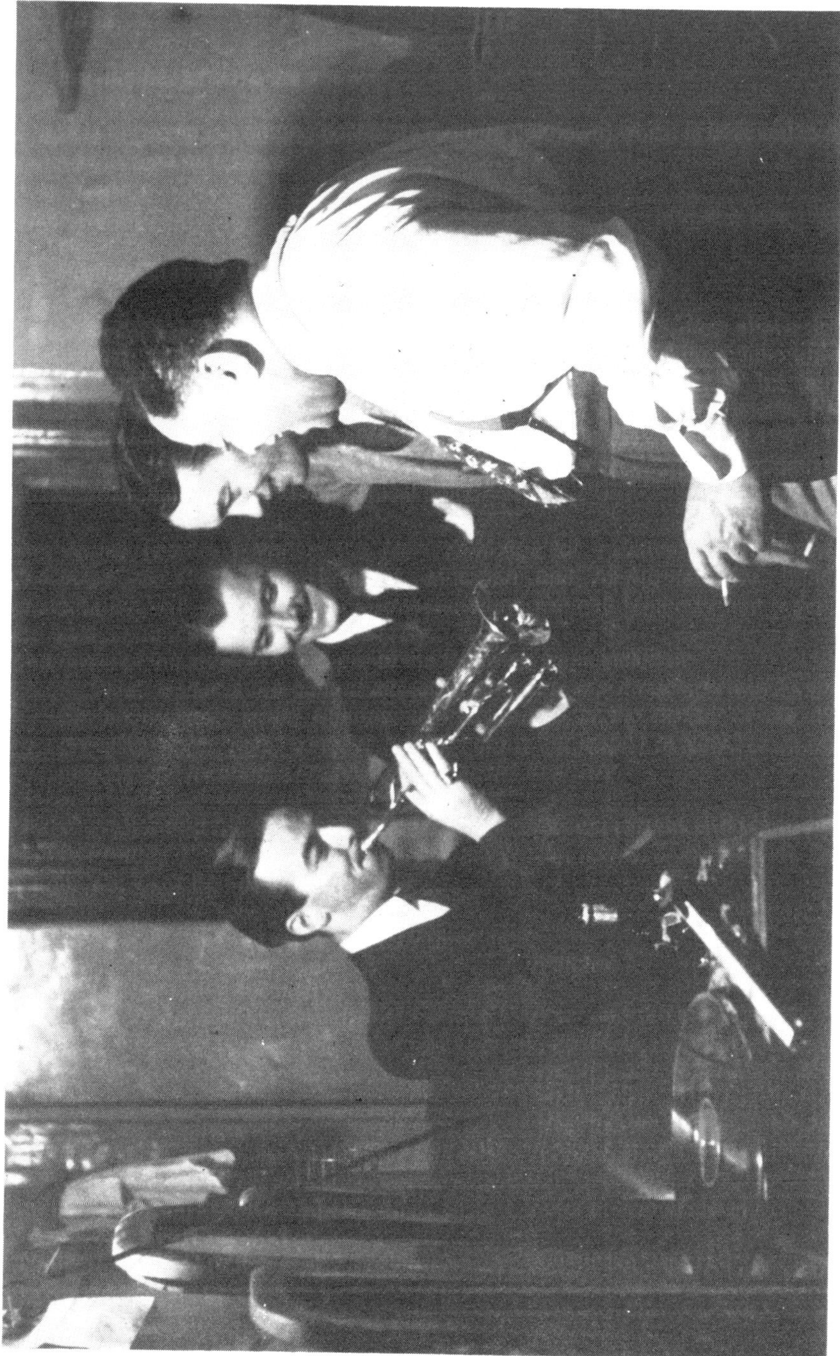

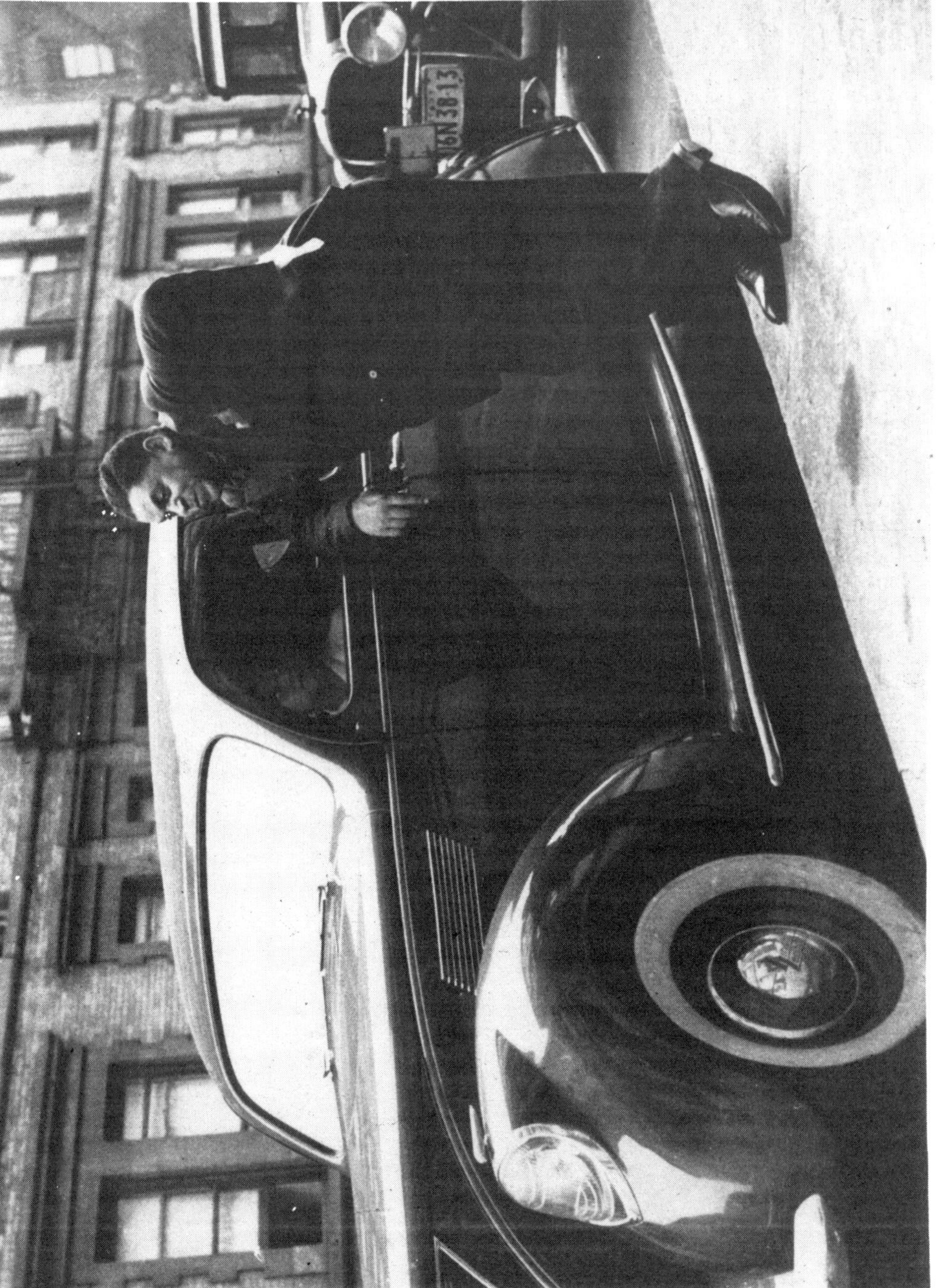

A somewhat ambiguous report, datelined New York City. June 3, appeared in the *Pittsburgh Courier* of 5 June:

> *Fats Waller ... started south this week for another short tour. The date for Waller's first summer tour of Dixie has been set through arrangements with Phil Ponce by Harry Moss, for whom the aggregation is touring.*
>
> *Opening date has been set for June 4, at V.M.I.'s annual Cotillion dance.*
>
> *After three weeks in the Southland, the band will trek north to New England for another short tour, after which a week's vacation will be the next mode of important business.*

I don't know the meaning of the V.M.I. inittials and the location of the dance is not given. The stay in the south was certainly much shorter than the three weeks noted and the 'Rhythm' were recording in New York on 11 June, presumably passing through on their way to New England.

*****

"Fats" Waller and his Rhythm -Fox Trot **Vocal refrain and piano by "Fats" Waller**

Herman Autrey, t; Gene Sedric, cl-1/ts-2; Fats Waller, p/v-3; Al Casey, g; Charles Turner, sb; Slick Jones, d.

Studio No 3, New York City, New York Friday, 11 June 1937
2:00 p.m. to 5:00 p.m. Mr. Eli. Oberstein directing

010647-1*	(You Know It All) SMARTY -1,-2,-3 (Ralph Freed-Burton Lane)	Vi 25608-A, HMV B.10168, HMVAu EA1976, HMVSw HE3043, HMVFr SG410,
010647-2	(You Know It All) SMARTY *-1,-2,-3*	Victor unissued, 'Hold'
010648-1*	DON'T YOU KNOW OR DON'T YOU CARE? -1,-3 (Irving Kahal-Sammy Fain)	Vi 25604-A, 20-2642-B, HMV B.D.5258, HMVAu EA2045
010649-1*	LOST LOVE -1,-3 (Andy Razaf-Thomas "Fats" Waller)	Vi 25604-B, HMV B.D.5258
010650-1*	I'M GONNA PUT YOU IN YOUR PLACE (And Your Place Is In My Arms) -1,-3 (Bob Rothberg-Joseph Meyer)	Vi 25608-B, BB B10008-B, HMV B.D.5493, HMVAu EA2260
010651-1*	BLUE, TURNING GREY OVER YOU -2 (Andy Razaf-Thomas Waller)	Vi 36206-B, *25779-A* (see note), ViJJB185, NB6004, HMV C.2937, HMVAu EB114, HMVSw FKX121, HMVFr L1041, HMVIt S10610, ASR LC2937

The recording sheet notes that the personnel is the same as for the previous date. Vi 25608-A bears the additional credit **(From the Paramount film "Double Or Nothing")**; and Vi 25604-A has **(From the "Pan American Casino Revue")**, and on this side 'Fox Trot' is abbreviated to **F.T.** As with the previous session, the final title is a 12" recording and as previously this issue bears no performance credit. An edited version to fit a 10" record was prepared and given the dubbed matrix number 17689 and issued in this form on Victor 25779 with the performance credit **Piano by "Fats" Waller**. Note the recording date which is as given on the recording sheet. The session then continued as below. Italian HMV HN 3043 -1st title shown in *Jazz Records* is almost certainly a misprint for the Swiss HE issue.

*****

"Fats" Waller Piano solo -Fox Trot (BB B-10099)
"Fats" Waller and his/His Piano Piano Solo -Fox Trot (VI 25631)

Fats Waller, p

Studio No 3, New York City, New York — Friday, 11 June 1937

5:00 p.m. to 6:15 p.m. Mr. Eli. Oberstein directing

010652-1*	KEEPIN' OUT OF MISCHIEF NOW (Andy Razaf-Thomas "Fats" Waller)	Vi/C 25618-B, 27767-B, ViAr 68-0499, ViJ A1047-B, BB B-10099-B, HMV B.8625, HMVAu E.A.2382, HMVSw HE2290, HMVScX4479, *HMVIn N.4479*, El EG6757
010653-1*	STAR DUST (Michael Parish-Hoagy Carmichael)	BB B-10099-A, Vi 20-2638-A, HMVEx JO.132, HMVAu E.A.2382, HMVSw HE2290, HMVIn N.14051, HMVSc AL5020, El EG6757
010654-1*	BASIN STREET BLUES (Spencer Williams)	Vi 25631-B, 27767-A, ViJ A1263, BB B-10115-A, HMV B.8636, HMVAu E.A.1985, HMVSw HE2289, HMVSc X4479, *HMVIn N.4479*
010655-1*	TEA FOR TWO (Irving Caesar-Vincent Youmans)	Vi/C 25618-A, 27766-A, ViJ A1047-A, ViAr 68-0499, RCA 420-0238, HMV B.8625, HMVAu EA3685, *HMVIn N.4478*
010656-1*	I AIN'T GOT NOBODY (And Nobody Cares For Me) (Roger Graham-Spencer Williams)	Vi 25631-A, 27766-B, ViJ A1263, BB B-10133- , HMV B.8636, HMVAu E.A.1985, *HMVIn N.4478*

This double session illustrates as clearly as possible the unbounding talent of Waller who, after a three-hour session with his rhythm, was able to toss off five superb piano solos in the space of one hour and a quarter, and all in an acceptable single take.

Labels of the reissue Victors quote a recording date of 9 June 1937 in error. HMV B.8636 omits the sub title on 010656. There are numerous minor variants on the labels from this session. The *New York Age* began reviewing records in its issue of 14 August 1937, and Victor 25618 was included in the first batch covered.

*****

Fats and his band were apparently on tour soon after this date, for Frank Driggs found the advert reproduced opposite from a Milwaukee paper (actual source not noted) dated 17 July 1937, which showed him booked to play in the Modernistic Ballroom in the city on Sunday with his famous orchestra This was assumably 18 July, and probably with his big band.

The only other date known is at Beckley, West Virginia, where Waller was booked in the Armory on Saturday, 28 August by impresario George Morton (*Pittsbugh Courier,* 28 August 1937) in what was said to be his only engagement in that area..

*****

WORLD'S LARGEST BALLROOM

MODERNISTIC

STARLIGHT TERRACE

STATE FAIR PARK

TONITE EVERYBODY WELCOME!
I. U. UNITED AUTO WORKERS OF AMERICA LOCAL NO. 336 DANCE

Many Surprise Features

Bill Carlsen's Music

Admission 35c All Evening

Saturday—Everybody Welcome

ALLIS-CHALMERS DANCE

Bill Carlsen's Music

SUNDAY
IN PERSON!

World's
Greatest
Entertainer

★ STAGE
★ SCREEN
★ RADIO
★ RECORDINGS

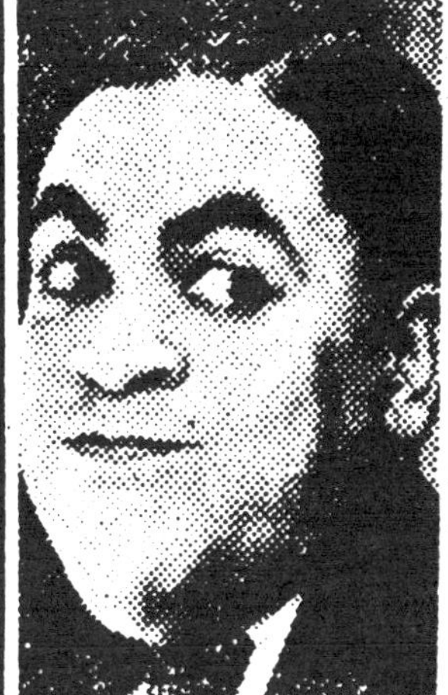

"FATS"

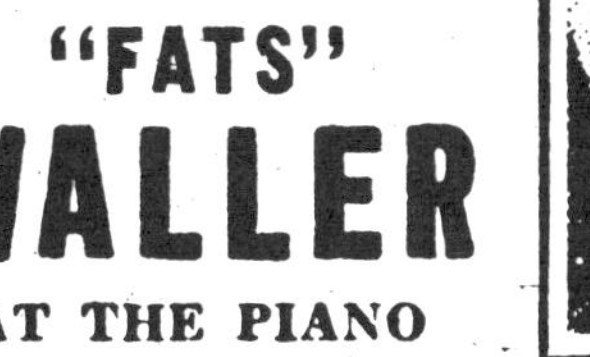

WALLER

AT THE PIANO

AND HIS FAMOUS ORCHESTRA

Plus ● BILL CARLSEN'S MUSIC

40c to 8:30; 50c, plus 5c tax after.

The youthful, cherubic photo of Fats used here dates from a much earlier period but, oddly, continued to be used in advertising almost until his death, even though later shots were available in abundance.

Further reports in the *International Musician* give the same personnel as noted in the Local 40 report of April present in Local 257, Nashville, Tenn. (June issue) and Local 294, Lancaster, Pa. (July issue). The July issue also notes the Waller band in Local 3, Indianapolis, Ind., but no personnel is listed. In the August issue they are reported by Local 543, Baltimore, Md., and 587, Milwaukee, Wis., where Myra Johnson, vocalist is added and Washington's first name is shown as 'Wilbert', as in most of the following. September has a long list: Sub 2 St. Louis; 26 Peoria, Ill.; 30 St. Paul, Minn.; 71, Memphis, Tenn.; 122, Newark, Ohio (Myra Johnson added here and Mathews omitted); 257, Nashville, Tenn.; 265, Quincy, Ill.; 344, Meadowville, Pa.; and 382, Fargo, N.D.

*****

"Fats" Waller and his Rhythm -Fox Trot **Vocal refrain and piano by "Fats" Waller**
Herman Autrey, t; Gene Sedric, cl-1/ts-2; Fats Waller, p/v; Al Casey, g; Charles Turner, sb; Slick Jones, d.

Studio No 2, New York City, New York — Tuesday, 7 September 1937
12:30 p.m. to 7:00 p.m. Leonard Joy directing

013344-1*	YOU'VE GOT ME UNDER YOUR THUMB -1,-2 (Livernash-Brooks-Hudgens)	Vi 25672-B, HMV B.D.5310
013344-2	YOU'VE GOT ME UNDER YOUR THUMB *-1,-2*	Victor unissued, 'Hold'
013345-1*	BEAT IT OUT -2 (Buddy Bernier-Bob Emmerich)	Vi 25672-A, HMV B.D.5377, HMVF K8174, SG.91, El EG6445
013346-1*	OUR LOVE WAS MEANT TO BE -1 (Hill-Davis-Waller)	Vi 25681-B, *20-2643-B,* HMV B.D.5310, HMVAu EA2033
013347-1*	I'D RATHER CALL YOU BABY -1 (Tot Seymour-Vee Lawnhurst)	Vi 25681-A, HMVAu EA2033
013347-2	I'D RATHER CALL YOU BABY -1	Victor unissued, 'Hold'
013348-1*	I'M ALWAYS IN THE MOOD FOR YOU -2 (Benny Davis-J. Fred Coots)	Vi 25671-A, HMV B.D.5297
013349-1*	SHE'S TALL, SHE'S TAN, SHE'S TERRIFIC -2 (Benny Davis-J. Fred Coots)	Vi 25671-B, HMV B.D.5297, HMVAu EA2045
013350-1*	YOU'RE MY DISH -2 (Harold Admason-Jimmy McHugh)	Vi 25679-A, HMVAu EA1990
013350-2	YOU'RE MY DISH *-2*	Victor unissued, 'Process'
013351-1*	MORE POWER TO YOU -2 (Harold Adamson-Jimmy McHugh)	Vi 25679-B, HMV B.D.5314, HMVAu EA1990, HMVIt GW1621, GW1900, El EG6294
013351-2	MORE POWER TO YOU *-2*	Victor unissued, 'Process'. Issued on LP

013351: Fourth line of vocal: -1" You changed your heart, oh, you cheated on me".
-2 "You changed your heart."

There is handclapping on the second title. The recording sheet names the personnel and has the note *(This To Be Specialed!)* against matrices 013348/013349. Both sides of Victor 25671 bear the additonal credit **(From the 3rd Edition of the "Cotton Club Parade")**, and both sides of Victor 25679 have **(From the Universal film "Merry-Go-Round of 1938")**, and this is shortened on HMV B.D.5314.

*****

The French magazine *Jazz Hot No. 20* of September-October 1937 gives the personnel of Fats Waller's regular big band as: *Clarence Smith, Herman Autry, Ed Anderson, t; George Wilson, Fred Robinson, tb; George James, Emmett Mathews, Al Washington, Gene Mikell, Gene Sedric, saxes, Hank Duncan, Fats Waller, p; Al Casey, g; Charlie Turner, sb; Slick Jones, d.* This presumably refers to the summer period of that year.

*****

According to Ed Kirkeby in *Ain't Misbehavin'*, the band was booked into a Boston theatre at the beginning of October and Fats took along Andy Razaf and J.C. Johnson. On the train ride up from New York the three men wrote a number of tunes for a forthcoming recording session, of which the best known is *The Joint Is Jumping.*

*****

"Fats" Waller and his Rhythm -Fox Trot **Vocal refrain and piano by "Fats" Waller**
Herman Autrey, t (except -5); Gene Sedric, cl-1/ts-2; Fats Waller, p/v-3; Al Casey, g; Charles Turner, sb; Slick Jones, d, Dorothea Driver, v-4
Studio No 2, New York City, New York Thursday, 7 October 1937
9:00 a.m. to 1:45 p.m. Leonard Joy directing

014645-1* HOW CAN I? -2,-3 Vi 25864-B, HMVAu EA2263
(J.C. Johnson-Thomas "Fats" Waller)
014646-1* THE JOINT IS JUMPIN' -1,-2,-3 Vi 25689-A, *20-1582-B,* HMV B.D.1079, El EG7860
(Razaf-Waller-Johnson)
014647-1* A HOPELESS LOVE AFFAIR -2,-3,-5 Vi 25689-B, HMV B.D.5314, HMVIn B.D.5354, HMVAu EA2068, *HMVIt GW1621,* El EG6294
(Andy Razaf-Thomas "Fats" Waller)
014648-1* WHAT WILL I DO IN THE MORNING? -1,-3 (J.C. Johnson- Thomas "Fats" Waller) Vi 25712-A
014649-1* HOW YA BABY? -1,-3 Vi 25712-B, *HMV B.D.5354,* HMV/In B.D.5354, HMVAu EA2128, HMVSw HE2345, El EG6383
(J.C. Johnson- Thomas "Fats" Waller)
014650-1* JEALOUS OF ME -2,-3 Vi 25864-A, HMV B.D.1079
(Andy Razaf-Thomas "Fats" Waller)
014651-1 CALL ME DARLING -?,-4 Victor unissued, 'Hold'; issued on LP

Police whistle and siren effects are heard on the second title and, according to Ed Kirkeby, Andy Razaf, J.C. Johnson (who were along to hear their new composition recorded) and a couple of girls as well as some of the studio staff added voices to provide the right sort of riotous atmosphere. The recording sheet shows the first title as *How Can I, With You In My Heart* and notes that the final title is *(Held In New York).*

Jazz Records shows JK 2345 for 014649-1 in addition to the HE number, but according to a Swiss HMV catalogue held here, JK 2345 couples Sidney Bechet's *Slippin' And Slidin'/Egyptian Fantasy* and, in fact, this issue is shown thus in the Bechet section. Jehangir Dalal reported that the Indian B.D.5354 issue coupled *A Hopeless Love Affair/How Ya Baby?* whilst copies of the U.K. issue couple the second title with *Paswonky.*

*****

The above was Charlie "Fat Man" Turner's last recording session with the Waller Rhythm and possibly his last engagement with Waller. With his Arcadians and Emmett Mathews his was the resident band at the newly-opened West End Theatre in New York from 18 November 1937 until at least 17 December, after which no further adverts appeared. Soon after that, he retired from music to open a chicken and turkey farm in up-state New York and a restaurant/bar on St. Nicholas Avenue in Harlem. His replacement in both the Rhythm and Orchestra was Cedric Wallace.

Following the above date the Waller aggregation must have gone straight to Chicago as a report from Ted Watson dated Oct. 14 (Thursday) in the *Pittsburgh Courier* has the following under the heading *'Fats' Waller And Brilliant Revue Wowed 'Em At RKO Palace:*

> *Chicago theatergoers were given something to go back home talking about the past week-end when "Fats" Waller and an all-star revue closed a record-breaking week at*

> *Palace theater in the loop.*
>
> *... Myra Johnson stood out ... a "jam session" with the "Fats"* (sic) *... sent plaudits to the rafters.*
>
> *Waller's band showed unique class in their terrific arrangements of the song hits; "Marie", "Don't You Know", "Caravan", "Honeysuckle Rose", and "That Old Feeling".*

*****

Further reports in the *International Musician* may be related to the Boston and Chicago engagements above. A personnel of Thomas (Fats) Waller, Albert Aloysius Casey, Wilmore Jones, Herman Autrey, Eugene P. Sedric, Alvin Cobb, Nathaniel C. Williams, William Alsop, John Hamilton, George O. Robinson, Cedric Wallace, Alfred A. Skerritt, James T. Powell and John Haughton are listed by Local 9, Boston, Mass. (November) and Local 10, Chicago, Ill. (December) plus Local 4, Cleveland, Ohio (December, but omitting Sedric).

*****

Reference should also be made here to Snub Mosley's recollection of having played with Waller's big band (see the note at the end of 1935 for further details). In *The World Of Count Basie* he says *...I was with Louis a bit over a year ... I went out on a tour with Fletcher Henderson for a few weeks ... Chu Berry was in that band ... Then I went with Fats Waller's big band for a few months. The first engagement was at the Howard Theater in Washington, and after that we had a lot more theater dates ... when I left Fats I organized my own band of six pieces ...* This suggests a period in late 1937, but I have been unable to trace any independent sources to allocate a more precise dating.

*****

However it was not very late in 1937 as, in *Really The Blues,* Mezz Mezzrow recalls that he sold Eli Oberstein on the idea of a racially mixed band. The plan was that Mezzrow would put together a 15-piece mixed band to open the Harlem Uproar House on 20 November 1937, which was also the night that RCA were resuming their "Magic Key of Radio" programme. Oberstein would ensure that the band was highlighted over the air; which would lead to further promotion and recordings. It took a little time to assemble the band and Mezzrow goes on to give the personnel and says: *Eugene Cedric* (sic), *clarinetist and tenor saxophonist, was with Fats Waller, but Fats was doing a single then, and his band was laying off, so Cedric was tickled to come with us.* This implies that Fats must have started out as a solo performer by early November, given the time taken for Mezzrow to assemble and rehearse the band ready for the 20 November opening. In fact, Fats had gone to Hollywood where he had been engaged to appear with bassist Al Morgan's band at the 'Famous Door' cabaret.

He appears to have been in residence for a time before the following, datelined New York Nov. 24, appeared in the *Pittsburgh Courier* of 27 November:

> *"Fats" Waller ... entrained for the coast after several theatrical and recording engagements in the East. Immediately after arriving on the coast, Waller was assigned to the post of maestro at the "Famous Door" in Hollywood, which had its fall opening recently.*
>
> *Besides leading the orchestra, for which he has already composed special dance arrangements of the swing variety, Waller will entertain at the piano ...*

Given the date of this report and the fact that the train journey took some three days, Waller probably left New York around the 10th of November at the latest. Also note that the Turner band which Waller had been using opened at the West End Theatre on 18 November.

According to Morgan, Fats was with the band for three and a half months which, given the confirmed dates, is just about possible. Whilst in Hollywood, Waller made some test recordings and the following day took the Morgan band into the studios to record as 'Fats Waller and his Rhythm':

*****

A quotation should also be inserted at this point with no further comment. It comes from the *New York Age* of 16 October 1937 and under the heading *Wife Sues 'Fats' Waller* has:

> *Rosalind Marquis, movie actress, took steps in Hollywood last week to annul her marriage to Louis 'Fats' Waller, swing pianist and orchestra leader. She charges he deserted her shortly after their marriage in New York in 1936.*

*****

Peggy Dade

Peggy Dade, v, acc: unknown group of t; cl/as; Fats Waller, p/vocal comments; g; sb; d -1.
Peggy Dade, v, acc: Fats Waller, p/vocal comments -2

Hollywood Recording Studio — Wednesday, 15 December 1937

1445	On The Sunny Side Of The Street -1	Victor test recording. Issued on LP
1446	Georgia -2	Victor test recording. Issued on LP

These are apparently audition recordings for which no recording sheet was available. They are known from a two-sided test owned by a collector in Salisbury, England. I have not heard them, but reliable reports indicate the instrumentation given above which, in the light of the session below, suggests the same group.

*****

"Fats" Waller and his Rhythm -Fox Trot **Vocal refrain and piano by "Fats" Waller**

Paul Campbell, t; Caughey Roberts, cl-1/as-2; Fats Waller, p/v; Ceele Burke g-3/stg-4; Al Morgan, sb; Lee Young, d.

Hollywood Recording Studio — Thursday, 16 December 1937
1:00 p.m. to 6:00 p.m.

09884-1	EVERY DAY'S A HOLIDAY -1,-3 (Sam Coslow-Larry Trivers)	Vi/C 25749-A, HMV B.D.5333, HMVAu EA2068
09884-2	EVERY DAY'S A HOLIDAY *-1,-3*	Victor unissued, 'Hold'. Issued on LP

09884: Eighth line of vocal: -1 "They ought to close those banks, yeah!"
-2 "They ought to close the banks."

09885-1	NEGLECTED -1,-4 (Johnny Marks-Joe Davis)	Vi/C 25749-B, HMB B.D.5342, El EG6369
09885-2	NEGLECTED *-1,-4*	Victor unissued, no disposition noted
09886-1	MY WINDOW FACES THE SOUTH -1,-4 (Silver-Parish-Livingston)	Vi 25762-B
09886-2	MY WINDOW FACES THE SOUTH *-1,-4*	Victor unissued, 'Hold'
09887-1	AM I IN ANOTHER WORLD? -1,-3,-4 (Ted Koehler-Johnny Green)	Vi 25753-A, HMV B.D.5360
09887-2	AM I IN ANOTHER WORLD? *-1,-3,-4*	Victor unissued, 'Hold'
09888-1	WHY DO HAWAIIANS SING ALOHA -2,-4 (Meskill-Raskin-Stept)	Vi 25762-A. HMV B.D.5342
09888-2	WHY DO HAWAIIANS SING ALOHA *-2,-4*	Victor unissued, 'Hold'
09889-1	MY FIRST IMPRESSION OF YOU-1,-3 (Charlie Tobias-Sam H. Stept)	Vi 25753-B
09889-2	MY FIRST IMPRESSION OF YOU *-1,-3*	Victor unissued, no dispostion noted

The recording sheet names the musicians (Lee Young is Lester's brother) and has the heading

Fats Waller and his orchestra typed in. The last word is then crossed out and "Rhythm" substituted in manuscript. This was certainly done for commercial reasons, for although the first description would have been more accurate, the familiar artist credit would be more inducive to record buyers. Vi 25749-A bears the additional credit **From Paramount film "Every Day's A Holiday"**, and the recording sheet notes that 09887 is *From Columbia film "Start Cheering" and 09889 is* From RKO film "Having Wonderful Time". 'Fox Trot' is abbreviated to **-F.T.** on Vi 25762-A. Roberts is almost inaudible on 09885 and 09888.

*****

The termination date for Waller's Hollywood engagement is unknown, but he was back in New York by mid-January 1938 for an article in the *New York World-Telegram* of Saturday, 15 January has Fats in his Morningside Avenue apartment talking about his stint in Hollywood and how he'd played from 7:30 p.m. until 4:00 a.m. seven nights a week at the 'Famous Door'. It also mentions that Fats was to take part in a jam session over station WABC that night and concludes by saying that his wife's name was Anita and their family comprised Maurice, 10, Ronald 9, and Carolyn, 8 — the only mention I've ever found of a third offspring and one which must be treated with caution.

*****

Early in 1938, Ed Kirkeby left RCA Victor and took over management of Fats Waller from an ailing Phil Ponce. According to Kirkeby's own account in *Ain't Misbehavin',* he organised a new band and sent Waller out on the road on a series of one-nighters which caused him a number of problems. Waller's reputation for unreliablity meant that the first part of the tour was a flop and Kirkeby cancelled it after an engagement in Columbia, South Carolina, after which Waller jumped a date in Durham. This led to further problems and on arriving at the Earle Theatre in Philadelphia, the band found that the Durham promoter had taken legal steps to secure the first $850.00 from the takings at the Earle. The Earle theatre engagement may be dated from a report in the *Pittsburgh Courier* of 12 March which has a report datelined Philadelphia, Mar. 10, which states that Waller and his group were at the theatre 'last week'. At the final engagement in Newark, Fats decided he'd had enough and called the Kirkeby office to say he was coming straight back without playing and only completed the tour after threats and a pleading phone call from Kirkeby. A report in the *International Musician* of March 1938 from Local, 16, Newark, N.J. lists the personel quoted previously on page 144, and may refer to this final engagement. These events presumably all took place prior to the next session in New York. George James also recalled a tour in 1938:

> *In the spring of 1938 the whole band, Charlie Turner's fronted by Fats, went out on a tour in a show with Buck and Bubbles, and 'Bojangles' Robinson. I remember we had three pianists in that; Fats was playing and singing, and we also had Hank Duncan, and then there was Buck Washington too. The show didn't last too long, but I seem to recall we played Boston ...we certainly played the 'Harlem Opera House' and we got as far as Indianapolis, where we played the 'Lyric Theater'.*

Note that although George James refers to the band as Charlie Turner's, and he had worked on and off with Turner for some years, Turner, as noted above, had actually quit music about this time. Alternatively (and more likely), George's memory of the date may be in error.

*****

A belated report in the March 1938 *International Musician* for January quotes the summer tour personnel of 1937 in Local 136, Charleston, V.Va., and probably belongs with that tour.

*****

Right: Ed Kirkeby, who took over from Phil Ponce as Waller's manager

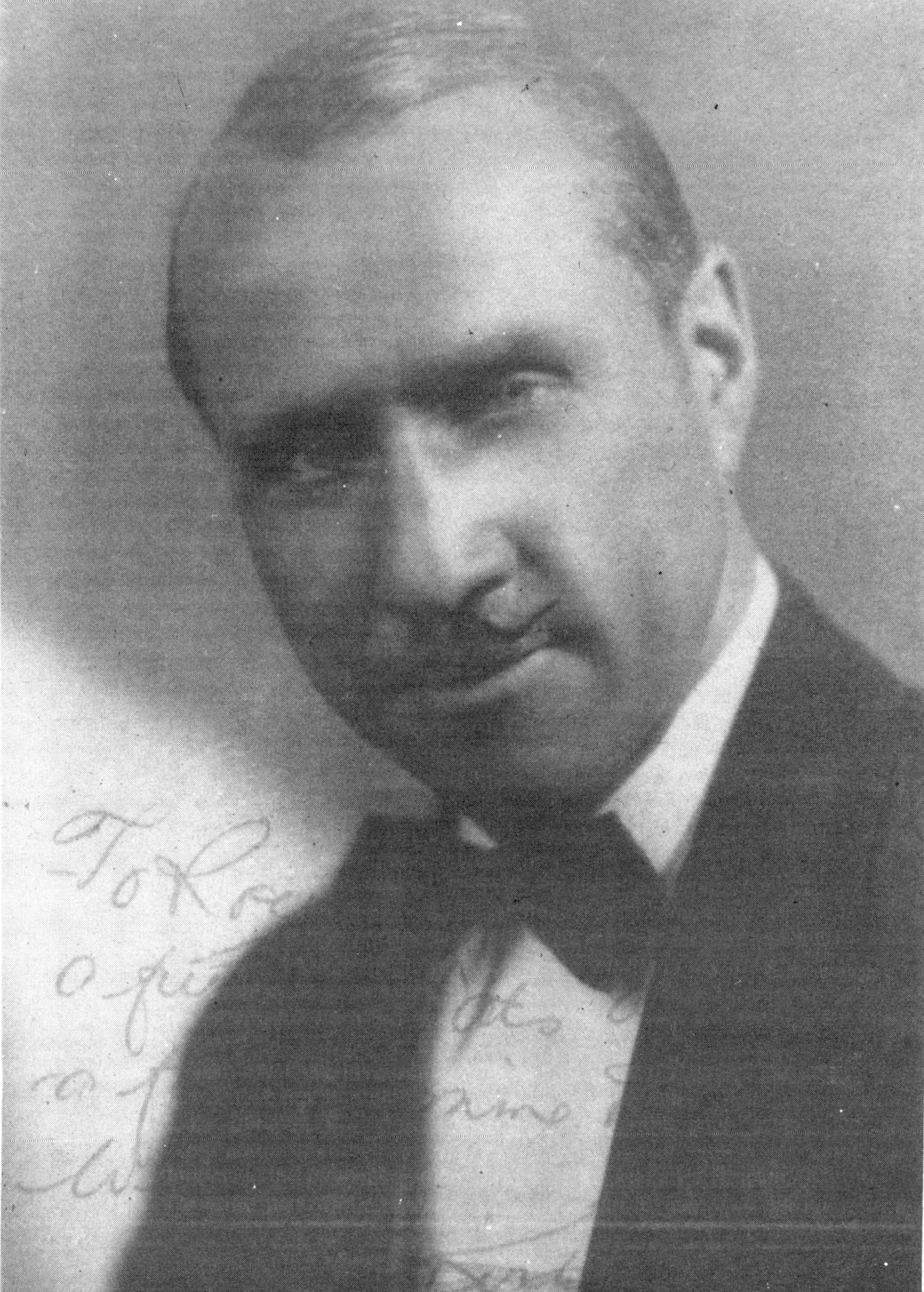

"Fats" Waller and his Rhythm -Fox Trot **Vocal refrain and piano by "Fats" Waller**

Herman Autrey, t; Gene Sedric, cl-1/ts-2; Fats Waller, p/v/cel-3; Al Casey, g; Cedric Wallace, sb; Slick Jones, d.

Studio No 2, New York City, New York — Friday, 11 March 1938
12:00a.m to 6:30 p.m.

021150-1*	SOMETHING TELLS ME -2,-3 (Johnny Mercer-Harry Warren)	Vi 25817-A, HMV B.D.5387, J.O.92, HMVIn N14038, El EG6540
021150-2	SOMETHING TELLS ME *-2,-3*	Victor unissued, 'Hold'
021151-1*	I LOVE TO WHISTLE -1 (Harold Adamson-JimmyMcHugh)	Vi 25806-A, HMV B.D.5360, J.O.273, HMVAu EA2083, HMVIn NE.699, El EG7727, ASR L25652
021152-1*	YOU WENT TO MY HEAD -2 (Meyer-Bernier-Emmerich)	Vi 25812-B, HMVAu EA2128
021153-1*	FLORIDA FLO -2 (Howard Johnson-Joe Sivad)	Vi 25806-B, HMV J.O.110, HMVF SG154, HMVSw HE2702
021154-1*	LOST AND FOUND -2 (Pinky Tomlin)	Vi 25812-A, HMV B.D.5377, El EG6445
021154-2	LOST AND FOUND *-2*	Victor unissued, 'Hold'
021155-1*	DON'T TRY TO CRY YOUR WAY BACK TO ME -2 (Phil Kelly-Henry Welling)	Vi 25817-B, HMV B.10495
021156-1	IF YOU'RE A VIPER -3 (See Note)	Victor unissued, master probably destroyed
2451-1	Marie FT. Vocal by Fats Waller	(Test for E.E. Oberstein)

Fats whistles and yodels on Victor 25806-A, and the label of this bears the additional credit **(From Universal film "Mad About Music").** There is no mention on the recording sheet of matrix 021156 which first appeared in Waller listings in the original compilation by John R.T. Davies and which has appeared in all subsequent listings. The source for this information is not now known but, since the fact that Waller played celeste on it was known it would appear that some firm information was forthcoming at that time and the side is therefore listed as before in the session above. The recording sheet shows that the Rhythm session finished at 5:45 p.m. and that the test, for which no instrumentation is given, was made between that time and 6:30 p.m. It features a well-rehearsed big band with a Waller vocal, and aurally is Waller's own big band, and Waller had been featuring the number in his stage presentation for several months.. The idea has been put forward that it was by another band which followed Waller into the studio with Fats playing piano and singing with them, but in fact this was the final session of the day which therefore rules that out.

*****

Les Airey sent a quote from the October 1939 issue of *Orchestra World* which may have some bearing on the final title above:

> *Don Donaldson is arranger for Fats Waller. He was born in Boston and studied at the New England Conservatory of Music. About 15 years ago he had a three-piece band and he was only 12. He later went to New York and worked with Jelly Roll Morton. His travelling took him to Montreal and then back to New York in 1934. His arrangements were noticed by Fats Waller, especailly 'Marie' and 'I Need Lovin''. Fats called him in and immediately*

placed an order for anything he could write and as fast as he could write it. There are two pianos in the band and Don plays the other one. He also conducts the band. He's been with the band for five years.

*****

The personnel for *Marie* above may be the band that Courtney Williams joined (see his piece elsewhere in this volume) and, if so, the second tenor player may be Al Cobb. Alternatively, the band may be a composite drawn from the band recalled by George James which had just finished a tour and the new one being formed as remembered by Courtney Williams.

*****

According to Ed Kirkeby in *Ain't Misbehavin',* two days before the next Victor record session, Fats took part in a jam session over at the Criterion Theatre on Times square hosted by Martin Block and broadcast over station WNEW. All other sources place this broadcast on 19 October, a Wednesday, or 12 December, a Monday, but Kirkeby says it took place on a Sunday (which fits) and that Waller and the band had returned from an engagement in the Capitol Theatre, Scranton, Pennsylvania that had finished on the Saturday night, arriving back in New York on the Sunday morning. I have not been able to establish the time of day the broadcast took place but if in the evening, as seems most likely, then Ed Kirkeby's recollection would, on a first examination appear to be probably correct as Waller and his group were working regularly at the Yacht Club from early October 1938 until mid-January 1939 and he and Casey would hardly be available for a broadcast on a Wednesday or a Monday evening — unless the broadcast were from a pre-recorded acetate.

Martin Block's own account also confirms a Sunday morning for the actual perfomance and gives the impression that it was transmitted 'live', although "just before we went on the air" might not have to be taken literally. The account is worth quoting in full:

"I arrived at the Criterion at about 9 o'clock, and at the stage door, seated on the doorstep was a very big man wearing a black derby hat and an overcoat with the collar turned up around his neck. I took one look and exclaimed, 'Fats Waller, what are you doing here at this hour?' Fats replied, 'Well Mr. Block, the train just got in and I didn't have no place else to go, so I thought I'd come over here and mix things up a bit.' He said, 'By the way, where can I get a drink?' I said, 'Fats, this is Sunday morning, it's impossible to get a drink.' He said, 'Oh man, nothing's impossible; you must have a friend who can come up with some liquid ham and eggs!' Well, I did have a friend to call upon in the 'emergency' and soon we had provided a bottle of White Horse scotch. When Fats was served his 'breakfast' I saw something that I never saw before in my life. Fats proceeded to consume the entire fifth of scotch straight down, without even bothering to stop to catch his breath. And, amazingly, this only served to enhance his thirst!

Just before we went on the air Fats called out that he was in need of further 'lubricating', and asked if we could come up with a bottle of sauternes. This was provided ... and I don't think that Fats ever performed better in his life than he did that Sunday morning in the Criterion."

Everything seems to fit nicely except that, as far as I am aware, the title *Jeepers Creepers* was written specifically for the film *'Going Places'* which was made in the autumn of 1938 and, even had it been available at this early date, it is extremely unlikely that permission would have been given for it to be used. Details are therefore shown against the date 19 October 1938.

*****

"Fats" Waller, his Rhythm and Orch. -Fox Trot Vocal refrain and piano by "Fats"Waller
"Fats" Waller, his Rhythm and Orch. -Fox Trot Piano by "Fats" Waller
"Fats" Waller & his Rhythm and Orch. -Fox Trot
Vocal refrain and piano by "Fats" Waller

Herman Autrey, John Hamilton, Nathaniel Williams, t; George Robinson, John Haughton, tb; William Alsop, James Powell, Freddy Skerritt, as; Gene Sedric, cl-1/ts; Lonnie Simmons, ts; Fats Waller, p/v-2; Albert Casey, g; Cedric Wallace, sb; Slick Jones, d.

New York City, New York — Tuesday, 12 April 1938

022429-1 IN THE GLOAMING — Victor unissued, 'Hold'. Issued on LP
022429-2 IN THE GLOAMING — Vi 25847-A, HMVAu EA2167
(Old Traditional Melody—Arr. by Thomas "Fats" Waller)
022429: Last four bars of piano solo:
-1 Fats plays from the middle of the keyboard down with heavy string bass acc.
-2 With sustain pedal on, Fats plays from top of keyboard down to the middle with barely audible string bass, thus achieving a light, almost celeste-like sound.

022430-1 YOU HAD AN EVENING TO SPARE -2 (Stanley Adams-Oscar Levant) — Vi 25834-B, *HMV J.O.397,* HMVAu EA2263
022431-1 LET'S BREAK THE GOOD NEWS -2 (Paul Denniker-Joe Davis) — Vi 25830-B, *HMVSw HE2357,* HMVAu EA2155
022432-1 "SKRONTCH" -2 (Mills-Nemo-Ellington) — Vi 25834-A, HMV B.D.5387, HMVF SG.91, K8174, El EG6540
022433-1 I SIMPLY ADORE YOU -2 (Ned Wever-Paul Mann) — Vi 25830-A, *HMVSw HE2357,* HMVAu EA2155
022433-2 I SIMPLY ADORE YOU -2 — Victor unissued, 'Hold'. Issued on LP
022433: Last line of vocal chorus: -1 "I simply adore you, my adorable one."
-2 "I simply adore you, ah, you say it, rascal, you adorable one."

022434-1 THE SHEIK OF ARABY -2 — Victor unissued, 'Hold'. Issued on LP
022434-2 THE SHEIK OF ARABY -2 — Vi 25847-B, HMVAu EA2167
(Smith-Wheeler-Snyder)
022434: Opening piano solo: -1 Right hand trills in first half of solo which ends in a descending phrase as a lead-in for the band.
-2 Right hand trills in second half of solo which ends with drum beat, one beat tacit, then descending phrase as lead-in for band.

022435-1 HOLD MY HAND -1,-2 — Victor unissued, 'Hold'. Issued on LP
022435-2 HOLD MY HAND -1,-2 — Vi 26045-A, HMV JO.89, HMVF SG56, HMVAu E.A.2296, HMVIn N14030
(J.C. Johnson-Thomas "Fats" Waller)
022435: Piano solo: -1 Melody picked out by one finger of left hand whilst right hand improvises
-2 Played fully by both hands

022436-1 INSIDE (This Heart Of Mine) -2 — Victor unissued, 'Hold'. Issued on LP
022436-2 INSIDE (This Heart Of Mine) -2 — Vi 26045-B
(J.C. Johnson-Thomas "Fats" Waller)
022436: End of fourth line of vocal: -1 "...Inside this heart of mine. Yeah. B-B-Blue skies..."
-2: "...Inside this heart of mine. C'mon Baby, let me tell you something. Blue skies...'

The recording sheet for this session was not available for study, so details of studio used, time and takes made are not known. HMV HE2357 and Electrola EG6540 are issued as **"FATS" WALLER AND HIS ORCHESTRA.** Victor 25834-A and HMVF SG.91 have the additional credit **(From 4th Edition Cotton Club Parade)**. Some copies of Victor 25834-A omit the inverted commas around the title.

First artist credit shown is used on Victor 25830, 25834 and 25847-B; second on Victor 25487-A and the third on Victor 26045.

Courtney Williams, who played lead trumpet with the band, has kindly supplied his recollections of the sides made, with comments and identifications from 78 r.p.m. recordings in his own collection as follows:

In The Gloaming: This was mainly a head arrangement, with the last chorus laid out by Don Donaldson, which was made up to feature trombone player 'Shorty' Haughton. I can remember, when I hear this, seeing 'Shorty' playing it with tears in his eyes because just before we went on stage that day in the theatre, he had just gotten word that his mother had died. I'll never forget that!

You Had An Evening To Spare: This was my arrangement and was built on a current stock.

Let's Break The Good News: Probably arranged by Don Donaldson. The trumpet obbligato sounds like Herman Autrey and the solos are by Gene Sedric, Johnny 'Buggs' and 'Shorty' Haughton.

Skrontch: This is another one for which I did the arrangement. As I recall, I built it on a current stock. The clarinet obbligato is by Gene Sedric, and the solos are by Herman Autrey, George Robinson on trombone and 'Lonnie' Simmons on tenor sax

I Simply Adore You: I remember that rather well as it was another of my own arrangements.

The Sheik Of Araby: It sounds as if this arrangement was done by Don Donaldson, but I'm not sure. The solos are by 'Shorty' Haughton and Johnny 'Buggs'.

Hold My Hand: Again, this arrangement sounds like Don Donaldson. This time the solos are by Gene Sedric and Herman Autrey, whose trumpet was featured on the out chorus.

Inside (This Heart Of Mine): Arrangement by Don in his typical style. He often featured sudden, spasmodic brass figures that Johnny 'Buggs' sometimes had trouble keeping up with. This sort of displays Fats's love to play, not always jazz or raucous music, but something serious. It might have been one of his favourites because he played it quite often on the job.

*****

It was presumably this band which played the Apollo Theatre in New York from 22 April to 28 April. They were billed as "Fats" Waller and his Sensational New Band and vocalist Myra Johnson and dancer "Rubberlegs" Williams were with them. The review in the *New York Age* the following week is enthusiastic and concludes with; *The same show which he presented at Loew's State Theatre on Broadway a few weeks ago is pleasing the Harlem fans.* I have been unable to date this latter engagement.

*****

According to BBC files, the Regional Service broadcast a CBS relay by Fats Waller and his Rhythm from 7:30 to 8:00 p.m. on Tuesday 17 May 1938. The titles played were: *Marie; I'm gonna write myself a letter; Hold my hand; St. Louis Blues* (Piano); *Sweet Sue; Rosetta; Tea For Two* (Piano); *The Joint is Jumping; Honeysuckle Rose; Ain't Misbehavin'* (Signing off tune). Allowing for time difference, this would have been broadcast by CBS in the early afternoon, and may have taken place immediately prior to the tour recalled by Ed Kirkeby below, or during it.

*****

Ed Kirkeby relates in *Ain't Misbehavin'* that another southern tour came up in May which, again was a financial disaster. Among the engagements he mentions are a week in Flint, Michigan; a rural location in MIssissippi; Rochester, Indiana in mid-June and Kansas City, where Waller met up with his old buddy Count Basie. The personnel on this tour is that of the band on the recording session above plus Don Donaldson as second pianist and arranger. Also note that Nathaniel and Courtney Williams are the same person. Reports in the *International Musician* suggest two tours either side of the New York theatre dates: Local 71, Memphis, Tenn, (April); Local 256, Birmingham, Ala.; Local 257, Nashville, Tenn.; Local 694, Greenville, S.C. (all May, but March reports held over from April). Also in May is a report from Local 38, Richmond, Va., which appears to add Ted Nixon. In all these reports Donaldson's first name is given as Lyman, so 'Don' may be a nickname derived from his surname. Realising that one-nighters were not the answer to his problems, Kirkeby asked Tommy Rockwell to try and book his client into Europe and was pleasantly surprised when his deliberately high price was accepted for a ten-week tour. A rush recording date was organised at Victor to provide funds for immediate needs and to ensure a supply of new issues while Fats was away.

*****

"Fats" Waller and his Rhythm -Fox Trot Vocal refrain and piano by "Fats" Waller

Herman Autrey, t; Gene Sedric, cl-1/ts-2; Fats Waller, p/v; Al Casey, g; Cedric Wallace, sb; Slick Jones, d.

Studio No 2, New York City, New York Friday, 1 July 1938

9:30 a.m. to 1:30 p.m. Leonard Joy directing

023760-1* THERE'S HONEY ON THE MOON TONIGHT -2 (Gillespie-Davis-Coots) — Vi 25891-A, HMV B.10297, HMVAu EA2199, HMVF SG502, HMVIt HN3079

023761-1* IF I WERE YOU -2 (Buddy Bernier-Bob Emmerich) — Vi 26002-A, HMV B.D.5452, HMVF K8281, SG.96, HMVIt GW1696, HMVAu EA2223, HMVSp GY417, HMVTu AX-4089

023762-1* (Take Me Back To) THE WIDE OPEN PLACES -1 (Stillman-Bloch-Simon) — Vi 26002-B

023763-1* ON THE BUMPY ROAD TO LOVE -1 (Hoffman-Lewis-Mencher) — Vi 25898-A, HMV B.D.5431, El EG6676 HMVTu AX-4089

023764-1* FAIR AND SQUARE -1,-2 (Andy Razaf-Ada Rubin) — Vi 25891-B, HMV B.10234, HMVAu EA2199, El EG7836, ASR L.BD.5415

023765-1* WE, THE PEOPLE -1,-2 (Razaf-Denniker-Davis) — Vi 25898-B, HMVAu EA2223

The personnel is named on the recording sheet. The composer credit on some copies of Victor 26002-B is shown entirely U/C.

*****

Billy Rowe had been complaining for some time about the better bands not playing New York any more and eventually named Fats Waller and Louis Armstrong in particular and the following week mentioned that Fats was to go to Europe. The editorial pages of the *Pittsburgh Courier* also picked this up and, in three separate news items, said that Waller was leaving his band, had recorded two new Andy Razaf hits (*Fair And Square In Love* and *We The People*) and the two men had written two new hits together; *I Had To Do It* and *Stayin' At Home*..

Following the above date, preparations went ahead for the forthcoming trip abroad; the band members sought other employment for the weeks ahead and eventually, Ed Kirkeby with Fats and his wife Anita boarded the Anchor line's *S.S. Transylvania* bound for Glasgow. Although the above was Waller's final recording date prior to his European trip, he continued to work almost until the day of his departure, and a number of broadcasts are known from this period, with portions of them issued on LP.

*****

Further reports in the *International Musician* list the 14 men on the 12 April 1938 recording date plus Don Donaldson, and apparently refer to the (second) tour: Local 543, Baltimore, Md. (June); Sub Local 2, St. Louis, Mo.; Local 257, Nashville, Tenn. (both August); Local 448, Hannibal, Mo. (August). Additional reports with no personnel listed are from Local 3, Indianapolis, Ind (August and September) and Local 166, Madison, Wis. (September).

*****

C.B.S. Saturday Night Swing Club (Broadcast)

James P. Johnson, Fats Waller, p duet, vocal by Waller, and comments by both men -1
Russ Case, t; 'Toots' Mondello, cl; Fats Waller, p/v; Frank Worrell, g; Lou Shoobe, sb; Bill Gussack, percussion -2.

C.B.S. Studios, New York City, New York — Saturday, 2 July 1938

I Found A New Baby -1	Issued on LP
Hold My Hand -2	Issued on LP

There is an unidentified M.C. on the above and on the complete version, the voices of Waller and Johnson are heard between the two numbers.

*****

Fats Waller and his Rhythm (Broadcast)

Herman Autrey, t; Gene Sedric, cl-1/ts-2; Fats Waller, p/p solo-3/o-4/v-5; Al Casey, g; Cedric Wallace, sb; Slick Jones, d.

N.B.C. Studios, New York City, New York — Tuesday, 5 July 1938

Ain't Misbehavin' -2	Issued on LP
I Simply Adore You -2,-5	Issued on LP
My Best Wishes -2,-4	Issued on LP
Handful Of Keys -3	Issued on LP
Hold My Hand -1,-2,-5	Issued on LP
The Sheik Of Araby -1,-2,-5	Issued on LP
Ain't Misbehavin' -2	Issued on LP

As above — Saturday, 16 July 1938

Ain't Misbehavin' -2	Issued on LP
Hold My Hand -1,-2,-5	Issued on LP
Stop Beatin' Around The Mulberry Bush -2,-5	Issued on LP
What's The Matter With You? -2,-5	Issued on LP
Hallelujah! -3	Issued on LP
What's Your Name -2,-5	Issued on LP
Hold My Hand -2	Issued on LP

*****

It should be noted at this point that Sheldon Harris notes a date in 1938 at the Capitol Palace Cafe, New York City when Lizzie Miles was featured along with Fats Waller. This was presumably in the first half of the year as Waller was resident at the Yacht Club from the time of his return from Europe and into 1939.

*****

Fats Waller's British visits have been well documented by Howard Rye and Jo Beaton in the 'Visiting Firemen' series in *Storyville,* and I am grateful to them for permission to use their work as a basis and for additonal help in documenting these periods.

*****

Ever since Waller's aborted visit to the U.K. in 1932, there had been mutterings in the British jazz fraternity and specialist press about a visit from him and eventually the *Melody Maker* of 4 June 38 was able to report:

Fats Waller Booked For London - World's No. 1 Jazz Ace Fixed At Last

After many false alarms and keen disappointments for British dance music fans, it seems that Fats Waller will really be coming to England this year to appear in London variety. .....sudden decision of Fats to entrust his European representation to M.P.M. Entertainments Corporation of London, who are associated with Rockwell O'Keefe in America.

Leslie Macdonnell, within twenty-four hours, functioned with his usual rapidity, notwithstanding the fact that he had been advised that it was no good offering Waller anything less than his American minimum price of $500 a week. That is tough going in England among bookers who often don't know A from a bull's foot.

The alert Paradise Club immediately made bid - hi-jacked by new Home Office ruling which precludes foreign artists from working at unlicensed British premises, effect, to postpone Fats's visit till later, when doubling dates between variety and licensed establishments more opportune. Bookers of Palladium and Holborn knew all about Fats Waller and quite receptive to MPM's representations. Ciro's eager for him. Should see him at the Palladium September 12, Holborn following week, further London dates to follow and August tour on continent to precede English visit.

As will be seen, things didn't quite work out that way.

*****

Eventually, advance notice of Waller's arrival was given by Leonard Feather in the *Melody Maker* and Leslie MacDonnell, who was acting as Fats's European agent had been doing his job well, as *The Performer* of 28 July had:

Fats Waller, heavyweight coloured swing pianist, known to radio and gramophone fans this side, makes his first personal appearance in Europe when he opens at the Empire, Glasgow on Monday. The following week he commences a headlining engagement at the London Palladium.

The Saturday supplement of the *Glasgow Evening News* carried an advertisement for Fat's appearance, including a standard photo saying:

Bach is the favourite composer of Fats Waller, the seventeen-stone Swing pianist who comes to the Empire next week. But as Fats said when he arrived in Glasgow on the Anchor liner 'Transylvania', anyone who plays Bach in America would starve to death — and Fats doesn't starve, as you can see from the picture below. His Swing selections next week will include the melodies which have made him famous and his own version of Loch Lomond.

On Friday, 29 July the *SS Transylvania* arrived at Greenock (the passenger list in the PRO files, ref: BT26/1142 gives 28 July and lists the travellers as Kirkeby, Wallace T., aged 46, manager; Waller Thomas, aged 34, composer; Waller, Anita, aged 27, housewife. The address for all three is given as Empire Theatre, Glasgow.

According to Ed Kirkeby (*Ain't Misbehavin'*), the Scottish press reporters boarded the boat for the journey to [Port] Glasgow where Fats was greeted by Billy Mason's Empirex Orchestra playing on the quayside. His movements on the following day are not documented, but it may be assumed that some sightseeing took place as well as wining and dining with the locals.

On Sunday, 31 July the American trio visited the Empire Exhibition and Loch Lomond in company with Billy Mason (*Melody Maker*, 6 August & *Ain't Misbehauin'*).

On Monday, 1 August Waller opened at Glasgow Empire for a one week engagement, and reviews in the Scottish press ranged from being very warm to the rave review from the *Glasgow Evening News*, quoted by Ed Kirkeby. According to the *Melody Maker* (6 August):

> *Fats was called upon for a speech by the first house, Monday, and said "It is the greatest reception I have ever had in my life, including my own country."*

The same report went on to say that, *The theatre was so crammed on Tuesday night that every permissible foot of standing room was occupied ... brilliant pianisms ... unique singing ... inspired touches of comedy ... His swing piano playing is as much to the taste of the uninitiated as it is to the, shall we say, intelligentsia.*

Waller's perfomances included most of his own famous compositions as well as others like *Tea For Two* and *I'm Gonna Sit Right Down And Write Myself A Letter* which were associated with him. *Marie* too, features in a number of press reports both in the U.K. and the U.S. as does *Loch Lomond* which, after the success of the first performance appears to have been an essential part of his act in Scotland.

After the last house at Glasgow Empire when, according to Ed Kirkeby, Fats had to take ten curtain calls, the trio made the short journey to visit Edinburgh to catch the overnight sleeper to London (Ed Kirkeby: *Ain't* Misbehavin') — and although Ed Kirkeby says that Waller had an engagement to fulfil in Edinburgh, it appears to have been a social rather than a playing engagement as no evidence has been found for an actual performance in the city. His recollections of an uphill journey up Princes Street in an ancient taxi during which Fats fell from the taxi on a "particularly sharp curve," also appear to be misplaced as Princes Street is virtually straight and level! The description does, however, fit the road up The Mount to the Castle.

Arriving at Euston station on the morning of 7 August, they were met by Spencer Williams, who took them to his home at Sunbury-on-Thames. Leonard Feather was also present. *A Cottage In The Rain* was composed. (*Melody Maker*, 20 Aug 38)

The first London engagement began at the London Palladium for one week commencing on Monday 8 August with two houses a night at 6.25 and 9.00 p.m., matinees on Wednesdays and Thursdays at 2.30 p.m. Reviews in the trade press were generally excellent as the following two examples will show:

> *The Performer*, dated 11 August "Palladium" review of 6.25 house, 8 Aug, by A.C.E.:
> *Billed as the World's Greatest Rhythm Pianist, Fats Waller, who comes here with a great reputation gained on the other side of the Atlantic, made his debut in London Variety at the Palladium on Monday, and right from the start justified his somewhat grandiloquent titling. Portly Waller, with beetling, swivelling eyebrows that never keep still, has hands like hams, but they caress the keyboard with a tender touch, whilst for his technique there can be nothing but praise. He plays such numbers as Ain't Misbehavin' and St. Louis Blues with the touch of a master, breaks into husky-voiced coaxing of his digits when least expected, essays a spot of double keyboard work when he plays piano and celeste simultaneously, but mainly clowns along as he charms with his flowing playing. His singing is typically Harlem, his strutting likewise, but there is no denying his great and immediate popularity and his attractiveness as a pianist of the modern rhythmic school. Business,*

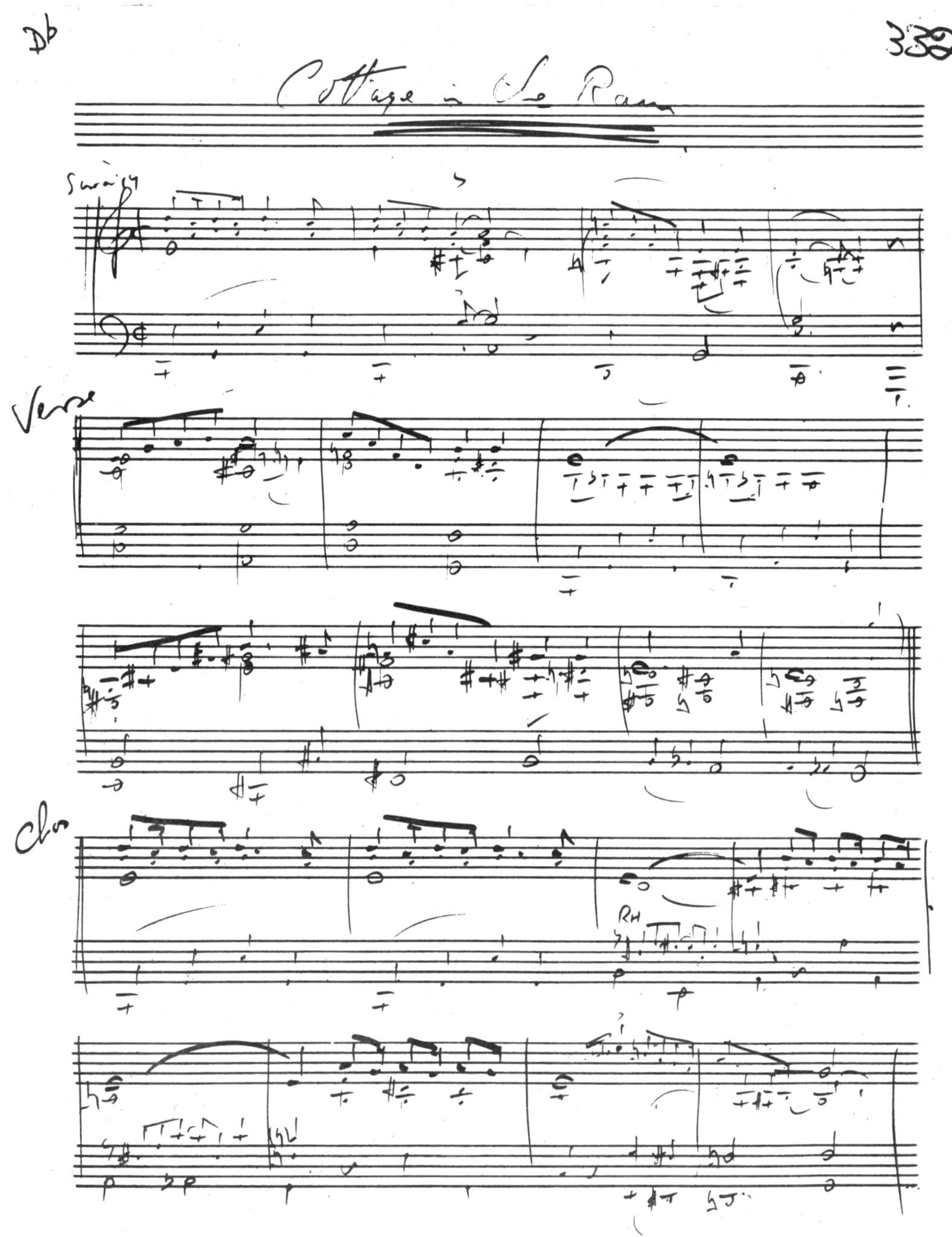

Above: Waller's original manuscript for *Cottage In The Rain.*
Right: On stage at the London Palladium during his second week.

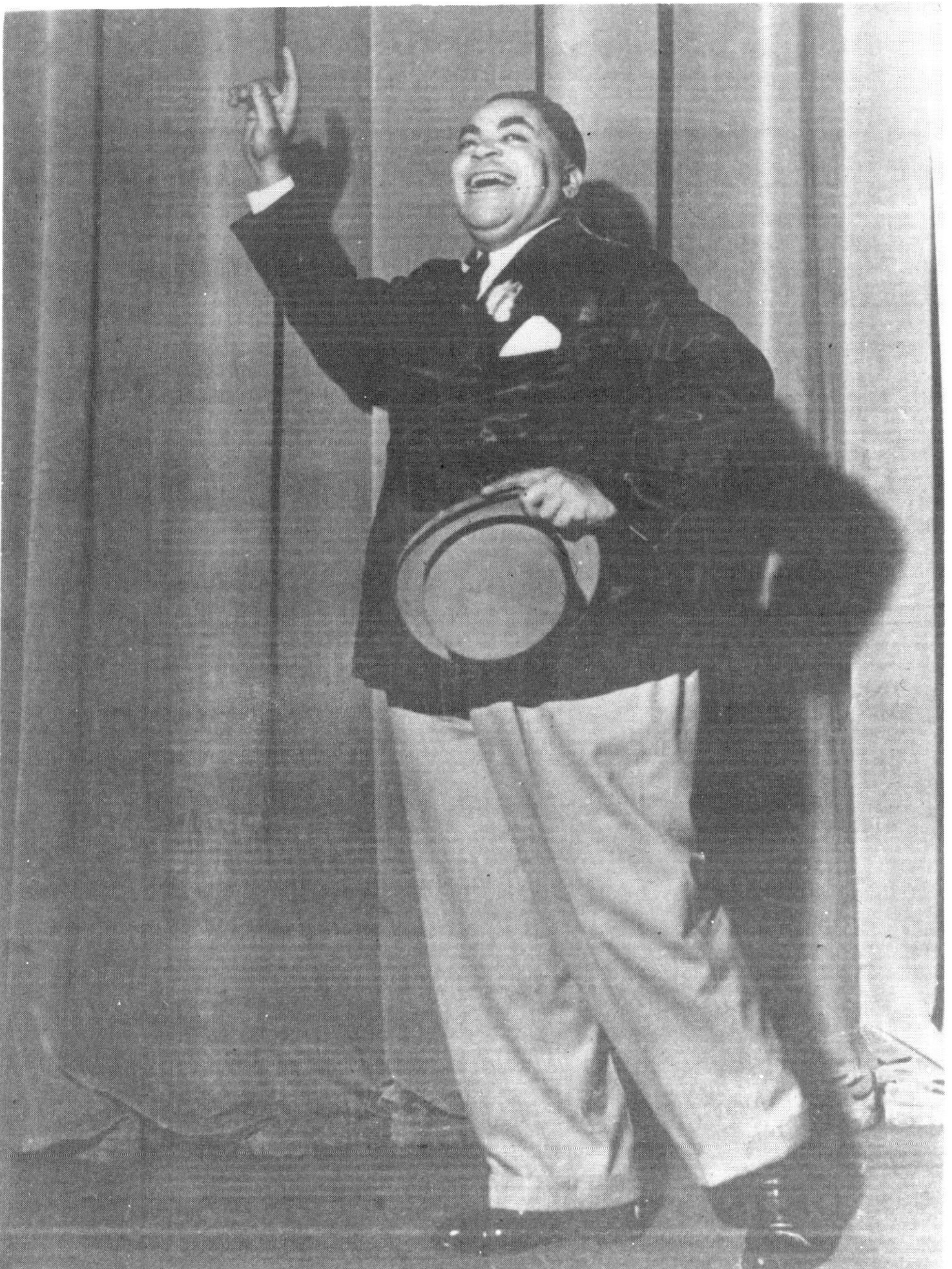

capacity, in spite of the humid weather.

The Era of the same date has a review by Frank Woolf under the heading:

Fats Waller Swings The Palladium

The long-awaited debut of Fats Waller, rhythm pianist and king of swing, was greeted with fanatical encores at the first house on Monday, and his apparently all-too-short programme was lengthened for the next house. His manner of disorganising the tune of a song is ineffably delightful, and his touch doubling on the celeste remarkably light. He is a genial fat Negro with the usual habit of muttering undertone while playing.

It should be remembered that both these reviews were for consumption by the non-jazz reader.

*****

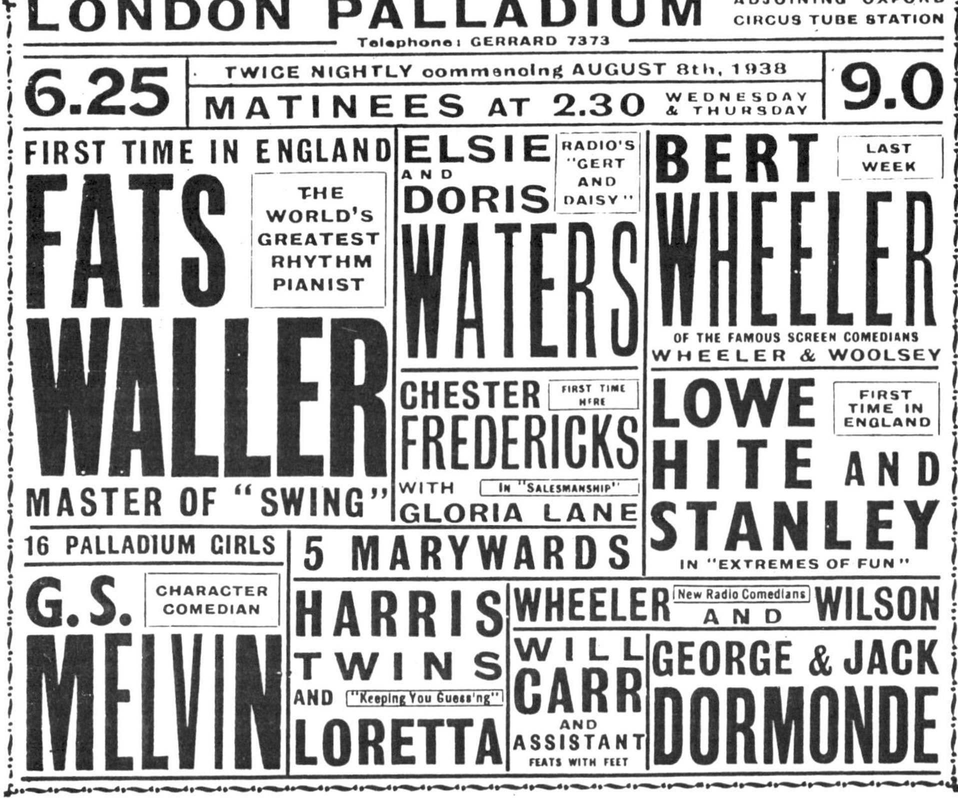
LONDON PALLADIUM
ADJOINING OXFORD CIRCUS TUBE STATION
Telephone: GERRARD 7373
6.25
TWICE NIGHTLY commencing AUGUST 8th, 1938
MATINEES AT 2.30 WEDNESDAY & THURSDAY
9.0
FIRST TIME IN ENGLAND
FATS WALLER
THE WORLD'S GREATEST RHYTHM PIANIST
MASTER OF "SWING"
ELSIE AND DORIS WATERS
RADIO'S "GERT AND DAISY"
BERT WHEELER
LAST WEEK
OF THE FAMOUS SCREEN COMEDIANS WHEELER & WOOLSEY
CHESTER FREDERICKS
FIRST TIME HERE
WITH GLORIA LANE
IN "SALESMANSHIP"
LOWE HITE AND STANLEY
FIRST TIME IN ENGLAND
IN "EXTREMES OF FUN"
16 PALLADIUM GIRLS
5 MARYWARDS
G.S. MELVIN
CHARACTER COMEDIAN
HARRIS TWINS AND LORETTA
"Keeping You Guessing"
WHEELER AND WILSON
New Radio Comedians
WILL CARR AND ASSISTANT
FEATS WITH FEET
GEORGE & JACK DORMONDE

A poster for the first week at the Palladium.

*****

Waller's first week at the Palladium proved to be so successful that he was held over for a further week: 15-20 August, and reviews were again excellent, although perhaps a little less fulsome in their praise, and the same two papers had in their 18 August editions the following:

The Performer, "Palladium" review of 6.25 house, 15 August, by A.C.E.

Fats Waller remains in the top-of-the-bill position for the second week in succession, which In itself is something of a breakdown in G.T.C. bill-spotting procedure of late. Mr. Waller is rather more subdued this week, and to the majority of variety patrons is all the more liked for it, although the rhythm fans will probably view the idea with distaste. He again coaxes melody from the white piano, goes all Harlem when he delves into song, and prances off stage this week with the additional embellishment of a grey topper. Whether you like him or not, as a rhythm pianist you have to admire his showmanship.

The Era, carries a Palladium advertisement for the 6.25 and 9.00 houses.

Sensational Hit! Fats Waller, World's Greatest Rhythm Pianist and master of swing. Change of programme this week.

And Frank Woolf in his "Palladium" review says:

Fats Waller, king of swing pianists, again roused enthusiasm amongst fans, and keen interest among others at his delightful piano playing.

*****

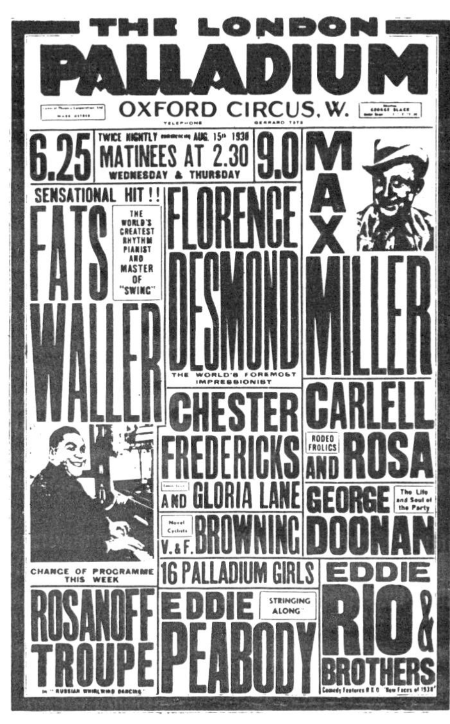

The bill for the second week at the London Palladium from15 to 20 August 1938.

"FATS" WALLER & HIS CONTINENTAL RHYTHM - SLOW FOX-TROT

(Vocal Refrain & Organ by "Fats" Waller)-9
With Vocal Ref. & Piano by "Fats" Waller -7

Dave Wilkins, t-1; George Chisholm, tb-2; Alfie Kahn, cl-3/ts-4; Ian Shepherd, ts-5/vn-6; Fats Waller, p-7/cel-8/po-9/v; Alan Ferguson,g; Len Harrison, sb; Hymie Schneider, d-10; Edmundo Ros, d-11

Abbey Road Studios, London — Sunday, 21 August 1938

6383-1	DON'T TRY YOUR JIVE ON ME -1, -2,-4,-9,-10 (Feather & Sampson)	HMV B.D.5415, HMVAu E.A.2189, HMVEi I.M.1020, El EG6839, EG7584, ASR L.BD.5415, *BB B-10100-A*
6384-1	AIN'T MISBEHAVIN' -1,-4,-9,-11	HMV Rejected. Issued on LP
6384-2	AIN'T MISBEHAVIN' -1,-4,-9,-11 (Razaf, Waller & Brooks)	HMV B.D.5415, HMVAu E.A.2189, HMVEi I.M.1020, El EG6839, EG7584, *BB/C B-10288-B*

6384: End of vocal: -1 "Savin' my love for you, for you, for you." Plus organ coda.
-2 "Savin' all my love for you, for you, for you, for you, for you, for you, for you."

6701-1	THE FLAT FOOT FLOOGEE -1,-2-3, -5,-7,-11 (Gaillard-Stewart-Green)	HMV/In B.D.5399, El EG6557
6702-1	PENT UP IN A PENTHOUSE -1,-2,-3 -6,-7,-11 (Connor & Williams)	HMV/In B.D.5399, HMVAu EA2245, El EG6557
6703-1	MUSIC, MAESTRO, PLEASE -3,-6, -7,-8,-11 (Magidson & Wrubel)	HMV/In B.D.5398, HMVAu EA2245, El EG6556
6704-1	A-TISKET, A-TASKET -1,-2,-4,-7,-11 (Ella Fitzgerald & Al Feldman)	HMV/In B.D.5398 El EG6556

The band join in the vocal chorus on the final title. Blue Bird issues as **"Fats" Waller and his Rhythm.** The issues of matrix 6384-1 all come from a test pressing 'junked' by Fred Hurlin, the original masters having been destroyed by EMI in 1964. 6703-1 bears the additional credit **(From "These Foolish Things")** and 6701 and 6704 are described as **QUICK STEP**; 6702 simply as **FOX TROT**. Copies of the EMI files held by NSA reveal that masters 6701/2/3/4 were destroyed on 16 December 1964. File cards for 6383/4 are missing. Canadian pressings of BB B-10288-B show the composer credit as (Razaf-Walter Brooks).

Irish HMV I.M.1020 is the only Irish issue inspected and, although I had assumed it would have been pressed at Hayes, it bears the legend "Pressed In Ireland".

This session was hurriedly put together with help from Leonard Feather and Leslie MacDonnell and the assistance of EMI, whose Abbey Road studios were actually closed at the time for the annual summer holiday. EMI agreed to open up for the occasion and a series of telephone calls and telegrams assembled the chosen musicians, some locally, others from very far afield. Dave Wilkins, much admired by Feather, was working with the Ken Johnson band at the Glasgow Empire, and caught the overnight sleeper to London. Others were musicians with whom Fats had jammed in visits to 'The Nest', a London night club popular with black artists and, it is claimed by Ed Kirkeby that George Chisholm even broke off his honeymoon briefly to be present. I talked at length with Dave Wilkins about the session, but his memories were a little hazy. He could recall hardly sleeping on the journey from Scotland, being met at the station and taken to Waller's apartment, where a crowd of musicians and assorted hangers-on had gathered, and then after a few drinks, going down to the studios by taxi. There was no rehearsal, no music, and the whole session was very informal and spontaneous with John Haig very much in evidence.

The first two titles were made in Studio 1, where the Compton organ was situated, then the musicians moved into studio 3 for the sides with piano, which explains the different matrix series on the session. After the session, the entire ensemble returned to the Waller apartment but Wilkins had to leave almost immediately to rejoin the Johnson band in Cardiff the next morning.

*****

Fats himself had a band call to meet on the Monday morning, for he was booked into Stratford Empire, in East London, for a one week engagement from 22 to 27 August with houses at 6.30 and 8.50 p.m. Reviews continue to be good as the following from *The Performer,* of 25 August illustrates:

> *"Stratford Empire" first house, 23 August. Upon reference to this week's programme we find that Walter Winchell, well-known American columnist, states that Fats Waller (top here this week) 'toys' with a piano. No one could have described the playing of this master of rhythm more aptly. The jovial Fats, who is a born humourist, talks cheerfully to his piano, seemingly to coax it to give of its best, scat sings with great gusto, and, best of all, plays in a manner which is entirely new to us, with a dexterous touch which seems to bring out a whole set of new sounds and shades of tone. He proves that 'Swing Music' does not necessarily mean a confused jumble of sound coming from half a dozen drums and a battery of brass. Emanating from his piano, at any rate, it is quite soothing to the ear. He is exceedingly popular here.*

*****

"FATS" WALLER (Organ Solo) -1
ADELAIDE HALL Organ Accompaniment played by "Fats" Waller -2

Fats Waller, po/vocal encouragement -2/v-3; Adelaide Hall, v-2

Studio 1, Abbey Road Studios, London — Sunday, 28 August 1938

6385-1	Swing Low, Sweet Chariot -3	HMV Rejected
6385-2	Swing Low, Sweet Chariot -3	HMV Rejected
6385-3	SWING LOW, SWEET CHARIOT -1 (Arr. Waller)	HMV/Au B.8818, El EG6647, Vi/C 27458-A
6386-1	All God's Chillun Got Wings -3	HMV Rejected
6386-2	All God's Chillun Got Wings -3	HMV Rejected
6386-3	ALL GOD'S CHILLUN GOT WINGS -1 (Arr. Waller)	HMV/Au B.8818, Vi/C/Ch 27460-B
6387-1	Go Down, Moses -3	HMV Rejected
6387-2	Go Down, Moses -3	HMV Rejected
6387-3	GO DOWN MOSES -1 (Arr. Waller)	HMV/Au B.8816, HMVF K8214, El EG6647, Vi/C 27458-B
6388-1	Deep River -3	HMV Rejected
6388-2	Deep River -3	HMV Rejected
6388-3	DEEP RIVER -1 (Arr. Waller)	HMV/Au B.8816, HMVF K8214, Vi/C 27459-A

6389-1	Water Boy -3 HMV Rejected	
6389-2	Water Boy -1 (Arr. Waller)	HMV/Au B.8845, Vi/C/Ch 27460-A
6390-1	Lonesome Road -1 (Austin & Shilkret, arr. Waller)	HMV/Au B.8845, Vi/C 27459-B
6390-2	Lonesome Road -3	HMV Rejected
6391-1	THAT OLD FEELING -2 (Brown-Fain)	HMV/Au B.8849
6392-1	I Can't Give You Anything But Love -2	HMV Rejected
6392-2	I CAN'T GIVE YOU ANYTHING BUT LOVE -2 (Fields-McHugh)	HMV/In/Au B.8849

Once again, HMV opened up the studios which were closed for the summer holiday and, as no recording had been done since Waller's visit the previous Sunday, the matrix numbers follow on consecutively. According to Ed Kirkeby, Fats been asked to record *Sometimes I Feel Like A Motherless Child*, but the emotion he felt at the loss of his mother caused him to break down and weep and he refused to attempt the title again but instead asked Adelaide Hall, who had accompanied him to the studios, to sing a couple of numbers.

In 1967, Bob Kumm wrote to EMI records asking if any of the unissued matrices from the 1938 Waller sessions had survived, and received the following in reply from Mr. R. Dockerill, then Repertoire Planning and Progress manager for the company, "The matrices of the unissued Fats Waller takes were considered redundant and therefore destroyed many years ago, and it therefore follows we are not in a position to supply copies of these." The copies of EMI files held by NSA reveal that 6389 was destroyed on 5 June 1939; 6391/2 on 23 August 1962, these latter were rejected on wear tests on 1 September 1938 (6391) and 12 January 1939 (6392), the reason in both cases being, "Vocal Blasts (20)". File cards for 6385/6/7/8 and 6390 are missing.

Victor (and Canadian Victor) reissues of these titles bear the credit **"Fats" Waller Pipe Organ Solo (Recorded in Europe)**. 27458-A has **(Old Negro Spritual)** added, and the B side has the sub title **(Let My People Go)** added. 27460-A has **(Convict Song)** added. All six sides were sold separately and also in Album P72, issued in both countries. The Chilean pressing of 27460-A shows a composer credit of (Avery Robinson).

*****

The following day, Fats began a week (29 August-3 September) doubling between Holborn Empire, London, and Finsbury Park Empire, North London. (Ed Kirkeby refers in *Ain't Misbehavin'* to "wild rides between theatres to make time schedules.") The two theatres were aproximately a ten-minute taxi-ride apart, and this involved four shows each night.

Life was hectic, even by the Waller standards, and details of two of his daytime engagements come from John Whittle, a long-time employee of EMI. His recollections of his long career were published in the April 1977 edition of *Recorded Sound* (The journal of the British Institute of Recorded Sound), and the portion concerning us is as follows:

One of my activities was to manage a company stand at the Ideal Home Exhibition. The authorities decided to let in the various musical firms and we were in an annexe hall right alongside the main exhibition, all one in effect. Earlier on I had got to know, through friends, the manager of the great jazz pianist entertainer, Thomas 'Fats Waller. We needed people of note to come to the stand to attract attention and create publicity and I managed to get 'Fats' Waller along. The occasion provided for me an unforgettable memory.

There I was, anxiously awaiting the great man, perched on the edge of the stand and peering along in the direction of the main exhibition. Suddenly I saw a cortège approaching. I should say at this juncture that whisky to 'Fats' Waller was like petrol to a car — absolutely essential. The procession approached, two by two. The first two were, of course 'Fats' Waller and the then Artists Manager of the English HMV company (you won't guess the name — unless you have heard me before) — Walter Legge. Yes, Walter Legge! He was carrying a tumbler of whisky (this was a public exhibition, remember) and the next pair included 'Fats's manager, Ed Kirkby, and he was carrying a bottle of whisky. Then came Mrs. Waller and sundry other females. There always seemed plenty of those in 'Fats' Waller's life.

I really must tell you another 'Fats' Waller story. About that time I also persuaded him to carry out the opening function of a very smart shop, The Gramophone Shop, at 130, Sloane Street, now gone alas, as also is its quixotic owner, Peter Taylor. Anyway the job was done properly. A good grand piano was hired, I greeted 'Fats' Waller outside who crashed down out of his taxi and nearly bore me to the ground (I was about ten stone then and he maybe was eighteen). He was happy, gay and generous, playing the piano for a long time, quite marvellously, I thought, as I leant on the piano watching him play. In due course he went off and it was many years before I learned the sequel to the events in Sloane Street.

Years later I again met 'Fats' Waller's manager, Ed Kirkby and he told me what happened. It seems that 'Fats' had been up all night before the shop opening and when they left (it was perhaps about 4.30), the great man had to go to the Holborn Empire, for the first house. He and his manager got into a taxi and on the way (Ed Kirkby told me) Tom (he always called him Tom) went into a great, great sleep: there was no waking him. Upon arrival at the theatre there were still some forty minutes to go so Ed told the stage door people 'stand by, don't worry, let him sleep'. And so the taxi meter ticked away and Thomas 'Fats' Waller slept. Some four or five minutes before the curtain went up, 'Fats' was somehow pummelled into consciousness, levered out of the taxi and semi-carried into the theatre, to the wings. Ed told me 'I said to Tom "Tom, you're on" and I pushed him', he said, in the direction of the piano. 'Fats' Waller went to the piano, sat down, straight away letting his fingers run over the keys. Ed said to himself 'Thank God' but (he told me) 'as I uttered that prayer of thankfulness I saw Tom fall asleep'. Fortunately he had just played enough or it was the welcoming applause that did it but he woke up and performed superbly, it appears. But I was considered the culprit for that rather terrifying incident!

Ed Kirkeby also relates the same anecdote in his book.

*****

However, there is still one, as yet undated, event which took place during this visit which may fit at this point. In a letter to a Mr. Nelson of uncertain date, but probably late 1960s, Eddie Pullen wrote from Brompton, Ontario as follows:

P.S. I recorded four titles with Fats Waller while he was over in England (I play guitar by the way) on H.M.V. label. "Honeysuckle" - "Mis-behavin'" - "Letter" - "Black & Blue" ...

Bob Kumm later corresponded with Mr. Pullen who, on searching his memory, confirmed that it was a radio broadcast for Radio Luxembourg, but he was unable to recall whether it was in 1938 or 1939. It is likely that Eddie Pullen is the "ex-professional guitarist" encountered by Jack Harvey and reported by him in *Storyville 1.* In that Jack reported that his acquaintance claimed to have recorded with Fats; that it was not at Abbey Road (i.e. not for E.M.I.) and that the records appeared with a reddish coloured label.

In a letter to *Storyville* dated 1 July 1979, Alex Andrew stated that his brother-in-law, Mickey Burberry had recalled making a transcription one Sunday morning at 9:00 a.m. at Bush House (!) with a personnel of Jack Doyle, t; Ellis Jackson, tb; himself, cl/as/bar; Frank Barnes, ts; Fats Waller, p; Eddie Pullen, g; Joe Gibson, sb; Arthur Blake, d.

Further research by Howard Rye reveals that this transcription was scheduled to be transmitted by Radio Luxembourg at 2:00 p.m. on 9 October 1938 and half an hour later by Radio Normandy. The entry in *Radio Pictorial* of 7 October 1938 lists this as:

The Kraft Show, dir by Billy Cotton, feat. Fred Duprez, with Phyllis Robins & Alan Breeze. Special Attraction: Fats Waller, America's King of Swing.

Thus, if memories are correct, we have the personnel and titles recorded, but not a firm date or place of recording, Bush House being the headquarters of the rival BBC. Doyle, Jackson, Burberry and Pullen were regular Billy Cotton bandsmen and Arthur Blake may be Arthur Baker who was his drummer. Frank Barnes had been a member of the Cotton band and thus it seems likely that he and Gibson were working the date in the orchestra. The most likely Sunday recording date, given other engagements which have been established, is 4 September, with 28 August (the date of the second visit to Abbey Road studios) also possible. It may also have taken place on 14 August, the Sunday between his two weeks at the London Palladium. It is extremely unlikely that the transcription(s) survived the war.

*****

Then for the week 5 September to 10 September, the two-theatre feat was repeated, doubling between New Cross Empire, South-East London, and Kilburn Empire, North-West London. (No reviews have been located of the Kilburn Empire appearances but they were advertised locally and there is no reason to suppose Fats did not appear.) This again involved four shows a night, but the distances involved were considerably greater. Fats was originally booked for this week at Leeds Empire (*Melody Maker,* 20 Aug 38) but this engagement was evidently cancelled. Also during this week, according to the *Melody Maker,* of 17 September, he composed *Please Find Me A Sweetheart* .

After the final show on the Saturday night (10 September), Fats broadcast to the United States over Post Office wireless telegraphy link at 0045 hours for relay by the N.B.C. network, and in the *Radio Times* of 23 September 1938, Leonard Feather reported that, *he enjoyed himself tremendously at the BBC Theatre Organ.* Adelaide Hall also appeared. (*Melody Maker,* 10 & 17 September). The broadcast was mentioned in a piece on Waller in the *Pittsburgh Courier* which, in common with other black newspapers, had commented on Waller's succes in Britain.

On Sunday, 11 September, the Wallers and Ed Kirkeby took the train to Harwich and caught the ferry from there to Vlissingen in Holland, travelling overnight en route to Scandinavia (*Melody Maker,* 3 & 17 September 1938).

*****

According to Ed Kirkeby's own account in *Ain't Misbehavin',* the trio journeyed by train through

Holland to Hamburg, where they changed trains for Copenhagen where Fats was to open his Scandinavian tour. I am deeply grateful to Morten Clausen for researching this period and the bulk of the information of the Scandinavian visit comes from him.

*****

Preparations for this tour had begun early in July when the Danish impresario Emilio G. Jacobsen had been commisioned to arrange a one week tour of Scandinavia for Fats Waller. Jacobsen, who incidentally had run his business from Spain for many years, had earlier in 1938 successfully introduced the Mills Brothers to the Scandinavians. The Danish part of that tour had been organised by Christen Sødring, who then worked for a music publishing firm called Skandinavisk og Borups Musikforlag. He and Knud Engstrøm, a former colleague, were now on the verge of establishing their own music house, the still active Engstrøm & Sødrings Musikforlag. Much of the information in this section is based on documents in the files of this firm and I'm deeply grateful to the staff for freely allowing use of this material.

The earliest document dealing with Waller in the files is a letter dated 13 July 1938, from Emilio G. Jacobsen to Christen Sødring. It's clearly not the first time the two men had discussed the coming tour, but it's also evident that no final plans had been made thus far. Jacobsen wrote:

> *...I must have Fats Waller placed in Scandinavia for at least one week. Now use your good head to find a suitable hall in Copenhagen or elsewhere, just for one day. I shall then fix the other six days in Sweden, or possibly Norway...*

The actual reason for writing the letter was however, Jacobsen wrote, a short notice in the same day's issue of the *B.T.* with the headlines: *The world's greatest jazz pianist is coming to Copenhagen - 'Fats' Waller, the brilliant show man and jazz acrobat* (sic) *announces a guest performance in Scandinavia.* The notice ends with the surprising information that: *'Fats' has applied for a work permit in England, but this has been refused. He has then decided that he'll first play in Holland, the home of the Continent's most loyal jazz youth, and subsequently he'll come to Scandinavia. If the odd thing happens that he can't get a work permit in Copenhagen either, there's always the possibility of going to Malmö to hear him - like at that time with Jimmie Lunceford. 'Fats' Waller will at all events be a huge sensation.*

'That time with Jimmie Lunceford' refers to Sunday 7 March 1937 when the *B.T.* and *Jac. Boesen's Music House* bought all 1200 tickets, and arranged transport, to Jimmie Lunceford's matinee in Malmö in Sweden.

Although most of the information in the notice, which was signed by the usually well-informed 'Maurice', proved to be wrong, it does seem to indicate that the plans for Waller's European tour were altered several times. However, on 26 July, when Fats was approaching Scotland, Sødring wrote to the State Police in Copenhagen requesting:

> *... permission for the American pianist Fats Waller, assisted by a Danish orchestra, presumably Winstrup Olesen and his Orchestra, to give four concerts on Tuesday the 13th and Thursday the 15th this year at the Odd Fellow Palæet's large auditorium.*
>
> *We can inform you that Fats Waller is regarded as the greatest living swing pianist, whose appearance in Scandinavia must be considered a first-rate sensation. His fee here is Kr. 1600 per day - regardless of the number of concerts per day.*

DKr 1600, which was about £71 or $343 in 1938, was an unusually high fee to be paid to a jazz musician in Denmark at that time. At the same time for example, Leon Abbey received only DKr 325 per day, and that was for a troupe consisting of thirteen people!

During the next month the outlines of the Scandinavian tour, which had been extended to two weeks, began to appear. On 13 August the manager of the Aarhus-Hallen in Aarhus, the second largest city in Denmark, applied for permission to present Fats Waller at a concert on 12 September on the same conditions as for the Copenhagen concerts. There were a couple of errors in his application: the date should really be 14 September and there would also be two concerts here. In Sweden the monthly paper *Orkester Journalen* reported in its September issue that Fats would give two concerts per day in Stockholm, Göteborg, Malmö, Hälsingborg, and Lund. He would play two days in Stockholm, 19 and 23 September, and would also visit Norway.

The work permit for the Copenhagen concerts was granted on 16 August, and for the Aarhus date on 12 September, both on condition that a Danish band participated.

On 20 August Emilio G. Jacobsen again wrote Christen Sødring. His long letter contained four enclosures:

l) A list of Fats Waller's repertoire, 20 numbers from which Sødring could select 10 to 12 to be played at each concert.

2) An overdue sheet of personal information to be attached to the applications for work permits. The sheet, which was never used for its intended purpose, discloses the following biographical details about Fats and his company:
Thomas Waller, born 21 May 1904 in New York, American, passport no. 570065.
Anita Waller, (his wife) born 11 October 1910 in New York, registered in her husband's passport.
Wallace Theodore Kirkeby, (Mr. Waller's manager) born 10 October 1891 in Brooklyn - New York, American, passport no. 9743.
Incidentally the name Kirkeby (meaning Church town in Danish) suggests that one of his forefathers came from Denmark or Norway.

3) The printed programme for an act called Steffani's 21 Silver Songsters.

4) A letter from Winstrup Olesen, the band leader who had been chosen to participate in the concerts.

This letter no longer exists, but it must have contained Olesen's salary claim; a claim that caused the following remarks from Jacobsen:

> *The price is sky high, which I immediately telephoned him. He said, however, that if the price was so high, it was because he expected there would be a large number of rehearsals, since he had understood that we would let him and the orchestra play with 'Fats' Waller. Accordingly he had looked for musicians who had the instruments the band on the gramophone records played. However, when he heard my explanation of the arrangement, he promised to consider the salary claim and give me the final answer in a couple of days.*

The final claim must still have been too high, for Winstrup Olesen's picked group was replaced by violinist Otto Lington and his so-called Swing Chamber Ensemble, a name apparently invented by Christen Sødring. Jacobsen continued the letter in his high-flown style by complaining about the lack of interest in Fats Waller shown by certain managers of establishments in the provinces when they heard the price. He concluded:

> *... I'm in no way what people call nervous, and it's certainly not my wish to make you*

unhappy, or paint a gale warning on the billboard but, as you probably will agree, our affairs are of that sort where you, not for one moment, must allow the various and sometimes large responsibilities to get out of sight.

I mean by this that 14 days are 14 days. Now, I'll only get 3 days in Denmark, where I had counted on at least 5 days. I have provisional arrangements for 6 or 7 days in the case of Sweden, and in all probability 2 days in Oslo; in all: 12 days. You see, I'm lacking the 2 days I thought were placed with manager Skaarup. Never mind, — it'll be all right, don't you agree?

Whether Sødring agreed or not, we don't know, but he certainly continued working on the practical side of the arrangement. One clever move was to get a large newspaper, the *Politiken,* to step in as co-organiser of the concerts. This, of course, had the great advantage of providing plenty of free publicity. The first reference to the coming event appeared in the 28 August issue of that paper:

The world's greatest jazz pianist Fats Waller to Copenhagen - The famous show man and jazz musician gives a concert on 13 September in the large auditorium of the Palace - The jazz concert is organised by the New Music House and manager Emilio G. Jacobsen in collaboration with the 'Politiken'.

The jazz youth will shout with joy at the announcement that the famous negro jazz pianist Fats Waller is coming here to give a concert in the Odd Fellow Palæet's large auditorium on Tuesday the 13th September.

It's the well-known music publisher Christen Sødring, who now has started his own independent New Music House, and the Spanish-Danish manager Emilio G. Jacobsen, who have caught Fats Waller for a tour of Scandinavia. The concert here is organized — like last year's memorable Mills Brothers performance — in co-operation with the Politiken.

Jazz enthusiasts don't need to be told who Fats Waller is, they all know him from his phenomenal gramophone records. They will immediately proclaim that he is the most famous coloured jazz pianist, a brilliant artist at the piano, a show man who is perfectly irresistible, one of the most outstanding exponents of swing music.

One only has to take a rapid glance at the picture of Fats Waller, to know that this is a gentleman who can hold our attention, and keep us in high spirits for an evening....

The paper had apparently been informed that Sødring had started a new music house, and erroneously assumed that this was the name of the firm. It also erred in stating that the Mills Brothers' concerts had taken place last year, while the fact is that they had performed in Copenhagen on 15 and 18 February and on 5 March the same year.

One week later, on 4 September, the publicity campaign really took off. This Sunday morning almost all Copenhagen's papers carried information about the forthcoming concerts.. The largest coverage was of course the *Politiken's,* whose two column article was headlined:

The greatest swing pianist of our time Fats Waller to Copenhagen — The world-famous show man will give two concerts at the large auditorium in the Palace on Tuesday the 13th September - The booking office opens tomorrow at 9 a.m. at Engstrøm & Sødring's Music House and at the Politiken's House.

The article consisted mainly of well-known information about Waller's career, obviously taken from publicity material provided by the impresario, who in turn must have received it from Ed

Kirkeby. Four sheets containing the first and rather clumsy translation of the press release still exist. They show that the material fell in two parts. The first consists of superficial descriptions of Waller's career; this came in three versions of varying length. The second part is classified 'foreword, anecdotes, and short stories'. Practically everything written about Fats in the Scandinavian papers during the tour came from this material, and practically everything is common knowledge, except perhaps the information that Fats was 5 feet 11 inches tall and weighed more than 200 lbs. An amusing error appears in the translation of the longest version of Waller's career where it claims that *he performed in piano roles for the Q.R.S. company.* Another obvious error, which however can't be blamed on the translation, is the assertion that, in the early thirties, Fats played in some of the leading night clubs in London, Paris, Berlin and Vienna. It even mentions two locations, the Kit Kat in London, and the Moulin Rouge in Paris.

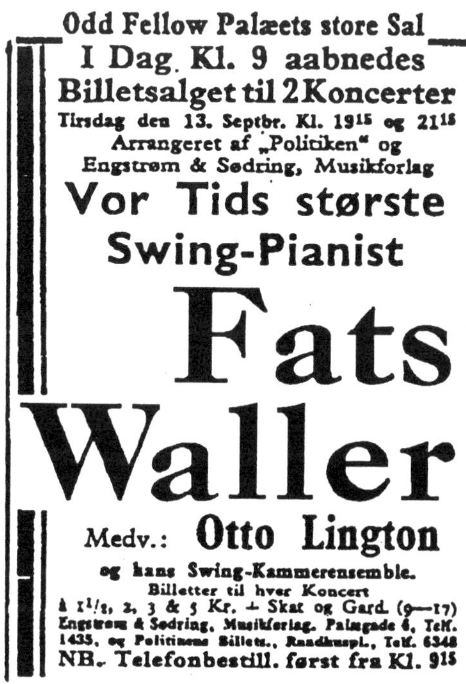

Right: Part of the advert which was placed in all the Copenhagen newspapers on 5 September 1938.

On 6 September the *Politiken* stated that soon after the booking offices had opened, almost all the tickets for the first concert, and the majority for the second, had been snapped up by the jazz interested youth. All tickets were reportedly sold by 10 September, but next day the paper proudly announced:

> *It has caused great difficulty, as Fats Waller is booked every day for a long time ahead, but his Scandinavian impresario, manager Emilio G. Jacobsen, has nevertheless managed to change the plans for the tour so that Fats Waller can return to Copenhagen*

for a single day.

This second evening — also with two concerts at 7.15 p.m. and 9.15 p.m. — takes place on Thursday the 15th in the Odd Fellow Palæet's large auditorium. On this occasion Fats Waller will also be assisted by Otto Lington's Swing Chamber Ensemble. Fats Waller will here sing a new repertoire...

The impresario's difficulties must have been negligible, since these two concerts had been planned all the time.

Then, at last, came the big day, Monday 12 September, when Fats would arrive in Copenhagen. The *Politiken* announced that:

It's expected that the Copenhagen jazz youth this afternoon will prepare a reception for Fats Waller, similar to that Louis Armstrong received some years ago. In any case, the reception at the railway station promises to be a festive occasion. Conductor Kai Ewans and his Orchestra will be playing on the platform when Fats arrives, and they will escort him with music to the Palace Hotel, where he will stay in the Prince Suite. It will undoubtedly draw many young people to the Copenhagen railway station, when the world-famous swing pianist arrives at 5.35 p.m., so the police will turn up in large numbers.

However, the *Politiken* reported next day that:

The world- famous swing pianist Fats Waller arrived in Copenhagen yesterday evening on the train from Hamburg and was greeted by many young people; but the reception was without festivity, because Kai Ewans' Orchestra didn't play, although they had promised to do so. Now Fats Waller was quickly guided through the crowd of people by policemen, and driven to the Palace Hotel in a cab.

The article finished with a small interview where the first question was about Waller's origins. He answered:

My father was a preacher in America, he preached in the Abyssinian Baptist Church in Harlem and in this church I played the organ and sang in the choir until I was 15 years old. But I had already played the piano since I was six.

Are you also a Baptist?

My father's religion has become mine too, I'm a devout believer. But chance has willed that I, being an artist, have had to perform wherever the secular life is lived. That's my bread, but back home in New York I never miss a service in my father's old church.

You play swing — what's that?

I don't know. I only know how I, myself, feel and understand swing and this I can't express, except when I'm sitting in front of the piano. But I've learned that Europe is full of swing music. This music is almost rated higher here than in America.

Fats found time to answer questions from other reporters too. To 'Prosit' from the *Social-Demokraten*, who also wanted to know what swing was, he gave a slightly different answer:

This can neither I nor any other human explain, swing is a matter of feeling, and it is with swing as it is with classical music — you either like it or you don't, it's the individual's own musical feeling that decides.

Do you like the classics?

Of course! I've been brought up on Mozart and Beethoven and this gives a jazz musician the best foundation for his art. The classics are the basis for all music since. When I have a little spare time at home I always play the classics, and my greatest joy is to play a fugue by Bach on the organ, preferably a cinema organ. Another thing is that jazz is the natural way for me to express my musical disposition, and it's more than any other music in harmony with our time.

When will jazz disappear?

Never! Today it has already created works that will live on, like 'Sweet Sue', 'Some Of These Days', 'St. Louis Blues', 'Dinah' and so on. And there will constantly appear new composers who'll write even better jazz music. It's ridiculous when people say that jazz is a passing phenomenon — it has only just begun.

To the reporter from the *Nationaltidende* Fats said that:

Symphonic jazz is nonsense, jazz can't be symphonic. We know so little about it. A hundred years from now jazz will be even more influential.

Ed Kirkeby recalled in *Ain't Misbehavin'* that the first concert in Copenhagen took place shortly after arrival, but this was clearly a slip of the memory. The first concert on the Scandinavian tour began at 7.15 p.m. on the next day, Tuesday 13 September 1938, at the Odd Fellow Palæet in Copenhagen. The printed programme shows that Sødring had selected 14 numbers to be played by Fats, the first being *Marie.*

In his sleeve notes to the 'Honeysuckle Rose' boxed set, Dan Morgenstern, then a young refugee from Austria recalls a concert in Copenhagen:

...opened by some of the better Danish jazz players, and then a huge black man came on stage, dressed in white tails and a silver top hat. He removed the hat, put it on top of the piano, and proceeded to play, sing and talk. I only knew a few words of English, but that posed no problems — Fats had me in a trance. I'd never seen anything remotely like this mountainous man in constant motion, or heard anything like the rhythms he produced with his hands, voice and whole body.

Next day almost all Copenhagen's newspapers praised Fats to the skies. It's of course not surprising that the *Politiken* critic was extremely enthusiastic in his review, which began: *The swing pianist Fats Waller had a fantastic success. A full house roared with enthusiasm for the cheerful and lovable Fats, who proved to be an outstanding jazz musician.* It's more interesting to read the review in one of the rivals, the *Nationaltidende,* who had sent its classical music expert, professor of music at the Copenhagen University Erik Abrahamsen, probably the most respected music scholar in Denmark at that time. He was definitely not known to be a jazz fan, but he could recognize talent when he heard it. He finished his review by stating that:

A competent pianist is Fats Waller, the technique is first-class, a totally superior pianist who seemed to be happier the more difficult the technical passages were. Captivating, incidentally, was his very differentiated attack, sometimes fat and heavy, as if all the stout man's weight lied in his fingers - sometimes so light and elegant that it could have been France Ellegaard playing the grand piano.

Lots of singing, lots of piano playing, lots of applause, more Lington, and more Fats Waller. A jolly evening; innocent, but of jazz pianistic interest. What a lovely left-hand technique Waller has. All the big tenth chords so beautifully clear and distinct, even in the most hazardous chromatic passages. There was a lot to learn for the jazz youth. (France Ellegaard was Denmark's leading pianist for many years.)

Right: Fats and Anita in thier Hotel room in Copenhagen on 12 September 1938

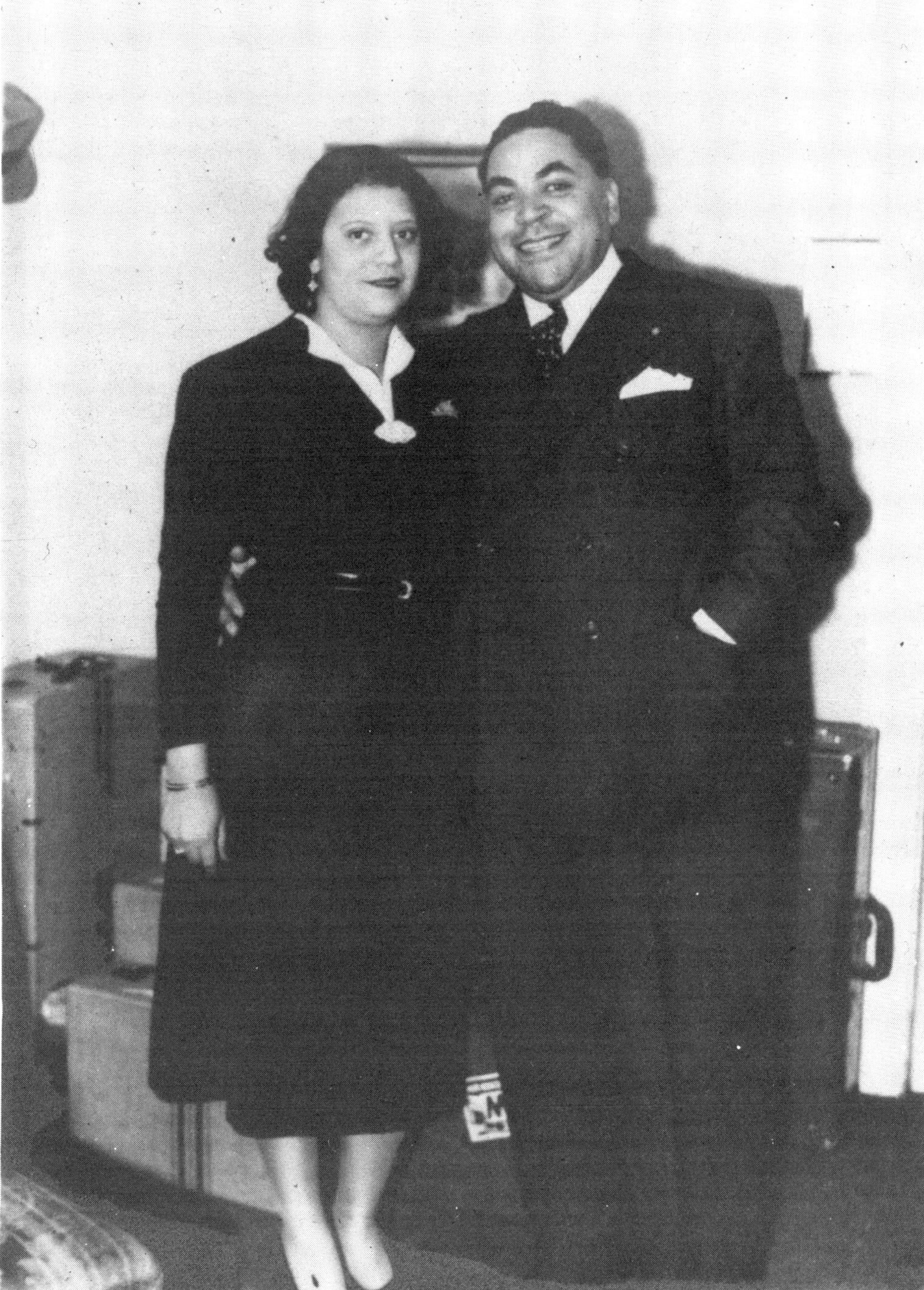

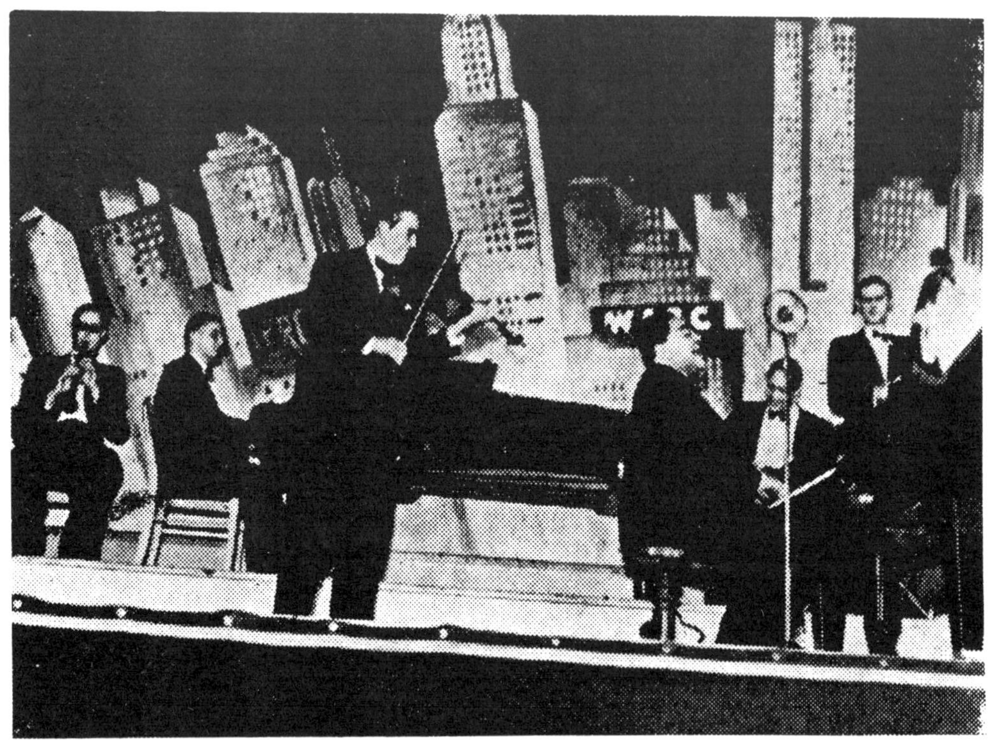

Above: Fats with Otto Lington's Swing Chamber Ensemble, probably 13 September 1938.

*****

Another interesting review was written by the well-known jazz critic Jørgen Rothenborg in the October issue of the monthly paper *Musik og Film.* He wrote, in part:

> *You cannot just include 'Fats' Waller under the more or less indeterminable host of jazz pianists; you must recognize in him the true piano virtuoso whose technique by no means is inferior to the interpreters of classical music. Those in the audience who were close to the bandstand, and who knew about these things, couldn't help noticing that Waller's fingering-, attacking-, and pedalling-technique in the more gentle passages of his performance was based entirely on the classical methods, which by and large are used and taught by Walther Gieseking, the famous Mozart interpreter, and it was extremely interesting to notice how little this fact weakened Waller's music in respect to its jazz value ... It would be pointless to enumerate all 'Fats's numbers, so I'll confine myself to mention only the few that were in the absolutely grand manner. First and foremost his interpretation of 'I Ain't Got Nobody', played the way it's played 'In Harlem at 5 in the morning when you mustn't wake the neighbours'; this was a number 'Fats' invented at his last concert, and I've never heard such elegance at a grand piano before. 'Fats' gave, with an incredibly soft and delicate attack, his hitherto best performance including all his*

> *countless records. This was worth the whole concert. Even the magnificent numbers 'Ain't Misbehavin'', 'Hallelujah', 'Basin Street Blues', and 'Loch Lomond' had to give up compared to this wonderful performance....*

The use of Otto Lington's Swing Chamber Ensemble as warm-up act, instead of Winstrup Olesen's Orchestra, was, according to Rothenborg, a total disaster:

> *Otto Lington, who once had a name as jazz conductor, albeit not quite justified, ventured to offer a performance, which in less friendly countries would have resulted in an immediate use of the hook which drags the duds off stage at amateur contests. You can't of course blame the musicians for not being able to do more than their abilities allow, but you can definitely demand that they've done some homework, and don't rattle off some rubbish which wouldn't even justify a placing at a second-rate amateur contest. Lack of accurate ensemble playing, bad and not thoroughly prepared solos, wrong chords and tedious attempts to be funny, seem to have been the standard of Otto Lington's performance.*

It must have been a relief to Fats that this band only accompanied him in one number, *Truckin'*, which was given as encore.

Among the newspapers that reviewed the concerts on the day after, only the *Aftenbladet* was a little negative. They wrote that:

> *... his playing reminded one a little too much of a competent — although very competent — bar pianist, rather than of a world-famous swinger. Perhaps he should have brought his own band along. As a soloist he fills — despite all his skill and outstanding technique — too little in a concert hall. He would have been brilliant in a night club.*

One of the more curious reviews appeared in the *B.T.*; perhaps it explains the origin of a still quite popular habit among Danish jazz buffs:

> *... I sat among the enthusiastic youth last night in the Odd Fellow Palæet and enjoyed 'Fats' Waller. It was fantastic. Enchanting was the modest, yet preposterously charming way in which he acted ... but what I really want to tell about here, was his performance of the number 'Sheik of Araby', one of the last.*
>
> *I don't think Copenhagen has ever witnessed a choir like the one that sang along on the refrain here. 'Fats' explained that 'The Sheik' wasn't one of his best things, but he did like it all the same. He just asked the audience to fall in with a certain refrain when he gave the signal. It turned out that we should all yell: 'He ain't got no pants on', each time 'Fats' had mentioned the sheik.*
>
> *It had a most strange effect. Our own 'Fats' Cornelius (who has a certain resemblance to Waller at the piano) led the singing from the second row and was bravely seconded by the entire neighbourhood. When 'Fats' finally sang with his wheezing voice about the sheik, who advanced through the desert sand, and the choir again went: 'ain't got no pants on', the atmosphere in the auditorium was comparable to what can be experienced in Harlem on the big nights.*

There seems thus to be no question about the success of Waller's Scandinavian debut, and a statement from the box office furthermore shows that close to 1500 tickets were sold for each concert, which means full house.

Wednesday morning the trio travelled by train and boat to Aarhus, on the east coast of Jutland, where Fats was to play two concerts in the evening. The reception this time was definitely a festive occasion. Several hundred people greeted Fats as soon as he went ashore, and Svend Asmussen's Five Swing Fans provided hot music. The well-known photo of Fats and Svend (below) comes from this occasion.

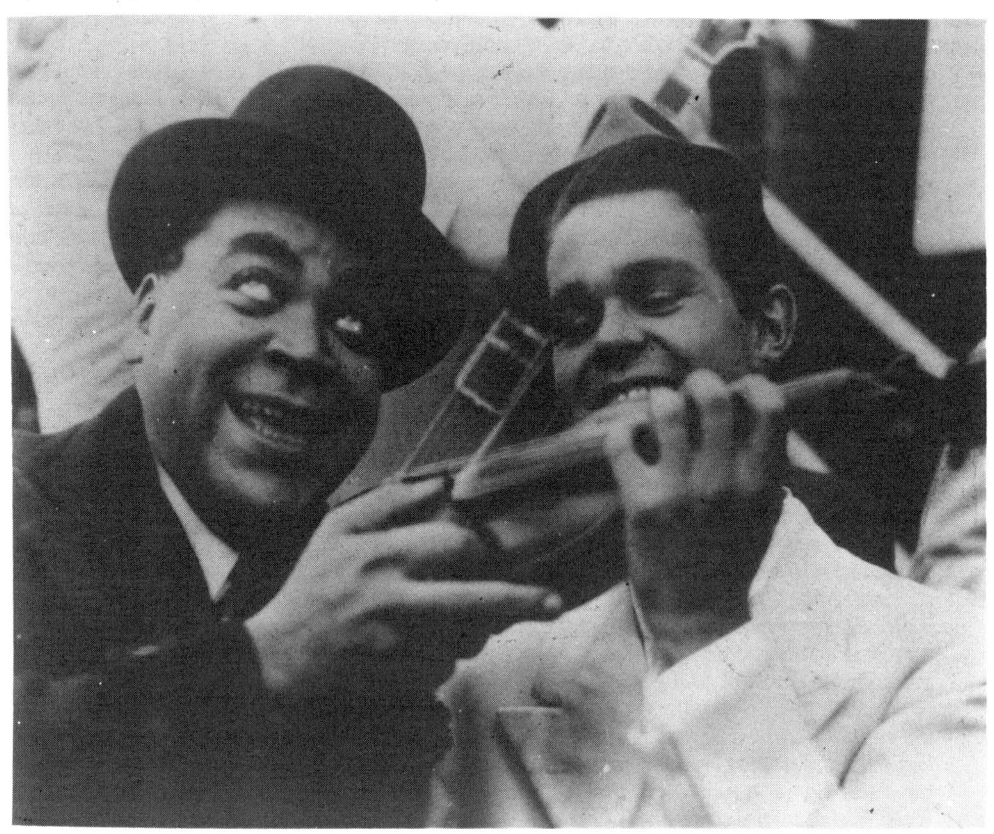

*****

The Aarhus public had been informed about Waller's arrival on 4 September when the *Aarhus Stiftstidende* wrote:

> *World-famous jazz pianist to Aarhus. Wednesday the 14th this month manager Westergaard Hansen presents the first of the planned world attractions in the first 'real' season at the Aarhus-Hallen: The world's best jazz pianist, Fats Waller ... Fats Waller himself is at the piano and he is accompanied by the Svend Asmussen Quintet, who will accompany the negro star on his Scandinavian tour....*

The last piece of information supports Ed Kirkeby's statement in *Ain't Misbehavin'*, that violinist Svend Asmussen backed Waller for two weeks through Norway and Sweden, but it's not correct. It is, however, quite possible that that had been the original intention. Asmussen, who had been playing in Aarhus-Hallen's Restaurant since 1 August and was to finish his engagement there on 15 September, seems to have had no engagements lined up for the following weeks, and he had previously assisted the Mills Brothers on their tour. He was however in Copenhagen while Fats toured Norway and Sweden.

There was incidentally some confusion as to who should actually perform with Waller in Aarhus, as the following extracts from a letter, dated 3 September 1938, from Christen Sødring to Svend Asmussen indicate:

Well, everything is now settled as you wished, but it's a mere coincidence that it worked out this way, and only because of willingness from all sides. Why on earth haven't you sent me one single word informing me that you had got permission? ... I had only understood from Aarhus that there were certain difficulties and doubts. Furthermore, when I heard that you'd recently suggested the negro orchestra from the National Scala, I felt convinced that you'd given up the thought. We had neither discussed the conditions, the programme, and the form, not even a single word, so I had come to believe that it wasn't topical anymore.

Luckily I hadn't definitely promised Lington Aarhus, but I had told him that I considered it very likely that we would ask him to come along ...

Now I ask you to let me know your programme as soon as possible. The duration will be as with the Mills Brothers, you can count on 15 - 16 minutes twice per concert. Perhaps a little less. Your salary will be Kr. 250 for both concerts.

A probable reason for the confusion may have been that, although the concerts were organized by the manager in Aarhus in co-operation with Engstrøm & Sødring in Copenhagen, the impresario had promised Svend Asmussen that his band should assist, and neglected to inform Sødring. The negro orchestra mentioned was Bobby Martin's, which had played at the National Scala in Copenhagen from 16 to 31 August. From 1 September they had played at the Roxy in Aalborg, about 100 kms north of Aarhus. It was an interesting idea to have them back Fats, but unfortunately not realistic, since they had their own job to take care of.

On 6 September the manager from the Aarhus-Hallen wrote a short note to Sødring, to inform him that the booking office would open next morning and that he'd written to six newspapers in other cities in Jutland and offered them 200 tickets each, so that they could arrange party tours to 'the titbit Fats Waller'. The papers had reacted enthusiastically.

Six days later the *Aarhus Stiftstidende* reported that:

The American negro pianist Fats Waller, who'll give two concerts in the Aarhus-Hallen on Wednesday, is the first real jazz celebrity to visit Aarhus. Some years ago we heard a well-known saxophonist Coleman Hawkins, who was a big success. Now we have a visit from a fine Dutch-American band, Ady Rosner, but Fats Waller certainly surpasses all the others. Whatever you may think of him, no one can doubt the genuineness of his world success.

All tickets are already sold to Fats Waller's concerts in Copenhagen on Tuesday evening, but what will the people of Aarhus think about the 120 kg heavy, 5 feet 11 inches tall negro pianist?

The answer was in the papers on 15 September. Under the signature 'dix' the critic from the *Jyllandsposten* wrote a bizarre, but well-intentioned review:

It was mainly the young people who'd shown up, of course. It is after all to the youth that

PROGRAM:

1. Rhythm is our business.
   Stardust.
   My blue heaven.

Svend Asmussens five Swing-fans.

---

2. Marie.
   Write myself a letter.
   St. Louis Blues.
   I ain't got nobody.
   Flat Foot Floogee.
   Lock Lomond.
   Sweet Sue.

FATS WALLER

Pause.

---

3. Snake charmer.
   Medley over Melodierne fra »Snehvide«.
   I got rhythm.

Svend Asmussens five Swing-fans.

---

4. Tea for Two.
   Ain't misbehavin'.
   Basin St. Blues.
   Hallelujah.
   Honeysuckle Rose.
   Handfull of Keys.
   Sheik of Araby.

FATS WALLER

Part of the programme for the Aarhus-Hallen concert on 14 September 1938. The programme is a single folded sheet using the photo on page 116 as a cover and the remainder taken up with advertising. It sold for 25 Øre.

jazz appeals the most. The more mature generation was however also represented, and it looked as if it surrendered during the evening, in company with the young people who were carried away from the first minute. ...

Fats Waller won the audience with a musicality quite out of the ordinary, which makes us understand the three stars the American music world has put above his name. A soft and delicate execution, followed by the queerest triads and discords, was forced into the captivating 4/4 rhythm, which hypnotizes because it speaks to the mind's most primitive music perception. Now and then he sang with a hoarse, but friendly voice, and sitting in the hall were Ady Rosner's American musicians who helped him with the refrain to the 'Sheik of Araby'.

For Svend Asmussen and his small competent swing orchestra, the evening was a great victory. The jazz experts in the audience understood that it was a union of colleagues in the — to us still — dark realm of jazz, when Fats Waller and Asmussen's orchestra played together in the finale.

Apart from Asmussen on violin, the band consisted of Knut Knutssøn, cl/ts; Børge Nordlund, p; Helge Jacobsen, g; and Alfred Rasmussen, sb. Ady Rosner's Orchestra played at the Regina Caféen from 9 to 15 September.

The reporter from the *Aarhus Stiftstidende* was however not entirely satisfied:

... Fats Waller is a jazz pianist, known and admired for a long line of records where his playing usually has been part of a brilliant ensemble, with occasional solo performances. We got him as soloist, and although the soloist Fats Waller was both extremely competent and funny, he wasn't unforgettable. He is in reality less of a swing man — as the term is nowadays — he is rather a sumptuous piano player. Time and time again there was more classicism and 'salon' than real jazz in his playing. You felt this in, for example, his own excellent and very jazzy 'Ain't Misbehavin'', where the entire introduction strongly reminded one of Rachmaninoff. Likewise Waller displayed a technical skill in other numbers which could easily cope with the most difficult of Chopin's etudes. There were magnificent details — primarily in 'St. Louis Blues', Waller's most perfect performance at the first concert, but also in 'Tea For Two' and 'Basin St. Blues'....

The same issue carried a small informative notice which told the readers that:

Fats Waller has left. After his concerts last night Fats Waller celebrated in the Aarhus-Hallen's Restaurant with his wife, his American impresario Wallace T. Kirkeby, and his Danish impresario Emilio G. Jacobsen.

The patrons forced the stout vigorous musician to play for them, which he did with much willingness. Early this morning Fats caught the express train to Copenhagen where he will give two farewell concerts tonight.

There may have been good reasons for Fats and the impresarios to celebrate, but for the organizers there wasn't, as Westergaard Hansen wrote, with poorly concealed bitterness, to Christen Sødring on 19 September:

Enclosed I send the interim accounts for Fats Waller's concert and I must say that it's a colossal disappointment to me. I believe you're right when you say in the letter I received today, and for which I thank you, that it was the fear of war and unrest in general, that made people run completely amuck, so that we in reality didn't sell anything.

I assure you that we have done our best over here, our conscience is clear in that respect....

The interim accounts show that out of 6000 tickets only 1388 had been sold. The management had however given away a rather large number of free tickets, so that in all 2330 Aarhusians had heard Fats play, which wasn't a bad result seen from his side. However, when the final accounts were presented on 31 October, they showed that the two concerts only had given the organizers a profit of Kr. o.49, less than 6 pence!

As already mentioned, the trio returned to Copenhagen by train on 15 September. With a bit of luck they could have run into Leon Abbey's 'Swing-Time 1938 Show' at the Central Railway Station, for this troupe arrived the same afternoon from Stockholm on their way to Vejle, about 70 kms south west of Aarhus.

Waller's two concerts that evening took place without much publicity. Apart from advertisements only the *Politiken* carried a little information:

There has probably never been such uproarious applause in the Palace's large over-crowded auditorium as to Fats Waller's first two concerts, and now tonight the famous swing pianist takes leave of Copenhagen and sets out to new triumphs in the world. The chances are that we'll probably never hear him again. So we'll have to make use of this occasion. ...

Tonight Fats Waller will present a new repertoire and will again be assisted by Otto Lington and his Swing Chamber Ensemble.

The top story in the papers that day was Chamberlain's meeting with Hitler at Berchtesgaden, and it seems that the unstable political situation affected Copenhagen too and kept many people at home, listening to the news on the radio. For the first house at 7.15 p.m. only half of the tickets were sold, and for the second at 9.15 p.m. two thirds.

Despite the threat of war Fats continued the tour as planned and next morning the trio journeyed by train up through Sweden to Oslo in Norway. That same day *Dagbladet* reported:

Fats Waller arrives this evening. It will probably be a youthful crowd that today will go down to the Lodge's large auditorium to listen to the greatest swing pianist ever seen — as the Copenhagen papers have characterised Fats Waller. It's just too bad, his Danish impresario says, that the famous negro has made such a tight plan for his tour that he's unable to exploit the success. Tonight at 7.15 p.m. he jumps off the Copenhagen train and goes directly to the Lodge, where no less than two concerts, one at 8 p.m. and one at 10 p.m. awaits him. Now we're curious to know if Oslo will become equally enthusiastic. Oslo is known to be a good jazz city — so why not?

It seems likely that Ed Kirkeby's recollection of having had to hurry from the railway station to the concert hall, took place here in Oslo instead of in Copenhagen, as he wrote in *Ain't Misbehavin'.*

The organizers of the concerts in Oslo, *Brødrene Hals Konsertbureau,* had hired the large auditorium at the Logen for Friday the 16th and Saturday the 17th. There were two concerts planned each day; Friday, as already mentioned, at 8 p.m. and 10 p.m. and Saturday at 7 p.m. and 9 p.m. Two jazz singers, Cecil Aagaard ('the biggest thing in swing') and Freddy Valier, who also played the guitar, were on the bill with Fats, but no orchestra was mentioned, neither in advertisements nor in reviews. It's likely, though, that a small unit accompanied the two singers.

The first house Friday evening was reviewed next day in the *Aftenposten*:

One thing is clear: It was a jazz concert of higher quality than previously heard in Oslo. At the moment Fats Waller stepped on the platform a roar of applause broke out — and with his first number 'Marie' he swept the audience off their feet — as a comedian. For, to tell the truth, one has to search a long time to find such charm and such a funny face. When he plays it looks as if he's sitting having a pleasant time in his own double chin, and his eyebrows go up and down like drumsticks.

He could safely have put the comedy part aside - for his triumph was first and last gained by his outstanding piano playing. Old chestnuts like 'St. Louis Blues' and 'I Ain't Got Nobody' were performed with fresh and personal liberty and a superior technique. A little Scottish song 'Loch Lomond' reminded one of the clear transparent sound of a spinet. Or 'Sweet Sue' - sophisticated and sparklingly clear — from the softest soft pianissimo to the heaviest fortissimo — he has striking power in his hands, Fats Waller.

We could name more, for example 'Tea For Two'; his own composition 'Ain't Misbehavin''; and last but not least 'Honeysuckle Rose' where he really displays his skill and demonstrates his versatility.

The publicity material mentioned that he plays classical music. We would love to hear that.

Cecil Aagaard and Freddy Valier assisted at the concert.

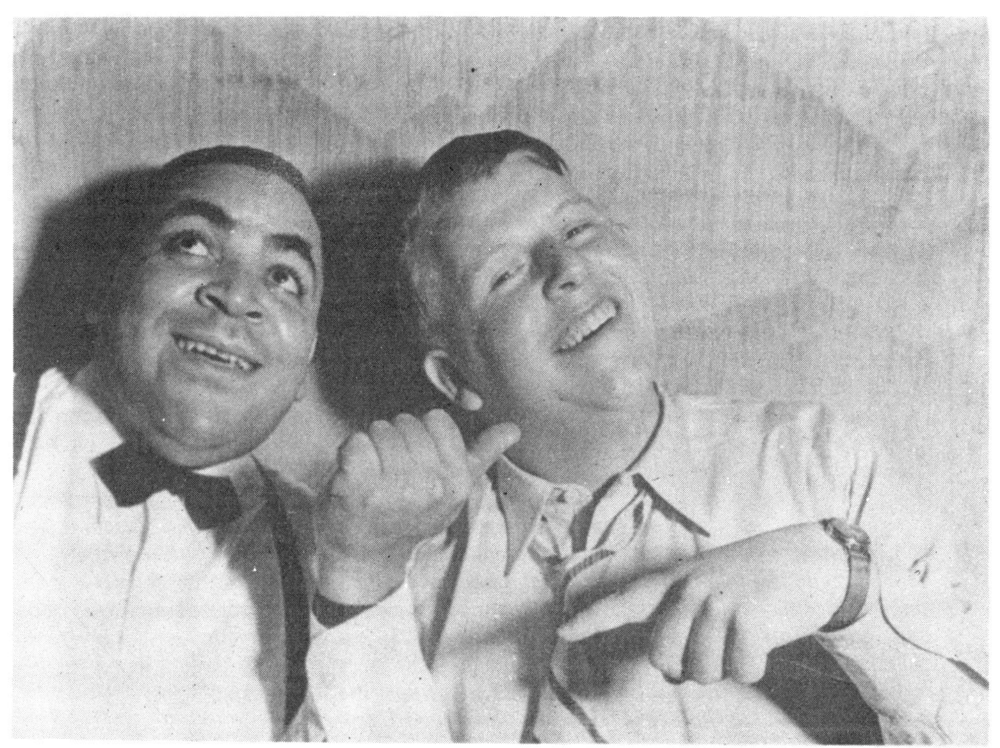

The second house Friday evening was reviewed by Pauline Hall who came directly from a classical concert. Her opinion appeared in the next day's issue of the *Dagbladet*:

> *Late last night after the orchestral concert a music critic's way led to the Logen where Fats Waller had his fling. He's called 'the world's greatest swing pianist', but he usually makes a show of not knowing what swing is, and this may bring some comfort to other ignorants.*
>
> *Fats is first of all a fantastic pianist, he could probably play the majority of his serious colleagues under the grand piano if he wanted. Secondly, he is a musician of the finest sort, his piano execution is so beautiful and discreet that one has to be a monomaniac jazz hater to deny it.*
>
> *He also sings, hoarse and pleasant — and yet very musical. And of course, he's a comedian from top to toe, and from the first second in contact with his audience. Fats is something of an oddity with his fantastic joy of music. He's worth hearing, this brown gentleman of swing.*

Fats repeated the two concerts next day and then departed for Stockholm where he was to open the Swedish part of the tour at 7.15 p.m. on Monday 19 September at the large concert hall the Auditorium. The intervening Sunday is the only day of the tour where no performances have been located. The probability of an unknown engagement on that day is however very small and the odds are that most of the Sunday was spent on the train from Oslo to Stockholm.

The organizers of the Swedish tour were an agency called *Konsertbolaget.* On 1 September they had made an application to the Kungl. Socialstyrelsen in Stockholm requesting permission for Thomas Waller to take up employment in Sweden between 17 and 29 September 1938. The applicant explained that 'Thomas Waller will give a number of concerts in Stockholm, Göteborg and some provincial towns during the said period'. The application was granted on 5 September and one week later the work permit was sent to the Swedish Legation in Copenhagen so that Fats could pick it up before leaving Denmark.

As warm-up act on the tour the *Konsertbolaget* presented a popular Swedish singer, Sonia Estelle, who seems to have been completely misplaced in this connection, according to reviews. Gösta Wallenius' Swing Band was added for the Stockholm concerts only.

The opening performance was reviewed in the Stockholm papers on 20 September. The *Dagens Nyheter* reported that:

> *Both Fats Waller's seances were well attended. We have heard him time and time again on the gramophone in combination with different orchestras. That's where he's best; as a soloist he's a little monotonous in the long run because of his limited harmonics. But otherwise he's a brilliant pianist of his kind. His greatest virtue is his delicate rhythm, easy, flexible and elastic in a way which is in astonishing contrast to his stout body. Moreover, apart from one or two sketchy digressions, his playing has nothing of the 'tempo di-sturb the neighbours' as he noted one of his compositions; it's in general quite subdued. That he nevertheless managed to keep the listeners in suspense shows his qualifications.*
>
> *He could however disturb the neighbours by means of his so-called singing; when he sings one of his songs about love's all-conquering powers, it's reminiscent of the sounds one could imagine uttered by a middle-aged jovial, but somewhat boisterous chimpanzee....*

The review in the *Svenska Dagbladet* was also written with mixed feelings:

> *It can be noted that Mr. Waller occasionally played jazz which even to reluctant ears was*

quite enjoyable, and where the rhythm even submitted to, or in a pleasant way mingled with, the melodic element. But I doubt that the voluminous and broadly grinning negro pianist has been elected 'radio- and swing-star' only by virtue of his musical talents. In any case he won over the solid majority of the young people at the Auditorium just as much by his grotesque — but too stereotyped — facial expressions, his smug yells and his highly-strung appearance.

It was in other words negro amusement for big children, who wanted to be entertained by all means — even the most simple tricks. And fun we had, so the applause washed like a foaming sea over the big woolly haired child on the platform....

Fats continued to Göteborg (Gothenburg) on the west coast of Sweden where he gave two poorly-attended concerts at 7.15 p.m. and 9.15 p.m. at the Konserthuset on 20 September. The review in the *Göteborgs Handels- och Sjöfarts-Tidning* was on a level with the Stockholm reviews:

The King of Swing proved to be a grimacing and hooting cabaret star of the most vigorous kind. He has composed a great deal of his numbers himself and is technically full-grown. That he has a feeling for rhythm was demonstrated incessantly. The singing, or whatever his affectation shall be called, was anything else but pretty, but the audience seemed to enjoy his clown act. Even his parodies of Beethoven and Brahms were appreciated. It was woolly haired and broadly grimacing negro amusement at the Konserthuset, and not just normal entertainment.

Next day Fats played two concerts at the Hippodromteatern in Malmö, the Swedish city just opposite Copenhagen. One of the houses was reviewed by Sten Broman in the 22 September issue of the *Sydsvenska Dagbladet.* Broman was a well-known figure on the Swedish music scene. A viola playing composer of both orchestral works and of chamber music, as well as a much respected scholar of music, and for many years chairman of the Swedish section of the International Society of Contemporary Music. He demonstrated his educational faculties in the 70's when he managed to make a classical music quiz one of the most popular TV programmes in Scandinavia. Part of his review read:

The jazz performance yesterday at the Hipp had a bad start. The audience was surprisingly small and the atmosphere not exactly high during the first part of the programme, which was singing by Sonia Estelle. It was a small act. ...

But then came the pleasant Fats Waller who turned up the atmosphere all at once. Such a big negro (or half ditto?) will of course smash up the keys immediately, one thought. Negroes usually play with extreme power, especially on the trumpet. But this Waller was completely different. He played soft and discreet, had an astonishingly elegant technique and furthermore, gave examples of a most unusually well-developed sense of rhythmical finesses. ...

We have seldomly heard such fluent jazz piano playing. The rhythm was broken and accentuated in an absolutely masterly way with surprisingly small and accurate means, and it's also evident that Waller is not only an excellent performer but also a gifted creator. He played variations on familiar jazz themes, even on own compositions as for example the excellent 'Ain't Misbehavin", and exactly this ability to vary the harmonics and the rhythm made us listen to his playing with sincere delight. He also tried to play variations in the style of Bach, Beethoven and Brahms (according to his own statement), but this was not successful. All these 'variations' reminded a bit of, was Chopin. But never mind. When it all reminded of Waller himself, it was excellent. The audience stamped their feet and applauded enthusiastically. If Fats Waller returns to Malmö, there will certainly be a full house.

Fats never returned, but there was a full house at his next concert, and as it took place in Lund only 16 kms north east of Malmö, it's possible that Broman's prophecy was of some importance after all. The concert, which took place at 8 p.m. on 22 September at the Universitetets Aula (the University's Assembly Hall), was favourably reviewed by the *Lunds Dagblad* next day:

Fats Waller is a glorious revelation. With his brilliant fingering-technique he is in total control of his instrument and with an incredible attacking-technique he manages to produce an endless number of shades. And all this technique is an obedient servant to his phenomenal and imaginative timbre.

On 23 September Fats was back in Stockholm where he once again gave two concerts at the Auditorium. Nils Hellström, the then editor of the *Orkester Journalen* wrote a review of these and the previous concerts, which appeared in the October issue of that paper. I'm grateful to Alf Lavér for translating this:

A Clown - but an outstanding pianist.

Fats Waller made a great success - but to a small audience.

We, who already knew Mr Waller's great record output, possibly feared a let down, but on the contrary, it was not so. After his performances one left the Auditorium in the best of spirits, very sure that one had heard one of the world's truly great jazz personalities.

Fats Waller's name appears so often in this paper, that it seems hardly necessary to write a review of his performance, as one knows almost every number in his programme. Someone has said that Fats is not an improvisor in the recognised sense, but that he very carefully rehearses his solos before his appearances before the public. That may be so, because his solos on both performances were exactly the same; this is unimportant if the final result is satisfactory. And that it is when Fats is at the piano.

Unfortunately, his concerts in Stockholm were not very well attended The first day was quite good, but the second day was very poorly attended indeed. A pity. It is not difficult to find explanations for that sorry state, because September is a dull month for concerts in Stockholm and a solo pianist always finds it harder to draw a good audience, even if it is Fats. Possibly a large orchestra might and, as a third drawback, the supporting orchestra meant nothing to the jazz-going public. I'm afraid to say that although Gösta Wallenius is respected in music circles here in Sweden, no one has ever heard of him connected with Swing before. The paying public knows exactly what it wants for its money, so there you are. The band was not even a regular organisation, but a "pick-up band" just for this tour. Furthermore Miss Sonja Estelle is not a swing-artist, the public knew this and, although she is well known from radio and records, there's no swing. You can't fool an audience with ads that a "Swing Artist" is on the stage. That she is a competent singer when it comes to popular songs is another matter. I do hope that the arranger of these concerts takes note that the public at jazz concerts is just as discerning as any other music audience. It is impossible to put an popular song artist into the jazz idiom. The acoustics in the Auditorium are definitely bad, no matter where you are, the

Right: The Auditorium programme showing all four pages

OPERAKÄLLAREN
STOCKHOLM
Lunch från kr. 2: 10.
Middag från kr. 2: 65.
Supé från kr. 2: 40.
Dans tisdag, torsdag.

GRAND HÔTEL
STOCKHOLM
Enkelrum fr. kr. 6:-. Dubbelrum fr. kr. 12:- 15 % reduktion vid längre eller ofta upprepad vistelse. Betjäningsavgift. Lunch fr. kr. 2: 10. Middag fr. kr. 4: —.
Supé från kr. 2: 40
Dans onsdag och fredag.

HASSELBACKEN
STOCKHOLM
Under vintern
endast för fester.

Tel.: 10 43 50, 20 78 59, 10 78 59

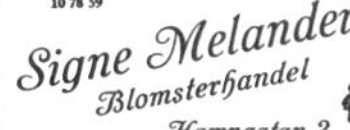

Signe Melanders
Blomsterhandel
Hamngatan 2

Edra trycksaker
beställas med fördel hos
Soneson & Rydells Boktryckeri
Stureg. 17, Sundbyberg. Tel. 280445, 281000

BOKTRYCK
OFFSET
STÅLTRYCK

Ivar Hæggströms Boktryckeri A.B.
Gamla Brogatan 26, Stockholm
Telefon Namnanrop: Ivar Hæggströms

Nästa konsert

Auditorium
Fred. den 23 kl. 7.15 o. 9.15

"Fats" Waller

Sista konserterna!

Bilj. i Konserthuset, hos Elkan & Schildknecht, tidn. depeschbyråer och N. K.

För musiker med världsrykte är
PAM SAMSONS ljudsystem
oumbärligt. Hör det i kväll.
Levererat av **AMPERITE CORP. A. B.**
Vartavägen 33. Tel. 61 22 62 o. 62 65 27.

Centrum RADIO
– mottagaren med den underbara tonen

RATIONELL REKLAM

För att i förväg kunna räkna med ett ekonomiskt lönande resultat måste reklamen utarbetas rationellt. Vi analysera marknaden och varan, sedan utarbeta vi de olika reklamenheterna och placera dem där de nå konsumenterna. Vi bygga upp kampanjer på basis av erfarenheter och ständigt förnyade studier.

A.-B. SVENSKA TELEGRAMBYRÅNS ANNONSAVDELNING
STOCKHOLM / GÖTEBORG / MALMÖ / HÄLSINGBORG

SÅNGPEDAGOGEN
GERTRUD GRUBBSTRÖM(-GRÖNBERG)
STOCKHOLM, ODENGATAN 45.
Telefon 33 10 00 (helst kl. 12–13)
Individuell röstutbildning.
Kyrkosång, Romans,
Opera, Operett.
★ *Talteknik. Röststörningar (heshet, sveda, slembildning, stämbandsknutar o. dyl.) bortarbetas.*

NYMAN & SCHULTZ
RESEBUREAU A/B

NAMNANROP:
NYMANS RESEBYRÅ
ARSENALSGATAN 9,
STOCKHOLM.

ordnar alla Edra resor. Tåg-, båt- o. flygbiljetter över hela världen. Kostnadsfria reseförslag. Växelkontor.

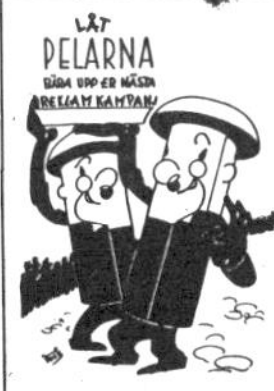

Affischplatserna som »hela Stockholm» ser.

FOTOGRAFISKA AKTIEBOLAGET
KUNGSGATAN 17, STOCKHOLM
Ring KARLÉN!
Tel. 230515

Program

"Fats" Waller

Konsertbolaget
Säsong 1938—1939

STOCKHOLMS PRIVATA KONSERVATORIUM

SVEAVÄGEN 33. Ledning: **TEL. 10 42 69**
Gurli Krüger / Felix Saul / Stina Sundell

★ *Undervisning på alla stadier, i alla stadsdelar, på alla instrument.*
Studiecirklar i sång. Uppfostran till musikalitet. Intressanta föreläsningar.

Låt barnen börja i tid i våra roliga, effektiva gruppiektioner.

Pressomdömen: »... ganska förbluffande saker, som presterades.» *(Aftonbladet.)* • »Det var en glädje att höra de säkra ungdomarna och se att musiken var dem själva till verklig glädje.» *(Soc.-Dem.)*

Strand Hotell
Stockholm
Trevligaste hotell *Intimaste matsal*

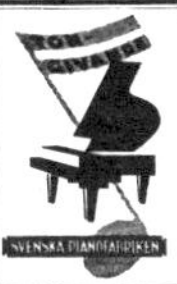

Generalagent för
AUGUST FÖRSTER
sedan mer än 80 år världsmärket inom flygel- och pianobranschen.
STOCKHOLM
AUDITORIUM
Tel. 10 28 82. 10 28 85.

BLÜTHNER

De senaste modellerna – Mignon och Baby – äga trots de små dimensionerna den världsberömda, säreget charmfulla Blüthner-klangen.
Ensamförsäljare: Kungl. Hovleverantör.
A/B J. LUDV. OHLSONS PIANOMAGASIN
Etabl. 1856. Verkst. dir.: Disponent George Lindahl
KONSERTHUSET

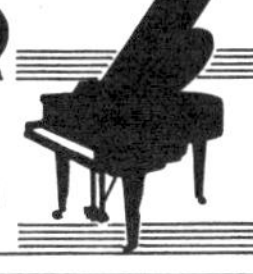

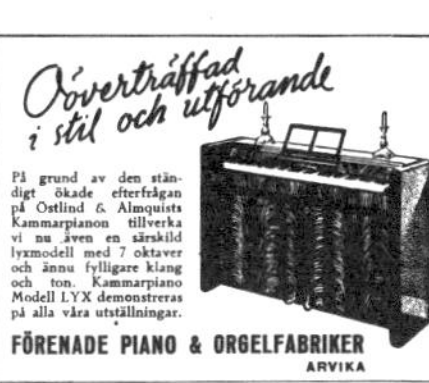

Oöverträffad i stil och utförande

På grund av den ständigt ökade efterfrågan på Östlind & Almquists Kammarpianon tillverka vi nu även en särskild lyxmodell med 7 oktaver och ännu fylligare klang och ton. Kammarpiano Modell LYX demonstreras på alla våra utställningar.

FÖRENADE PIANO & ORGELFABRIKER
ARVIKA

HÖR
Alla Världens Stora Konstnärer
på

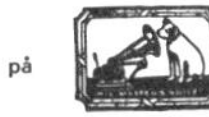

"HUSBONDENS RÖST"
HIS MASTER'S VOICE

AUDITORIUM

»FATS» WALLER

(»THE KING OF SWING»)

Medverkande: GÖSTA WALLENIUS' SWING-BAND

Chinatown .. .. *Schwarz*
You can't swing a love song .. .. *Gaby Rogers*
I'm a ding dong daddy *Phill Baxter*
Ain't misbegavin' .. .. *»Fats» Waller*

Marie .. .. *Irwing Berlin*
Write myself a letter *Young & Ahlert*
St. Louis Blues .. .. .. *W. C. Handy*
I ain't got nobody .. *Spencer Williams*
Flat Foot Floogee .. .. *Slim & Slam*

Lock Lomond .. .. .. *Folkvisa*
Sweet Sue .. .. *Victor Young*

– Kort paus –

If I had You .. .. .. *Reg Conelly*
Mr. Jinx .. .. *Larry Clinton*
Ja – Da .. .. *Bob Carleton*
Rhythm in my nursery rhymes .. .. *Lunceford*

Tea for Two .. .. *V. Youmans*
Ain't misbehavin' .. *»Fats» Waller*
Basin St. Blues .. .. *Spencer Williams*
Halleluja .. .. *V. Youmans*
Honeysuckle Rose .. *»Fats» Waller*

Handfull of Keys .. .. *»Fats» Waller*
Sheik of Araby .. .. *Ted Snyder*

Steinway-flygel från Lundholms

HÆGGSTRÖMS, STHLM 383719

Se sista sidan!

»Fats» Waller spelar endast för »HUSBONDENS RÖST.»
PAM SAMSONS LJUDSYSTEM användes.

Ni som älskar musik — unna Er glädjen av att äga en **Centrum RADIO**

Köp värdefull musik på skivor!
Kompletta verk ur klassiska repertoaren av världens förnämsta mästare föras ständigt i lager, även för automatiska skivbytare.
REGERINGSGATAN 26, STOCKHOLM

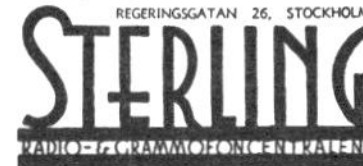

KARL WOHLFARTS MUSIKSKOLA

Läroämnen: Piano, sång, violin, violoncell, harmoni, orgel, allmän musiklära, kontrapunkt, komposition, instrumentation, musikdiktat, fraseringslära, solfège, musikhistoria.
Lärareutbildningskurser i piano finnas.

Överlärare vid skolan äro:
i piano **Karl Wohlfart;**
i violin **Professor Julius Ruthström;**
i violoncell **Bror Persfelt;**
i orgel **Gustaf Nordqvist.**

HUVUDLOKAL: **SKEPPAREGATAN 3.**
Telefoner: 61 11 01, 61 11 02.
Mottagning för anmälningar varje dag kl. 12–1.

Rich. Anderssons Musikskola

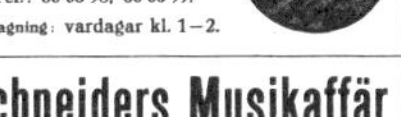

Förest.: ASTRID BERWALD
Huvudavdelning:
Humlegårdsgat. 11, 1 tr.
Tel.: 60 03 98, 60 03 99.
Mottagning: vardagar kl. 1–2.

Schneiders Musikaffär
Fiolbyggare
JAKOBSBERGSGATAN 6 (invid Biblioteksg.)
Tel. 10 60 17. Grundad 1885.
Stråk- och Stränginstrument
Ensamförsäljare av Thomastik-strängar.

STEINWAY
FLYGLAR PIANON

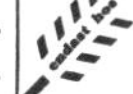

PIANO-
LUNDHOLMS
REGERINGSGATAN 9

BECHSTEIN

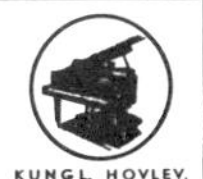

AUG. HOFFMANN FLYGEL- OCH PIANOFABRIK MALMSKILLNADSGATAN 33. KUNGL. HOVLEV. Tel. 20 16 06, 10 16 61

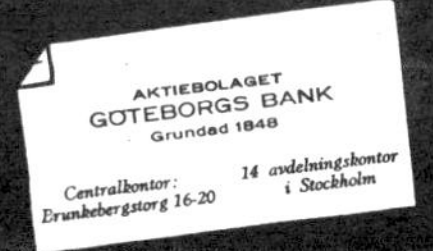

orchestra will sound like thunder. The orchestra played 8 swing arrangements, all of them up-tempo. The trumpeter, Mr Rune Ander took some very nice solos, and thereby put some raisins into the cake.

The personel of the Orchestra is: Rune Ander, t; Folke Emanuelsson, Carl Erik Jaerde and Olle Henriksson, saxes; Gösta Wallenius, p; Torsten Johansson, sb; Sven Mattesson, g; Sture Åberg, d.

The orchestra performed stock arrangements of Chinatown, My Chinatown; You Can't Swing A Love Song, I'm A Ding Dong Daddy, Ain't Misbehavin, If I Had You, Mr Jinx, Ja-da, and Rhythm In My Nursery Rhymes.

Following this domestic performance by the orchestra, we arrived at Fats Waller's programme. He performed the following tunes in his own special style:

Marie, Write Myself A Letter, St. Louis Blues, I Ain't Got Nobody, Flat Foot Floogee, Loch Lomond, Sweet Sue, Tea For Two, Ain't Misbehavin', Basin Street Blues, Hallelujah, Honeysuckle Rose, Handful Of Keys, and with the orchestra Sheik Of Araby and Dinah.

Fats's style on the piano is well known and he's not taking things too seriously, as we all know; he's scatting, making funny faces, telling jokes and so forth while playing. He's a clown, maybe it is a part of himself, but also that he knows that it pays well in the end. But if you ignore all this nonsense he played some wonderful solos. Maybe because he had to concentrate more, the best was his Loch Lomond, performed in utmost pianissimo. Most of the numbers were performed with real swing, so massive but floating. When it comes to the more stompy numbers he was shouting and displayed his fast licks on the keyboard. We all know this from most of his recordings.

Fats backstage was a real comedian with robust clowning with all and sundry. A very likeable person. He told me something which I did not know before; that he had studied piano in Vienna around 1920. He arrived there together with his friend and trombone player Herbert Flemming, and another boy who was playing violin. All the three boys were not more than 15 years old, and the teacher was very severe towards them. Fats got so many hits on his fingers that he barely managed the scales, and the violinist got his violin banged on his head, and the violin was broken in smithereens. "It didn't matter," commented Fats, "he got a new and much better one."

Fats was very surprised that the audience was so enthusiastic and gave him such an ovation. He told me that in The States he didn't get such a response.

It seems certain that the report of Fats having studied in Vienna is the result of a language problem in the noise of the back-stage revelries. What Fats probably said was that he had studied piano with a professor from Vienna. Actually, the press release states that Fats had studied music for eight years under Godowsky from Vienna and Carl Bohn from New York (other sources spell the latter's name as Bohm). It seems extremely unlikely that the Waller family could have afforded the transatlantic fare for their son at that time and, given Edward Waller's resistance to his son's wish to become a musician, it seems unlikely even had funds been available; there is no other reference known to me for this excursion and Herb Flemming was certainly in New York during the period given by Fats.

The Swedish part of the Scandinavian tour finished on 24 September with two concerts at the Konserthuset in Hälsingborg just opposite Helsingør (Elsinore) in Denmark. One of the houses, which weren't too well-attended, was reviewed next day under the headline 'Swing party at the Konserthuset yesterday' in the *Helsingborgs Dagblad.* The commendatory review concluded that:

> *Fats Waller had to give several encores and we went home without having in any way regretted the visit. On the contrary, we could have stayed for another hour and still have had a pleasant time.*

After the last house the trio travelled by boat and train to Copenhagen where Fats was to give no less than three concerts in one day. It seems that the plans for these were made rather late and it's possible that they only came about because Fats didn't want to travel through Germany. Clearly, some changes of plan had occured as the advert overleaf for an appearance in Belgium indicates. It comes from a programme by Ambrose and his Orchestra (courtesy of Robert Pernet, Léon Dierckx and Georges Debroe) which took place on 7 August 1938 in the Théatre des Variétés in Brussels so that Waller's appearance had been contracted prior to that date. However, the concert with the Ramblers never took place.

Whatever the reason, on 21 September Christen Sødring had mailed the following application to the State Police in Copenhagen:

> *We hereby permit ourselves to apply for permission to give 3 concerts on Sunday the 25th September at 4,7 and 9.15 p.m. with the American pianist Fats Waller, assisted by conductor Otto Lington and his Swing Ensemble.*
>
> *Fats Waller's fee is Kr. 1600 for all three concerts.*
>
> *Since the Fats Waller concerts Thursday 15 this month disappointed, because of the threatening foreign situation which made people stay at home, we would very much like to make use of an opportunity that has appeared because Fats Waller will come here on his return journey to England.*
>
> *As the concerts, if permission is granted, will take place already on Sunday, we will be very grateful for an immediate handling of the matter. The concerts will, like the previous concerts, take place in co-operation with the 'Politiken'.*

The permission was granted two days later so that Fats could finish his Scandinavian tour where it had begun, at the Odd Fellow Palæet in Copenhagen. The *Social-Demokraten* reported on 26 September that:

> *Yesterday the vigorous and cheerful swing pianist Fats Waller took final leave of the Copenhagen jazz audience with 3 concerts at the Odd Fellow Palæet, and all 3 concerts were well-attended. As previously he took the crowds by storm with his eminent piano playing and his impressive rhythm, and he displayed a sparkling humour which infected the listeners. After the last concert he thanked the audience for their kind reception and said that the Copenhagen crowds were the best he had played to in Scandinavia.*

The Wallers and Kirkeby left Copenhagen on Monday 26 September, exactly two weeks after their arrival. The original intention had probably been to travel overland through Germany, play the Brussels date and maybe tour Belgium and the Netherlands, and then cross the Channel, but, taking the unstable political situation into consideration, the odds are that they chose to travel directly to England from Denmark. The most likely way would be to catch the train to Esbjerg, on the west coast of Jutland, and then board the daily ferry to Harwich which sailed at 5.45 p.m. By using this method of transportation the trio could have been in London on the evening of Tuesday 27 September.

*****

Amateurs de Jazz
une date à retenir !

Lundi 26 Septembre proch.
en la grande salle de la
Zoologie à Anvers

Unique soirée en Belgique avec :

Le célèbre pianiste Américain

Fatts WALLER

et l'Orchestre

The RAMBLER'S

Places de Frs. 10.- à 40.-
Location ovuerte à partir du 1 septembre à la Maison FAES - 16, Marché aux Souliers, Anvers
(On peut inscrire pour des places dès à présent)

According to Ed Kirkeby, the threat of war in Europe was such that the party decided to cut short their tour, playing three dance hall jobs before returning to Britain and fitting in three more dance hall appearances and Fats's first ever TV programme whilst waiting for their ship.

Clearly, as noted above, some changes of plan had occurred. It may have been the original intention to travel overland from Stockholm; play the Belgian concert on the 26th September; cross the Channel to Dover and then on to Brighton. All that is known for the moment is that the trio were back in Britain by Wednesday, 28 September for a cabaret appearance in Brighton on the south coast and, since no port of arrival nor any departure point from the continent has been confirmed (passenger lists, if they ever existed, no longer survive), it is possible that they flew rather than travelled by boat. At that time, Croydon was the airport for London and it was but a short journey from there to Brighton, where Waller appeared in cabaret at Sherry's, Middle Street, Brighton, with Sherry's Swing Quintet. As noted above, had the journey from Scandinavia been by ship, the nearest port of arrival would have been Harwich and although train connections were good from Copenhagen to Esbjerg and from Harwich to London, they would not have arrived before evening and would presumably have stayed the night in the city. Had they arrived at Croydon, they would most likely have gone straight on to Brighton. Waller's appearance in Brighton is confirmed by the following report in the *Brighton Evening Argus* of 29 September:

> *Great Reception For 'King of Swing' at Sherry's, Middle Street, Brighton, yesterday evening.*
>
> *The hall was packed and the large crowd of dancers and spectators simply would not let him go. He gave encore after encore, and ended with a session of swing music, accompanied by Sherry's swing quintet.*
>
> *Among the songs he sang was Pent Up In A Penthouse, one that he has made famous. Fats returned from Scandinavia to play at Sherry's and it is the first ballroom in which he has played since he came to Europe.*
>
> *Not only is Fats Waller a wonderful pianist, he is also a great comedian and singer.*

Sherry's was presumably the first of the three dance hall bookings recalled by Ed Kirkeby and Streatham Locarno and the Royal in Tottenham (announced in the *Melody Maker* of 3 September) are presumably the others. However, his statement that the threat of war caused the Scandinavian tour to be cut short is called into question as arrangements for a number of engagements seem to have been concluded prior to the departure for the continent and the party seem to have returned as scheduled. Likewise with the case of the broadcast with Jay Wilbur, copy would have had to be submitted some time in advance for it to have appeared in the *Radio Times* — a weekly BBC publication detailing the forthcoming programmes, and the same is true of the advert appearing in the *Tottenham and Edmonton Weekly Herald.* On the other hand, the European trip in toto may well have been curtailed because of the Munich crisis, but even that may be queried in the light of the following.

The entry in the *Radio Times* issue of 23 September for 29 September is:

> *Thursday Regional 8.00 Jay Wilbur and his band in Melody Out Of The Sky with Sam Costa, The Mad Hatters, Charles Smart at the organ. Guest Artist Thomas 'Fats' Waller (The King of Swing). Fats Waller returns to the US this week after a highly successful visit here. Those listeners who have admired, from gramophone records, the style of this master of rhythmic piano playing will perhaps be interested to known that his musical*

career began as a church organist. Tonight it is hoped that he may be induced to play one number on the organ.

Although this broadcast was scheduled for the Regional Programme at 8.00 p.m.it was actually transmitted on the National Programme at 5.00 p.m. according to Charles Fox (*Fats Waller).* The BBC's Broadcast Log Sheet shows that the programme was from 4.45$^1/_2$ - 5.30 p.m. so that Charles Fox's diary may well be correct that Fats actually came on the air at 5.00 p.m. The Log Sheet shows that he was down to play *Marie* (piano & vocal); *Hallelujah* (piano); *Pent up in a penthouse* (piano with orchestra & vocal) and *Flat Foot Floogie* (piano with orchestra & vocal). The personnel of the orchestra is shown as "14 instrumentalists + Jay Wilbur".

No confirmation that Waller actually made the scheduled appearance at Streatham Locarno has been found, nor for that at the Royal in Tottenham although for the latter he was clearly expected as an advert for the dance hall in the *Tottenham and Edmonton Weekly Herald* of 23 September has:

Thursday next. Personal appearance of Fats Waller, World's Greatest Rhythm Pianist. Also Rumba Competition with Norman Binick and Vera Stickland.

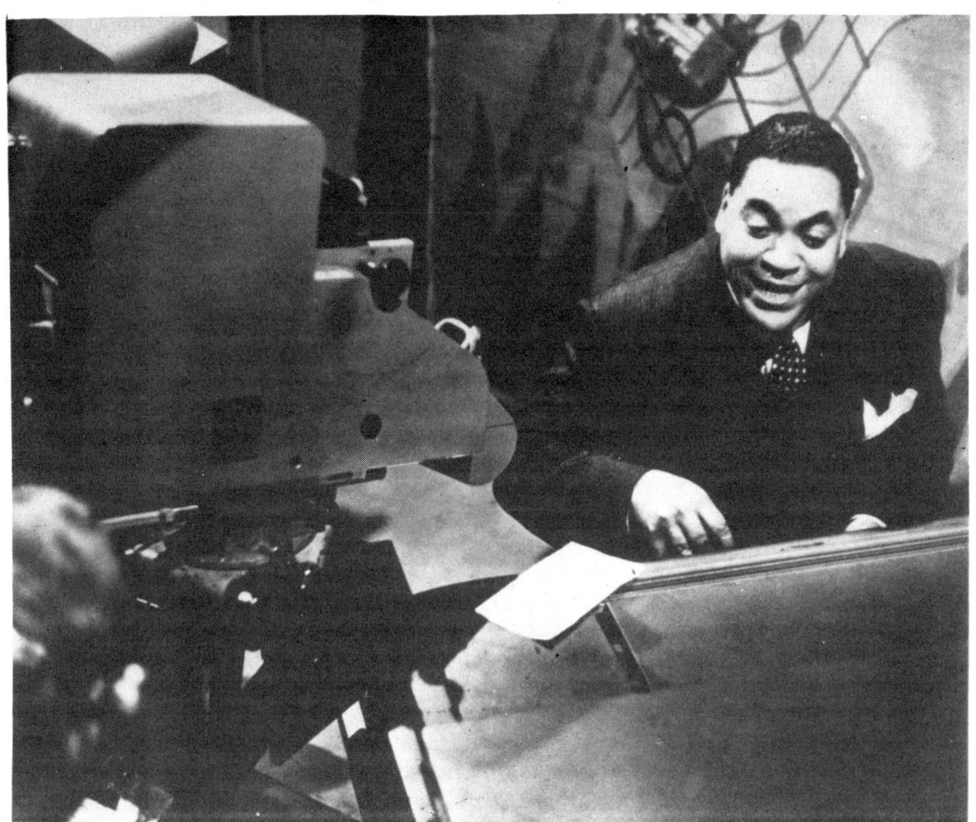

Two shots of Fats in the Alexandra Palace studios

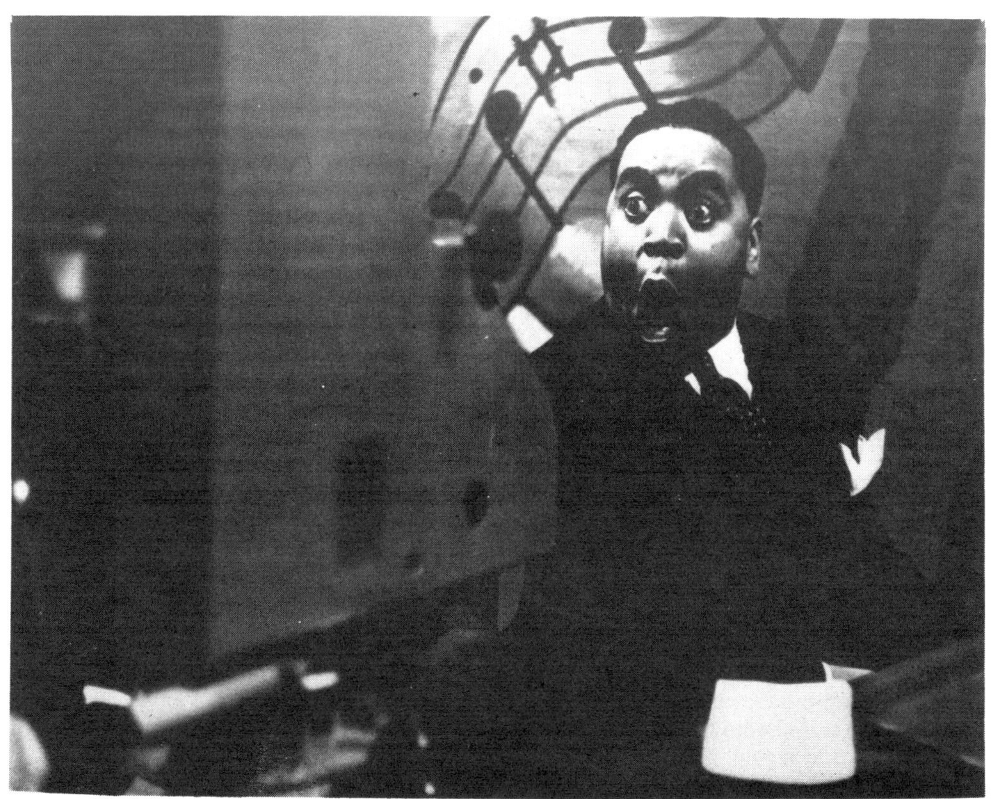

Fats appeared on Television for the first time during his British visit. Ed Kirkeby told Bob Kumm that the appearance was on the 'Starlight' programme, hosted by Dallas Bower and transmitted from the Alexandra Palace studios at 9.00 p.m. on Friday, 30 September 1938. However, the *Radio Times* indicates that the scheduled programme for that time was a news film and investigation shows that no 'Starlight' programme was scheduled for that week. In fact, the only scheduled 'Starlight' programme during Waller's stay in Britain was on 7 September and, since Waller was dashing back and forth between New Cross and Kilburn and videotape was a thing of the future, that can safely be ruled out. Subsequent investigation of the BBC's own files by Howard Rye confirms Kirkeby's recollections in all respects and it appears that the BBC schedule was changed at short notice to take advantage of Waller's presence after the *Radio Times* had gone to press. The rearranged timing sheet for the programme shows that the programme opened at 21.00 with the chimes of Big Ben and a time signal which took 1 minute and 6 seconds, and then Waller, shown as *Songs at the Piano*, was listed to play five numbers: *I'm crazy about my Baby; Honeysuckle Rose; Neglected; Hallelujah* and *Truckin'*. Since the BBC worked to very strictly timed schedules in those days, it may be presumed that Waller had been present for a rehearsal earlier in the day.

This TV show was Waller's final public appearance on this European tour, and the following day, Saturday, 1 October, the party boarded the *Ile de France* at Southampton for the journey back to the United States. The PRO, ref: BT27/1528 confirms the date, and notes the departure address for all three as 32 Duke Street, London, W.1.

*****

Whilst he had been away, there had been numerous reports of Waller's successes in Europe in the American black press, which merely echoed the reports in the European papers, and there had also been concern expressed at the deteriorating international situation and the threat of war. Waller's return was first mentioned by Billy Rowe on 8 October when he said that Fats would return 'this week and round up his orchestra for an immediate engagement at the Yacht Club', which he said would be his first 'nitery engagement in the Broadway locality'. The actual return date was reported in the *Pittsburgh Courier* of 15 October which, in a piece datelined New York Oct. 13, stated that he had returned 'Friday nite' (7 October), and would shortly be taking a band into the Yacht Club which was 'seemingly going colored with a vengeance this year.'

Back in New York, Fats enjoyed a few days rest and then re-assembled his little group and went into the Yacht Club in its new location at 150 West 52nd Street, near Seventh Avenue, for what was to be his longest stand in any one place. According to Bill Chase in his column 'All Ears' in the *New York Amsterdam News* of 15 October, Fats was scheduled to open there on 21 October and was resident there until mid-January 1939. In *The Street That Never Slept,* Arnold Shaw describes the place and says that it was decorated like a pleasure yacht with the ceiling representing the night sky ablaze with stars, and it was whilst working there that Fats, spotting Art Tatum in the audience one night, made his celebrated tribute to the partially-sighted pianist: "Ladies and gentlemen, I just play the piano, but God is in the house tonight." But Tatum too, was equally complimentary towards Waller and, in one interview when asked about his musical derivation he answered, "Fats, man, that's where I come from." Then, as an afterthought, "Quite a place to come from." The Yacht Club had a line from it enabling broadcasts to be made direct from the club, and it was not long before Fats and his group were heard over the air. But prior to the Yacht Club debut, Victor were in need of new recordings to meet the constant demand.

*****

"Fats" Waller and his Rhythm - Fox Trot **Vocal refrain and piano by "Fats" Waller -3**
Herman Autrey, t; Gene Sedric, cl-1/ts-2; Fats Waller, p/v-3/o-4; Albert Casey, g; Cedric Wallace, sb; Slick Jones, d.

Studio No.2, New York City, New York — Thursday, 13 October 1938
1:30 to 7:00 p.m. Leonard Joy directing

027289-1*	TWO SLEEPY PEOPLE -2,-3 (Frank Loesser-Hoagy Carmichael)	BB B-10000-A, *Vi/C 20-1583-A,* ViJ A1464, MW M7787-A, HMV B.D.5452, HMVF K8281, SG.96, HMVIt GW1696
027290-1*	SHAME! SHAME! (Everybody Knows Knows Your Game) -1,-3 (Joe Davis)	BB B-7885-B, HMVAu EA2261
027291-1*	I'LL NEVER FORGIVE MYSELF (For Not Forgiving You) -1,-3,-4 (Redmond-Sanford-David)	BB B-10000-B, MW M7787-B, HMVAu EA2302
027291-2	I'LL NEVER FORGIVE MYSELF -1,-3,-4	Victor unissued, 'Hold'. Issued on LP

027291: Last line of vocal: -1 "I'll never forgive myself, no baby, for not forgiving you."
-2 "I'll never forgive myself, no I'll never forgive myself, for not forgiving you."

027292-1*	YOU LOOK GOOD TO ME -1,-3 (Billy Rose-Walter Donaldson)	BB B-10008-A, HMV B.10297, HMVF SG502, HMVAu EA2260, HMVIt HN3070
027292-2	YOU LOOK GOOD TO ME -1,-3	Victor unissued, no disposition noted. Issued on LP

027292 -1 Vocal after introduction and 32-bar piano solo
-2 Vocal begins in bar 9 and is followed by 32-bar piano solo

027293-1*	TELL ME WITH YOUR KISSES -2,-3 (Cliff Friend-Dave Franklin)	BB B-7885-A, HMVAu EA2261
027293-2	TELL ME WITH YOUR KISSES -2,-3	Victor unissued, 'Hold'. Issued on LP

027293: Second line of vocal: -1 "Just how much you care; tell me how much you cáre baby."
-2 "Just how much, just how much you care."

027294-1*	YACHT CLUB SWING -1,-2 (Autry-Johnson-Waller)	BB B-10035-A, HMVAu EA2279

This is the first session recorded specifically for release on the cheaper Bluebird label and for the first time on a Waller session Victor are using "flowed" and "cast" waxes for recording; all the -1A takes except 027291-1A being on "cast" waxes, with that and all the other takes on "flowed" wax masters. The recording sheet (as usual at this time) notes the personnel and the fact that these are "Wide Range Recordings". *Yacht Club Swing* had been written by Fats and Herman Autrey as a tribute to their new place of work and was used as a theme to open and close sets. The recording sheet shows the sub title of 027290 as *(Everybody Knows Your Name).* Bluebird B-10000-A bears the additional credit **(From Paramount film "Thanks for the Memory")**, shortened on HMV B.D.5452 and SG.96. The reverse of Bluebird B-10035 is by **Eddie DeLange and his Orch.**

*****

Yacht Club Broadcast

Herman Autrey, t; Gene Sedric, cl-1/ts-2; Fats Waller, p/p solo3/v-4; Albert Casey, g; Cedric Wallace, sb; Slick Jones, d.

Yacht Club, 150 W. 52nd Street, New York City, New York — Friday 14 October 1938

Yacht Club Swing -1	Issued on LP
Hold My Hand -1,-2,-4	Issued on LP
Pent Up In A Penthouse -1,-2,-4	Issued on LP
Honeysuckle Rose -1,-2	Issued on LP
Yacht Club Swing -1,-2	Issued on LP
You Look Good To Me -2,-4	Issued on LP
Hallelujah -3	Issued on LP
St Louis Blues -2	Issued on LP
Flat Foot Floogie -1,-2,-4	Issued on LP
After You've Gone -2	Issued on LP
Yacht Club Swing -1	Issued on LP

Although the above all apparently come from the same date, they probably represent the product of two sets. Note that Waller is featuring two of the titles he cut whilst in England which Victor issued in the U.S. Hugues Panassié had arrived in New York on 12 October and recounted in his book *Cinq Mois A New York* that he finished up the night of 14 October in the Yacht Club in the company of Mezz Mezzrow:

First of all I met my old friend Gene Sedric. Then Fats came towards me, moving his eyebrows up and down in a funny way, and spoke several words to me in what he took to be French. The swing of Fats's orchestra, with Sedric, Slick Jones and Albert Casey is "formidable". Then a piano was rolled out onto the floor and Fats played a number on his own, as a special turn. His enormous head had a tiny bowler hat on top of it, and the movements of his eyebrows moved it around in a comical way. He announced, "I"m gonna play 'Tea For Two', in other words, 'Milk For Six' ...

*****

Yacht Club Broadcast

Herman Autrey, t; Gene Sedric, cl-1/ts-2; Fats Waller, p/v-3; Albert Casey, g; Cedric Wallace, sb; Slick Jones, d.

Yacht Club, 150 W. 52nd Street, New York City, New York — Tuesday 18 October 1938

Yacht Club Swing -1	Issued on LP
You Can't Be Mine And Somebody Elses Too -1,-2,-3	Issued on LP
Monday Mornin' -2	Issued on LP
What Do You Know About Love? -1,-2	Issued on LP
I Had To Do It -2,-3	Issued on LP

The final title is a Waller composition and Waller's only known recording of it.

*****

Martin Block Jam Session

Louis Armstrong,t/v-1; Jack Teagarden, tb/v-2; Bud Freeman, ts; Fats Waller, p/v-2; Al Casey, g; George Wettling, d.

Station WNEW, New York City, New York — Wednesday, 19 October 1938

Tiger Rag	Issued on LP
Jeepers Creepers -1	Issued on LP
On The Sunny Side Of The Street -1	Issued on LP
Honeysuckle Rose	Issued on LP
The Blues -1,-2	Issued on LP
I Got Rhythm (incomplete)	Issued on LP

For further information please refer back to April 1938. Ed Kirkeby names *The Blues* as *In The Crack Blues.* It is probable that the programme was recorded in advance of the transmission date, which might explain how the musicians (presumably all working elsewhere) were able to be available. If this is the case, then the recollections by Ed Kirkeby and Martin Block of a Sunday may well be correct and Kirkeby is just confusing the sequence of events and the period in which it took place.

However, a piece in the *Pittsburgh Courier* of 12 November stated that Martin Block 'further endeared himself in the hearts of jitterbugs far and near when a few weeks ago he inaugurated a "live in person" jam session every Wednesday', and goes on to name recent participants. No mention is made of the session with Waller, but this does at least support the October date and although it is claimed the performance was 'live', this is not neccessarily so.

Although many have identified the drummer as Slick Jones on aural evidence, Bud Freeman and Al Casey have independently named Wettling. Unfortunately, though, neither is able to provide any clarification on the time of recording. Louis Armstrong also named Wettling when interviewed by Gösta Hägglöf.

*****

Hugues Panassié had become a fairly regular visitor to the Yacht Club, and several quotations from his book add a little to our knowledge of New York night life of the period and of Waller himself. For Friday 21 October he recalls:

> *Soon after 9 p.m., Mezzrow and Benny Carter arrived. We all go together to the Yacht Club, where I'm to be photographed with Fats. Fats Is fast asleep on a seat, his head resting on a table, whilst his "understudy" Hank Duncan, is playing the piano in his orchestra. As soon as he spotted us, Fats made a stupendous effort to say a few words. He explained that he hadn't been to bed for the last 24 hours. He then went straight back to sleep. Nevertheless, at half past midnight, the hour when he was due to make his appearance, he leapt over to his piano and started to play and sing with such gusto that he had us all in fits...*

This is the only indication I have found that Waller used Duncan as a relief pianist when working with his small group. Just over a week later, on Saturday, 29 October, Panassié was again a visitor to the club:

> *After dinner, I make my way to the Yacht Club where I found Fats in a very lively mood. As Sedric improvises a superb chorus on his tenor sax., Fats calls out to him, "One more, Sedric" and makes the piano boom out. As Sedric's next chorus is even better than the last, Fats again calls out, "One more, Sedric, one more". This time it's like a hurricane. ... Even the most hardened customers of the Yacht Club; those who have drunk too much; those who are fast asleep; are obliged to straighten themselves up and to take note that something that Is most unusual is happening. Fats must be possessed of some vitality in order to wake up that lot! During the breaks, the orchestra goes downstairs, just beneath the dance floor. Above our heads, the noise made by the dancers' feet is exactly like the woodwork of a ship which is combined with the noise of the waves beating against the sides of the boat. ... I leave the Yacht Club about 3 a.m.*

On Saturday, 12 November:

> *From the Kit-Kat Club, I go along to the Yacht Club at about one o'clock in the morning. As I go in, Fats is busy doing his number at the piano. When he spotted me, he called out, "The Joint is Jumpin', Hugues Panassié is here tonight." ... I then showed Fats a coin that had been given to me that afternoon which I suspect is a forgery. "You're quite right," said Fats, "I'll take it from you — here's a good one In exchange. No, don't refuse to take it — I collect dud coins." Towards 4 a.m., Fats, having finished his work at the Yacht Club, took me along to the nearby studios where he was due to make a broadcast. It was the opening night for the station, and all the orchestras came to play for a few minutes, once they had finished their work. Fats seated himself at the piano and played two lovely solos. I was then asked to say a few words at the microphone. The announcer asked me the usual question "Are you pleased to be in New York?" I replied, "I'm pleased to be here with Fats." Fats then played some more at the piano and got up to leave. As the next lot of musicians that were awaited to follow Fats had not arrived, one of the organisers begged him to play some more. Fats very kindly seated himself at the piano once more. As the wait went on, Fats asked for some whisky, which they hurried to bring to him, and he started to drink it neat. Sometimes he played, and sometimes he went over to the microphone and made a few jokes. He told the listeners, "See how much whisky I'm going to take in." Then he got hold of the whisky bottle and poured himself a glassful right by the*

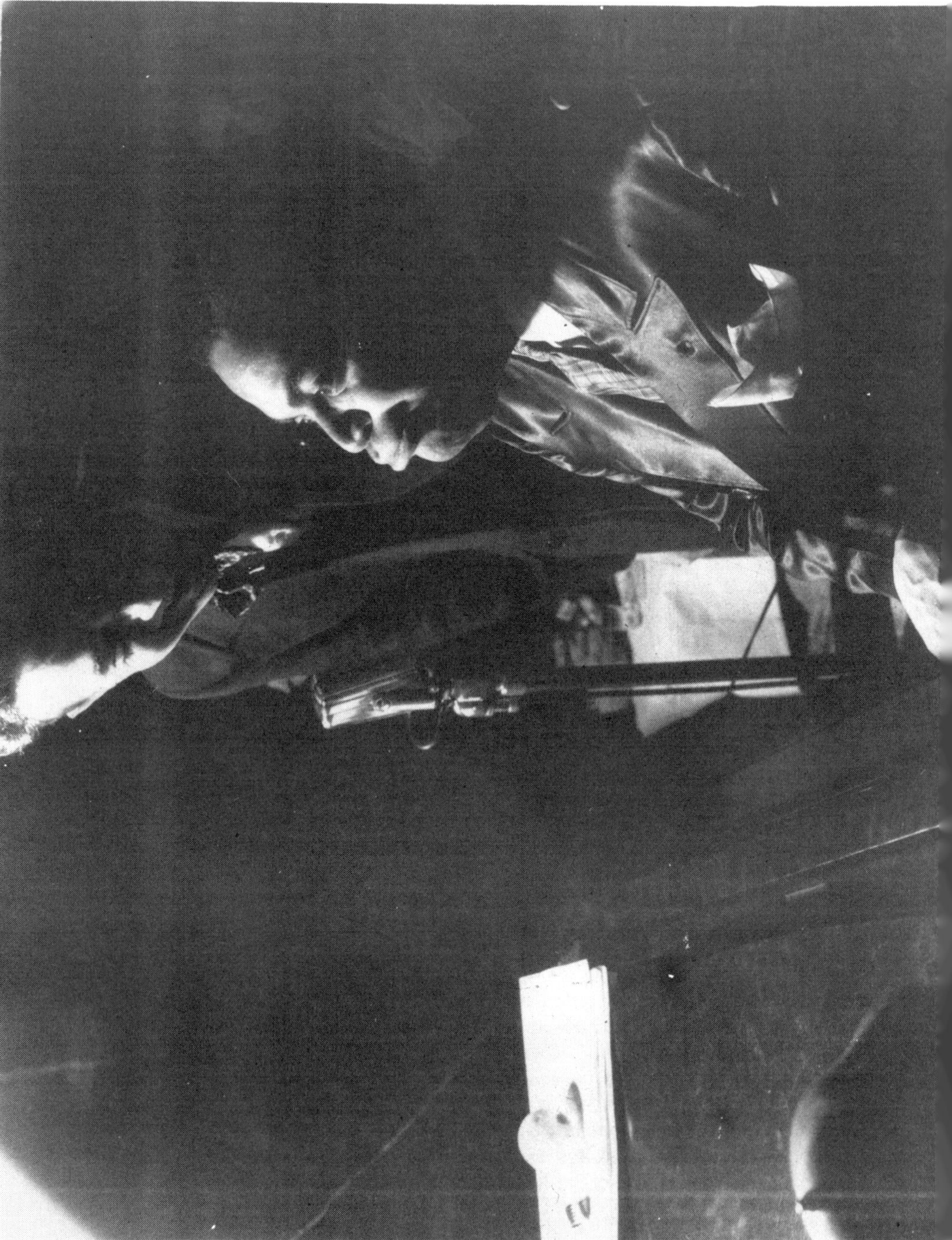

microphone, so that his audience could hear the whisky being poured, saying, "Listen carefully" He swallowed the contents of his glass in one go and made noises with his tongue. Then he let out a tremendous belch into the microphone, then said, "Wait a minute, I'm not there yet ... Be patient, here we are!" This was followed by two or three belches that were even bigger, which he followed by several amusing "Yes's..." Only Fats could get away with such goings-on on the radio and in public. Fats comes back with me about five o'clock in the morning, with all sorts of kind attentions for me. It's quite impossible to give you an idea of the warm heart and kindness of the man ...

It seems most unlikely that Fats did collect dud coins. and was probably more concerned that Panassié should not be out of pocket. The radio station has not been identified but may have been WABC for Bill Chace had the following to say in his column in the *New York Amsterdam News* of that same date in a ghastly bit of writing:

Three cheers to Fats Waller's grand pianology of the WABC Saturday Night Swing Club ... Gad, but how that man does come on! Incidentally, have you seen Fats new figure since he returned from London ... Swelegant, no doubt, but we'll bet it's no more easily wear those Bond Street clothes.

*****

Under the heading *"Fats" Waller To Be Featured On W.C. Handy Concert*, the *New York Age* of 12 November 1938, after saying that Waller was newly returned from a triumphal tour of Europe, has:

...will be one of the featured artists of the William C. Handy Concert to be held in Carnegie Hall on Monday evening, November 21 in honor of the 65th birthday of William C. Handy, father of the blues.

It goes on with some details of the proposed concert and a long list of artists who will appear. The paper of the following week has a similar paragraph in which Waller is just included in the list of artists. A review of the concert, which was sponsored by the 'Harlem Musicians' Committee To Aid Spanish Democracy' for the 'Spanish Children's Milk Fund', did not appear until the issue of 3 December and, although considerable coverage is given, Waller's contribution is covered by; *..."Fats" Waller and his orchestra were much in evidence.*

Waller also makes the front page of this issue in a secondary role, where a whole column is devoted to the shooting of his brother by a thug. Edward L. Waller, "Fats", and Lucky Millinder were leaving the Turf Club, 113 West 136th Street at 3:00 a.m. on the morning of Sunday, 27 November when the incident happened. Waller's own account, which was very similar to that in the paper, was later given to an English reporter and published in *Radio Pictorial* of 19 May 1939:

"Fats" Waller, sensational thirty-five year old coloured pianist-scat singer, told me an exciting story of a New York shooting drama he figured in before he left for this country.

"Fats", his brother Lawrence and a fellow bandleader named Lucky Millinder were waiting for a cab under the brilliantly lit Harlem Turf Club Foyer.

A taxi pulled up. As the three approached it, a white girl jumped out and rushed to "Fats" with an autograph and pen.

"Fats" was obliging, when suddenly:—

"Bang! Bang!"

Orange flame spurted from the cab and Lawrence Waller slumped to the pavement, clutching his stomach.

Cab driver and policeman rushed the gunman, who turned out to be Ed Kohoe, a notorious underworld figure.

Appears it was the work of a "shake-down" gang who staged the shooting to have the Turf Club, which did not pay for "protection", shut down.

Anyway, Lawrence is as right as rain again, and neither "Fats" nor Lucky Millinder were hurt. Just the same, as "Fats" put it: "It wasn't any Sunday school picnic!"

*****

"Fats" Waller and his Rhythm - Fox Trot **Vocal refrain and piano by "Fats" Waller**

Herman Autrey, t; Gene Sedric, cl-1/ts-2; Fats Waller, p/v; Albert Casey, g; Cedric Wallace, sb; Slick Jones, d; band vocal -3

Studio No.2, New York City, New York — Wednesday, 7 December 1938

1:30 to 5:00 p.m. Joy and Shoals (sic) directing

Matrix	Title	Issues
030363-1*	LOVE, I'D GIVE MY LIFE FOR YOU -2 (Oppenheim-Palmer-Jacobs)	BB B-10070-A, MW M-7797-A, HMV B.10495, RZAu G24244
030364-1*	I WISH I HAD YOU -2 (Green-Stillman-Thornhill)	BB B-10078-A, HMVEx J.O.397, RZAu G24308
030365-1*	I'LL DANCE AT YOUR WEDDING -2 (Joe Davis)	BB B-10070-B, MW M-7797-B, HMVEx/H J.O.196, HMVSw HE2896, HMVIn N14065, RZAu G24244
030365-2	I'LL DANCE AT YOUR WEDDING -2	Victor unissued, no designation noted. Issued on LP

030365 Second vocal, second line -1 "Realising some other cat has won your heart, yes!"
-2 "Realising some other cat baby has won your heart, yeah!"
Vocal tag -1 "Go on get mad again" -2 No vocal tag

Matrix	Title	Issues
030366-1*	IMAGINE MY SURPRISE -1,-2 (Hotchkiss-Fitch-Phillips)	BB B-10062-B, MW M-7792-B, HMV B.D.1073, RZAu G24194
030367-1*	I WON'T BELIEVE IT (Till I Hear It From You) -1,-2 (Block-Selsman-Robinson)	BB B-10062-A, MW M-7792-A, HMV B.10168, HMVF SG410, HMVSw HE3043, RZAu G24346
030368-1*	THE SPIDER AND THE FLY -1,-4 (Waller-Razaf-.Johnson)	BB B-10205-A, HMV B.D.5486, HMVSp GY541
030369-1*	PATTY CAKE, PATTY CAKE (Baker Man) -2 (WallerRazaf-Johnson)	BB B-10149-A, HMV B.D.5476, HMVF K-8328, ASR L.BD.5476

Once again the recording sheet lists the personnel and notes the use of "Flowed" and "Cast" waxes, the latter only used on the -1A takes. Bluebird B-10070-A bears the additional credit **(From "The Hollywood Revue Production")**. "Shoals" is Steven Sholes who was to play a significant role in the Waller story a few years later.

Jazz Records also lists HMV HN3043, an Italian issue, against 030367-1, but this is thought to be a typo, and also shows GY394 against 030368-1 in error. This issue will be found on pages 131/2. HMV B.D.5476 omits the sub title.

*****

Fats Waller and Andy Razaf with the Leith Stevens Orchestra

Fats Waller, p-1/v-2; Andy Razaf, v-3; Studio Orchestra with Gilbert Seldes, compere

WABC Studio, New York City, New York — Sunday, 11 December 1938

Introduction -1	Issued on LP
Harlem -1	Issued on LP
The Joint Is Jumpin' -1,-2,-3	Issued on LP
Summertime -2	Issued on LP
Stompin' At The Savoy -1,-2,-3	Issued on LP

This is from one of the weekly "This Is New York" broadcasts.

*****

Hugues Panassié recalls that after dinner, on Monday, 19 December he went to the Yacht Club, where Fats welcomed him with the usual big smile and up and down movements of the eyebrows. As soon as he had finished playing, Fats joined him at his table and told him that on the previous day he had gone to Sing-Sing Prison to play to the inmates.

*****

In the *Defender* of 24 December 1938 under the heading "Orchestras", George Dixon reported that: *"Fats" Waller, the muggin' pianist, and his swingsters will do a week at the Apollo in New York the week of December 30.* However, he appears to have jumped the gun, for Waller did not appear at the Apollo again until 3 February and the headliner for the week he mentions was Jimmie Lunceford.

*****

Back to Panassié, and for Tuesday, 12 January 1939 he writes:

> *Coming out of the Cafe Society, I made my way along to the Yacht Club, where Fats is still playing. His greeting is so kind that I tell him about several problems I've had, several difficulties that I'd like to clear up. As he could see how upset I was, he said to me, "Wait here a few minutes; I'll soon have finished work, then I'll take you back home with me, and we'll spend the rest of the night together — a suggestion that I'm delighted to accept. When we were about ready to leave, I could see Fats in the distance going towards the bar and stuffing some bulky objects into his pockets. His chauffeur quickly drove us to his home. As soon as we were in the main room of his apartment, Fats took out two bottles from the pockets of his overcoat, one of gin and one of whisky. He showed me an enormous quantity of records which had no covers on them and which were unwisely heaped one upon another to dizzy heights ... Fats played for me a little while on the piano, then we listened to records for a long time. ... About six o'clock in the morning, guessing that I might be hungry, Fats took me into the kitchen and treated me to a great big stew that his servant had reheated for him. Finally, at 7 a.m. he gets his chauffeur to take me back to Mezz Mezzrow's apartment, after having given me an affectionate hug. You wouldn't normally guess how kind and thoughtful Fats was.*

*****

On 15th January, 1939, Fats took part in a pioneer television presentation that was transmitted by N.B.C. from the outdoor ice skating rink and the adjoining Café Français at Rockefeller Center in New York. The television apparatus was mounted on a ten ton truck located in the sub-basement of the RCA building and, according to NBC, this was the first-ever programme in which an entertainment bill was transmitted from a building other than the one occupied by the experimental studio.

The programme started with an exhibition of ice skating televised from the outdoor rink and then a pickup was made to the floor show at the café. Featured in the show, along with Fats, was Frank Gaby the ventriloquist and comedienne Shelia Barrett.

*****

"Fats" Waller and his Rhythm - Fox Trot **Vocal refrain and piano by "Fats" Waller**
or **Piano and vocal refrain by "Fats" Waller**

Herman Autrey, t; Gene Sedric, cl-1/ts-2; Fats Waller, p/v/o-3; Albert Casey, g; Cedric Wallace, sb; Slick Jones, d; band vocal -4

Studio No.3, New York City, New York — Thursday, 19 January 1939
1:30 to 6:30 p.m. Leonard Joy directing

031530-1* A GOOD MAN IS HARD TO FIND -1,-2 (Eddie Green) — BB B10143-A, HMV B.10439, HMVFi TG156, HMVN ALS5040
031530-2* A GOOD MAN IS HARD TO FIND -1,-2 — Victor unissued, 'Process'. Issued on LP
031530: Vocal: -1 ...Give him plenty lovin', you know what I mean, and treat him right...
-2 ...Give him plenty lovin', yes, and treat him right...
031531-1* YOU OUTSMARTED YOURSELF -2 (Razaf-Davis-Sears) — BB B-10116-B, RZAu G24346
031532-1* LAST NIGHT A MIRACLE HAPPENED -2 (Oscar Levant-Jack Lawrence) — BB B-10136-A, HMB B.D.5469, B.10050, HMVSw HE2976, HMVIt HN3042, HMVSp GY474, RZAu G24563, ASR L.BD.5469
031533-1* GOOD FOR NOTHIN' BUT LOVE -2 (Eddie De Lange-Jimmie Van Heusen) — BB B-10129-A, HMV B.D.5476, HMVF K-8328, ASR L.BD.5476
031533-2* GOOD FOR NUTHIN' BUT LOVE -2 — Victor unissued, 'Process'. Issued on LP
031533: First vocal: -1 "But I can tell the world how wonderful you are — yes baby; I'm good for nuthin' but love."
-2 "But I can tell the world how wonderful you are, yeah, but I'm good for nuthin' but love — you hear me talkin' to you baby, don't you?"
031534-1* HOLD TIGHT (Want Some Sea Food, Mama) -2,-4) (Kent Brandow-Robinson Ware Spotswood — BB B-10116-A, *Vi 20-1581-B*, HMV B.D.5469, HMVSp GY474, ASR L.BD.5469
031534-2* HOLD TIGHT (Want Some Sea Food, Mama) *-2,-4* — Victor unissued, 'Process'.
031535-1* KISS ME WITH YOUR EYES -1,-3 — Victor unissued, 'Process'. Issued on LP
031535-2 KISS ME WITH YOUR EYES -1,-3 — BB B-10136-B, HMVAu E.A.2296
(Frank Loesser-Burton Lane)
031535: Last line of vocal -1 "Darling, kiss me with your eyes."
-2 "Darling, kiss me, kiss me with your eyes."

Once again, the recording sheet gives the personnel and notes the use of "flowed" and "cast" waxes; the latter for the -1A masters, all of which are marked 'Hold'. The composer credit for 031534 is shown as: Sidney Bechet, Leonard Ware, Edw. Robinson, Willie Spottswood and Ben Smith. The use of the Hammond organ on the last title is not noted. Both issues of 031535-2 bear the additional credit **(From Paramount film "Cafe Society")**. "Fox Trot" is abbreviated to **F.T.** on BB B-10116-B and B-10136-B.

*****

Hugues Panassié was present at the above recording session and his account is as follows:

> *In the early afternoon I went along to the Victor Studios to be present at a recording session of Fats Waller and His Rhythm There was a relaxed atmosphere there, as pleasant as was possible. In complete contrast to most musicians, Fats showed no nervousness at all in the recording studio. You could feel that he was as much at ease as when he's playing at home or late at night in a night club. From time to time, he would take hold of the bottle of whisky that was permanently placed on his piano, and take a big swig for himself. You get the impression that he is only there to amuse himself, and not for a delicate job of work. After the first few sides, one of the Victor bosses asks Fats to record 'Hold Tight', which was the current hit. Fats refuses, but they pushed him so hard that he agreed to do so in the end. He then set off in his own humorous interpretation, with such comical vocal effects that several of those present were in stitches with laughing. He asked his little group to repeat all together some of the words. I, of course, joined in the fun. On one of the titles recorded, Fats played on an Electric Hammond organ.*

*****

On Sunday 22 January 1939, Panassié was rushed to The Harlem Eye And Ear Hospital with a very serious throat infection, and was not expected to live. He recalls:

> *On Tuesday, 24 January 1939, Fats Waller came to visit me, despite his dread of hospitals. He was wearing a grey suit and a scarlet carnation. When the nurses heard the name "Waller" they exclaimed, "What? Is that the famous Fats Waller?" When he noticed them, Fats put his hand in front of his mouth and muttered, "Just the sight of nurses makes me feel bad." As he was leaving, he informed me that the next day he would bring me a radio to keep me company, and told me to let him know if I was short of money.*

*****

It was presumably shortly after the above Victor recording date that Fats Waller and his Rhythm left the Yacht Club. Ed Kirkeby recalls in *Ain't Misbehavin':*

> *But all runs must end sometime, and this one, owing to some disagreement with the club managers, ended even before it had to, during mid-January. I pulled the band out in mid-week but luckily got them bookings at the Apollo Theatre in Harlem and, the following that, at the Howard in Washington.*

*****

However, before moving on there is a small anecdote from a rather unlikely source that fits into the Yacht Club period. In his sleeve note to his own album on Progressive PRO 7042, Harry "The Hipster" Gibson recalls how when he first started out he had been digging Fats Waller's records and had learned to play some of them note for note. In line with the image he was trying to build he would describe himself to anyone who asked as "Waller's star pupil'. One night a big guy came into the place where he was working, dropped five dollars into the kitty and asked for *Sit Right Down And Write Myself A Letter.* Gibson obliged, the big man asked how he'd learned to play like that and Gibson went into his spiel whereupon *the guy just about broke up, stuck out his hand and said, "Sonny, say hello to your old professor, Thomas Waller".* Gibson goes on to relate how Waller kept dropping bills into the kitty and asking for more of his numbers and, at the end of the night, asked Gibson if he'd like to work at the Yacht Club. Waller got Gibson a job at the club as intermission pianist playing a small piano on wheels and often took him to Grant's, an after hours club where all the top pianists would hang out.

*****

By the time Fats quit the Yacht Club, the Wallers had moved to St. Albans, a part of Queens Borough at the New York end of Long Island. I recall on one visit to New York, flying down from Canada and being met by Spencer Williams (Clarence Williams's son). It was afternoon rush hour and, to avoid the traffic Spencer said, "we'll keep off the freeway and I'll show you where we used to live." We eventually pulled up at a cross-roads with a cul-de-sac as one arm and Spencer pointed down it and said, "My father owned those houses, James P. Johnson lived in one, then us, then Hank Duncan and Willie 'The Lion' Smith. This was Fats Waller's house (pointing to a big house on the junction) and Fats used to hang out of that window and bawl 'Anita!' if she was out talking and he wanted her ... and this house here (on the opposite side) is Count Basie's, but he's not often here now, he lives in the Bahamas." That was some collection of pianists and explains some of the great parties that went on in that little street.

*****

The appearance at the Apollo was for the week commencing Friday, 3 February and also on the bill were Jeni Le Gon and Myra Johnson, both as featured performers rather that as vocalists with the band. Unfortunately, the *New York Age* had ceased reviewing the Apollo shows at this point, so nothing is known of the performance.

*****

Bob Kumm supplied details of a tape which is in circulation among collectors, but which is dated only as "1939". It may come from this period and known details are as follows:

Broadcast "Magic Key Of Radio"

Fats Waller, p/v

New York City, New York — 1939

What's The Matter With You

*****

Reputedly on Monday, 6 February 1939 **"The Broadway Showcase"** broadcast from New York City included *Old Grand Dad* by Fats Waller. However, this broadcast is, in fact, only the Bluebird recording of this tune with audience applause dubbed in, and should not be treated as a separate entity. It is issued on LP. However, since the recording was not made until the following year, the date quoted for the broadcast is clearly in error.

*****

In its issue of 18 February, the *Pittsburgh Courier* has a paragraph headed **'Fats' Is A Riot At Howard.** Unfortunately, the paper has been microfilmed in its case and the item disappears into the fold between the pages so that it is impossible to read. However, enough is legible to determine that it is Waller and that he opened at the Howard Theatre, Washington, D.C. 'last Friday' (presumably 10 February as the item is datelined 15 February); that Myra Johnson was with him and that he also had a Hammond organ. If the engagement was for a week, as was normal, then the broadcast that follows was either pre-recorded, or Waller had dashed back to New York to participate, which seems unlikely.

*****

Broadcast. "George Jessel's Celebrity Program"

George Jessel sp-1; Fats Waller, sp-1/p-2

New York City, New York — Sunday, 12 February 1939

Theme (Stompin' At The Savoy) -1	Issued on LP
Hallelujah -2	Issued on LP

The first number is by the studio orchestra, but Waller and Jessell are heard over the closing bars. Although *By The Light Of The Silvery Moon* (with Waller on organ) is presented on CD as being part of this Jessel broadcast, this seems unlikely for a number of reasons: The tune, although written in 1909, had been out of the common repertoire for twenty years or more and was not revived until several years after this date when Waller was among those who featured it; it seems unlikely that a Hammond Organ would have been on hand for a single item to be performed by a guest; Waller had in fact recorded the title as the last item at his V-Disc session and, given his comments: "Are you having fun over there?" "...chicks over there" 'Thanks, fellers, for joining me in the chorus." and the fact that he sings of "the victory moon", it seems probable that a V-Disc test has been found and tacked on to the end of the Jessel broadcast.

*****

Panassié's New York visit was coming to a close, and on Wednesday, 22 February he called to see Fats to say "Goodbye" but Waller was ill and was unable to see him. The following day, he sailed on the *Ile de France*.

*****

There was already speculation that Waller was to return to Europe and, datelined New York City, Feb. 23, the *Pittsburgh Courier* has:

> *Rumor has it that Fats Waller has nixed his proposed European tour in favor of an appearance at the Famous Door. If Fats does go in, he will be accompanied by his piano and his organ, but not his orchestra. The capacity of the nitery wouldn't accomodate all of them and an audience too.*

*****

"Fats" Waller & Gene Austin

Gene Austin, v, acc: Fats Waller, o/vocal comments; Otto "Coco" Heimel, g; Russell "Candy" Hall, sb.

Studio 3, New York City, New York — Monday, 6 March 1939
9:15 to 10:30 a.m. Ed. Kirkeby present

033993-1*	Sweet Sue (Victor Yourng-Will J. Harris)	Victor unissued, 'Hold'. Issued on LP
033993-2*	Sweet Sue	Victor unissued, 'Hold'
033994-1*	I Can't Give You Anything But Love (Dorothy Fields-Jimmy McHugh)	Victor unissued, 'Hold'. Issued on LP

The personnel for the above was finally established by Tor Magnusson who, in his 1976 study of the Gene Austin recordings with Waller said, "It is not clear if these recordings were ever meant to be released. They were made in connection with a Thesaurus radio transcription session that Gene Austin made with Candy & Coco in the Victor studios, but the recordings were never issued as 78 rpm records." Subsequently, Tor interviewed Russell Hall who confirmed himself and Heimel in the accompaniment and said that the session took place at 10:00 a.m. He had no knowledge of any transcription recordings. The recording sheet which, until recent years had been missed by researchers as it was filed in a separate folder under the session heading name, reveals the details given above. The titles were apparently originally intended for Bluebird, and take -1 of each title is marked as accepted. Heimel played four-string guitar. Composer credits are as on the recording sheet.

*****

Soon after the departure from the Yacht Club, Ed Kirkeby must have begun negotiations for a return to England and indications in the British press were that Waller was due to arrive in the U.K. on 27 March 1939 but, for reasons not yet explained, the party set sail earlier and arrived well ahead of that date. As at the time of the first trip, a visit to the Victor studios was made to ensure that releases could be made in Waller's absence.

*****

"Fats" Waller and his Rhythm - Fox Trot **Vocal refrain and piano by "Fats" Waller**

Herman Autrey, t; Gene Sedric, cl-1/ts-2; Fats Waller, p/v; Albert Casey, g; Cedric Wallace, sb; Slick Jones, d.

Studio No.2, New York City, New York Thursday, 9 March 1939

7:30 to 11:30 p.m. Leonard Joy directing

032942-1*	YOU ASKED FOR IT — YOU GOT IT -1,-2 (Charlie Tobias-Abel Baer)	BB B-10170-A, HMV/In B.D.1036, RZAu G24859
032943-1*	SOME RAINY DAY -1 (Carmen Lombardo-John Jacob Loeb)	BB B-10192-B
032944-1*	'TAIN'T WHAT YOU DO (It's The Way That Cha Do It) -1,-2 (Sy Oliver-James Young)	BB B-10192-A, HMV B.D.5486, HMVSp GY541
032945-1*	GOT NO TIME -2 (Ted Koehler-Rube Bloom)	BB B-10170-B, HMV B.D.5493, RZAu G24938
032946-1*	STEP UP AND SHAKE MY HAND -2 (Mack David Jerry Livingston)	BB B-10184-A
032947-1*	UNDECIDED -1 (Sid Robin-Charles Shavers)	BB B-10184-B
032948-1*	REMEMBER WHO YOU'RE PROMISED TO -2 (Whiting-Burton-Johnson)	BB B-10205-B (See note)
032948-2*	REMEMBER WHO YOU'RE PROMISED TO -2	Victor unissued, 'Hold'. Issued on LP

032948: -1 (Bluebird take) Sedric's tenor sax solo is followed by a vocal.
-2 (LP issues) Sedric's tenor sax solo is followed by a piano solo, then a vocal.

As before, the recording sheet notes the personnel and the use of "flowed" and "cast" waxes in the normal manner. All the -A masters are marked 'Hold'. In the case of the final title, both -1 and -2 are marked for issue, but no indication is given as to which was actually used and no take number is visible in the wax, although LP issues indicate that it was -1. This was Waller's first recording session for Victor after leaving the Yacht Club and reverts to an evening call and studio No.2.

Bluebird B-10170-B and HMV B.D.5493 bear the additional credit **(From World's Fair Edition of "The Cotton Club Parade")** and B.D.5486 omits the sub-title. "Fox Trot' on Bluebird B-10205-B is abbreviated to **F.T.**

*****

Ed Kirkeby says that they sailed the following day (10 March) aboard the *Queen Mary*. However, as so often, his recollection of dates and chronology is suspect and a report in the *Southern Daily Echo* of 17 March says:

> *It was only last evening that the Queen Mary concluded a voyage from the States, having crossed from the Ambrose Channel Light Vessel to Cherbourg Breakwater in 4 days, 14 hours, 33 minutes at an average speed of 28.31 knots.*

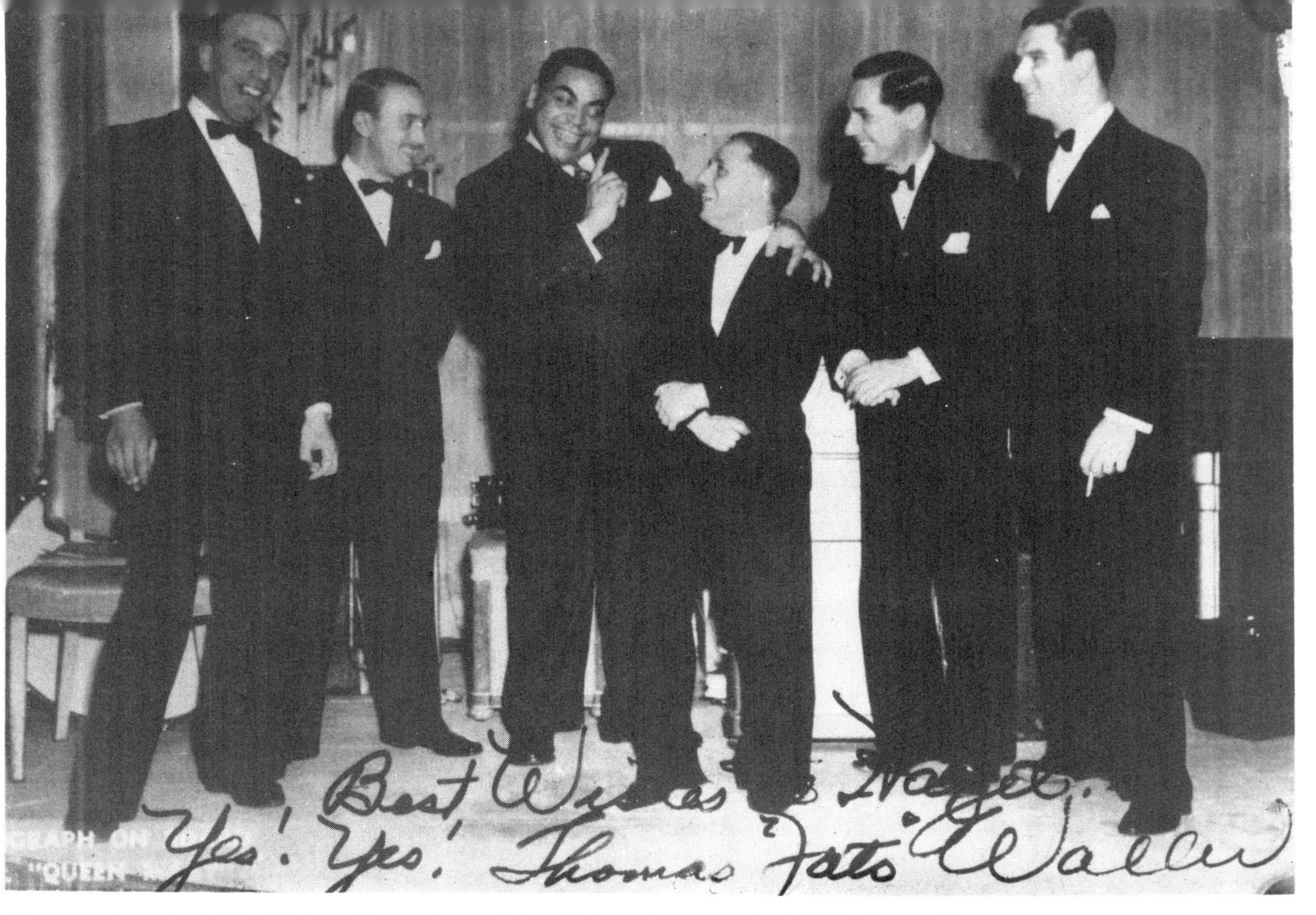

Above and overleaf: Fats Waller with members of the ship's orchestra on the *R.M.S. Queen Mary.*

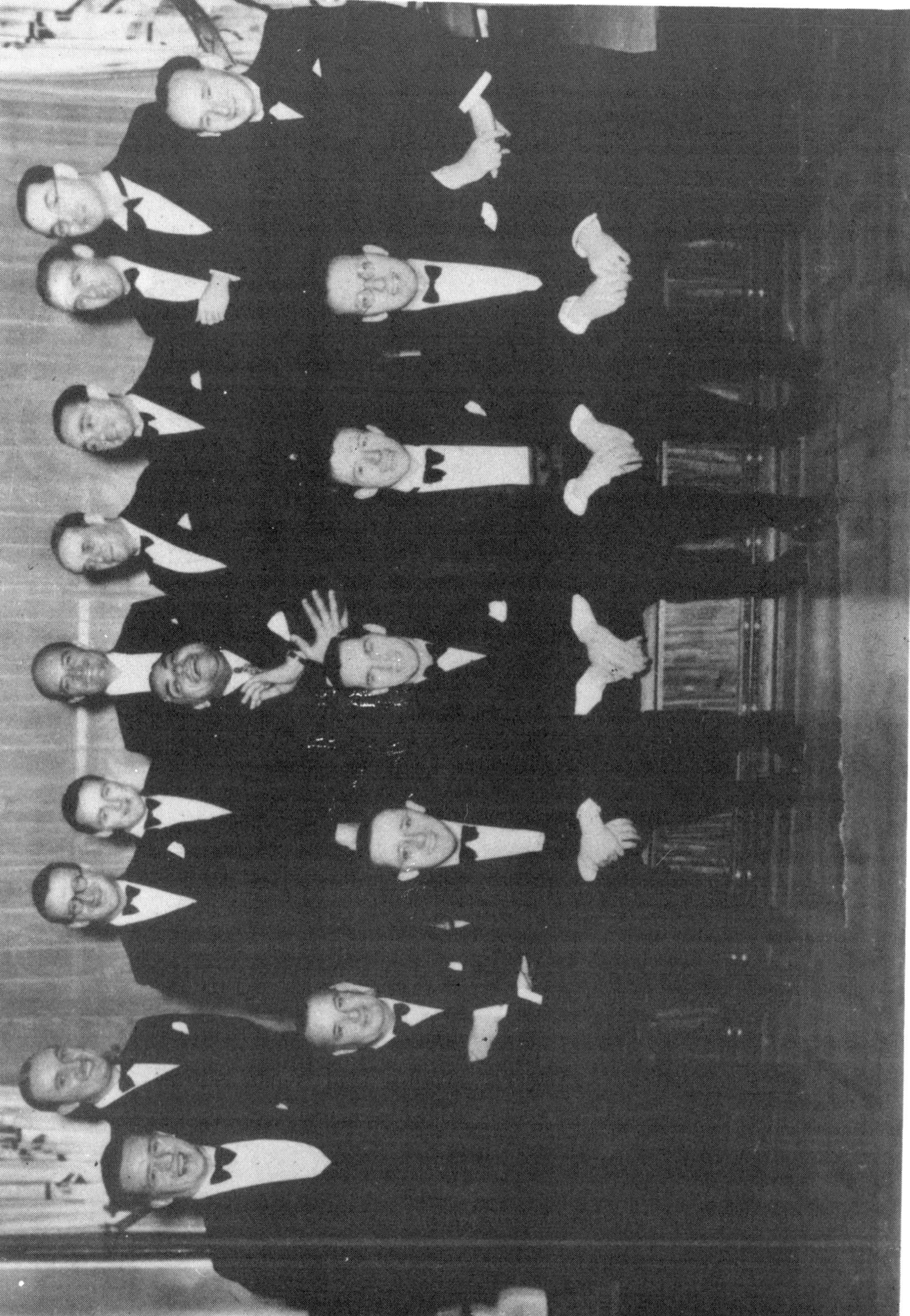

Howard Rye has checked the Public Record Office reference for this voyage which also confirms the arrival of the *Queen Mary* at Southampton on 16 March 1939 (Ref. BT 26/1182) and shows Kirkeby aged 40 — he'd lost a few years since his trip in 1938 (!) as an artist and Waller aged 34 as a pianist. Their address was given as 199 Piccadilly, London. Fast transatlantic passages by the luxury liners were, in those days, a matter of considerable national pride and were often reported in the press. It is evident from the above report that Ed Kirkeby is a couple of days out in his departure date, which indicates that the *Queen Mary* left New York in the morning of Sunday, 12 March and arrived in Southampton, having crossed the Channel from Cherburg, late in the evening of Thursday, 16 March, and provides a more reasonable schedule prior to departure. The *Pittsburgh Courier* has two items covering Waller's departure, both of which place it on the Saturday. One states that he is to tour and will pick up an orchestra in Europe to accompany him where necessary and that his return before the late fall is unlikely; the other has a photo of Fats with Anita and Mrs. M. Rutherford (Anita's mother) and states that Fats is taking his family to Europe for a vacation. From these reports is seems likely that Anita and her mother had come to see Fats off and that passengers had boarded the liner the night before departure, which may also explain discrepancies in the reported departure date from New York (*Lloyd's List* of 13 March 1939 quotes 11 March as the departure date).

Arriving in London, the visitors found that agent Leslie McDonnell had again been very active and Fats was due to begin another week of doubling at two theatres beginning on Monday, 20 March. He opened at Holborn Empire and was teamed with the Mills Brothers, who were the headliners with Fats second in a bill which also featured English comedian Ted

HOLBORN EMPIRE 6.30 & 9.0

MONDAY, MARCH 20th TWICE NIGHTLY 'Phone: Holborn 5367-8-9

BIG VARIETY BILL—Including

MILLS BROS
4 Boys and a Guitar

'FATS' WALLER
THE GREAT RHYTHM PIANIST
MASTER OF SWING

STONE & LEE
Crazy Wisecrackers

TED RAY
Fiddling & Fooling

WRIGHT AND MARION
Nitwits of Satire

THREE DIXI BROS
COMEDY IN DANCE

3 ABERDONIANS

DICK HENDERSON
Yorkshire Comedian

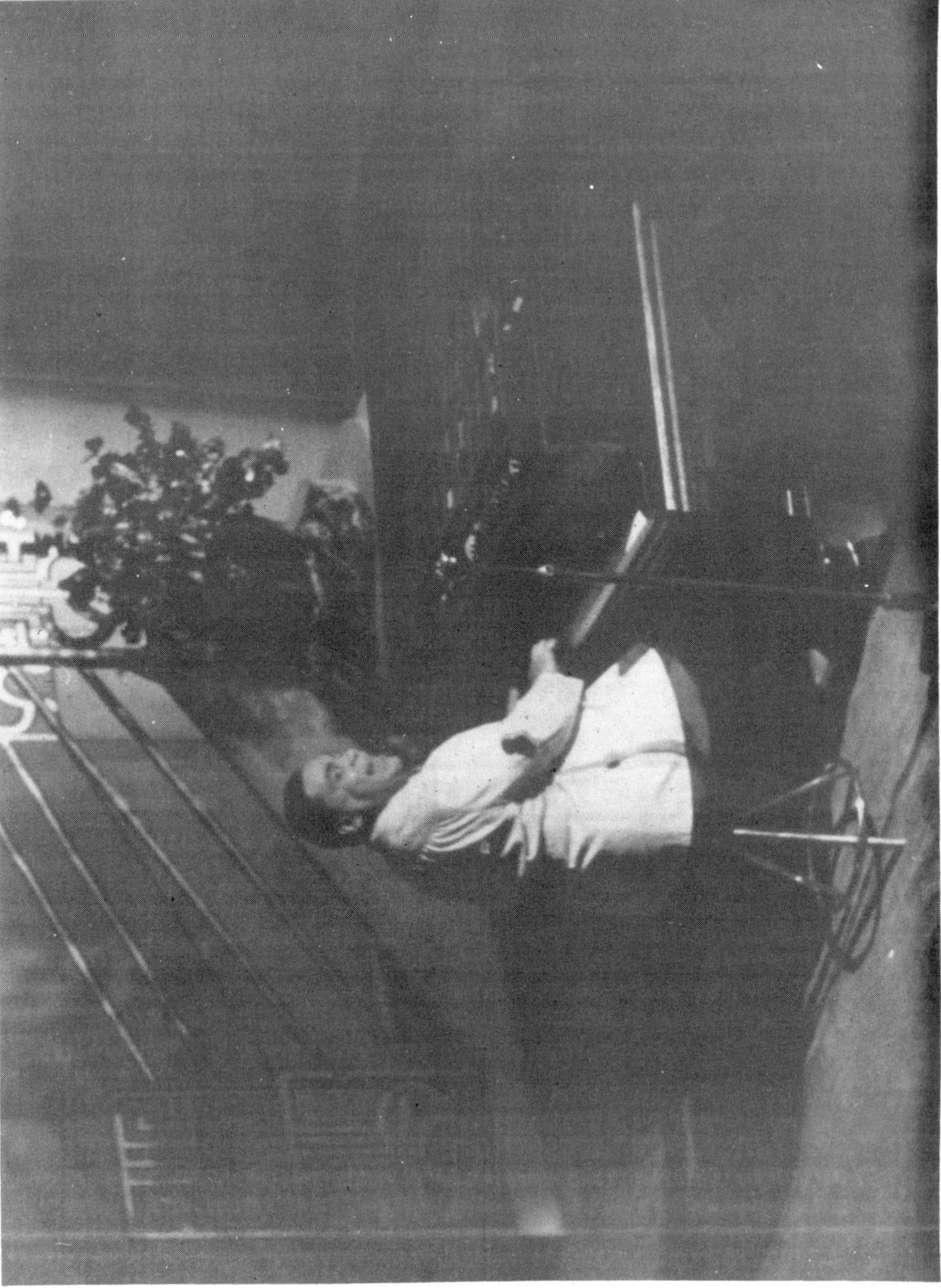

Ray. The second theatre, also in North London, was Finsbury Park Empire and, since both headliners were appearing at both theatres, some hectic taxi journeys to get to and from the theatres for the two houses at each location must have taken place. Ted Ray, who featured a violin in his act, achieved greater fame in post war years and in 1967 I telephoned him to see what recollections he had of working with Waller. "Oh yes, those were the golden days of variety, and I was only just coming up then. We did quite a few shows together and I usually followed Fats on the bill, so I would be standing in the wings during his act. He could see me, of course, and would throw out remarks like 'you wanna get rid of that thing and get a piano and get in business boy!' — referring to my violin." The *Pittsburgh Courier* reported this doubling and explained to its readers that it was because there was insufficient talent available to meet the demand, especially as many Americans were loathe to make the transatlatic crossing in the worsening international situation.

During that week, Fats discovered that his protégé Una Mae Carlisle, who had taken up residence in England, was sick in hospital. According to Ed Kirkeby, on Sunday 26 March, the Gaumont State Theatre, Kilburn was hosting a musicians' benefit at which all the top bands of the day were playing. Fats invited a large number of friends to be his guests, bought tickets and told everyone to meet him at the stage door. Everyone except Fats turned up on time and Ed had quite a job persuading the management to let the crowd in. A remorseful Fats later explained that he had gone to visit Una Mae and forgotten the time.

On Monday, 27 March, the two-theatre act moved to South London, opening at Croydon Empire, and doubling at Clapham Grand for a one-week engagement at each. The Mills Brothers were top of the bill at Croydon, with Fats second, but at Clapham they headlined jointly, and were to do so for most of their subsequent joint variety engagements.

Perhaps Waller's return was a little too soon, for the London reviewers covering the first two weeks were not quite as welcoming as in the previous year, and two examples will suffice to give the general tone.

Melody Maker, 25 March 1939:

> *When Fats Waller came bounding out of the wings at the Holborn Empire last Monday a lot of jazz fans unbent their ears and settled down for a session of Waller piano.*
>
> *But they got more for their eyes than their ears in the fifteen minutes that followed.*
>
> *Fats has improved his technical powers. His touch and his dexterity have improved enormously. But the necessity of playing from a stage for an audience which seems to expect to see Fats wriggle his scalp and roll his eyes at the antics of his active right hand, seems to take the fifteen-minute programme into the field of an exhibition rather than a jazz recital.*
>
> *For a moment or two in his first number, Two Sleepy People, the old Waller satirical touch was there. He managed to knock the last ounce of sentiment from that particular ditty.*
>
> *But in St. Louis Blues, Flat Foot Floogee and I'm Gonna Sit Right Down And Write Myself A Letter there didn't seem to be much of anything except the usual bunch of licks, with a few arpeggios and things which the audience is usually spared.*
>
> *It is hardly fair, however, to accuse Fats of not playing good jazz. He isn't doing that kind of a show.*

The Stage, 30 March 1939 under the heading "Grand, Clapham":

> *The Mills Brothers share the head with Fats Waller, both of whom give typical*

Transatlantic ideas with all the smartness one expects from them... Fats Waller's reputation as a swing pianist has preceded him, and he secures full attention throughout in an arresting turn that embraces other entertaining things apart from his pianoforte playing, amongst them being gay snatches of song interpolated between his musical selections. A genial personality is also of considerable help to him.

*****

Fats Waller — Piano Solo (TeE A-76)
THOMAS "FATS" WALLER (Ri)

Fats Waller, p/v-1; Johnny Marks, d-1.

Billy Higgs recording studio, London — *Sunday, 2 April 1939*

Title	Issues
YOU CAN'T HAVE YOUR CAKE AND EAT IT -1 FATS WALLER	*TeE A-76, Ci R305, JSo AA576, El Disc A.1*
NOT THERE, RIGHT THERE -1 FATS WALLER	*TeE A-76, Ci R305, JSo AA576, El Disc A.1*
Cottage In The Rain -1 (*Waller*)	*Ri 8, Les Amis de Fats* (unnumbered)
WHAT A PRETTY MISS -1	Unissued
London Suite - Piccadilly	Unissued
London Suite - Chelsea	Unissued
London Suite - Soho	Unissued
London Suite - Bond Street	Unissued
London Suite - Limehouse	Unissued
London Suite - Whitechapel	Unissued

These are all acetate recordings and the first four sides were owned by Sinclair Traill who told me that they were double sided and that he still had them in a trunk (!) until the time of his removal from 27 Willow Vale to Brighton, when he lost track of them. He thought the fourth side was as given above, but it is a mystery why this was never issued to provide a coupling with the third side. Some copies of Tempo A 76 are without the hyphen (thus) and on these the composer credit appears in brackets.

The above is the original version of the London Suite and was owned by Ed Kirkeby. Bob Kumm heard them in 1967 and noted that there were substantial differences between them and the version subsequently issued by HMV. Ed Kirkeby declined to have them issued and their present whereabouts is unknown, and although some of his musical effects were donated to Rutgers these were, at the time I was there, not among them. Ed Kirkeby's recollections of how they came to be made and the date has caused considerable confusion and is clearly in error. (See the note after the 13 June 1939 session).

The *Melody Maker* of 8 April 1939 has:

Fats Waller has had a terrific burst of composition in the last few weeks. He has written four new songs, with lyrics by Spencer Williams, and a suite of six piano solos.

In a recording session at Billy Higgs' last week, Fats put the whole ten compositions down on wax, aided by Johnny Marks at the drums.

To save himself the trouble of writing out his new tunes on manuscript, Fats decided it would be faster just to do a recording session and get them all down at once. The tunes could then be transcribed when wanted for publication...

The first is Fats' Not There Right There... As for the six piano solos, these are six parts of a London Suite in which Fats gave his impressions of London in piano music. He has caught the atmosphere of the various districts in London...

At the recording session, without any previous preparation, Fats just sat down and improvised, and as he thought of the locality concerned played his own impressions of it.

This clearly establishes that the ten titles were made at the same time and that Ed Kirkeby's June date, derived from his interview with Bob Kumm published in *Storyville 13,* for the *London Suite* is in error. The part of the interview that concerns us is as follows:

"On the Sunday morning before our scheduled return, I called Fats at his hotel and reminded him that we were committed to do a set of hot piano recordings to fulfil a contract on which I'd taken a substantial payment when we first arrived in Britain. Fats had been out on the town the night before. Nevertheless, after a hearty breakfast of his liquid 'ham and eggs' he arrived at the small studio in a state of lucidity and obviously was 'feeling no pain' thanks to his magnanimous imbibing. I was quite apprehensive about how the session would go, but after a few minutes at the keyboard Fats demonstrated that in spite of, or perhaps because of his libations, he was rarin' to go and the session would run smoothly. Fats ran through a number which we tentatively titled PICCADILLY PARTY, but his temperament that day didn't seem to be inclined to hot piano stylings, so I suggested that he do a series of tone poems about London, that we had first discussed on the boat coming over. I described to Fats my sentiments about the different sectors of London. He would interpret my thoughts into an improvised melody and immediately recorded each number. The entire session was finished in less than two hours. Since the recordings were made only on acetate discs and the acoustics of the small studio were somewhat inadequate, I set up a session at the HMV studio the following day, where Fats could do a remake of the entire session. These recordings from the second session are the ones that were finally released, though twelve years and the ravages of war were to intercede before the LONDON SUITE would ever be pressed on to a commercial gramophone record."

Ed Kirkeby still has the acetates from the first session in his possession. He feels that the rhythm and tonal structure is somewhat superior to the version that was released. He stated that since the HMV recordings were done to fulfil a business contract, and those from the first session merely as improvisational-compositional recordings, he feels that it would be unethical to have the first LONDON SUITE released at this time.

It will be noted that Kirkeby's reason for not releasing the acetates it at odds with his opening statement which is assumably true as he would hardly have known about the Billy Higgs studio, nor found it open on a Sunday unless by prior arrangement, but the question arises of to whom he was contracted, and what happened about the 'hot piano recordings'?

The exact date is a problem. The *Melody Maker* report merely says "last week" and, since Fats was working constantly, a Sunday afternoon, which is what Ed Kirkeby said it was, was most likely, and hence probably 2 April. The 3 April date given in *Jazz Records* is obviously wrong as Fats was due in Birmingham for a rehearsal at 11:00 a.m. So, once again Kirkeby's recollections of details seem to fit, but his dates do not.

*****

According to reports in the 8 April *Melody Maker,* Fats appeared at a Geraldo Sunday Night Swing Concert at St. Martin's Theatre, London in the evening of 2 April. Also on the bill were

The Heralds of Swing, Una Mae Carlisle, Don and Jimmy Macaffer, George Shearing, and The Radio Revellers. Una Mae had obviously made a quick recovery from whatever had put her in hospital.

> *The intimate little theatre, instead of being packed for a really thrilling show, was a third empty, a great disappointment, if not discouragement for the sponsors... and the artists...The three hundred old faithfuls in the stalls and circle had the time of their lives the band is grand... so was Fats Waller, but then he always is. Artists who enjoy their work as Fats does nearly always are that good, anyway.*

Among the tunes played by Fats at the concert was *Not There — Right There* accompanied by the Heralds of Swing Rhythm section. After the concert, Fats jammed at The Nest, Kingly Street, with George Chisholm and Tiny Winters, both of whom were members of The Heralds of Swing. The *Melody Maker* report went on:

> *Fats had another burst of composition last Sunday night down at the Nest. With George Chisholm on trombone and Tiny Winters on bass, he played the blues for half an hour and between George and Fats the amount of original ideas flying around the night club was tremendous.*

The *Melody Maker*, 15 April in "Music-Go-Round" enlarged on this:

> *It was around dawnish the other morning at The Nest that the M.C. stepped onto the postage-stamp dance floor and announced that the next 'surprise' would be a jam session featuring Fats Waller on piano, Tiny Winters on bass, Chisholm on trombone, and the one and only Hawkins on tenor. But the Hawk wasn't having any, being beat right down to his chops after a twenty-one day grind, which had him playing a new town every night and playing the Phoenix show and the Gig Club on the day of his arrival in London.*
>
> *Can you blame him - like some people did - for sitting that one out.*

*****

But did Hawkins sit that one out or did the *Melody Maker* reporter just leave too early? In an interview published in Coda, George Shearing recalled:

> *We were in a club in London and we heard that Fats Waller and/or Coleman Hawkins were coming by, and they both did. When everybody left they both got up and played. By the time we left the club the sun was shining brightly.*

This may not have been the occasion referred to in the Melody Maker, but there appears to be no other occasion when the two men were in London at the same time.

*****

Following that late night at The Nest, the party must have caught an early morning train for Birmingham to make the 11:00 a.m. rehearsal and Fats opened at Birmingham Hippodrome for a one week engagement, excluding Friday, 7 April, which was Good Friday.

*****

From Birmingham, he headed north and on Monday, 10 April opened at Glasgow Empire for a one week engagement as featured artist in the Will Collins and Lew Grade Ltd., *'Runnin' Wild'*. This revue, which also included Joe Daniels and Teddy Foster with the Hot Shots, was touring independently and Fats was withdrawn from the joint tour with the Mills Brothers to headline the revue for this week only.

*****

An advert appeared in the Hull *Daily Mail* of 6 April 1939 for a Swing Concert to take place in

Hull City Hall on Sunday, 16 April featuring "40 Minutes' Entertainment by the WORLD'S GREATEST SWING PIANIST, FATS WALLER". The Monday edition of the paper (17 April) carried a review, parts of which read:

> *...Thomas "Fats" Waller who delighted the audience for over 40 minutes ... attendance was good ... Mr. Waller responded to encores generously. He has a style of his own, and whether one is watching his fingers glide over the the piano keybopard, or one is watching his comical facial expressions, his act always holds the attention of the audience.*
>
> *His programme included such "hot" numbers as "St. Louis Blues", "Honeysuckle Rose" (his own composition), and "Flat Foot Floogie" down to the more melodious "Two Sleepy People", Irving Berlin"s "Marie" and "Write Myself A Letter", finishing the evening with Louis Gold and his Monarchs of Melody on the tune "Sweet Sue".*

*****

Two further one week engagements with the original tour followed; the first from Monday, 17 April to Saturday, 22 April was at Sunderland Empire, then, from Monday, 24 April to Saturday, 29 April at Edinburgh Empire.

*****

Following this, Fats again left the tour and headed to the south coast and, on Monday, 1 May began a one week engagement at Portsmouth Hippodrome for one week engagement. In a letter to me, Alan Turner recalled, *I saw Fats at the Portsmouth Hippodrome at an afternoon matinee which most probably was on Saturday 6 May 1939. I particularly remember him telling the audience to be very quiet during his next number — the audience expecting something pretty quiet from Fats instead got a rip-roaring version of the 'Flat Foot Floogie'. Wish I could remember more about the occasion, but the whole thing went like some glorious dream and was over before I could be thinking of just what he had played.*

The Mills Brothers remained in the North of England during this week. Initially, Fats was scheduled to rejoin them at Bradford Alhambra the following week according to the *Melody Maker,* of 6 May 1939, but there is no doubt that he did not. Instead he moved along the south coast to Brighton and opened at Brighton Hippodrome for a one week engagement, commencing Monday, 8 May and headlining jointly with comedian Tommy Trinder. In the evening of Monday, 8 May, Fats jammed at Sherry's, Brighton, with Nat Gonella and his Augmented Band as reported in *Melody Maker,* 20 May 1939. "A week ago last Monday" (i.e. 8 May):

> *Fats Waller together with Nat Gonella and his bunch of boys in an evening of glorious jamming, was the unexpected treat given at Sherry's, Brighton. ....Mecca had engaged Nat and his augmented band... When the portly figure of Fats Waller, who was making a current appearance at the Hippodrome, strolled in and was induced to come on the stand there was a minor riot and the crowd went crazy with excitement at the glorious jam session that resulted.*

In *Georgia On My Mind,* Nat Gonella recalled that Fats had just dropped into Sherry's to hear the band, but over a bottle of gin was persuaded to sit in on a jam session. They only played one tune, Waller's *Honeysuckle Rose,* but they played it for nearly an hour! Nat says that the management of the Hippodrome got to hear of this impromptu jam session and, interpreting this as a breach of contract, fined Fats £50, which almost caused Waller to explode with anger as £50 represented about two crates of gin in those days, and it was only Ed Kirkeby's tact and powers of persuasion that averted an immediate cancellation of the tour.

*****

Hazel Mundell recalled going to see Fats:

> *The week he was appearing at the Hippodrome, I used to catch a bus from Steyning (a 12-mile journey) to see the show and rush to catch the last bus home. The first night of that week, I went backstage for his autograph and to show him the photographs taken on the Queen Mary. He was so kind and interested and wanted to know how I came to have them. When he knew I was hoping to come in each night to watch and listen to him, he very kindly arranged with the manager for me to watch from the wings each time I came. I remember he came dancing off one night and reached up and swung with one arm from one of the beams overhead (I thought the old hip would collapse!) and said, "Well, how was I?"*
>
> *The following week a parcel arrived for me from "Fats"; a large signed photograph saying, "To my good girl friend Hazel, may you always be blessed from above. Your Friend, Sincerely, Thomas "Fats" Waller". Also a beautiful tie, brown silk with musical instruments all over it and bars of music; the one he is wearing in the photo on the pier! I was so proud of it, I nearly wore it out during the war.*

*****

Fats then headed north again to rejoin the tour with the Mills Brothers, and the following one-week engagements took place:

Monday, 15 May — Saturday, 20 May at Nottingham Empire.

Monday, 22 May — Saturday, 27 May at Sheffield Empire. It was during this week that Fats composed *Honey Hush*, according to Ed Kirkeby.

Monday, 29 May — Saturday, 3 June at Manchester Palace.

Monday, 5 June — Saturday, 10 June at Newcastle Empire. Fats and the Mills Brothers were evidently added late to this bill as initial local announcements show 'Cecil Lyle & Co' top of the bill.

*****

Reviews in the Provinces had generally been very good and warmly welcoming as the following small selection will show.

Birmingham Gazette, 4 April 1939

> *...Then there's Fats Waller, a man who would make a very useful Rugby scrum set all on his own, but who handles the piano so delicately and so delightfully that one is fully prepared not to quibble about his description as 'the world's greatest rhythm pianist and master of swing' You'll like Fats, even if, as a rule, you don't like rhythm and you have a dislike for 'swing'.*

Glasgow Evening News, 8 April 1939:

> *From the moment immense, jovial Fats Waller swung into a typical version of Two Sleepy People until he trucked smilingly off the stage at the Empire last night, he demonstrated that he is in an entertainment class by himself.*

The Evening Despatch (Edinburgh), 25 April 1939:

> *...This individualist of the piano is one of the cleverest in the world of 'jazz' and his performance this week leaves little doubt about that ... able technique, great concentration, and an acute sense of rhythm... Fats possesses these three qualities, and*

Right: Fats on Brighton Pier

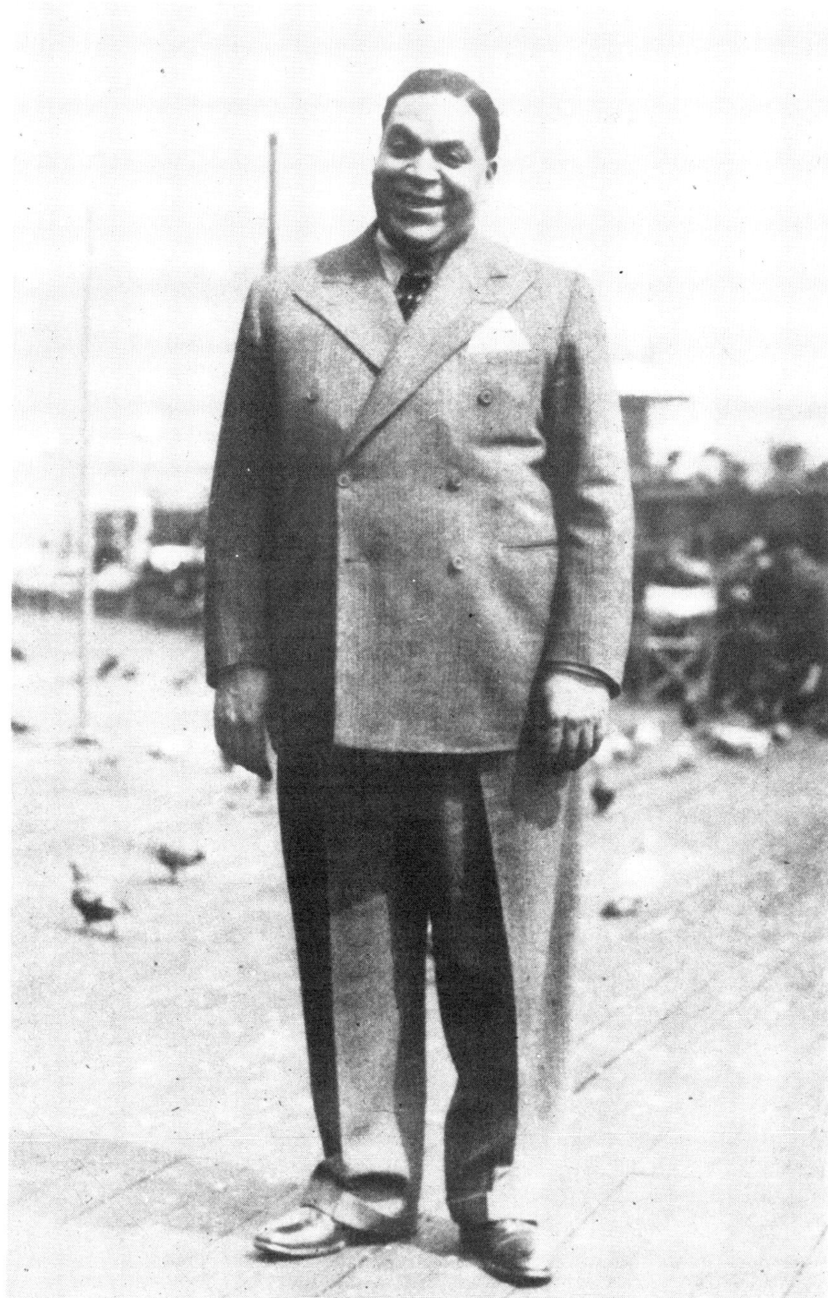

last night the audience showed their appreciation by demanding an encore.

Nottingham Journal, 16 May 1939:

Another great Negro artiste, who is making his first appearance in Nottingham this week is Fats Waller ... he gives a most varied selection of numbers at the piano including Hallelujah (from Hit The Deck), the popular Two Sleepy People, and his own composition Honeysuckle Rose. His grin alone is worth the price of your seat.

The Star (Sheffield), 23 May 1939 printed a cartoon of Fats and had:

...Twenty-stone Fats Waller, the great 'swing' pianist and composer, has not been here before, but Sheffield gave him a splendid reception on his first appearance. Rolling his big eyes at the audience, Fats played some well-known dance numbers...

The tour completed, the visitors headed back to London for a few days before joining their boat for the journey back to the States.

*****

Private Recording

Fats Waller, p

HMV Studios, Abbey Road, London — Monday, 12 June 1939

Reminiscing Through England No.2, Part 2 Issued on LP

There is a dull rhythmical noise during part of the above which might indicate the presence of a drummer, or possibly the microphone has picked up the noise of the Waller foot. The only evidence for this session is a test pressing in Waller's private collection sent by Bill Krasilovsky, the lawyer acting for the Waller estate, to John R.T. Davies and issued by him on Ristic LP 22. It is dated 12/6/39 and bears the inscription "Reminiscing Through England No.2, Part 2". It might be assumed from this that there was a number 1, possibly in one or more parts, and a part 1 to accompany the disc that has survived. It is possibly this session that Ed Kirkeby has recalled and joined in his memory to the Billy Higgs recordings when he said that he set up a recording with HMV the following day. It may be this session that singer Zaza Geldray (then Zaza Peters) recalled to Val Wilmer in conversation in August and September 1991 (see pages 302/3 for the full text).

*****

Piano Solo by "FATS" WALLER With Drums (Max Lewin) -1
(Organ Solo with Vocal by "Fats" Waller) -2
"FATS" WALLER (Vocal and Organ by "Fats" Waller) -3

Fats Waller, p-1/v-2/po-2; Max Lewin, d-4

HMV Studios, Abbey Road, London — Tuesday, 13 June 1939

LONDON SUITE (WALLER)

7878-1	1. Piccadilly -1	*HMV/In/D B.10059, HMVSw JK2721, El EG7630*
7879-1	2. Chelsea -1	*HMV/In/D B.10059, HMVSw JK2721, El EG7630*
7880-1	3. Soho -1	*HMV/In/D B.10060, HMVSw JK2722, El EG7631*
7881-1	4. Bond Street -1,-4	*HMV/In/D B.10060, HMVSw JK2722, El EG7631*
7882-1	5. Limehouse -1	*HMV/In/D B.10061, HMVSw JK2723, El EG7632*

7883-1	6. Whitechapel -1	*HMV/In/D B.10061, HMVSw JK2723, El EG7632*
7884-1	Hallelujah -1	HMV Rejected
7884-2	Hallelujah -1	HMV Rejected
7885-1	Signing On At H.M.V. -1	HMV Rejected
7885-2	Signing On At H.M.V. -1	HMV Rejected
7982-1	SMOKE DREAMS OF YOU -2,-3 (Gibsone—De Greville)	HMV/In B.8967
7983-1	YOU CAN'T HAVE YOUR CAKE AND EAT IT -2,-3 (Williams—"Fats" Waller)	HMV/In B.8967

As with the 1938 sessions the sides with organ were made in studio 1 and the remainder in studio 3, which explains the jump in matrix numbers. The masters for the London Suite were unissued prior to the war and, according to Ed Kirkeby, were lost during the blitz. A set of tests were found in a music publisher's office, dubbed masters made, and release finally achieved twelve years after recording. Although all the labels for the suite note the presence of Max Lewin on drums, and he is named on the relevant file cards, he is heard only as indicated.

Previous listings show the Swiss issues with the HE prefix, but a Swiss HMV catalogue held here shows them as above which is also confirmed by the file cards. Copies of the EMI files held by NSA reveal that the original masters for the 'London Suite' were destroyed on 12 January 1942. Dubbed masters (suffixed -1A) of all were made on 1 January 1951, plus a second master of the first title (-1B). 7883-1A was found to be damaged, and -1B was made on 17 January 1951. All of these were destroyed by the end of 1964. 7884/5 were also destroyed on 12 January 1942; 7982/3 on 30 October 1945. The file cards for 7884/5 do not name an artist, and that for 7886 is missing.

Victor had apparently intended issuing the London Suite and had prepared their own dub masters prefixed D6-VB- and having the following numbers respectively: 2885-1; 2882-1; 2881-1; 2883-1; (*Bond Street* not seen); 2884-1A.

Although Kirkeby's explanation of what happened to the masters to achieve release has been accepted without question, one might query why a set of HMV masters should have been in a music publisher's office. It seems equally likely that the version which eventually achieved release was a set of dubbings of the Billy Higgs acetates, but that for obvious reasons no one involved was going to reveal the truth.

*****

The following day, Wednesday, 14 June 1939 with the war clouds gathering in Europe, Fats and Ed Kirkeby boarded the *Ile de France* for the return journey to the United States, and the final word on the British tour rests with the Melody Maker of 10 June 1939:

> *One of the most brilliant true jazz artists ever to come from America to Britain, he returns a more popular idol than ever, and will long be remembered with great affection.*

*****

According to *Lloyd's List*, the *Ile de France* arrived in New York on 20 June 1939, and after a short rest at home, Fats reassembled his Rhythm for a recording session at Victor. But there were problems. Al Casey was sick, Gene Sedric had taken work with Don Redman and was not immediately available, nor was Slick Jones, so replacements had to be found.

*****

"Fats" Waller and his Rhythm -Fox Trot **Vocal refrain and piano by "Fats" Waller**

Herman Autrey, t; Chauncey Graham, ts; Fats Waller, p/v; John Smith, g; Cedric Wallace, sb; Larry Hinton, d.

Studio 2, New York City, New York — Wednesday, 28 June 1939

1:30 to 5:30 p.m. Ed Kirkeby directing

038207-1*	HONEY HUSH (Ed. Kirkeby-"Fats" Waller)	BB B-10346-B, ViC B-10346-B, MW M-8394, HMV B.10191, HMVEx J.O.274, HMVF SG357, HMVSw HE2997, HMVIt HN3128, HMVIn N.14080, El EG7719, RZAu G24220
038207-2*	HONEY HUSH	Bluebird unissued (see note). Issued on LP.

038207: 5th line of vocal: -1 "Oh how I love you Honey Hush, Yeah."
-2 "Oh how I love you Honey Hush."

038208-1*	I USED TO LOVE YOU (But It's All Over Now) (Lew Brown- Albert von Tilzer)	BB B-10369-A, Vi 20-2219-B, MW M-8393, HMV/In B.D.5533, HMVF K8469, RZAu G24274
038209-1*	WAIT AND SEE (Andy Razaf-Thomas "Fats" Waller)	BB B-10405-B, HMVSp GY552
038210-1*	YOU MEET THE NICEST PEOPLE IN YOUR DREAMS (Hoffman-Goodhart-Kurtz)	BB B-10346-A, ViC B-10346-B, HMVAu G24220
038311-1*	ANITA (Thomas "Fats" Waller)	BB B-10369-B, MW M-8393, HMV/In B.D.5533, HMVF K8469, RZAu G24938
038912-1*	WHAT A PRETTY MISS (Thomas "Fats" Waller-Spencer Williams)	BB B-10437-A, HMV B.10050, HMVIt HN3042, *HMVIn NE810*

Note that Ed Kirkeby is mentioned here, and for the next few sessions, in the position on the recording sheet normally used to note the session director. Included in this session are two of the compositions Waller had written in Britain, and the composer credit for the final title suggests that Sinclair Traill's memory of this being the unknown fourth title at Billy Higgs's studio may well be correct.

Both takes of the first title are marked as suitable for issue on the recording sheet which also notes the personnel (with some of the usual mis-spellings) and the use of flowed and cast waxes.

*****

Al Casey's replacement of John Smith proved to be very much to Waller's liking, so much so that when Al was fit enough to resume work he joined Teddy Wilson's big band and didn't rejoin Fats until late 1940. Ed Kirkeby states that Waller's first engagement back in New York was a week at the Apollo followed by an appearance at the World's Fair and then into Loew's State Theatre, during which time he made a record session for Muzak. This was followed by a "long series of one nighters" of which he mentions Washington, D.C., Atlantic City, Millsboro, Delaware and then back to New York for another Victor date. Available evidence suggests that he has his chronology wrong and that the tour of one-nighters actually took place between the engagement at Loew's and the Muzak recording session.

*****

The appearance at the Apollo was for the week commencing Friday, 30 June and for the first time the billing was for **"Fats" Waller His Organ His Band And Revue** and among the artists listed was Myra Johnson. This was the first time that mention had been made of an organ and this is presumably the occasion recalled by Bob Hall who was the Apollo's stage electrician, as related in Jack Schiffman's book on the history of the Apollo:

Fats was always a big drinker. He'd always come to the theater with a case of whiskey and he'd invite everybody to drink with him, and I mean everybody. He just didn't like being alone or without a drink for very long.

The first time he brought a Hammond Organ into the theater, he moved it in around eleven o'clock at night, just as we were starting to hang the new show, which ordinarily took a few hours. We set up his organ on its platform and started to hang some drops when Fats brought in not one but three cases of whiskey. I mean, there was all kinds of whiskey.

We stopped hanging the show and Fats started playing that organ. He'd play a few songs and we'd all have a drink. Then he'd play some more and we'd sing along with him. Then we'd have another drink. In a little while, we were all half-potted. Suddenly we looked through the fog and saw Mr. Schiffman standing there, looking kind of stern. Know what time it was? Nine-thirty in the morning, and we hadn't hung the scenery yet! And the show went on early in those days — about noontime. Well, we got the scenery hung all right, but none too soon. That Fats, he sure was somethin' else.

I have found no review of the performances for this week.

*****

Assuming that Kirkeby is correct, the appearance at the World's Fair would have been during the week between ending at the Apollo and commencing at Loew's, which can be dated from adverts in the New York papers as being from 14 - 20 July 1939. Thereafter, no engagements have been found until the session for Associated below, and it is probably during this period that Kirkeby's "long series of one nighters" took place.

*****

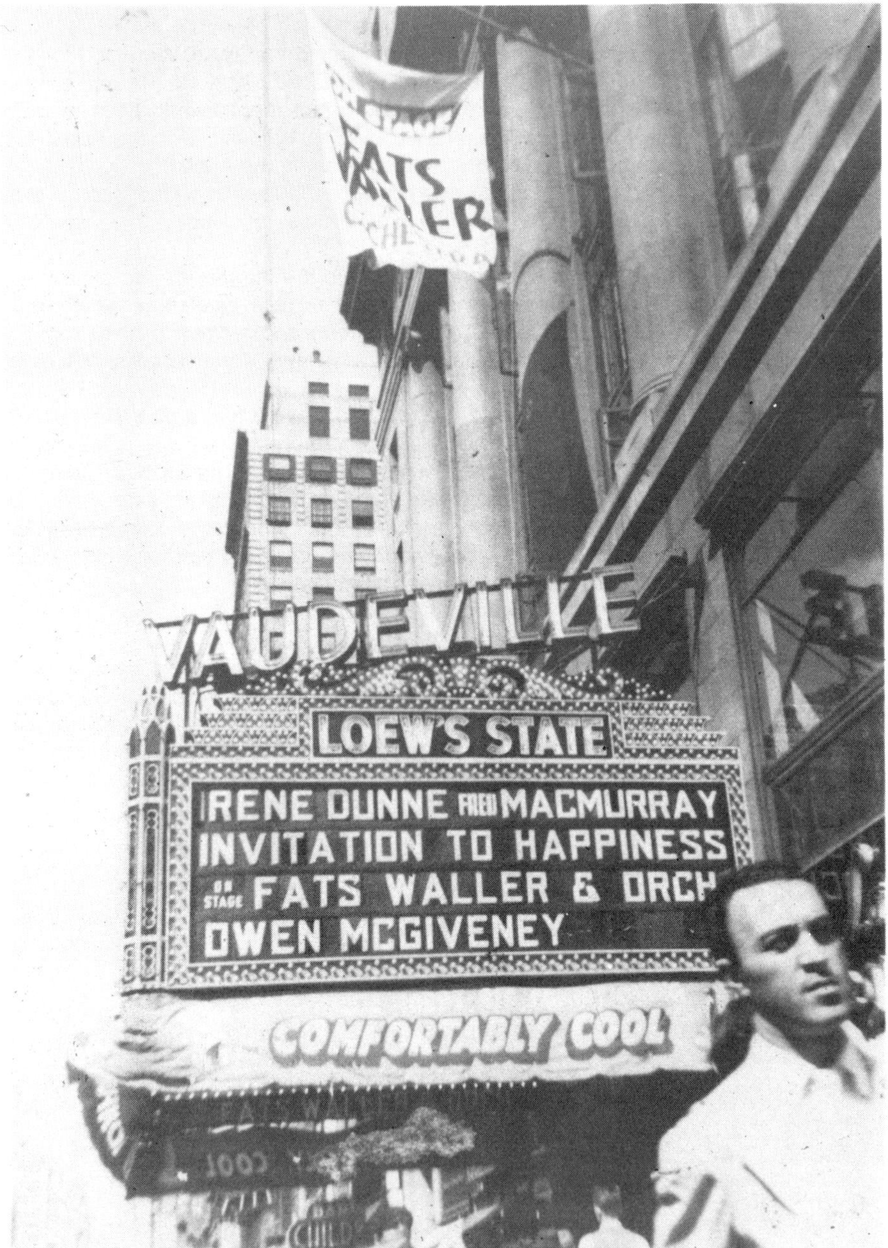

FATS WALLER
VAUDEVILLE
LOEW'S STATE
IRENE DUNNE FRED MACMURRAY
INVITATION TO HAPPINESS
ON STAGE FATS WALLER & ORCH
OWEN MCGIVENEY
COMFORTABLY COOL

THOMAS "FATS" WALLER AND HIS ORCHESTRA

John Hamilton, t; Gene Sedric, cl-1/ts-2; Fats Waller, p/v-3; John Smith, g; Cedric Wallace, sb; Slick Jones, d.

Electrical Research Products Inc. Studio, Bronx, New York — Monday, 7 August 1939

2143 The Moon Is Low #1 -2 — Issued on LP
THE MOON IS LOW #2 -1,-2 — Associated No. 60,130-B
From Picture "Montana Moon"
THE SHEIK OF ARABY -1,-3 — Associated No. 60,130-B
(Vocal introduction by "Fats" Waller)

2144 E Flat Blues (incomplete) -3 — Issued on LP
"E" FLAT BLUES -1,-3 — Associated No. 60,130-B
(Spoken introduction by "Fats" Waller)
Introductory patter: Incomplete version: "...Be careful now..."
Complete version: "...Take it easy now"
Honeysuckle Rose #1 -2,-3 — Issued on LP
HONEYSUCKLE ROSE #2 -2,-3 — Associated No. 60,130-B
From "Load Of Coal" (Spoken introduction and vocal by "Fats" Waller)
Introductory patter: #1 "And now we bring one of the originals by the Fatsy Watsy..."
#2 "...by yours truly, little Fatsy Watsy Waller."
AIN'T MISBEHAVIN' -1,-2,-3 — Associated No. 60,133-A, R6,023-B, 60,493-B, *JSo AA536*
From "Connie's Hot Chocolates'

2145 SWEET SUE, JUST YOU -2,-3 — Associated No. 60,133-A, R6,023-B, 60,493-B, *JSo AA535*
Nagasaki (breakdown) — Issued on LP (see note)
NAGASAKI — Associated No. 60,133-A, R6,023-B, 60,493-B, *JSo AA536*
I'm Crazy 'Bout My Baby (incomplete) -3 — Issued on LP
I'M CRAZY 'BOUT MY BABY -2,-3 — Associated No. 60,134-A
THE SPIDER AND THE FLY -1,-3 — Associated No. 60,134-A

2146 LONESOME ME -2,-3 — Associated 60,133-A, R6,023-B, 60,493-B, *JSo AA535*
After You've Gone #1 -2,-3 — Issued on LP
AFTER YOU'VE GONE #2 -2,-3 — Associated No. 60,134-A
First vocal #1 ...the bestest pal that you've ever had... and Fats messes up the vocal
#2 ...the bestest pal you've ever had... and Fats sings the lyrics more or less as written

Fats Waller — Hammond Organ Solo

2147 Dinah (incomplete) — Issued on LP

THOMAS "FATS" WALLER — Piano Solo

POOR BUTTERFLY — Associated No. 60,133-B
ST. LOUIS BLUES — Associated No. 60,133-B
HALLELUJAH From "Hit the Deck" — Associated No. 60,133-B

2148 TEA FOR TWO From "No, No, Nanette" — Associated No. 60,134-A
HANDFUL OF KEYS — Associated No. 60,133-B

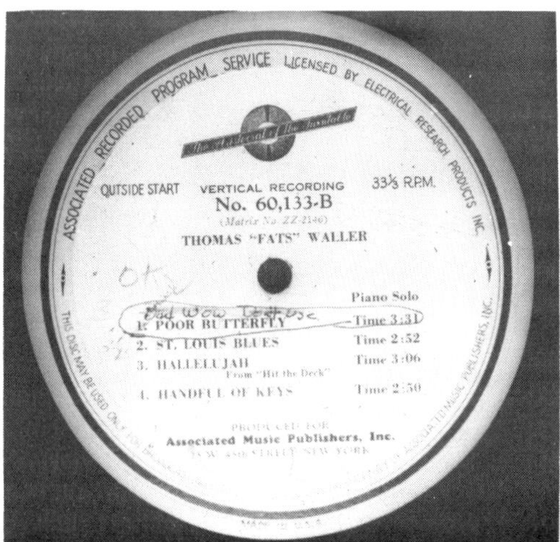

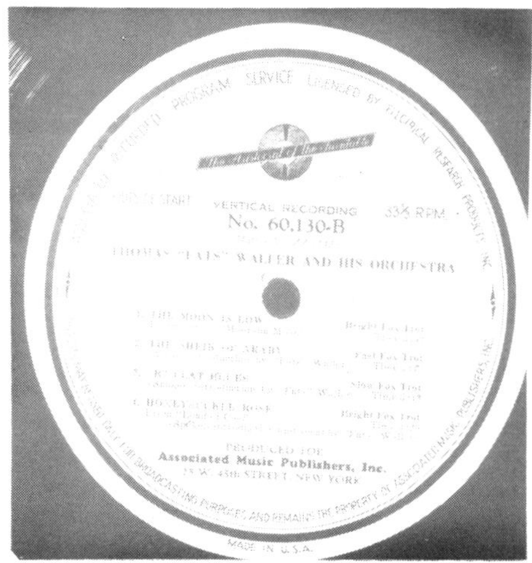

The recording engineer seems to have had some difficulty in getting the right balance and the bass is barely audible on the first title; is a little better on the second and comes into focus on the third. Although *E Flat Blues* is so labelled (it has been manually altered on the label illustrated), Fats distinctly says "B Flat..." in his introductory patter to both versions and the tune is played in that key. On the aborted first take, Fats can be heard muttering to himself as it cuts off and on this, the cut-off point occurs before the entry of Sedric or Hamilton, and the same thing happens on the very short aborted take of *I'm Crazy 'Bout My Baby.* Many of the titles have vocal patter and/or spoken introductions and these are all shown marked -3. A number of the tunes are ones that Fats had featured heavily during his British tour and, since these had been well received and he was apparently given a more than usually free hand at this session, he obviously took the opportunity to get them on to wax.

These recordings were made for radio use and edited versions of the programmes appeared on vertically-cut 16" 33⅓ r.p.m. Associated Program Service recordings. Ken Crawford has kindly supplied much of the information included and also explains the method of recording and issue as follows: Originally, a 'direct mastering system' was used by Associated Muzak in which everything recorded, including false starts, etc. got issued. In 1938 the company began to use an 'Acetate first system' and the content of the original acetates is that given above in recording order, using the original acetate numbers. The content of these acetates was then selected for issue and the same acetate numbers, but prefixed ZZ, were used as matrices for the issued records. This means that selections which were recorded on one number might be issued under a different number which is confusing if this is not understood. The content of the issued discs is as follows:

ZZ-2143 The Moon Is Low/The Sheik Of Araby/"E" Flat Blues/Honeysuckle Rose
ZZ-2144 Ain't Misbehavin'/Sweet Sue, Just You/Nagasaki/ Lonesome Me
ZZ-2145 I'm Crazy 'Bout My Baby/The Spider And The Fly/After You've Gone/Tea For Two
ZZ-2146 Poor Butterfly/St. Louis Blues/Hallelujah/Handful Of Keys

There are no composer credits shown on any of the issued discs.

Reverses: 60,130 is by **TEDDY POWELL ORCHESTRA**; 60,134-B is by **BEN SELVIN AND HIS COCKTAIL ORCHESTRA**; 60,493 and R6,023 by **ROSARIO BOURDON AND**

CONCERT ORCHESTRA with all titles on 60,493 u/c.

These recordings were never intended for 78 r.p.m. issue. Jazz Society 535 is a 12" issue showing the title of the first side as simply *Sweet Sue* with composer credit Harris and the reverse showing a composer credit of Waller. It is issued as **THOMAS "FATS" WALLER AND HIS ORCHESTRA** . Jazz Society 536 is 10", labelled **Fats Waller and his Orchestra** and shows composer credits of Waller and Dixon respectively. In 1981, Jerry Valburn gained access to the original recordings, complete with false starts, etc. and issued the complete set except for the breakdown of *Nagasaki,* along with the 1935 Muzak recordings in a boxed set of LPs. The breakdown of *Nagasaki,* which lasts for only five seconds, appears on LP elsewhere. It is not known whether it preceded or followed the complete version in recording order.

*****

Fats Waller and his Rhythm - Fox Trot **Piano by "Fats" Waller (B-10437-B)**
John Hamilton, t; Gene Sedric, cl-1/ts-2; Fats Waller, p/v-3; Cedric Wallace, sb; John Smith, g; Slick Jones, d.

Studio 2, New York City, New York Thursday, 10 August 1939
10:00 a.m. to 1:00 p.m. Ed Kirkeby present

041528-1*	(When You) SQUEEZE ME -2,-3 (Razaf-Williams-Waller)	BB B-10405-A, Vi 20-2217-B, MW M-4892, HMVEx JO.132, HMVSp GY552, HMVSc AL5020, HMVIn N14051
041529-1*	BLESS YOU -2,-3 (Eddie Lane-Don Baker)	BB B-10393-A, HMVH MH.52
041530-1*	IT'S THE TUNE THAT COUNTS -1,-3 (Don Raye-Jan Savitt)	BB B-10393-B, HMV JO.89, HMVF SG56, HMVIn N14030
041531-1*	ABDULLAH -1,-2,-3 (Neal Laurence-"Slick" Jones)	BB B-10419-B, *Vi 20-2639-B,* MW M-8391, *HMVIn NE724,* RZAu G24166
041532-1*	WHO'LL TAKE MY PLACE (When I'm Gone) -1,-3 (Raymond-Klagis-Billy Fazioli)	BB-B10419-A, Vi 20-2642-A, MW M-8391, *HMVIn NE724,* RZAu G24166
041533-1*	BOND STREET -1 (Thomas "Fats" Waller)	BB B-10437-B, *HMVIn NE810,* RZAu G24274

As usual, the recording sheet notes the use of flowed and cast waxes, but that the former are "Wide Range". The final title has the sub-title *(from The London Suite)* added. It is something of a mystery why this is the only part of the suite to receive further attention from Fats, given the prominence that Ed Kirkeby seems to have attached to it.

*****

A photo of Fats with the caption 'Sued Again' appears in the *Pittsburgh Courier* of 19 August. A brief paragraph explains that he is being sued by the owner of Rosedale Beach, Millsboro, Delaware, for failure to turn up for an engagement. No indication of when this should have taken place is given, but it was presumably at least a week or two prior to the legal action. Note that Ed Kirkeby had mentioned Millsboro in his list of 'one-nighters'.

*****

Back on 22 July, the *Piittsburgh Courier* had reported that the William Morris agency, booking Waller, had a contract for him to open in the Panther Room of the Hotel Sherman in Chicago with a six-piece band on or about the 10th August and running through to September. Presumably he left for the Windy City immediately after the session above and according to Ed Kirkeby's account in *Ain't Misbehavin',* Waller spent four weeks in Chicago at College Inn, where for at least part of the time he shared the bill with Muggsy Spanier and his Ragtime Band and harpist Casper Reardon as indicated by the poster outside the Hotel Sherman below; then to Salt Lake Theatre and then back to the Regal in Chicago before returning to New York and the Adams theatre in Newark, New Jersey. Whilst in Chicago, Waller and his band had been booked as headliners for the annual Musicians' Picnic organised by Local 208 along with a selection of other top-flight attractions as shown in the advertising reproduced opposite. The picnic took place from noon until midnight on Monday, 21 August and, as far as is known, Waller did fulfil his obligation. Additional news of the stay in Chicago is given by Ted Watson in his column in the Pittsburgh Courier. Datelined Aug. 31, he says, 'Fats Waller, who won Thursday's Washington Park daily double race, is basking at the Ritz after a reported closing at the Grand Hotel.' Further on in the same column he says, 'Fats Waller is playing in the Panther Room of the Hotel Sherman'.

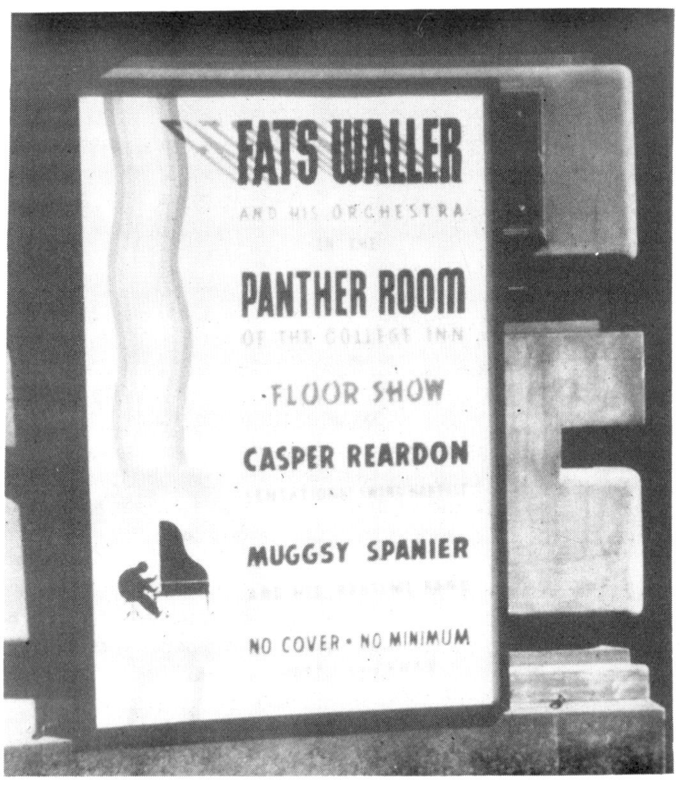

*****

The week spent at the Regal in Chicago, on South Parkway at 47th Street, was that described by Ernie Anderson elsewhere in this book. This was reported in the *Pittsburgh Courier* which added that the band had been playing in the loop, and this information is amplified by another in the October *International Musician* which says that Waller had played the State Lake Theatre for the week beginning 22 September. According to an advert in the *Defender* of 30

FATS WALLER

and HIS ORCHESTRA

IN PERSON

HORACE HENDERSON

JOHNNY LONG

FLOYD CAMPBELL

JIMMIE NOONE

"KING" KOLAX

WILL POSITIVELY APPEAR

— at the —

MUSICIANS'

ANNUAL PICNIC

MONDAY

AUGUST 21st, 1939

— at —

BERGMAN'S GROVE

24th and Desplaines Avenue

NORTH RIVERSIDE, ILLINOIS

CONTINUOUS

DANCING

12 NOON UNTIL 12 MIDNIGHT

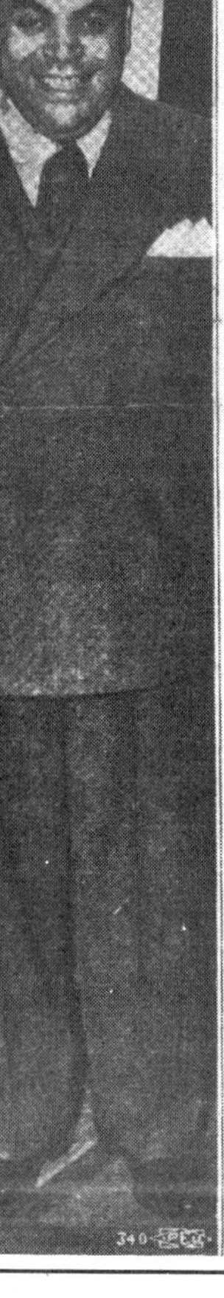

DIRECTIONS

GARFIELD BLVD. AUTO ROUTE:

Garfield Boulevard (55th St.) West to Harlem Avenue North on Harlem to Cermak Road west to Desplaines Avenue. Then South to Grove.

STREET CAR ROUTE:

Take 22nd Street Car to 48th Ave. and 22nd Street and then La Grange car to Grove. Take Douglas Park Met. "L" Branch to 48th Avenue and then La Grange car to BERGMAN'S GROVE, Desplaines Avenue, North Riverside, Ill.

ADVANCE SALE TICKETS **25c**

ADMISSION AT GATE **35c**

LOCAL 208, A. F. of M. 3934 SOUTH STATE STREET

September 1939, the week began on Friday, 29 September and the advert proclaimed:

Today, Sept. 29 — In Person — All Week
2 — Great Orchestras —2
"Fats" Waller And His Orch.
Versus
"Muggsy" Spanier And His Orch.
In A Giant "Battle Of Swing"

Under the heading "Regal Gets "Fats' Midnight Show At "Met', Fats Waller's Band Opens Regal Stage' the same issue of the *Defender* reviewed the confrontation as follows:

> *The Regal Theater stage might well be considered a 'battleground of swing' this week inasmuch as it is the meeting place of "Fats' Waller and His Harlem Orchestra and 'Muggsy' Spanier and His Ragtime Band. The contest opened Friday, Sept. 29th and will continue all through the week.*
>
> *In the 'swing-heat' conducted between both those bands at the State-Lake theater, 'Fats' and his tunesmiths were conceded the edge. The battle was 'nip and tuck' at the loop house until the very last day when Waller and his 'swingeroos' broke in the lead and kept their distance.*
>
> *'Fats' and 'Muggsy' are palsy-walsy between shows backstage, but the very minute the stage lights come up the feud commences. Waller takes his place at the helm of his group and breaks into a fast swing arrangement of a currently popular tune. When he finishes, 'Muggsy' Spanier raises his baton and plays the same number, substituting slow, sweet music for swing.*
>
> *In addition to 'The Battle of Swing', the Regal is also presenting an extravagant stage revue featuring a long list of singers, dancers and comedians. These performers help break the tension of the sizzling orchestras.*

*****

The photograph opposite (dated Newark, 1939) of what appears to be a broadcast by Fats with Pee Wee Russell and Max Kaminsky and an unidentified bass player may have been taken during his spell at the Adams Theatre. Following which, according to Kirkeby's account, Waller went to the Southland night club in Boston for two weeks and a one-nighter in New Haven before going into the Famous Door on 52nd Street. This engagement can be dated independently from various issues of *Jazz Information* which gave advance news of the booking: *Fats Waller goes into the Famous Door in a few weeks* (26 September); *Fats Waller replaces Teddy Powell at the Famous Door October 22* (3 October); *Fats Waller and his Band opened at the Famous Door tonight (Tuesday) sharing Billing with Maxine Sullivan...* (24 October). The issue of 31 October said they were still there with Kirby Walker as relief pianist, whilst the issue of 7 November has, *Fats Waller left the Famous Door Tuesday and was replaced by Jack Jenny and his Orchestra. Fats goes into the Apollo for a week on November 10.* The appearance at the Apollo was confirmed the following week. The November *International Musician* noted the starting date at the Famous Door as 24 October and also reported transfers deposited in Chicago for Hamilton, Sedric, Waller, Smith, Wallace and Jones, thus confirming the group which played the two theatres in the city. During the Famous Door engagement, another Victor record date took place:

*****

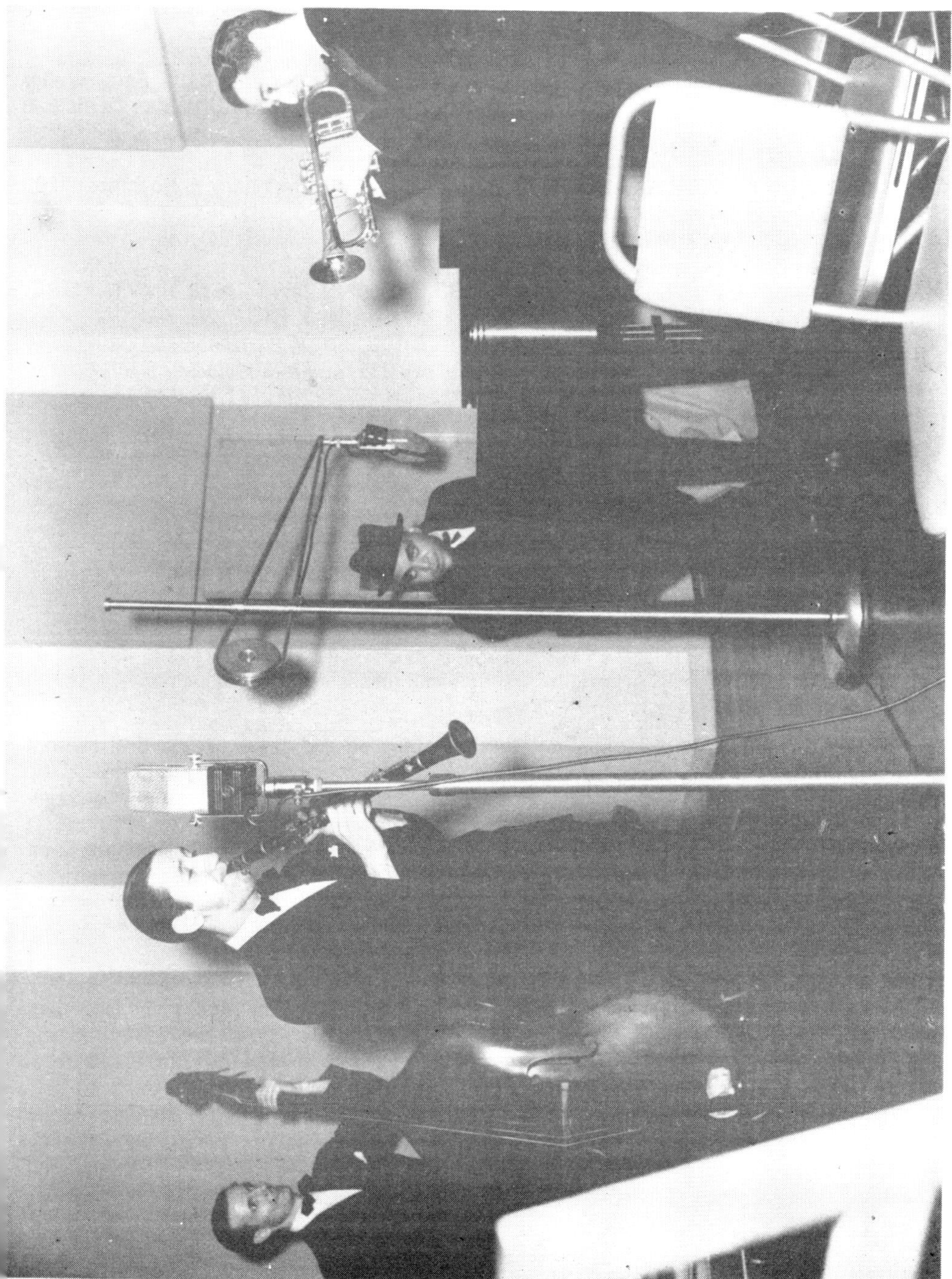

"Fats" Waller and his Rhythm - Fox Trot **Vocal refrain and piano by "Fats" Waller** or **Vocal refrain by "Fats Waller" and Una Mae Carlisle -5**

John Hamilton, t; Gene Sedric, cl-1/ts-2; Fats Waller, p/v; Cedric Wallace, sb; John Smith, g; Slick Jones, d; band vocal -4; Una Mae Carlisle, v-5.

Studio 2, New York City, New York — Friday, 3 November 1939
1:45 to 5:45 p.m. Ed Kirkeby present

043346-1*	IT'S YOU WHO TAUGHT IT TO ME -1,-2 (Harley-Razaf-Davis)	BB B-10527-B, HMVEx JO.128, HMVSW HE2731
043347-1*	SUITCASE SUSIE -1,-2 (Reubens-French-LaFreniere)	BB B-10500-B, MW M-8648, HMV/H J.O.81, HMVIt HN2426, *HMVIn NE.790*
043348-1*	YOUR FEET'S TOO BIG -1 (Ada Benson-Fred Fisher)	BB B-10500-A, *Vi 20-1580-B, 44-0009,* 244, 420-0235, MW M-8648, HMV B.9582, HMVH MH.52, HMVIt HN2359, *HMVIn NE.790, V-D 308*
043349-1*	YOU'RE LETTIN' THE GRASS GROW UNDER YOUR FEET -1,-2 (Ager-Selsman-Livingston)	BB B-10527-A, HMV J.O.273, EI EG7727
043350-1*	DARKTOWN STRUTTERS' BALL -1,-2 (Shelton Brooks)	BB B-10573-A, *BBC B-10573-A,* Vi 20-2220-B, HMVEx JO.116, HMVF SG388, HMVIn N14045
043351-1*	I CAN'T GIVE YOU ANYTHING BUT LOVE, BABY -2,-5 (Dorothy Fields-Jimmy McHugh)	BB B-10573-B, *BBC B-10573-B, Vi 20-1582-A,* 420-0237, ViJ A1464, HMVEi IW341, HMVSp GY417
043351-2*	I CAN'T GIVE YOU ANYTHING BUT LOVE, BABY	Victor unissued, 'Hold'. Issued on LP

The recording sheet shows personnel and the use of flowed and cast waxes and at the foot, *NOTE:- On BS043351-2 & 2A vocal was by Fats Waller alone* and, despite the entry in *Jazz Records,* it is Waller's voice alone that is heard. Apparently, Una Mae Carlisle had walked into the studio during the session and been invited to join in the vocal on one take.

Victor 44-0009 is a special pressing by the company for coin operators and has the same performance on both sides; Victor 244 (backed by 243) is a demonstration record pressed on vinyl. It credits the performance to "**Fats" Waller, his Rhythm and his Buddies** and incorrectly notes Una Mae Carlisle as a vocalist.

*****

"Fats" Waller and his Band with Myra Johnson were advertised as headliners at the Apollo for the week commencing Friday, 10 November, and the *New York Age* of 11 November carried a photo of Waller, the caption to which said, *"Fats" Waller, perennial Harlem favorite, who is doubling at "The Open Door" and the Apollo where he is presenting the same revue which recently closed a record-breaking week at Loew's State on Broadway.*

*****

Mon. Night
JITTERBUG
Contest

Wed. Night
AMATEURS

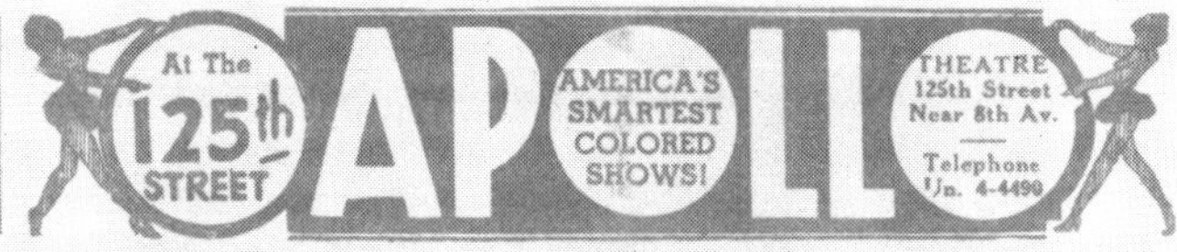

Saturday
MIDNIGHT
SHOW

Reserved Seats
Now On Sale

ONE BIG WEEK – BEGINNING FRIDAY, NOV. 3rd

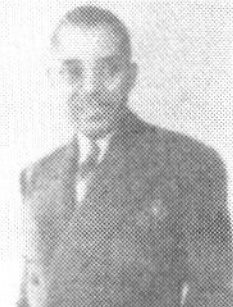

NOBLE SISSLE AND HIS BAND

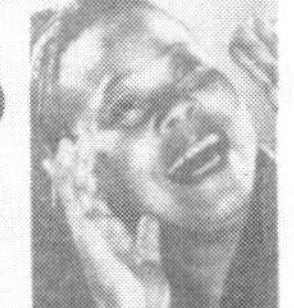

ADA BROWN

RUBY HILL
BILLY BANKS

JERRY TAPS – 5 BUDDS – CLAUDE & CORINNE

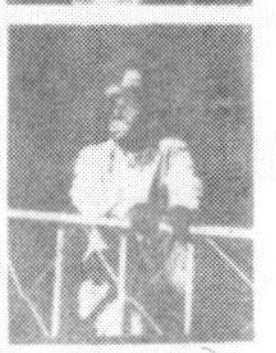

JOHN MASON SANDY BURNS GEO. WILTSHIRE **20** DANCING GIRLS & BOYS

ALSO — THE DRAMATIC SCREEN HIT **"ISLAND OF LOST MEN"** with ANNA MAY WONG

ONE WEEK ONLY – BEGINNING FRIDAY, NOV. 10th

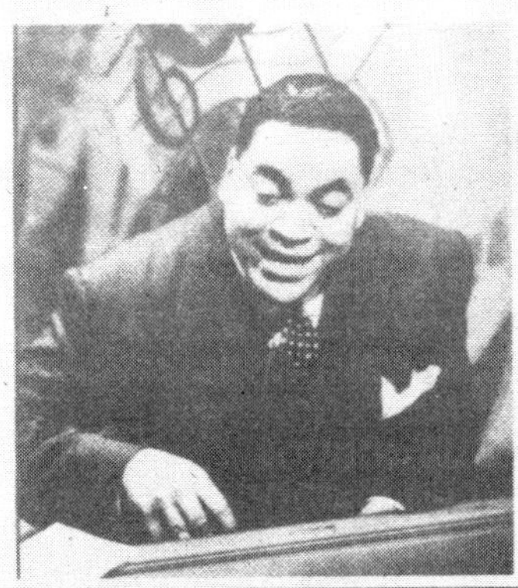

"FATS" WALLER

AND HIS BAND

with

MYRA JOHNSON

AND A REVUE CAST OF 45

COMING SOON – Another Delightful Surprise

THE QUEEN OF HI-DEE-HO

BLANCHE CALLOWAY

AND HER BAND AND REVUE

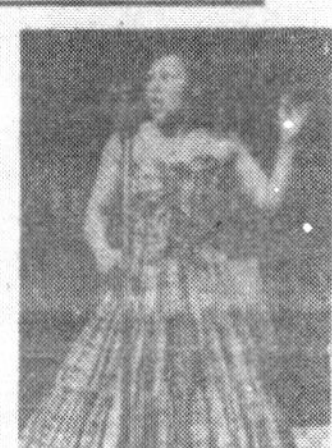

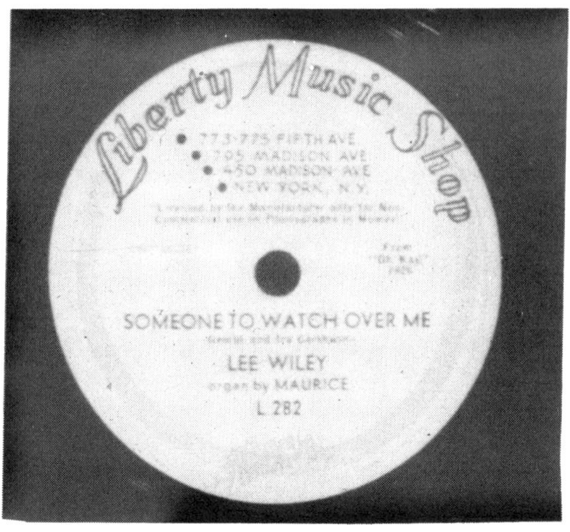

LEE WILEY with Max Kaminsky's Orchestra -1
LEE WILEY organ by Maurice -2
Lee Wiley, v, acc: Max Kaminsky, t; Pee Wee Russell, cl; Bud Freeman, ts; Fats Waller, p-1/o-2/cel-3; Eddie Condon, g; Artie Shapiro, sb; George Wettling, d.

Liederkranz Hall, New York City, New York — Wednesday, 15 November 1939

26270-A I'VE GOT A CRUSH ON YOU -1 — LMS L282
-George and Ira Gershwin-

26271-A SOMEONE TO WATCH OVER ME -2 — LMS L282
-George and Ira Gershwin-

26272-A HOW LONG HAS THIS BEEN GOING ON? -George and Ira Gershwin- -1,-3 — LMS L281

26273-A BUT NOT FOR ME — LMS L284
-George and Ira Gershwin- -1

The reverses of Liberty Music Shop L281 and L284 are by **LEE WILEY with JOE BUSHKIN'S ORCHESTRA**. Each side notes the original show from which the composition came.

Please refer to Ernie Anderson's account elsewhere in this volume for the story behind this session. The arranger for the session was Brad Gowans.

*****

The session above was made during Waller's week at the Apollo and, before leaving for an engagement with his Rhythm at the Sherman Hotel's Panther Room in Chicago, he visited the Victor Studios to record a number of programmes for radio use. Other news of his activities was given in the *Pittsburgh Courier,* as the following extracts from a report datelined New York City, Nov. 16 indicate:

> *Fats Waller ... was shown through the eyes of fame in yet another light Sunday (12 November) as a hobbyist on the widely heard Hobby Lobby commercial program ... Waller's hobby is the collecting of rabbit's feet and he has several varieties.*

*****

Completing his duties here which also included a week's engagement at the Apollo ... will entrain for Pittsburgh where he has been contracted to play an exclusive private party. On the 24th he will take the band into Washington for a session at the Howard theatre headlining an all-star colored revue. After his date in the Capitol City ... will return to Chicago and his second engagement at the College Inn, Panther Room of the Hotel Sherman where he broke attendance records during his engagement there last season.

With his band cut down to five pieces ... still as popular as when he batoned fourteen or more pieces.

*****

The Lang-Worth Recordings

Fats Waller, p-1/o-2/v-3

Victor Studios, New York City, New York — Monday, 20 November 1939

043185-1	Go Down Moses -2,-3	Program: No. 517
	Swing Low, Sweet Chariot -2,-3	FATS WALLER
	I'm A Bum -2,-3	Swing Singin' With a Hammond
	Hand Me Down My Walkin' Cane -2,-3	
043186-1	Frankie And Johnnie -2,-3	Program: No. 518
	She'll Be Comin' Round The Mountain -2,-3	FATS WALLER
		Swing Singin' With a Hammond
	Deep River -2,-3	
	Lord Delivered Daniel -2,-3	
043187-1	Ah So Pure -1	Program: No. 521
	Then You'll Remember Me -1	FATS WALLER
	Lucia di Lammamore (Sextette)	Swinging With a Steinway
	My Heart At Thy Sweet Voice	
043188-1	Cavalleria Rusticana (Intermezzo) (No Vocal) -1	Program No. 519
		FATS WALLER
	When You And I Were Young, Maggie -1,-3	Swing Singin' With a Steinway
	Loch Lomond -1,-3	
	Oh, Susannah -1,-3	
043189-1	Old Oaken Bucket -1,-3	Program No. 520
	Oh Dem Golden Slippers -1,-3	FATS WALLER
	Faust Waltz (No Vocal) -1	Swing Singin' With A Steinway
	Annie Laurie -1	

The above are all 16" transcription discs intended for radio broadcast. Although these bear Victor-style matrix numbers and would seem to be 'custom' recordings, Ed Kirkeby told Bob Kumm that they were made in a small studio on 57th Street, New York, and said that Lang-Worth was not connected to Victor in any way. After Fats died, Lang-Worth offered to sell the masters to Victor for commercial release, but the deal was never finalised and eventually Bill Grauer and Orin Keepnews acquired the right to issue the material on their Riverside label.

From photographs supplied, two types of label and two pressing sources were used and

Ken Crawford advises that *all* Lang-Worth issues from Program 1/2 until shortly after these Waller recordings were made were issued by Lang-Worth in identical form on both their own label and the Planned Program Services label. Programs 519 and 520 on the 'Planned Program Service' label bear at the foot the legend 'RCA Manufacturing Co. Inc.' with address; Program 521 has 'Pressed But Not Recorded By COLUMBIA RECORDING CORPORATION' with address. Program 521 has a reverse by **THE BOB HAMILTON TRIO** (Program 522). Programs 517 and 518 are coupled, as are 519 and 520. The grids printed on the NAB-LANG-WORTH label are to record the number of airplays given to each number and on both types of label the tunes are numbered and timings for each given.

*****

Soon after this, Fats and his Rhythm presumably fulfilled the engagements noted in the report above and then returned to Chicago for a six-week engagement at the Hotel Sherman's Panther Room as recalled by guitarist John Smith and during which, according to Ed Kirkeby, *Jitterbug Waltz* was written. Ed Kirkeby also relates how Waller played organ in his hotel room after the show on Christmas Eve, presumably as related to him by Fats. Another version appears in *An Autobiography Of Black Jazz* in the recollections of Franz Jackson:

> *Waller usually had a portable organ in his room. He often told me the story about the Christmas Eve he spent in Chicago at the Ritz Hotel located on South Parkway (King Drive) and Oakwood Boulevard. That night after he finished work he went to his room with a friend and started working out on the organ. The room was literally rocking when it slowly began filling up with piano players. Duke Ellington, who was staying in the hotel, was the first to drift into Waller's room, followed by Earl Hines, who was working next door at the Terrace. Billy Kyle, the pianist with John Kirby's orchestra, was also staying at the hotel, and he came downstairs to Waller's room feeling good and just flopped down on the bed. Not too much time had passed before Duke pulled out his handkerchief, pretending to wipe his nose. Earl Hines started rubbing his eyes as though they itched. There was not a dry eye in that room because all the "cats" had become homesick and were moved by Waller's sensitive renditions of "Silent Night" and other holiday songs.*

There are a number of other accounts extant of this occasion, including one from Earl Hines who says it was the College Room in the Hotel Sherman that Fats was playing. He says that Fats was missing the following day and the Hotel proprietors contacted him to see if he knew of Waller's whereabouts. The following morning he received a telegram saying, *I'm on my way to New York. Call the College Room. Fats.* Hines says that Waller became so homesick after playing the Christmas songs that he just took off to be with his family.

The termination date at the Panther Room is given in *Jazz Information* of 8 December 1939, which says, *Fats Waller and Jimmy McPartland continue at the Hotel Sherman's Panther Room until Jimmy Dorsey arrives on Dec. 29.* However, the issue of 5 January 1940 states, *Fats Waller and Jimmy McPartland at the Sherman,* so presumably they had been held over.

Whatever the truth of the matter with all these conflicting reports, Fats was still in (or back in) Chicago the following week for a date in Victor's studios there.

*****

NAB·LANG-WORTH

TAX-FREE MUSIC SERVICE

PRODUCED BY

LANG-WORTH FEATURE PROGRAMS INC.

42 MADISON AVE., NEW YORK, N. Y.

IN COOPERATION WITH

NATIONAL ASSOCIATION OF BROADCASTERS

PROGRAM: No. 5 MASTER: 043187

FATS WALLER

Swinging With a Steinway

SELECTIONS (numbered outside in)

1: Ah So Pure - - - - - 2:40
2: Then You'll Remember Me - - - - - 2:40
3: Lucia di Lammamore (Sextette) - - - - 2:10
4: My Heart At Thy Sweet Voice - - - - - 3:20

PLANNED PROGRAM SERVICE

PRODUCED BY

LANG-WORTH FEATURE PROGRAMS

INCORPORATED

420 MADISON AVE., NEW YORK

A DIVISION OF LANGLOIS & WENTWORTH, INC.

MUSICAL CONTENT IN THIS RECORDING HAS BEEN CHECKED BY THE MUSIC PUBLISHERS' PROTECTIVE ASSOCIATION AND FOUND TO BE FREE FROM COPYRIGHT IN THE U. S. A.

Program No. 520 MS 043189

FATS WALLER

Swing Singin' With A Steinway

Selections:

1 – Old Oaken Bucket – 3:15
2 – Oh Dem Golden Slippers – 2:45
3 – Faust Waltz (No Vocal) – 2:55
4 – Annie Laurie – 2:45

THIS PROGRAM IS SOLD WITH THE AGREEMENT THAT IT WILL NOT BE RESOLD, RENTED OR LOANED, NOR BROADCAST FROM ANY RADIO STATION OTHER THAN THE ONE TO WHICH IT IS SOLD.

RECORDED, PROCESSED AND MANUFACTURED BY

RCA Manufacturing Co., Inc.

Camden, N. J., U. S. A.

"Fats" Waller and his Rhythm — Fox Trot **Vocal refrain and piano by "Fats" Waller -3**
or **Hammond Organ by "Fats" Waller -4**
or **Piano by "Fats" Waller -6**

John Hamilton, t; Gene Sedric, cl-1/ts-2; Fats Waller, p-3/o-4/v-5; John Smith, g; Cedric Wallace, sb; Slick Jones, d/vb-6.

Studio A, Chicago, Illinois — Friday, 12 January 1940
1:30 to 5:15 p.m.

044597-1*	SWINGA-DILLA STREET -2,-4 (Razaf-Johnson-Silver)	BB B-10858-B, RZAu G24504
044598-1*	AT TWILIGHT -2,-3,-5 ("Fats" and Anita Waller)	BB B-10803-B, HMVEx J.O.96, HMVIn N14033
044598-2	AT TWILIGHT *-2,-3,-5*	Victor unissued, 'Hold'
044599-1*	OH! FRENCHY -1,-2,-3,-5 (Sam Ehrlich-Con Conrad)	BB B-10658-B, *Vi 20-1595-A, V-D 359B*, HMVSw HE2291, HMVSc X6543,
044599-2	OH! FRENCHY -1,-2,-3,-5	Victor unissued, 'Process'
044600-1*	CHEATIN' ON ME -1,-3,-5,-6 (Jack Yellen-Lou Pollack)	BB B-10658-A, HMVSw HE2291, HMVSc X6543, RZAu G24563
044601-1*	BLACK MARIA -1,-3,-5 (Razaf-Johnson-Rose)	BB B-10624-B
044601-2	BLACK MARIA *-1,-3,-5*	Victor unissued, 'Hold'
044602-1*	MIGHTY FINE -2,-3,-5 (Andy Razaf-Thomas "Fats" Waller)	BB B-10744-A, HMVSp GY447, HMVEi IW339
044602-2*	MIGHTY FINE -2,-3,-5	Victor unissued, 'Process'
044603-1*	THE MOON IS LOW -2,-3,-6 (Arthur Freed-Nacio Herb Brown)	BB B-10624-A, HMVAu EA2571
044604-1*	THE MOON IS LOW PART #2 -2,-4	Victor unissued, 'Hold'. Issued on LP

The final title has a note in manuscript "N.G. Steven Sholes" and "D" (=Destroy) written against the masters and another note, added much later "No parts on hand since 1947". 044601 is credited to (Rose) alone on the recording sheet. V Disc 359B has two Waller titles (see 5 June 1936 session) on one side and on the reverse two titles by **The King Cole Trio.**

*****

Picking up Ed Kirkeby's account, the band then went to Detroit's Colonial Theatre (presumably for a week), where they broke all records. This is confirmed by a report datelined Detroit, Feb. 1 in the *Pittsburgh Courier* which says, 'Fats Waller's opening day at Ray Schribner's Colonial Theatre set an all-time record for the house, when the famous pianist and his band drew 9,034 people in the 1,455-seat house.'

From there they travelled on to Toronto to Shea's Theatre. Art Pilkington has checked the Toronto papers and is able to date this as 19 to 24 February. Waller's appearance was advertised in the *Toronto Daily Star* of 20 February stating that he would be featured on "the amazing Northern Hammond Electric Organ ... supplied by Simpson's" (a local department store). A review in same issue of the same paper by Jack Karr has:

> *For some unknown reason, we went to Shea's this week expecting to find a unit show. We were slightly surprised, therefore, to see the regulation five acts with Fats Waller, the headliner, merely occupying the last stanza. His swing aggregation keep the hep cats and*

alligators in a perfect lather for the all-too-short time they're on stage. Just happened to wonder if all the fans who know Waller best for his jump and jive, realize that he is an accomplished musician, that he started his musical career as an organist and worked for several years at theatre consoles. At the conclusion of his act he shows that he is no novice at the instrument when he mounts the Hammond electric for a spot of sweet fingering of the keyboard.

The theatre featured three shows a day including the movie *'Remember The Night'*, at 2:40, 5:45 and 8:50 p.m. and Waller's appearance was also reviewed in *The Evening Telegraph* of Toronto under the heading "Jitterbugs Fill Shea's "Fats" Waller's program makes them happy".

Don Loudon grew up in Toronto and recalled seeing this show and remembers that Valaida was also on the bill and he recalls her *charging on stage, lifting her golden trumpet to a 45° angle and playing St. Louis Blues in her best Armstrong manner. ... Ted Reeves was Canada's premier sport columnist and lived opposite us on Glenmanor Drive and Fats visited him when in Toronto for late night parties and also on Sundays as the 'Blue Laws' didn't allow Sunday shows. I was well aware of these and my father was invited along, but I was not, due to my tender years.*

Despite all this evidence from local sources, there are some conflicting reports in the *International Musician:* March 1940 states that Waller was at the Hippodrome Theatre, Toronto, the week of February 19th; January says "Fats Waller and his band were warmly welcomed at Blatz's Palm Gardens, Milwaukee, January 21st for a fortnight's stay" and April (held over from March) notes Waller, Jones, Sedric, Wallace, Hamilton and Smith in Local 587, Milwaukee. The February issue also has a report (held over from January and thus probably relating to December 1939) for the same group in Local 710, Washington, D.C. (see Addenda)

From Toronto, the group headed for New York with a stopover at Worcester, Massachusetts on the way back. Kirkeby says a month was spent in the city before the band headed south for Florida for a series of one-nighters. There are reports that this tour was by the Rhythm only, but a snapshot in Freddie Skerritt's files, reproduced overleaf, indicates that it was the big band. It is out of focus, making identifications difficult, but is dated "Palm Beach, Mar. 29, 40" and shows four men in bathing gear at the edge of the sea. Fats is clearly indentifiable and Skerritt appears to be next to him.

*****

However the "month" in New York was not a rest cure and *Jazz Information* of 1 March 1940 states: *Fats Waller plays the 125th Street Apollo for a week beginning tonight.* This is confirmed by the Apollo advert in the *New York Age* of 2 March which bills Waller as the headline attraction as **"Fats" Waller, His Piano, His Organ, His Band with Myra Johnson.**

*****

The itinerary of the tour of Florida by the band is given by the *Pittsburgh Courier's* correspondent in a report datelined Miami, Fla. Mar 26 as follows:

Monday, 25 March	New York Club, Jacksonville
Tuesday, 26 March	Florence Villa
(no engagements given for the 27th and 28th March)	
Friday, 29 March	Sunset Auditorium, West Palm Beach
Saturday, 30 March	Fort Lauderdale (for whites)
Sunday, 31 March	Bill Davie's Rockland Palace
Monday, 1 April	St. Petersburg
Tuesday, 2 April	Jacksonville (dance for whites)

Kirkeby mentions Jacksonville, Miami and Fort Lauderdale and recounts some of the racial prejudice they encountered. They were back in New York early in April and during a ten-day rest, the Rhythm visited the Victor studios once more and cut "eight good sides":

*****

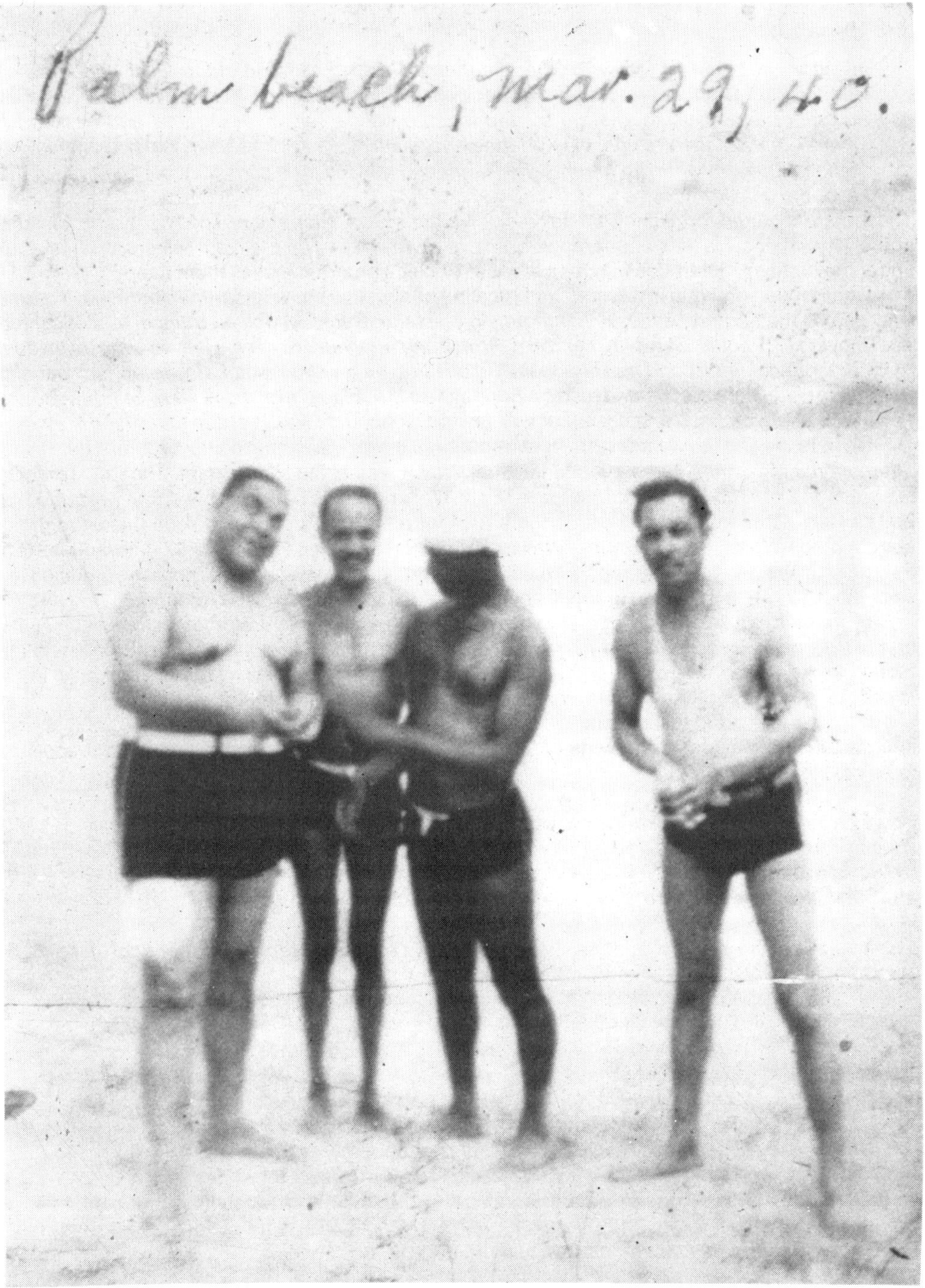

Palm beach, mar. 29, 40.

"Fats" Waller and his Rhythm — Fox Trot **Vocal refrain and piano by "Fats" Waller**

John Hamilton, t (except on 048777); Gene Sedric, cl-1/ts-2; Fats Waller, p/v; John Smith, g; Cedric Wallace, sb; Slick Jones, d.

Studio 2, New York City, New York — Thursday, 11 April 1940
6:00 to 12:00 p.m.

048775-1*	OLD GRAND DAD -1,-2 (Thomas "Fats" Waller)	BB B-10698-B, HMV B.10262, HMVIt HN3013, HMVSp GY547
048776-1*	FAT AND GREASY -2 (Porter Grainger-Charlie Johnson)	BB B-10803-A, HMVEx JO.116, HMVIn N 14045
048777-1*	LITTLE CURLY HAIR IN A HIGH CHAIR -2 (Charles Tobias-Nat Simon)	BB B-10698-A, HMV B.D.1235, HMVF/Sw SG 363, HMVSp GY 547, GY 897, HMVAu EA2571
048778-1*	(You're A) SQUARE FROM DELAWARE -2 (Leonard Feather)	BB B-10730-B, HMVSp GY553, HMVEi IW341
048779-1*	YOU RUN YOUR MOUTH, I'LL RUN MY BUSINESS -1	Victor unissued, 'Hold'. Issued on LP
048779-2	YOU RUN YOUR MOUTH, I'LL RUN MY BUSINESS -1 (Lillian Armstrong)	BB B-10779-B, HMVSp GY512

048779: 2nd line of second vocal:
-1 "You run your office and I'll handle my transactions brother."
-2 "You run your mouth and I'll run my business brother."

048780-1*	TOO TIRED-2 (Little-Sizemore-Shay)	BB B-10779-A, HMV B.10406, HMVIt HN3120, HMVSp GY512, HMVSA S.A.B.169, HMVFi TG157
048781-1*	"SEND ME" JACKSON -1,-2 (Cliff Friend-Jack Reynolds)	BB B-10730-A, HMV B.D.1229, HMVF SG65, HMVSw HE2672, HMVSp GY553, HMVIt HN2599, HMVEi IW342, EI EG7860
048782-1	EEP, IPE, WANNA PIECE OF PIE -1 (Jerry Blaine-Artie Dann)	BB B-10744-B, HMV B.D.906, HMVEi IW343
048782-2*	EEP, IPE WANNA PIECE OF PIE -1	Victor unissued, 'Hold'

For the first time on a Waller Victor recordings sheet, timings of the titles to the nearest five seconds are noted. Take -1 of 048779 (marked 'hold') is shown as 3:25 and take -2 as 3:10. LP reissues of this title have variously claimed either take -1 or take -2 as previously unissued, but timings confirm the markings on the recording sheet and issues as given above. Timing for take -1 of 048782 is given as 2:45 but take -2 is not indicated, the only one for the entire session for which this is omitted. Blue Bird B-10698-A has the additional credit **(From the M-G-M film "Forty Little Mothers")**.

*****

Hints of further Waller engagements were given in an article on the 'New Artists Service', booking agents for Moe Gale, Inc. in the *Pittsburgh Courier* of 13 April. It stated that Lee Mathews, director of the company, had Fats Waller on his date pad and had booked him and a 13-piece band for a choice series of one-nighters in the last week of April and the first week of May after Waller's run at the Howard theater in Washington. One of these engagements was confirmed by the *Pittsburgh Courier* which stated that:

"Fats" Waller ... will be doing his bit for the youngsters of St. Louis ... when he brings

> *himself and his famous Victor Recording Rhythm band to St. Louis for an appearance at the Sixth Annual "Y" Camp Benefit Circus to be staged in the huge Municipal Auditorium Friday and Saturday nights*

It is not clear from this report whether Fats played both nights or only one in this event staged to give deprived youngsters a vacation.

*****

It seems likely that the big band used for the above engagements was similar to that which soon after left on a coast-to-coast tour. A note in the *Pittsburgh Courier* on 4 May from Ed Kirkeby's office stated that Fats was fully booked, big band and small band, right through to August, and the personnel which undertook the trip was:

> John Hamilton, Bob Williams, Francis Williams, t; George Wilson, Alton Moore, tb; Dave McRae, Jimmy Powell, as; Franz Jackson, Freddie Skerritt, ts; Gene Sedric, cl/ts; Fats Waller, Don Donaldson, p; John Smith, g; Cedric Wallace, sb; Slick Jones, d.

Whilst researching his article on Freddie Skerritt which appeared in *Storyville 66,* David Griffiths went through Freddie's scrapbooks. One of these contained a number of dated photographs taken whilst a member of Fats Waller's big band (for the second time), and give us exact locations which were not necessarily places where the band played, but merely indicate the route followed, most of the photographs being of typical tourist sights. However, by combining this information with Ed Kirkeby's account and with interviews with Franc Williams, Bobby Williams (not related) and John Smith and additional notes in the newspapers it has been possible to build up a fairly detailed picture of this tour. Where exact dates are quoted, these are from Freddie Skerrit's photographs.

The tour left New York for Danville, Virginia and then continued on through North and South Carolina, Virginia, West Virginia, Ohio and Michigan playing a long series of one-nighters.They left their bus in Gull Lake, Michigan and travelled to St. Louis by rail. Then down into Mississippi to Jackson and Greenville. On Saturday and Sunday May 18 and 19 they played at the Blossom Health Night Club in Oklahoma City to a "standing room only" audience. By Monday, 20 May they were in Dallas Texas and two days later in nearby Fort Worth, where they played the 400 Club. Then on to Wichita Falls, Texas on 23 May. The following day to Carlsbad in New Mexico, where they played at the Armory and to Liberty Auditorium in El Paso, Texas for two days. On Monday, 27 May they were in Phoenix, Arizona, at Riverside Park, where Kirkeby recalled it was so hot that eggs could be fried on the sidewalk; too hot for dancing and the dance that night was a flop with the promotor losing heavily.

From Phoenix they chartered a bus for the 400 mile trip across the desert to Balboa Park, San Diego for an engagement on 29 May, then north for the opening at the Paramount theatre in Los Angeles on Saturday, 1 June where Fats shared top billing with Rochester from the Jack Benny show for two weeks. The stay is partially confirmed by Skerritt photographs of the Paramount Theatre (1 June); Los Angeles (3 and 5 June) and Hollywood (4 June).

From there they headed north and made their base in Oakland while they played a series of one-nighters in the Bay area and two local dances at Sweet's Ballroom in Oakland itself. Freddie has photos taken in Oakland on Saturday 15, June and on the following day when he also visited the San Francisco Fair, and another in San Francisco on 17 June. A paragraph in

Freddie has photos taken in Oakland on Saturday 15, June and on the following day when he also visited the San Francisco Fair, and another in San Francisco on 17 June. A paragraph in the *Pittsburgh Courier* says that Waller is booked to play Sweets Ballroom on Monday night (June 17).

An overnight trip to Salt Lake City (Freddie has a photo dated Monday 24 June, 'Utah'), and then a long haul through the Rocky Mountains to Denver, Colorado for a single engagement and on to Kansas City, Missouri where, arriving exhausted after a six hundred plus mile journey, they found the booking had been cancelled. Finding that Count Basie was in town, Fats took off to find him and "have a little drink" together. Homesickness surfaced and Fats headed for the railway station and New York, but Kirkeby found him just as he was boarding the train. However, as the final dates in St. Louis and Indianapolis had been booked by the same promotor who had cancelled in Kansas City and no deposits paid, they decided to cut these. Fats went back to New York via Chicago and Kirkeby and the band headed back home in the bus. Franc Williams and John Smith recalled that they roomed together most of the time on this trip, striking up a friendship which was to last for many years and they were colleagues together with Panama Francis in the re-constituted Savoy Sultans. On returning to New York, John Smith left to join the Mills Brothers and Al Casey finally came back into the Rhythm.

*****

Franc Williams recalls that this coast to coast tour with Fats was one of the most arduous that he ever undertook, even in his much travelled life. He remembers one engagement 'out in the sticks' where they travelled as far as they could by bus. Then when the road became too twisting and narrow they transferred to a fleet of waiting cars. A few miles further on and the road had become no more than a track and they transferred once again to horses and Fats and the whole band, with their instruments (including drums and bass) completed the journey on horseback and played to a delighted and highly enthusiastic local community.

When they eventually reached the West Coast, Fats, who was always known to take good care of his men and realised what a tough time they'd had, took the whole band to a well known 'establishment' where good food and drink and female companionship was available and announced that everything was on him! Franc recalls that they partook freely of the delights on offer and spent the evening making up for lost time.

Franc also emphasised what a professional Fats was and that he insisted his men were likewise. "When you get on the stand, no-one wants to know you've got a back-ache, or your mother's ill — you're up there to give people a good time" was the sort of reminder he gave frequently.

Franc had a copy of the band photo with the bus taken in Texas on 21 May 1940 which all the band had autographed, but he so disliked Ed Kirkeby that he had cut him from the print. The identifications overleaf are from Franc's copy.

*****

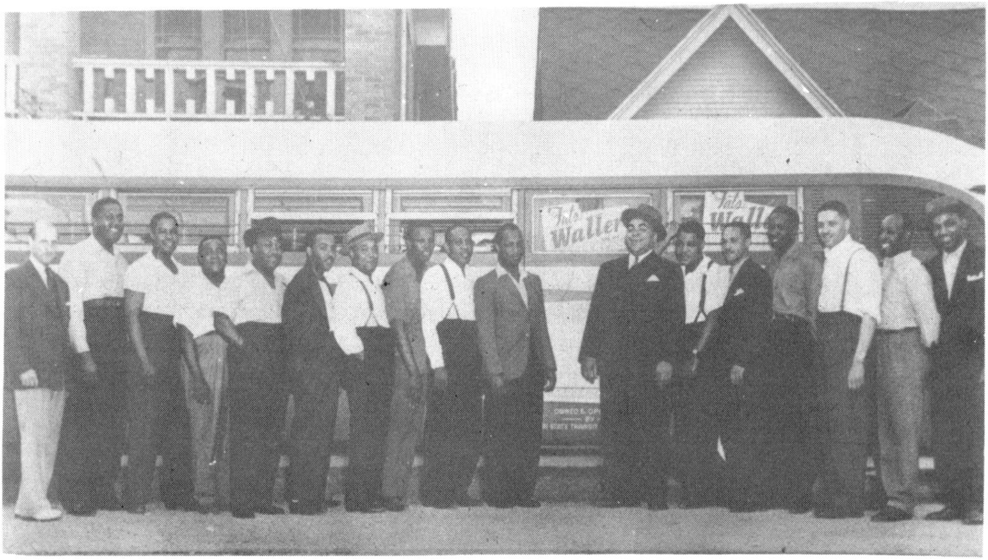

Above: The orchestra pose in front of their tour bus in Texas on 21 May 1940.
L to R: Ed Kirkeby, Alton Moore, Bobby Driver (band boy); Eugene Sedric, Don Donaldson, Jimmie Powell, George Wilson, Cedric Wallace, Slick Jones, Francis Williams, Fats Waller, John 'Bugs' Hamilton, Freddie Skerritt, Bob Williams, Franz Jackson, Dave McRae, and John Smith.
Below: Fats with twin girl fans in Wichita Falls, Texas on 23 May 1940

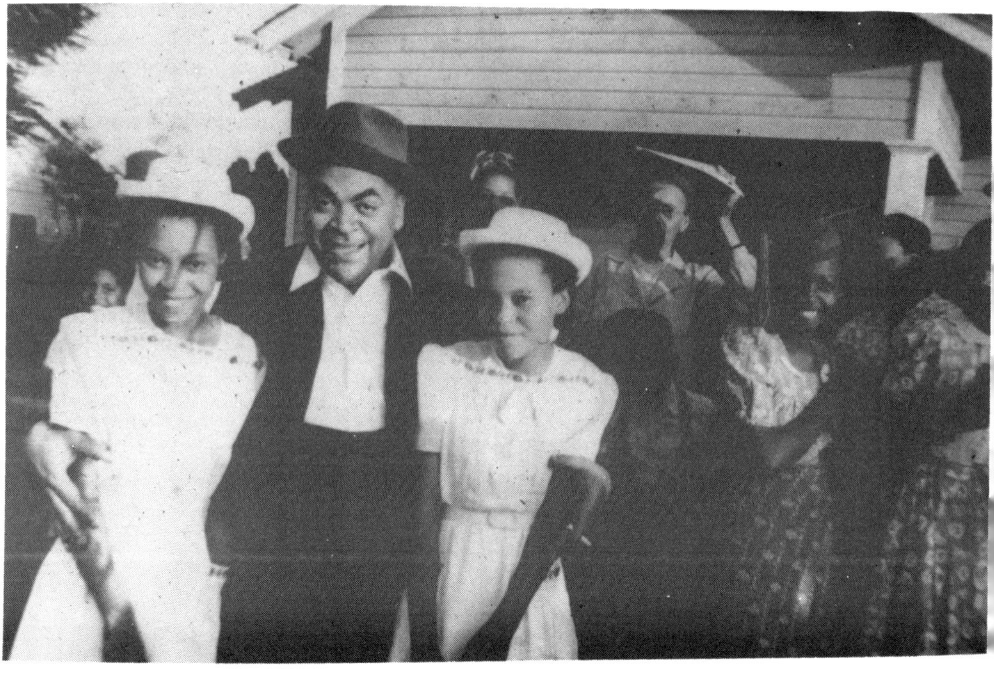

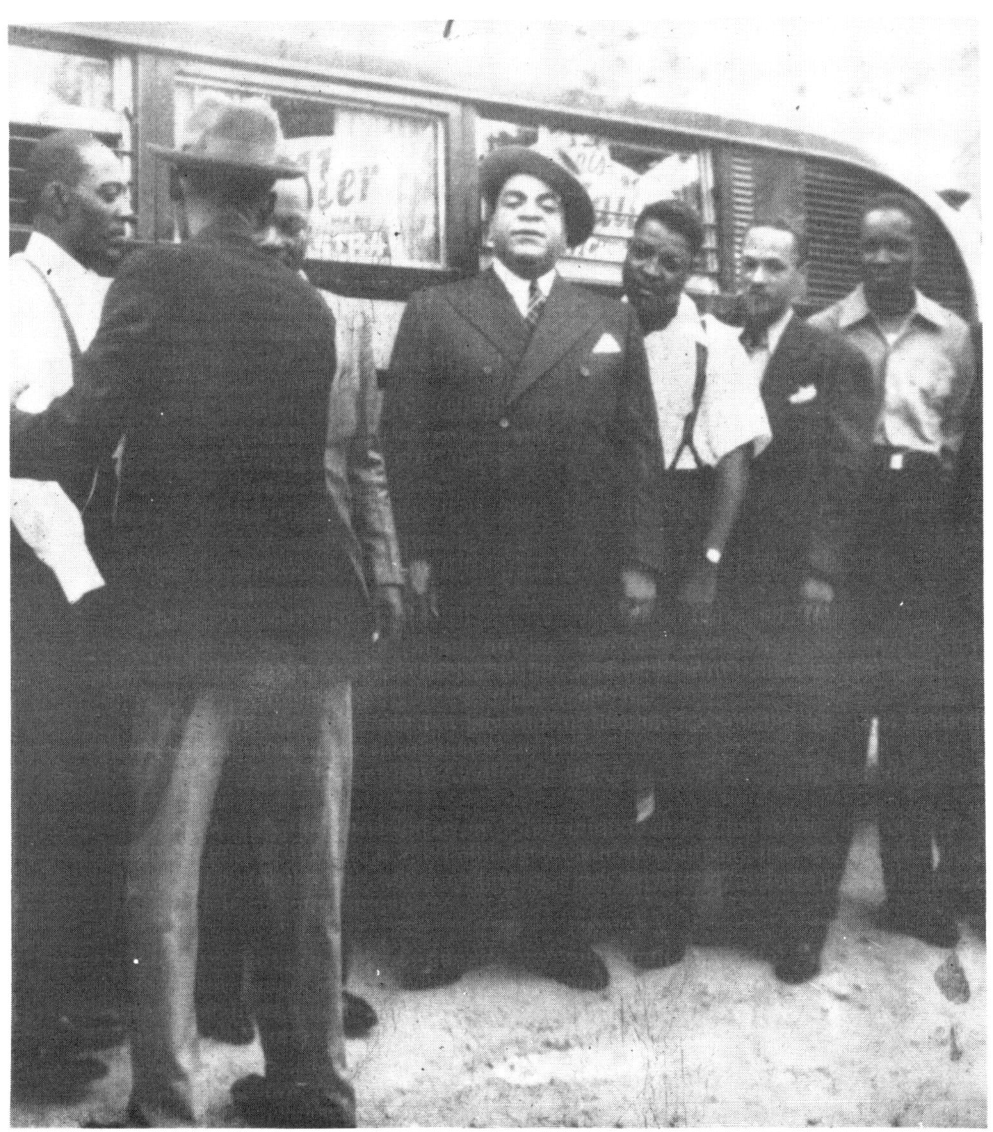

Above: In El Paso, Texas, on 25 May 1940. L to R: Slick Jones, possibly Bob Williams with back to camera, Francis Williams, Fats, John Hamilton, Freddie Skerritt and Cedric Wallace.

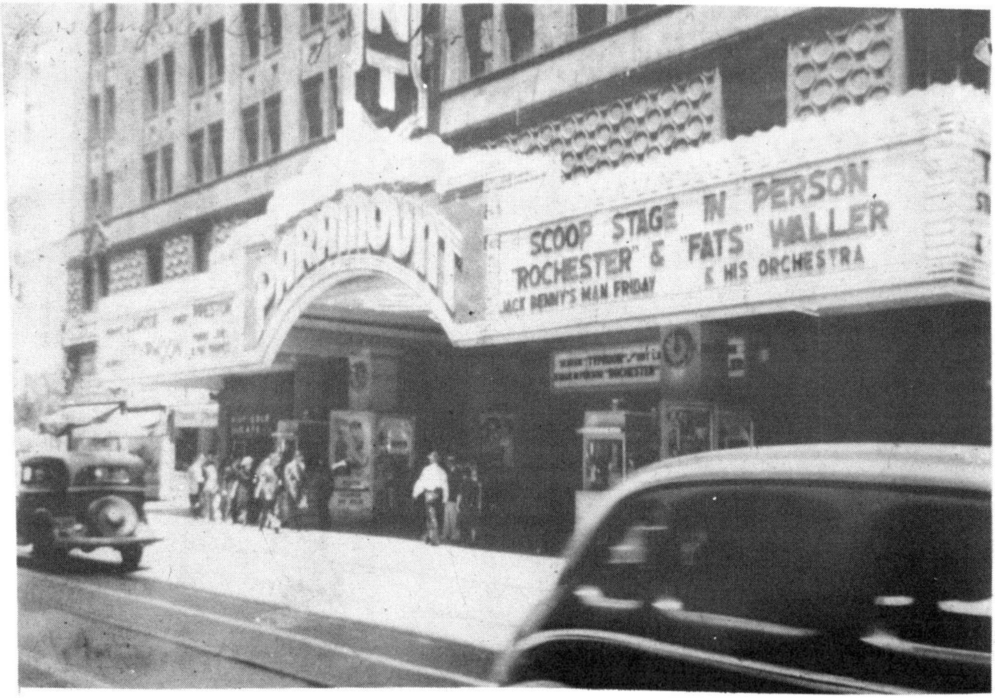

Above: The Paramount Theatre, Los Angeles on 1 June 1940.
Below: A trailer advertising the orchestra appearing at Sweets Ballroom, Oakland.

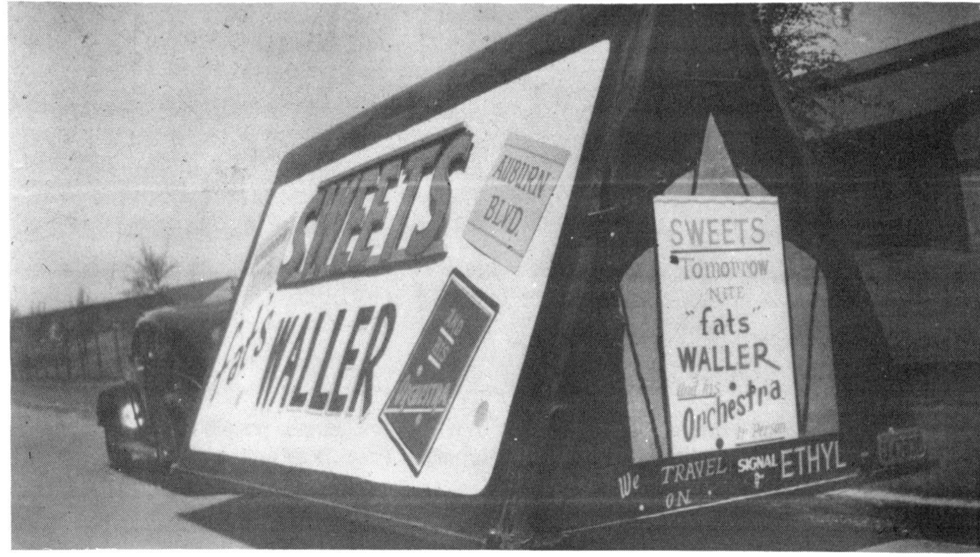

"Fats" Waller and his Rhythm — Fox Trot **Vocal refrain and piano by "Fats" Waller** or **Vocal Refrain by "Fats" Waller and Chorus -3**

John Hamilton, t; Gene Sedric, cl-1/ts-2; Fats Waller, p/v; Al Casey, g; Cedric Wallace, sb; Slick Jones, d; band vocal -3.

Studio 2, New York City, New York — Tuesday, 16 July 1940
1:30 to 6:45 p.m. Ed Kirkeby present

Matrix	Title	Issues
051865-1*	STOP PRETENDING -1,-3 (Buddy Johnson)	BB B-10829-A, HMV B.10406, HMVF SG515, HMVIt HN3120, HMVSA S.A.B.169, HMVFi TG157, RZAu G24859
051866-1*	I'LL NEVER SMILE AGAIN -1 (Ruth Lowe)	BB B-10841-A
051867-1*	MY MOMMIE SENT ME TO THE STORE -2,-3 (Ken Hecht-Sid Bass)	BB B-10892-A, HMVEx JO.128, HMVSw HE2731, RZAu G24800
051868-1*	DRY BONES -1 (Dick Rogers-Will Osborne)	BB B-10892-B, HMV B.9885, J.O.133, HMVSw HE2813, HMVIt HN2763, HMVIn N14052, El EG7622, RZAu G24813
051869-1*	"FATS" WALLER'S ORIGINAL E FLAT BLUES -1 ("Fats" Waller)	BB B-10858-A, HMV B.D.906, GZAu G24504
051870-1*	STAYIN' AT HOME -2 (Andy Razaf-Thomas Waller)	BB B-10841-B, HMV B.D.1235, HMVF/Sw SG363
051871-1*	HEY! STOP KISSIN' MY SISTER -1,-2 (Eddie Peyton-Kay & Phil Coblin)	BB B-10829-B, HMV J.O.110. HMVF SG164, HMVSw HE2702, RZAu G24813

The recording sheet again notes playing times, but now to the nearest second. It also shows the composer credit for 051870 as (Andy Razaf-Joe Davis), but the record is as above.

*****

According to *Jazz Information,* 23 August 1940: *Fats Waller is booked into the Blatz Gardens, Milwaukee for a month starting August 21.* The Blatz Palm Gardens was a night club and confirmation of Waller's presence is found in the 'Orchestra Routes' section of *The Billboard* (issues of 5 and 12 October 1940), which both report him there. However, Ed Kirkeby states in *Ain't Misbehavin'* that from August until the end of September the small band played a series of one nighters, so it may be that a number of short engagements were undertaken at this venue, interspersed with other gigs in other locations. This is also supported by an announcement in the *Pittsburgh Courier* which just states that Waller will play two days 'in this section of the country'. The microfilm is badly out of focus and it is difficult to read the date given, but it appears to be 9 September, and the report goes on to say 'the band will probably play one date at the Savoy Ballroom'. Alternatively, Kirkeby's memory of chronology is slightly at fault and an extended engagement at the Blatz Palm Gardens was followed by a series of one-nighters. Kirkeby certainly has vivid memories of one night a little later, in October, when the band were in Manitowoc in upper Wisconsin and it was freezing.

They were back in New York by the end of October for Waller was among the vast array of black and white talent which appeared at a midnight benefit concert at the Apollo Theatre on Sunday, 27 October. It was organised by Bill Robinson and Noble Sissle and was intended to feature artists who had played the British Isles and the *proceeds were for the purchase of a mobile kitchen to feed Britain's bomb disorganized citizens.*

*****

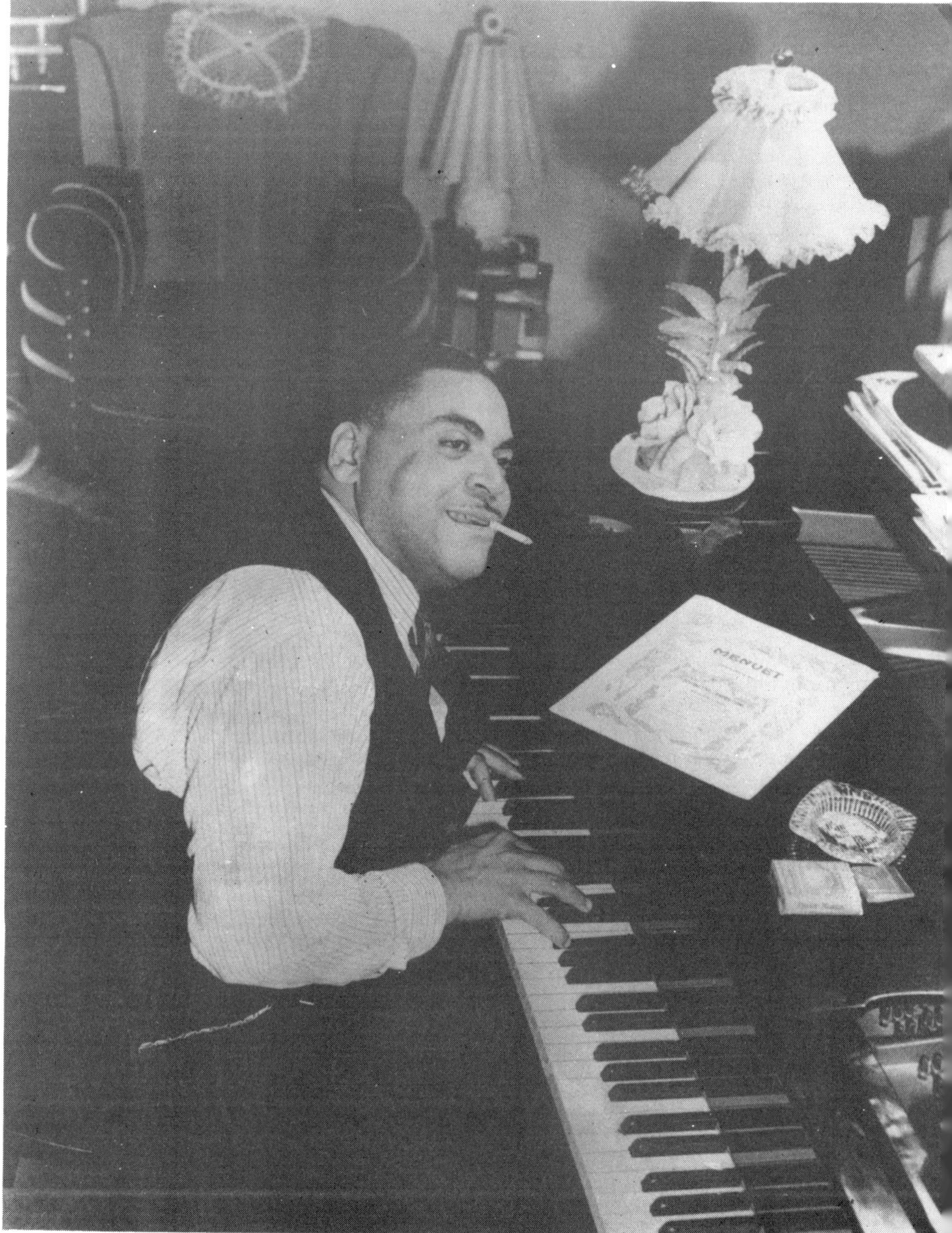
MENUET

"Fats" Waller and his Rhythm — Fox Trot **Vocal refrain and piano by "Fats" Waller -3 or Piano by "Fats" Waller -6**

John Hamilton, t (except on 057087); Gene Sedric, cl-1/ts-2; Fats Waller, p/v-3/cel-4; Al Casey, g; Cedric Wallace, sb; Slick Jones, d; Kathryn Perry, v-5.

Studio 2, New York City, New York — Wednesday, 6 November 1940
1:30 to 7:15 p.m. Ed Kirkeby present

057083-1*	EVERYBODY LOVES MY BABY (But My Baby Don't Love Nobody Bu tMe) -1,-3 (Jack Palmer-Spencer Williams)	BB-B10989-A, Vi 20-2217-A, HMV B.9935, HMVF SG304, RZAu G25009
057084-1*	I'M GONNA SALT AWAY SOME SUGAR (For My Sugar and Me) -1,-3 (Seymour-Davidson-Coots)	BB B-10943-A, HMV J.O.92, HMVIN N14038
057085-1*	'TAIN'T NOBODY'S BIZ-NEZZ IF I DO -2,-3 (Grainger-Prince-Williams)	BB B-10967-B, HMVEx J.O.96, HMVF SG388, HMVIn N14033
057086-1*	ABERCROMBIE HAD A ZOMBIE -1,-3 (Mort Green-Vee Lawnhurst)	BB B-10967-A
057087-1*	BLUE EYES -1,-3,-4 (Dave Ringle)	BB B-10943-B, HMVEx JO.123
057088-1*	SCRAM! -6 (Leonard Feather)	BB B-10989-B, RZAu G25009
057089-1	MELANCHOLY BABY -1,-3,-5	Victor unissued, 'Hold'. Issued on LP

The sides with the Rhythm were made between 1:30 and 6:30 p.m. and that with Kathryn Perry (so spelled on the recording sheet) between 6:30 and 7:15 p.m. On this Waller's vocal is more in the nature of speech. Miss Perry may have been auditioning with the band and, as Kay Perry, accompanied them to their Sherman Hotel residency later in the year. A line of text on the recording sheet beneath the entry for her title has been heavily X'd out, but my reading of it is "this last selection recorded with thxxx xxxxxx extra".

HMV JO.123 is credited simply to **FATS WALLER** with no mention of the band.

*****

Ed Kirkeby recalls "a knockout show at the Apollo" and *Jazz Information* of 25 October 1940 notes that Fats Waller was booked for the Apollo Theatre beginning Friday, November 8, and this is confirmed in the advert for the show in the *New York Age* of 9 November which shows Kathryn Perry with the band. Also on the bill was Louis Jordan's Band. The write-up in the paper stated that Waller had been on the road for almost a year and had grown enormously in popularity in that time.

*****

Left: Fats at home on his own piano. This shot was suggested as coming from 1940, but comparison with the shots taken with Condon and the Carnegie Hall Concert poster suggests that it was almost certainly taken at the same time as those — note the music on top of the piano and the fact that Fats appears to be wearing the same clothes.

EDDIE CONDON and his BAND

Marty Marsala, t; George Brunies, tb; Pee Wee Russell, cl; Fats Waller (as "Maurice"), p; Eddie Condon, g; Artie Shapiro, sb; George Wettling, d.

Liederkranz Hall, New York City, New York — Monday, 11 November 1940 or (see note) Thursday, 14 November 1940

29054-1 GEORGIA GRIND (Williams-Allen) Com 536-A
29054-1st alt. Georgia Grind Commodore rejected. Issued on LP
29054-2nd alt. Georgia Grind Commodore rejected. Issued on LP

29054: After piano intro:
-1: Band enters together with clarinet in high register; clarinet solo ends in descending phrase and trombone solo starts with ascending phrase.
1st alt: Band enters together with clarinet in mid register; first bar of clarinet solo is played by string bass and trombone with clarinet overlap at end of solo; trombone solo starts with high note.
2nd alt: Band entry preceded by trumpet and trombone slur; clarinet and trombone solos distinctly separated.

29055-1st alt. Oh, Sister! Ain't That Hot ? Commodore rejected. Issued on LP
29055-2 OH SISTER AIN'T THAT HOT (White-Donaldson) Com 535-B
29055-2nd alt. Oh, Sister! Ain't That Hot ? Commodore rejected. Issued on LP
29055-partial Oh, Sister! Ain't That Hot ? Commodore rejected. Issued on LP

29055 Second (clarinet) chorus:
1st alt. Clarinet enters with high register phrase. Chorus runs into next (piano) chorus, which is two-fisted
-2 Clarinet enters with series of staccato high notes. Next chorus starts with bass and high register accompanying piano chords.
2nd alt. Low register clarinet entry and ends in the low register. Next chorus starts with treble chords from piano with bass accompaniment.

29056-1 DANCING FOOL (Smith-Wheeler-Snyder) Com 536-B
29056-1st alt. Dancing Fool Commodore rejected. Issued on LP
29056-2nd alt. Dancing Fool Commodore rejected. Issued on LP

29056: -1 Trombone chorus punctuated by single note from piano, bars 4, 8 and 12; followed by high register trumpet chorus and two 16-bar piano choruses.
1st alt. Trombone chorus with piano and rhythm acc.; followed by muted trumpet chorus and two 16-bar piano choruses.
2nd alt. Trombone chorus with rhythm and no piano; followed by low-register open trumpet chorus and one 16-bar piano chorus.

29057-1 (You're Some) PRETTY DOLL (Clarence Williams) Com 535-A
29057-1st alt. (You're Some) Pretty Doll Commodore rejected. Issued on LP
29057-2nd alt. (You're Some) Pretty Doll Commodore rejected. Issued on LP

29057: Entry of band after piano solo:
-1 No trombone slur. Clarinet chorus entirely lower register.
1st alt. Trombone enters with slur. Clarinet chorus in low and middle register.
2nd alt. Pick-up by clarinet; clarinet chorus low register split by drum rattle.

Takes given for the issued items are those found in the wax of the Commodores. Bob Hilbert claims that the issued takes are all -3 — probably based on sequence of recording on a 16" safety. Hilbert quotes takes -1,-2 of first three titles as unissued, plus an unidentified take of the fourth. However, the matter is further complicated by the Mosaic boxed set of Commodore recordings, which claims a recording date of 14 November against the previously accepted one of 11 November, and includes additional takes plus a breakdown of the second title. Although the Mosaic notes make no claim to do so, the inclusion of this additional material, especially the breakdown, suggests that they had access to the "safety" recording, but the numbers allocated by Mosaic look suspiciously like their own invention and may not refer to the actual recording sequence. The 'breakdown' on the second title is in fact not a musical breakdown, but the recording equipment being switched off after 1'.54", presumably after running out of "wax".

The 14 November date claimed by Mosaic for this session looks suspect and may be the date on which the information was entered into the Commodore files or the result of a transcription error, as evidence from surrounding matrix numbers in the 29000 series supports the 11 November date, although it is always possible that the numbers for the session were pre-assigned. Matrices 29027-30 are by Goodman on 7 November; various non-jazz artists account for numbers between these and the Condon set which are followed by 29058-61 by the McFarland Twins (date unknown) and 29062-5 by Goodman on 13 November and 29066-9 by Frankie Masters on the same date. Then there are more non-jazz items and a Basie date on 19 November which accounts for 29087-90.

*****

The above session took place during Fats's week at the Apollo (and from this it may be deduced that it took place one morning) and he must have left New York almost immediately at the conclusion of that engagement and probably travelled overnight, for the 'Orchestra Routes' section of *The Billboard* for 16 November 1940 shows him at the Sherman Hotel, Chicago, where he opened on Friday 15 November, and this information was repeated weekly up to and including the issue of 27 December 1940. The *Pittsburgh Courier* had noted that Waller had left New York after a week at the Apollo 'with his small aggregation and featuring the voice of Katherine Perry' for an indefinite engagement at the Panther Room of the Hotel Sherman during which he would provide both dinner and dance music and would be broadcasting several times weekly on a national hook-up. *Jazz Information,* 6 December 1940 has the note:

> *Fats Waller's small Combo and Bob Zurke, soloing intermissions, make vigorous music for the Hotel Sherman's Panther Room in Chicago. Fats played a Waiter's Ball at the Savoy on November 18, his off-night downtown.*

In *The Billboard* of 30 November, Nat Green reviews the show, which took place in the Panther Room of the Hotel and, in line with the paper's policy, gives details of prices, etc. at the venue:

> *Talent Policy: Show and dance band; floorshows 9 p.m. and 12 midnight. Management: Ernest Byfield and Frank Bering, managers; Howard Mayer, publicity. Prices: Dinner from $2; drinks from 50 cents; minimum, $1 weekdays and $2 Saturdays.*
>
> *The Harlem note that has prevailed in several of the Hotel Sherman's shows this year continues in the new show that opened Friday (14). "Fats" Waller and his boys are on the bandstand and the way they whoop up the Harlem rhythm sets the jitterbugs agog. Waller is an accomplished showman and his mugging and ivory tickling are swell entertainment. On this trip Waller has brought with him Kay Perry and Kitty Murray, both artists in their line. Miss Perry has an appealing voice and scores solidly with her singing of 'I'm Nobody's Baby' and other sentimental ballads. Kitty Murray, a buxom brownskin gal, brings the house down with her grotesque dancing. ... Waller offers many favorites, including 'Bond Street', Ain't Misbehavin'', and 'Your Feet's Too Big'.*

Although this report gives "Friday (14)", 14 November 1940 was actually a Thursday. Also mentioned are other artists on the bill, including Bob Zurke, then working as a solo artist and, as noted above, playing the intermission spots. *Jazz Information* of 20 December 1940 shows

Waller and Zurke still at the Panther Room.

During this residency in Chicago the band were included in some of the broadcasts from the hotel and the following are known or are believed to come from this period.

*****

Broadcasts

John Hamilton, t; Gene Sedric, c-1/ts-2; Fats Waller, p/v-3; Al Casey, g; Cedric Wallace, sb; Slick Jones, d; Kay Perry, v-4

Panther Room, Hotel Sherman, Chicago Illinois		Tuesday, 3 December 1940
Yacht Club Swing -1	Issued on LP	
Watcha Know Joe? -1,-2,-3	Issued on LP	
I Give You My Word -2 -4	Issued on LP	
Lila Lou -2	Issued on LP	
Frenesi -1,-2	Issued on LP (see note)	
So You're The One -2,-4	Issued on LP	
Dark Eyes (Fats Waller arrangement) -2	Issued on LP	
Perfidia -1	Issued on LP	
When You And I Were Young Maggie -2	Issued on LP	
Yacht Club Swing -1	Issued on LP	

Maraccas are heard on *Frenesi,* both on the above and that from the next broadcast, possibly played by Hamilton as they are not heard during the trumpet solo, but equally they could be played by someone else.

As before		Tuesday, 10 December 1940
Yacht Club Swing -1	Issued on LP	
I Do, Do You? -2	Issued on LP	
Honolulu Bundle -2	Issued on LP	
Perfidia -1	Issued on LP	
There I Go -2,-4	Issued on LP	
Frenesi -2	Issued on LP	
I Give You My Word -2,-4	Issued on LP	
Watcha Know Joe? -2,-3	Issued on LP	

As before		Probably December 1940
Dark Eyes -2	Issued on LP	

As before		Tuesday, 31 December 1940
Dark Eyes -2	Issued on LP	
Jingle Bells -2,-3	Issued on LP	
Lila Lou -1,-2	Issued on LP	

Some of the above have shouts of encouragement by Waller which might be classified as vocals by some. *Lila Lou* is sometimes shown as *Lila Low* but it has not been possible to discover which is correct, although it is certainly announced as the former on the broadcasts here. The tune is based on the chorus of *Hold My Hand.* It is curious that Waller should be using *Yacht Club Swing* as his theme when playing the Sherman Hotel unless it is so named only on the issues of the broadcasts. It is common practice for a band to have a catchy theme which changes its title according to the venue being played and it is possible that when Waller first moved into the Panther Room it was announced as *Panther Room Swing*. According to *Who's Who Of Jazz,* Herb Flemming joined Waller at the Hotel Sherman on this date. However, there is no aural evidence for his presence on the above broadcast nor is he present on the recording session which follows, although he is believed to have been a member of the big band formed in February.

*****

"Fats" Waller and his Rhythm -Fox Trot **Vocal refrain and piano by "Fats" Waller**
or **Vocal refrain, piano and organ by "Fats" Waller**
or **Organ by "Fats" Waller**

John Hamilton, t; Gene Sedric, cl-1/ts-2; Fats Waller, p-3/v-4/o-5; Al Casey, g; Cedric Wallace, sb; Slick Jones, d; band vocal -6.

Victor Studio "A", Chicago, Illinois Thursday, 2 January 1941
1:30 to 6:00 p.m.

053794-1* MAMACITA -2,-5 BB B-11078-B
(Thomas "Fats" Waller-Anita Waller)
053794-2 MAMACITA *-2,-5* Victor unissued, 'Hold'
053795-1* LIVER LIP JONES -1,-3,-4 BB B-11010-B
(Irene Higginbotham)
053795-2 LIVER LIP JONES *-1,-3,-4* Victor unissued, 'Hold'
053796-1* BUCKIN' THE DICE -1,-2,-3,-4 BB B-11102-B, *Vi 20-2640-B,*
(Cedric Wallace-Tiny Parham) RZAu G24853
053797-1* PANTIN' IN THE PANTHER ROOM -1,-2,-3,-5 Victor unissued, 'Hold'. Issued on LP
053797-2* PANTIN' IN THE PANTHER ROOM -1,-2,-3,-5 (Casey-Cedric-Kirkeby) BB B-11175-B, HMV B.10262, HMVIt HN3013, RZAu G24836
053797 First piano passage: -1 With very prominent guitar
-2 Guitar as part of rhythm section
053798-1*COME DOWN TO EARTH, MY ANGEL -1,-3,-4,-5 (Sour-McRay-Gold) Victor unissued, 'Hold'. Issued on LP
053798-2*COME DOWN TO EARTH, MY ANGEL -1,-3,-4,-5 BB B-11010-A, HMV J.O.205
053798 Fourth line of vocal: -1 "Make you do so much, make you do so much if you'd only try"
-2 "Could do so much, if you only would try"
053799-1* SHORTNIN' BREAD -1,-2,-3,-4,-6 BB B-11078-A, HMV B.D.1218,
(Arranged by Thomas "Fats" Waller) HMVIt HN2584
053799-2* SHORTNIN' BREAD -1,-2,-3,-4,-6 Victor unissued, 'Hold'.Issued on LP
053799: Vocal after tenor sax solo:
-1 "Say delivery man where have you been?
Oh mercy, it sure is a sin,
Mama, mama, don't be fast, do not show your
big fa... — Shortnin' bread"
-2 "Say mama the man is here with the flour,
Say baby it's past the hour,
Look baby, don't take it too fast,
Mama, mama don't show him your — fine bread"
059100-1* I REPENT -2,-3,-5 (Thomas & Anita Waller) BB B-11188-B
059100-2 I REPENT *-2,-3,-5* Victor unissued, 'Hold'

There is some confusion over which takes of 053797 and 053798 were originaly selected for issue. The recording sheet is not helpful in that both takes as well as some of the simultaneous recordings of all titles were marked as "Process". However, only take -1 of each title plus take -2 of 053798 is actually marked with an "A". Bluebird issues normally have the take information in the wax suppressed, but B-11010-A bears a figure 2 in the expected place and microgroove issues claiming to use the previously unissued take -1 are quite different. The above therefore reverses previous listings as to which takes were used on the 78 issues.

*****

The termination date at the Sherman Hotel is not known, but a clue may be obtained from the fact that Kitty Murray was back in New York and on the bill at the Apollo for the week commencing Friday, 24 January 1941. Leaving the Sherman Hotel, the band spent a week in the State-Lake Theatre, also in Chicago and so named because of its location on the corner of State Street and Lake Street on the north edge of the loop in the downtown area, before returning to New York. Ed Kirkeby relates that the big band was booked into the RKO Strand Theatre in Syracuse, but this had to be cancelled as Fats was unwell with a bad cold. After a few days rest and a medical check-up, as his health was giving some cause for concern because of the hectic life style, the big band left in February for a six-week tour of the South. The tour was one of solidly booked one-nighters and Kirkeby recalls that it started in Maryland, through Washington. D.C., (the photo in the "Crystal Cavern" may date from this), Virginia, North and South Carolina, Georgia and down to Fort Lauderdale in Florida. Advance news that Waller would tour Florida in February had been given by Associated Promotors in an announcement in the *Pittsburgh Courier* of 28 December. Some weeks later the same paper reported that Waller was to play the colored auditorium, Lakeland, Florida on Thursday, 13 February and would then play Miami's Rockland Palace on Sunday, February 16. He would be featuring his band and his organ.

If the Crystal Cavern photo comes from this period, the personnel on this trip included: John Hamilton, t; George Wilson, tb; Herb Flemming, tb/v; Dave McRae, Scoville Brown, as; Gene Sedric, cl/ts; Fats Waller, p; Al Casey, g; Cedric Wallace, sb; Slick Jones, d; Myra Johnson, v.

*****

"Fats" Waller and his Rhythm -Fox Trot **Vocal refrain and piano by "Fats" Waller**
(Hammond Organ, Guitar and Drums) Vocal refrain by "Fats" Waller -4

John Hamilton, t; Gene Sedric, cl-1/ts-2; Fats Waller, p/v; Al Casey, g; Cedric Wallace, sb; Slick Jones, d; band vocal -3; Waller, o/Casey, g/Jones, d; only -4.

Studio 2, New York City, New York — Thursday, 20 March 1941
2:00 to 6:00 p.m. (see note)

062761-1* DO YOU HAVE TO GO? -2 (Anita and "Fats" Waller) — BB B-11222-B, HMV B.D.5787, HMVIn NE.699

062762-1* PAN-PAN -1,-3 (Jerry Daniels) — BB B-11383-B, HMV/In B.D.1011, HMVSw HE2416, HMV/H M.H.131

062763-1* I WANNA HEAR SWING SONGS -2 (Billy Moore-Sy Oliver) — BB B-11115-B, HMV B.D.1028, HMVSw HE2346

062764-1* YOU'RE GONNA BE SORRY -1,-2 (Clarence Gaskill) — Vi/Ar 20-1602-B, HMV B.10830, *HMVFi TG224*

062765-1* ALL THAT MEAT AND NO POTATOES -1 (Ed Kirkeby-"Fats" Waller) — BB B-11102-A, RZAu G24800, *V-D 308*

062766-1* LET'S GET AWAY FROM IT ALL -4 (Tom Adair-Matt Dennis) — BB B-11115-A

The recording of the final title may have been an on-the-spot decision as no mention of

Hammond Organ is made in the instrumentation at the head of the recording sheet. The session time is typed as given here, but the 00 of 6:00 is crossed through and 30 written in manuscript above it. Also typed in is: "NOTE:- Last selection (062766) Hammond Organ, Guitar & Traps ONLY (Vocal by Fats Waller)". According to Ed Kirkeby, the penultimate title derives from an aside made by Waller when he saw the large posterior of singer Kitty Murray.

Some copies of HMV B.D.1028 amend the title to *I WANNA HEAR SWING MUSIC SONGS.* The reverse of HMV B.D.5787 is by **SPIKE JONES AND HIS CITY SLICKERS.**

*****

Next on the Waller agenda came a return engagement at the Blatz Palm Gardens which Ed Kirkeby recalls was for three weeks. It is confirmed by a report in *Jazz Information* of 21 March 1941: *Fats Waller to Milwaukee's Blatz on* [Wednesday] *March 26 with Bugs Hamilton, Gene Sedric, Al Casey, Cedric Wallace and Slick Jones.* Three weeks would have taken them through to April 16, after which Kirkeby recalls three theatre dates, three days rest in New York and then a week the Howard Theatre, Washington which would have concluded around the end of April when the group returned to New York for a break before setting out on another coast-to-coast marathon with the big band

*****

FATS WALLER

John Hamilton, t; Gene Sedric, cl/ts; Fats Waller, p/v; Al Casey, g; Cedric Wallace, sb; Slick Jones, d; Vivian Brown, v-1; Myra Johnson, v-2

New York City, New York — unknown date, possibly in May 1941

4001 Honeysuckle Rose -1 — Program #1040, selection 1, released 3 November 1941
(M11731) © 3 November 1941. — Issued on LP

4203 Your Feet's Too Big — Program #1042, selection 3, released 17 November 1941
(M11776) © 17 November 1941. — Issued on LP

4403 The Joint Is Jumping -2 — Program #1044, selection 3
(M11871) © 1 December 1941. — Issued on LP

4607 Ain't Misbehavin' — Program #1046, selection 7, released 15 December 1941
(M11937) © 15 December 1941. — Issued on LP

The above are soundtrack recordings from short films of Fats Waller and his Rhythm, produced by Fred Waller (no relation) and directed by Warren Murray, made by Minoco Productions for the Soundies Distributing Corp. of America, Inc., Chicago, and the Soundie catalogue number is that appearing to the left of the title. These short films were normally assembled into programmes of eight items, and the original programme number, selection and release date (where known) is given. The copyright registration number and date of each is given below each title. 4001 was reissued as 11603 in program #1116 on 3 May 1943, and 4607 was reissued as the 8th selection in program #X995 on 15 November 1943. Complete information on reissues is not available, and there may have been other re-releases. The Soundie catalogue also lists a "Fats Waller Medley" under the number 4M which was copyrighted at the Library of Congress on 16 March 1945 under the number M15727. This is known to contain *Ain't Misbehavin'/Your Feet's Too Big/The Joint Is Jumpin',* but it has not been seen to ascertain whether the extracts used are drawn wholly from previously released complete versions. According to all previous listings, these films were made on Thursday, 7 November 1940, but the source of this is no longer known and in the light of present

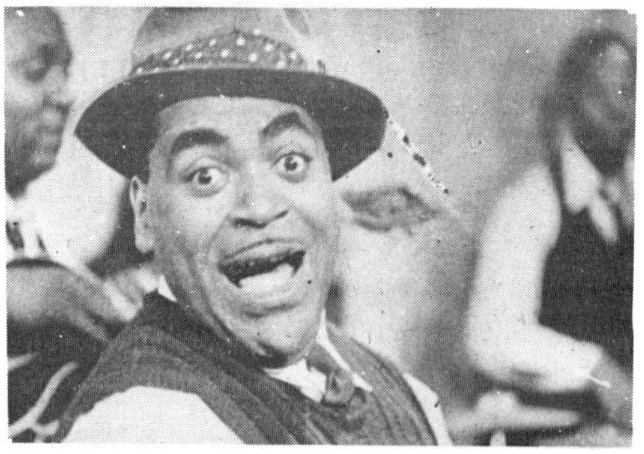

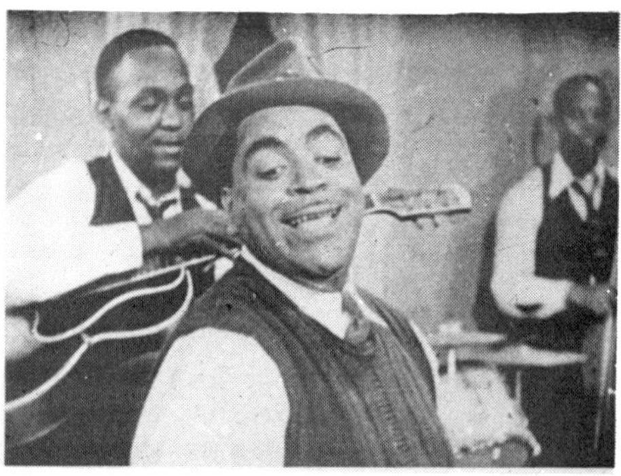

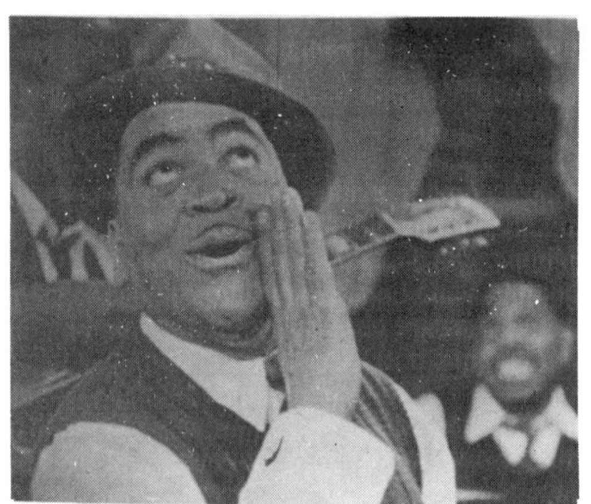

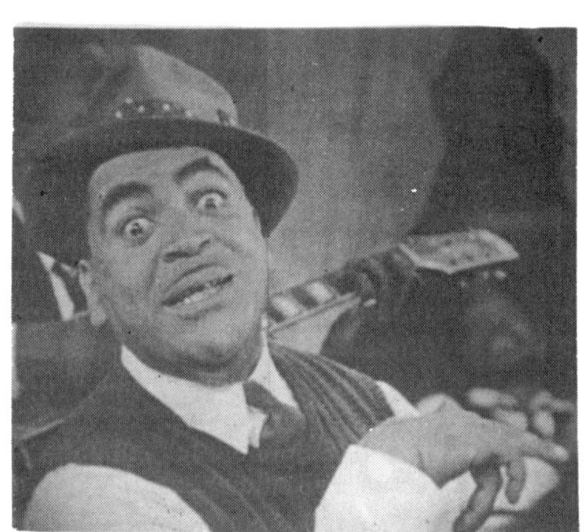

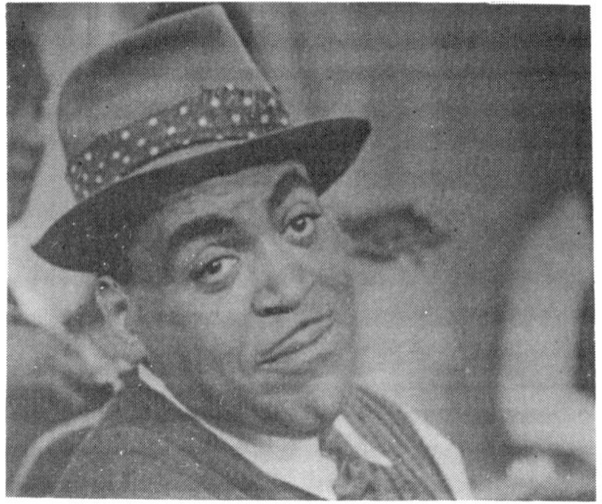

Five shots of Waller from the soundie *'The Joint Is Jumping.*

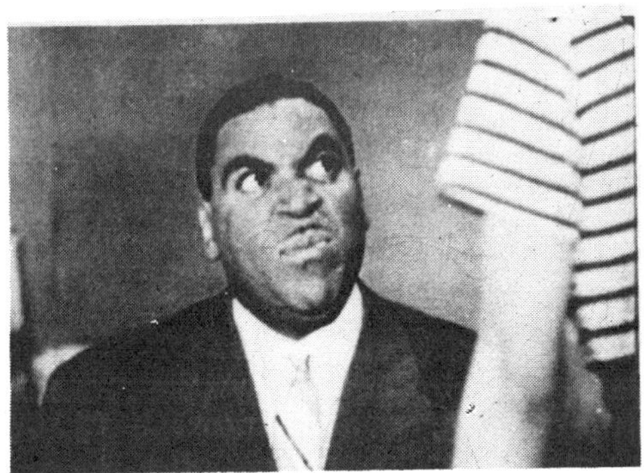

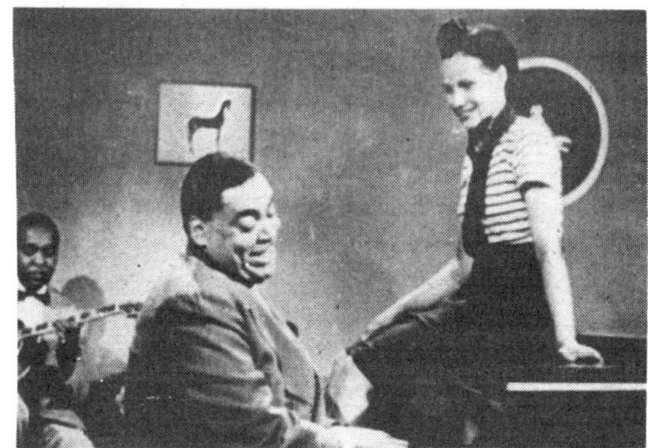

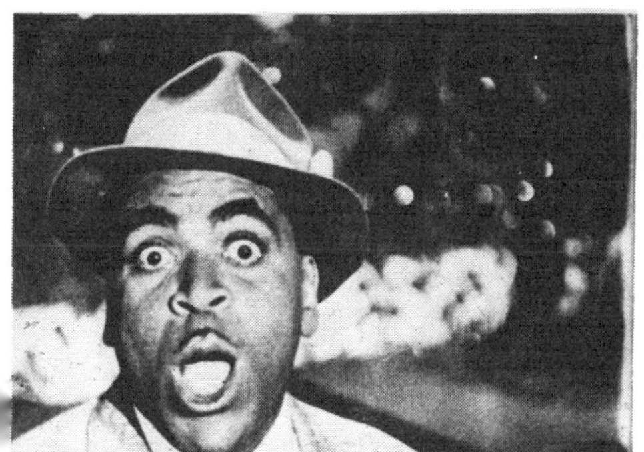

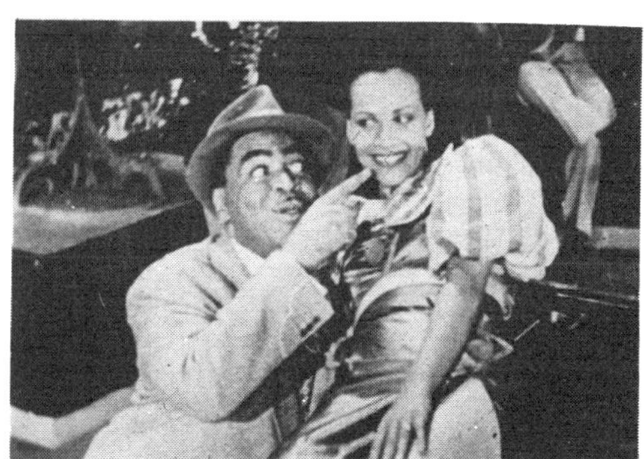

More shots from the soundie films. At top are two from *'Ain't Misbehavin''*, with Vivian Brown on the piano. In the middle are two from *'Honeysuckle Rose'* with Vivian Brown again on the piano, and on the right is one from *'Your Feet's Too Big'*.

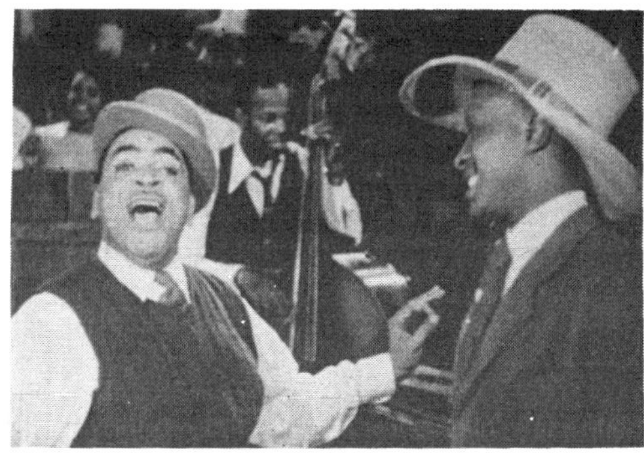

knowledge is probably almost a year too early as the Minoco company is not thought to have commenced operations prior to March 1941. Additional circumstantial evidence supports the date proposed here. Firstly, although reports in the black press mentioned that Minoco Productions had begun filming black bands, Waller's was not among those listed. Secondly, during his interview with Rochester in Hollywood on 19 June 1941 Fats said he had made "quite a few shorts". Since no others have ever been traced, it is reasonable to assume that it is this group of four to which he refers and they had to be made between the date the company began operations and Waller's departure on the coast to coast trip.

"Soundies" were made for use on a special type of coin-operated film projector about the size of a juke box known as a Panoram, in which the films were back-projected on to a screen opposite a small viewing window. From evidence available from prints seen, the films were shot, and a "live" soundtrack made. This was then followed by a second (at least) filming, known as a 'sidelining session', in which the musicians and cast mimed to the previously made sound recording. Prints were then spliced up from the resultant recordings and might conceivably be entirely "live"; "mimed", or a mixture of both. Many years ago, Reg Coldham told me that he had seen two versions of each of the films, and subsequently I have been able to confirm that visually different versions of the first and second titles do exist, but it is not known whether more than one version was released to Panorams.

I screened these for Al Casey in an effort to discover when they were made and the identity of the girl who sits on the piano in the first title and also sings. Al thought the films were made in a studio on Long Island (they were) and although he tried, could not remember the girl's name, only that she was the sister of one of the girls in the chorus line in which she herself appears in this and other films. Later, on a visit to Paris, I discussed these shorts with film collector Michel Pfau and he told me that he had interviewed Lee Gaines (the bass singer with the Delta Rhythm Boys) at length, and that Lee had told him that she was one of 'the Brown Twins'. She was named Vivian, and her sister who only dances was Lilian. Lee also said that Winnie Johnson was another of the chorines (she comes between the two quarreling men in *Your Feets Too Big*) and that she was also featured in other 'Soundies', notably *'Let's Scuffle'* and *'Take Me Back Baby'* with Jimmy Rushing. Lee also stated that Winnie Johnson's brother, Bobby, was one of the three policemen who enters at the end of *'The Joint Is Jumping'.* Howard Rye, during the course of his researches into 'Soundies' generally, has identified the girl who hands the outsize shoes to Fats in *'Your Feet's Too Big'* as Mabel Lee.

*****

"Fats" Waller - Piano Solo

Fats Waller, p.

Studio 2, New York City, New York — Tuesday, 13 May 1941

11:00 a.m. to 1:45 p.m. Ed Kirkeby present

063887-1* GEORGIA ON MY MIND (Hoagy Carmichael-Stewart Gorrell) — Vi 27765-B, HMVSw HE2975, HMVIn N.4477

063888-1* ROCKIN' CHAIR (Hoagy Carmichael) — Vi 27765-A, 243, HMVSw HE2975, HMVIn N.4477, HMVAu EA 3685

063889-1 CAROLINA SHOUT — Victor unissued, 'Hold'. Issued on LP

063889-2* CAROLINA SHOUT (James P. Johnson) — Vi/C 27563-B, HMVIt AV722

063889: See note

063890-1* HONEYSUCKLE ROSE (À la Bach-Beethoven-Brahms-Waller) (Thomas "Fats" Waller) — *Vi 20-1580-A, 420-0235*

063891-1* RING DEM BELLS (Duke Ellington-Irving Mills) — Vi/C 27563-A, HMVIt AV722

The recording sheet indicates that both takes of 063889 were accepted for issue and gives the timing for take -1 as 2:30 and for take -2 as 2:15. Although there are easily recognisable differences in the introduction and coda they have proved rather difficult to separate and describe for the non-musician and I again sought the help of pianist Louis Mazetier who comments: "*Carolina Shout* actually has five themes but in the two versions here Waller employs only four of them, but in different permutations. If we letter them in the order in which Fats introduces them we have the following:"

-1		-2	
	Introduction		Introduction
	A theme played twice		A theme played twice
	B theme followed by a a modified theme B		B theme played once
	C theme played once		C theme played once
	D theme followed by a modified theme D		D theme played once
	C theme in modified form		C theme in modified form
	A theme with the transition into this is by a series of four octaves played by left hand		D theme played once
	Piece ends on a single bass G note		A theme in modified form, the transition into this being by a single chord
			Piece ends with the final G note played twice

Victor 243 is a demonstration record (backed by 244) pressed on vinyl on a special orange, black and white label.

*****

"Fats" Waller and his Rhythm -Fox Trot **Vocal refrain and piano by "Fats" Waller**

John Hamilton, t; Gene Sedric, cl-1/ts-2; Fats Waller, p/v; Al Casey, g; Cedric Wallace, sb; Slick Jones, d; band vocal, -3.

Studio 2, New York City, New York Tuesday, 13 May 1941
2:00 to 5:15 p.m. Ed Kirkeby present

063892-1* TWENTY-FOUR ROBBERS -1,-3 BB B-11222-A, HMV/In B.D.1011, HMVSw JK2651, HMV/H M.H.131, RZAu G24853
(James Young-Ted Buckner)

063893-1 I UNDERSTAND -2 BB B-11175-A
(Kim Gannon-Mabel Wayne)

063893-2* I UNDERSTAND -2 Victor unissued, 'Hold'. Issued on LP?

063893: Note that although a number of LP issues have claimed to use take -2, all such issues which have been checked have proved to be identical with the original Bluebird issue.

063894-1* SAD SAP SUCKER AM I -1 BB B-11296-A, HMVSw HE2428 RZAu G24895
("Fats" Waller & Ed. Kirkeby)

063895-1* HEADLINES IN THE NEWS -1,-2 BB B-11188-A, RZAu G24836
(Milt Noel-Edgar Battle)

Note that the first session was recorded for Victor and the second for Bluebird with a 15-minute gap between them. The Indian pressing of HMV BD.1011 omits the first stop in the catalogue number (thus).

The reverse of HMV JK2651 is *Singin' The Blues* by **Brad Gowans' New York Nine**.

*****

Fats normally made records for Victor before departing on a lengthy tour and this time, he was booked for twelve weeks with his big band which comprised:

John Hamilton, Bob Williams, Herman Autrey, t; George Wilson, Ray Hogan, tb; Jimmy Powell, Dave McRae, as; Gene Sedric, cl/ts; Bob Carroll, ts; Fats Waller, p; Al Casey, g; Cedric Wallace, sb; Slick Jones, d.

No second pianist was carried which threw an even heavier load on Fats's shoulders. Ed

Kirkeby recalled that the tour was hectic, but was broken up by a couple of residencies, and mentions a week at the Tunetown Ballroom in St. Louis. This is confirmed in *The Billboard's* "Orchestra Routes" section in the edition of 24 May 1941 which shows Waller playing the Tunetown Ballroom in St. Louis, Missouri from 20 to 26 May; the *Pittsburgh Courier* just says May 30-week.

From there they headed to the West Coast for two weeks at the Paramount Theatre in Los Angeles and, whilst there, Fats made a broadcast and he and the band made some recordings for Victor.

*****

The broadcast took place on Thursday, 19 June 1941 from Hollywood and took the form of an interview between Fats and Rochester of the Jack Benny Program and the following are excerpts from a transcription by Roy Cooke of what took place:

R: Are any other members of your family musicians?
FW: No, no. Nobody else in the family, other than my grandfather, and he's long been gone.
R: Have you ever played with any other orchestras?
FW: Well, I've made records with quite a number of orchestras. Paul Whiteman for one; I made some with Fletcher Henderson. I also made some with Vincent Lopez.
R: What instruments do you play?
FW: Piano, violin, and organ.
R: Well, gee, that violin is ...
FW: No, no, no, no. Lemme tell you about that violin episode right now. I played violin in the school orchestra and played it so terribly that the boys used to ... when I start playin' a solo ... they'd say, "Hey! Get that rat some cheese."
R: Which is your favourite?
FW: My favourite is organ.
R: I thought so. Well, when did you organise your first band?
FW: In 1932. I was at a little radio station in Cincinnati.
R: How many members are there in your band at the present time?
FW: At the present time there is thirteen of us.
R: How many of your musicians are eligible for Selective Service?
FW: Well, we have three or four. There's John 'Bugs' Hamilton, our first trumpet player; we have Hogan, our first trombonist; we've got a couple of other 'cats' in there ...
R: When you organized your first band, did you pattern your style after any particular band of that time?
FW: No, when I started that first band, it was every man for hisself and every tub on its own bottom.
R: Why did you choose this particular selection?
FW: What selection?
R: The one that you call your theme song.
FW: Ohhhh — well, I'll tell you, that was written — our theme song bein' *Ain't Misbehavin'* — that was written while I was lodging, or, rather, incarcerated in the alimony jail, and I wasn't misbehavin'—you dig?
R: How many recordings have you made; can you give me an idea?
FW: Well, roughly between 800 and 1,000 records.
R: Do you remember what the title of your first recording was?
FW: The title of my first recording was *'Tain't Nobody's Biz-ness If I Do.*

R: Where do most of your musical engagements take place?
FW: Oh, all over the country. We just got though touring through Louisiana, Texas, Mississippi, and now we're hung in this good old sunny California and the flotilla-dilla from Manila.
R: Have you done any motion picture work?
FW: I made a couple of pictures. I made *'Hooray For Love'* and *'King Of Burlesque'* and made quite a few shorts.
R: What is your personal opinion of the boogie-woogie type of music?
FW: "Beat me, daddy, eight to the bar."
R: What has been the most outstanding incident in your musical career?
FW: The most outstanding incident ... let me see. Well, I'll tell you one thing; when I was over in Manchester, England, in 1939, I fell out of a cab door. We were doin' about thirty miles an hour. I didn't get a scratch.
R: Well, that was an incident. Do you have any hobbies?
FW: Hobbies? Ohhhh, yes. I got one hobby I can't tell the people about over this air ...

The interview is obviously a contrived tongue-in-cheek affair. However, it is worth examining some of the statements made by Fats, although clarification of the majority will be found elsewhere in this listing.

1. Recordings with Vincent Lopez: Vincent Lopez, when asked about this said that although he and Waller had been close personal friends and that Fats had sat in with his band on a number of occasions, he could not recall any actual recordings as such.
2. Writing *Ain't Misbehavin'* in the alimony jail: Although the story was untrue, it had been around for some years and delighted Fats's sense of humour, and he often referred to it jokingly. To ascertain the true facts, Bob Kumm wrote to Andy Razaf about this, and in a letter dated 5 October 1966, he replied:

   ...There is no truth to the widely circulated erroneous story about AIN'T MISBEHAVIN' being written while Fats was in prison. The song was written by Fats and myself at his West 133rd St. home in Harlem. The title and words are entirely mine. An hour after we wrote it we went to the 44th St. Theatre and demonstrated it for the show in rehearsal. It was selected to be the theme song of the show. After Paul Bass and Margaret Simms sang it as a love duet, I suggested that Louis (Satchmo) Armstrong sing and play a chorus from the orchestra pit. When he did it, it became a terrific hit.

   Thank you for giving me an opportunity to play this small part in the preparation of the book. Good luck and best wishes.

   Very sincerely,
   Andy Razaf

3. Fats's first recording: From documented evidence, Fats is in error here ... unless there are recordings of which we have no knowledge which predate *Muscle Shoals/Birmingham Blues.*
4. Fats mentions "quite a few shorts" in answer to the question on films. Only four are known.
5. The fall from the cab in England: Ed Kirkeby places this as Edinburgh in 1938. This is more likely, but not in Princes Street as he recalled. It was more likely on the road up to Edinburgh Castle.

*****

"Fats" Waller, his Rhythm and his Orchestra **Piano by "Fats" Waller**
or **Vocal refrain and piano by "Fats" Waller -3**

John Hamilton, Bob Williams, Herman Autrey, t; George Wilson, Ray Hogan, tb; Jimmy Powell, Dave McRae, as; Gene Sedric, Bob Carroll, ts; Fats Waller, p/v-1/sp-2; Al Casey, g; Cedric Wallace, sb; Slick Jones, d; band vocal -3

Hollywood Recording Studio, Hollywood, California Tuesday, 1 July 1941
1:45 to 4:45 p.m. Harry Meyerson directing

061334-1	CHANT OF THE GROOVE -2 (Robert Hicks)	BB/C B-11262-B, *Vi 20-2638-B* RZAu G24895
061335-1	COME AND GET IT -1,-2 (Thomas "Fats" Waller-Ed Kirkeby)	BB/C B-11262-A, Vi 20-2448-B
061336-1	RUMP STEAK SERENADE -1,-3 ("Fats" Waller-Ed. Kirkeby)	BB B-11296-B, HMV B.9582, HMVSw JK2475, HMVIt HN2359
061337-1	GETTIN' MUCH LATELY? (Aint Nothin' To It) (T. Waller- E. Kirkeby)	BB B-11262-A

Swiss HMV JK2475 as **New Orleans Feetwarmers,** HMV and Italian HMV isues as **"Fats" Waller and his Orchestra** the latter in Italian. The final title was originally accepted for issue on Bluebird, but then changed to "Hold". It is as shown on the recording sheet, but this is crossed through, leaving only the sub-title, which has a note in manuscript against it: "per letter C. Reddy 7-14-41". It was issued in error on some copies of Bluebird B-11262-A labelled as *COME AND GET IT.*

The reverse of HMV JK2475 is *Shag* by **Sidney Bechet & his Orch**.

*****

From Hollywood, the band presumably headed north. In his column in the *New York Age* of 12 July 1941, Floyd Snelson mentions *...Fats Waller in the Pacific northwest, at Seattle, Moore Theatre. The Billboard* of 27 September also mentions the Moore Theatre, Seattle in a list of "recent engagements" as well as the Hotel Sherman in Chicago. The *Pittsburgh Courier* is more specific and, in a report datelined Seattle, July 10, announces that, *Fats Waller and his orchestra, plus several additional musicians have been booked to play a swing concert at the Moore theater, July 13.* In a review of the concert, the same paper had this to say:

> *... near capacity crowd ... sweet side not overlooked and Waller did "Still Of The Night" and "Summertime" on the organ and the band gave "Two Sleepy People" and "Sometimes I'm Happy" ... but it was swing the crowd liked best ... cheered hot improvisations with John Hamilton, trumpet and Eugene Sedric, sax ... four reeds, five brass, four rhythm...*

Leaving the West Coast, the band carried on with the tour and Ed Kirkeby mentions stops at Idaho Falls, Denver, and St. Louis. After a month's vacation in New York, the band re-assembled and left on a another tour which went first to Grandview, Virginia, on to Maryland, and then headed north to Massachusetts and Maine, followed by according to Kirkeby, "a series of theatre dates". The advert for the Apollo Theatre for the week commencing Friday, 19 September shows *"Fats" Waller and his Band and Revue* featured with Myra Johnson among the artists listed. This engagement is reviewed by the *Pittsburgh Courier,* which noted that Waller had played "Summertime" and "Stardust", and mentioned in the report in *The Billboard Talent & Tunes Supplement* of 27 September 1941 (see above) which states that Fats is "Now appearing" at the Apollo Theater, New York City; following which he is scheduled to go on a 16-week theatre tour. His band is noted as comprising three trumpets, two trombones, four reeds, guitar, bass and drums in addition to Waller himself, but only Herb Fleming (sic) is mentioned by name. Recent engagements noted include Hotel Sherman, Chicago; Moore Theater, Seattle; Paramount Theatre, Los Angeles, and Loew's State, New York City. This last engagement presumably preceded the week at the Apollo and, at the completion of that Waller and his band played a one night stand at the Renaissance Casino at 138th Street and Seventh Avenue on Sunday, 29 September. They began at 5:30 p.m. and went on until late. Then before leaving on the tour recalled by Ed Kirkeby, there was another recording date for Victor:

*****

"Fats" Waller and his Rhythm -Fox Trot **Vocal refrain and piano by "Fats" Waller** or **Hammond Organ by "Fats" Waller -3**

John Hamilton, t; Gene Sedric, cl; Fats Waller, p-/v-1/bells-2/o-3; Al Casey, g; Cedric Wallace, sb; Slick Jones, d.

Studio 2, New York City, New York Wednesday, 1 October 1941
1:30 to 6:15 p.m. Ed Kirkeby present

067946-1*	OH BABY, SWEET BABY (What Are You Doin' To Me) -1 ("Fats" Waller-Ed Kirkeby)	BB B-11383-A, HMV/In B.D.1036, HMVSw HE2416
067947-1*	BUCK JUMPIN' (Albert Casey-Ed Kirkeby)	BB B-11324-B, HMVSw HE2446, HMVSc X8190, RZAu G25055
067948-1*	THAT GETS IT, MR. JOE -1 ("Fats" Waller-James P. Johnson)	BB B-11425-B, HMV B.D.1028, HMVSw HE2346, RZAu G25055
067949-1*	THE BELLS OF SAN RAQUEL -1,-2 (Wise-Leeds- Barcelata)	BB B-11324-A, HMVSw HE2446
067949-2	THE BELLS OF SAN RAQUEL -*1,-2*	Victor unissued, 'Hold'
067950-1*	BESSIE, BESSIE BESSIE -1	Victor unissued, 'Hold'. Issued on LP
067951-1*	CLARINET MARMALADE -3 (Larry Shields-H.W. Ragas)	BB/C B-11469-B, HMVSw HE2371, HMVIt Av750

Unusually, the recording sheet indicates which waxes were selected for issue, and they are respectively: -1; -1; -1; -1A; --; -1A. 067947 is a feature for Al Casey and, although there is no vocal in the accepted sense, Fats is heard giving encouragement to Casey. Al told me that this tune was often a feature of the stage show and was "really only a twelve bar blues". Kirkeby's name appeared as part-composer because, "he always took a piece to get something recorded or published."

The X-series HMV issues are normally for distribution throughout Scandinavia, but X8190 appears to have been specifically for Denmark. 067950 is shown on the recording sheet as composed by Thomas "Fats" Waller.

*****

The 16-week tour mentioned in *The Billboard Talent & Tunes Supplement* of 27 September 1941 was somewhat shorter than that as the band were back in the city well before the expiration of 16 weeks. However, as noted in *The Billboard's* "Orchestra Routes", one of Ed Kirkeby's recollections is confirmed by the issue of 11 October which notes Waller at the Howard Theater, Washington (snapshot of Waller outside the theatre taken by Herb

Flemming). Kirkeby also mentions the Royal Theatre; the RKO, Syracuse; the Colonial, Detroit, the Grand, Evansville and the Regal in Chicago for this tour.

Further information on the RKO engagement is found in the *Pittsburgh Courier* datelined Rochester, N.Y. Oct. 23 which stated that 'officials of the RKO Temple theatre will determine whether the theatre-going public will take to flesh shows when it will bring in Fats Waller and his band for a four-day stand beginning Thursday'. The report went on to explain that audiences in the area had not supported 'live' performances in the past. 23 October was a Thursday, so either the engagement ran from 23-26 October (most likely) or, if the report is taken literally, from 30 October to 2 November.

A photo of the husband and wife comedy team of Apus and Estrelita in the *Pittsburgh Courier* of 8 November is accompanied by a paragraph informing that they had been a great success 'with Maestro Fats Waller and his crew at the Roosevelt theatre' in Pittsburgh last week.

Herb Flemming recalled that Fats Waller gave him a trombone on stage at the Colonial Theatre, Detroit. He dated this as 1939 and played the instrument until the end of his life. However, Herb is not thought to have been a member of any Waller group as early as this, nor is any engagement traced for the Colonial in that year and, as he recalls playing the Apollo with Fats and several other locations mentioned above, he is probably thinking of the above tour. The personnel is not established, but it is known that Arthur Trappier replaced Slick Jones around this time and is present in a photo of the big band which may have been taken on stage at the Apollo. This includes:

John Hamilton, Joe Thomas, Courtney Williams, t; Herb Flemming, Fred Robinson, tb; Jimmy Powell, *Scoville Brown,* as; Gene Sedric, Bob Carroll, ts; Fats Waller, p/o; Al Casey, g; Cedric Wallace, sb; Arthur Trappier, d; Myra Johnson, v.

*****

Two entries in the *International Musician* for November 1941 may relate to engagements on the tour mentioned above. The reports are from Local 123, Richmond, Virginia and Local 543, Baltimore, Maryland. The first gives: Fats Waller, Eugene Sedric, David McRae, Theodore McCord, Herman Autry, J.B. Hamilton, Herbert Flemming, George Wilson, Albert Casey, Cedric Williams, Wilmore Jones, Bob Williams and Jimmy Powell (all of 802) and the second notes all the above names but substitutes Cedric Wallace for Cedric Williams which suggests that the latter is simply an error. Note that Slick Jones is still present.

*****

On 7 December 1941, Japan attacked Pearl Harbor and the United States entered World War II. Fats Waller immediately threw himself into entertaining the armed forces and to supporting the War Bonds drive and other patriotic activities.

*****

Broadcast

Fats Waller, p/v with large orchestra in which Gene Sedric, ts and Arthur Trappier, d. are identifiable.

Freedom's People Program, New York City, New York — Sunday, 21 December 1941

Honeysuckle Rose — Issued on LP

The orchestra is almost certainly Fats's own big band, playing an arrangement from their stage presentation.

*****

"Fats" Waller and his Rhythm -Fox Trot **Vocal refrain and piano by "Fats" Waller**

Herman Autrey, t; Gene Sedric, cl-1/ts-2; Fats Waller, p-/v; Al Casey, g; Cedric Wallace, sb; Arthur Trappier, d.

Studio 2, New York City, New York — Friday, 26 December 1941
11:00 a.m. to 2:30 p.m.

068810-1*	WINTER WEATHER -2 (Ted Shapiro)	BB/C B-11469-A, HMV B.10234, HMVSw HE2371, HMVIt HN3139, AV750, El EG7836
068811-1*	CASH FOR YOUR TRASH -1 (Ed Kirkeby-Fats Waller)	BB B-11425-A, HMVSw HE2428
068812-1*	DON'T GIVE ME THAT JIVE (Come On With The Come On) -1 (Ed Kirkeby-"Fats" Waller)	BB B-11539-B, *HMV/In B.D.1077*, RZAu G24989
068813-1*	YOUR SOCKS DON'T MATCH -2 (Leon Carr-Leo Corday)	BB 30-0814-A, HMV B.D.1073
068813-2*	YOUR SOCKS DON'T MATCH -2	Victor unissued, 'Hold'. Issued on LP

068813 Fourth line of second verse of vocal: -1 "Doggone you gal, your socks don't match"
-2 "Baby what happened? Your socks don't match"

The personnel, showing two changes from the previous "Rhythm" recording date, is shown on the recording sheet.

*****

Broadcast — Dave Elman's Hobby Lobby Program

Fats Waller, p/v/sp; Dave Elman, sp; studio orchestra -1

CBS studios, New York City, New York — Saturday, 10 January 1942

Go Down Moses	Issued on LP
Ain't Misbehavin' -1	Issued on LP

Waller made a guest appearance on this weekly show and attempted a brief history of jazz in the short period available to him.

*****

Concert by FATS WALLER with Assisting Artists

Fats Waller, p/v; acc: by Hot Lips Page, t -1 or 'The Chicagoans' -2: Max Kaminsky, t; Pee Wee Russell. cl; Bud Freeman, ts; Eddie Condon, g; John Kirby, sb; Gene Krupa, d.

Carnegie Hall, New York City, New York — Wednesday, 14 January 1942
Concert scheduled to begin at 8:30 p.m.

Blues In B Flat -1	Issued on LP
Honeysuckle Rose -2	Issued on LP

For full details of this concert, which was promoted by Ernie Anderson, please see his account elsewhere in this volume. It will be noted that the entire concert was recorded on acetates and it is possible that items other than the above have survived. In this connection, I have unconfirmed reports of tapes of *I'm Gonna Sit Right Down And Write Myself A Letter* and *St. Louis Blues.* The concert was previewed in the *New York Age* of 17 January with two columns of the worst possible journalese and inaccurate reporting which went as far as to claim that Waller had played in Berlin and Vienna. Despite this lavish preview no review appeared the following week.

*****

CARNEGIE HALL PROGRAM

SEASON 1941-1942

Wednesday Evening, January 14, at 8:30

Concert by

FATS WALLER

with Assisting Artists

•

THE PROGRAM

1. At the piano—THE SONGS OF FATS WALLER

In order to give Mr. Waller all possible liberty in selecting his material and in order to retain a maximum of spontaneity for his performance, no formal program has been arranged. In this, his first group of selections at the piano, he will play some of his own popular compositions. A list of the best known of them follows. He may be expected to play several of these items. Some of the best of Mr. Waller's popular songs (which are *not* included in this list) are not credited to him simply because he sold all rights to them to unscrupulous Tin Pan Alley authors.

1919 Squeeze Me

1926 Senorita Mine

1927 I'm More Than Satisfied
St. Louis Shuffle

1928 Candied Sweets
Willow Tree
Got Myself Another Jockey Now

1929 Ain't Misbehavin'
I've Got a Feelin' I'm Fallin'
Gone
My Fate is in your Hands
Zonky
Honeysuckle Rose
Black & Blue
How Jazz was Born
Dixie Cinderella
Sweet Savannah Sue
Can't We Get Together
Snakehip Dance
That Rhythm Man
Off-time
Why Am I Alone with No One To Love

1930 Rollin' Down the River
Blue Turning Grey over You
Keep a Song in your Soul
Little Brown Betty
Prisoner of Love

1931 I'm Crazy 'bout My Baby
Heart of Stone
Take It From Me
Concentratin' on You
The Iceman Lives in an Ice House

1932 Keepin' Out of Mischief Now
Buddy
If It Ain't Love
Radio Poppa, Broadcastin' Mamma
When Gabriel Blows His Horn
Lonesome Me
Gotta Be, Gonna Be Mine
Oh You Sweet Thing
Strange As It Seems
That Where the South Begins
Angeline
My Heart's at Ease
Sheltered by Stars
I Didn't Dream It Was Love
Old Yazoo

1933 Aintcha Glad
Tall Timber
Sittin' Up Waitin' For You
Doin' What I Please
I've Got You Where I Want You
Handful of Keys

1934 Swing On Mississippi
How Can You Fail Me
Piano Pranks

1935 Numb Fumblin'

1936 Smashin' Thirds
Stealin' Apples
I Can See You All Over the Place
The Panic Is On
Sugar Rose

1937 Our Love Was Meant To Be
Lost Love
Call the Plumber In
Crazy 'bout That Man of Mine
The Short Trail Became a Long Trail
Swingin' Hound
Any Day the Sun Don't Shine
Brother Ben
Lonesome One

1938 Inside This Heart of Mine
On Rainy Days
Hold My Hand
I Got Love
Bluer Than The Ocean Blues
I'm Gonna Fall in Love
Cottage in the Rain
What a Pretty Miss
Not There, Right Here
Moonlight Mood
The Spider and the Fly
Patty Cake, Patty Cake
I Can't Forgive You

1939 The Jitterbug Tree

1940 The Joint Is Jumpin'
Happy Feelin'
Stayin' at Home

1941 All That Meat and No Potatoes
Mamacita
Blue Velvet

2. At the organ—SPIRITUALS

Among the spirituals Mr. Waller may play are the following:

Go Down Moses
Swing Low, Sweet Chariot
Deep River
All God's Chillun Got Wings
Water Boy
Sometimes I Feel Like a Motherless Child
Lonesome Road

At the organ—A MELODY

This selection, says Mr. Waller, was inspired by 8 bars of Sir Edward Elgar's Pomp and Circumstance.

3. At the piano—IMPROVISATIONS

Mr. Waller may be expected to begin this part of the program by playing:

The Blues, in A

He will then improvise on some of the songs which he has recorded. For example:

I'm Gonna Sit Right Down And Write Myself A Letter

He will then play:

The Blues, in B flat

In this last improvisation Mr. Waller will be accompanied by Hot Lips Page, cornetist, who will sing and play his own blues.

— INTERMISSION —

4. At the piano—LONDON SUITE, 1939

This six part piano suite is an impressionistic sketch of pre-war London. Written in 1939 during Mr. Waller's last European tour, he first played it at the Salle Pleyel in Paris, and later recorded it as an album in London. The album has never been released in this country.

1. Soho
2. Mayfair
3. Bond Street
4. Whitechapel
5. Limehouse
6. Piccadilly Circus

At the piano—VARIATIONS ON A TCHAIKOVSKY THEME

5. At the organ—GERSHWINIANA

Musicologists often refer to the broad influence of the blues on the works of George Gershwin. This group of variations on Gershwin popular themes will provide illustration for this point. Among the Gershwin songs that may be played are:

Bidin' My Time
But Not For Me
Embraceable You
Feeling I'm Falling
How Long Has This Been Going On
I've Got A Crush On You
Liza
Luckiest Man In the World
Man I Love
My One and Only
Oh Lady Be Good
Sam and Delilah
Somebody Loves Me
Someone To Watch Over Me
Strike Up The Band
Summertime
Swanee
Sweet and Low Down
Who Cares
Why Do I Love You

At the piano—VARIATIONS ON A THEME BY GEORGE GERSHWIN

Assisted by Mr. Bud Freeman, Mr. Waller plays a composition inspired by Gershwin's I Got Rhythm.

6. Orchestral group—FATS WALLER AND THE CHICAGOANS. *Assisting Artists are*: Eddie Condon, Guitar; John Kirby, Bass; Gene Krupa, Drums; Bud Freeman, Tenor Saxophone; PeeWee Russell, Clarinet; Max Kaminsky, Cornet.

Mr. Waller will play a group of impromptu selections with the leaders of the Chicago style.

Among the tunes these musicians may play are:

China Boy
I Found a New Baby
Honeysuckle Rose
"Havin' a Ball at Carnegie Hall,"
an improvised fast blues.

Steinway Piano — Hammond Organ — Victor Records

Mr. Waller is presented in this recital by

ERNEST ANDERSON

485 Madison Avenue New York City

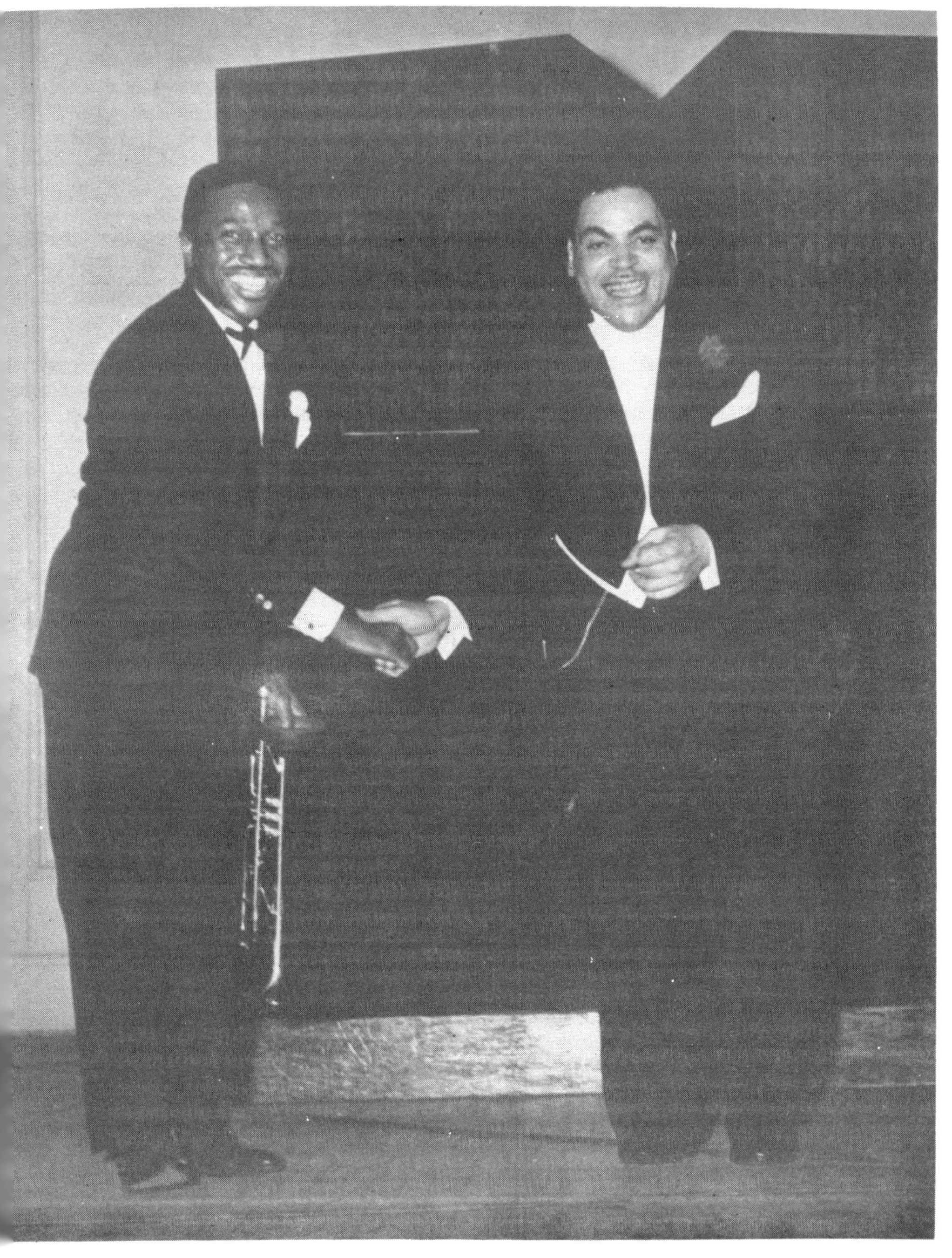

ɔove: Fats and 'Lips' Page take a bow at the end of the first half.
ɘft: The programme.

The Carnegie Concert had been previewed in the *Pittsburgh Courier* which indicated that Waller had replaced John Kirby on "Duffy's Tavern" for Thursday evenings and would be performing on 15 January. "Duffy's Tavern" was a commercial radio programme, sponsored by a razor manufacturer and broadcast over Station WABC of the CBS network. It was hosted by Ed Gardner and Shirley Booth and was virtually the only such programme to feature black artists.

However, Waller's tenure was brief and the *Pittsburgh Courier* reported that he had opened on Thursday, 29 January in the new Downbeat Room of the Garrick Stagebar in Chicago, where he was scheduled to play for at least four weeks, and would be broadcasting over the CBS network whilst there.

The Billboard's "Orchestra Routes" of 31 January 1942 also shows him at the Garrick Stagebar Café in Chicago, which information is repeated in the issues of 7 and 14 February. From these reports it follows that the broadcast of 2 February (below) came from this location rather than either New York or the Blatz Winter Hotel as reported previously. Ed Kirkeby also recalled a four-week engagement at the 'Down Beat Room' at this time, followed by a residency at the Sherman Hotel and other dates. It was during the Sherman Hotel residency that Waller featured the then up and coming singer Dinah Washington, aged eighteen, and she apparently worked with him for several weeks both in Chicago and after he left the city. Billy Rowe had advised his readers as far back as 8 November that Waller was 'set for a January fling at the Sherman hotel' and would be taking the band and a show on a five-night-a-week tour of the south. He added that the show Fats was to put together was to include Candi and Pepper, Clyde Barrie and the Apus and Estrelita act. He seems to have been very well informed.

*****

Broadcast — Fats Waller and his Rhythm

John Hamilton, t; Gene Sedric, ts; Fats Waller, p/v; Al Casey, g; Cedric Wallace, sb; Arthur Trappier, d.

Garrick Stagebar Café, Chicago, Illinois — Monday, 2 February 1942

Winter Weather	Issued on LP
Cash For Your Trash	Issued on LP

Herman Autrey is normally listed for this date, but aurally Hamilton seems more likely and his presence is confirmed by the note below.

Waller's Bluebird recording of *Cash For Your Trash* had been selected by the Waste Paper Conservation Campaign Committee to promote their activities and they purchased 100 copies for distribution to their various campaign offices.

*****

A report from Local 208, Chicago (held over from March) in the April *International Musician* shows transfers deposited for Fats Waller, Eugene Sedric, John Hamilton, Cedric Wallace, Albert Casey and Arthur Trappier and probably refers to the Sherman Hotel engagement and broadcast above.

*****

Leaving Chicago, Ed Kirkeby says they next went to Flint, Michigan, probably for a week, after which they headed to Minneapolis for an engagement at the 'Happy Hour'. Whilst there Fats played a benefit with Dimitri Mitropoulos on a Sunday. However, from other evidence it

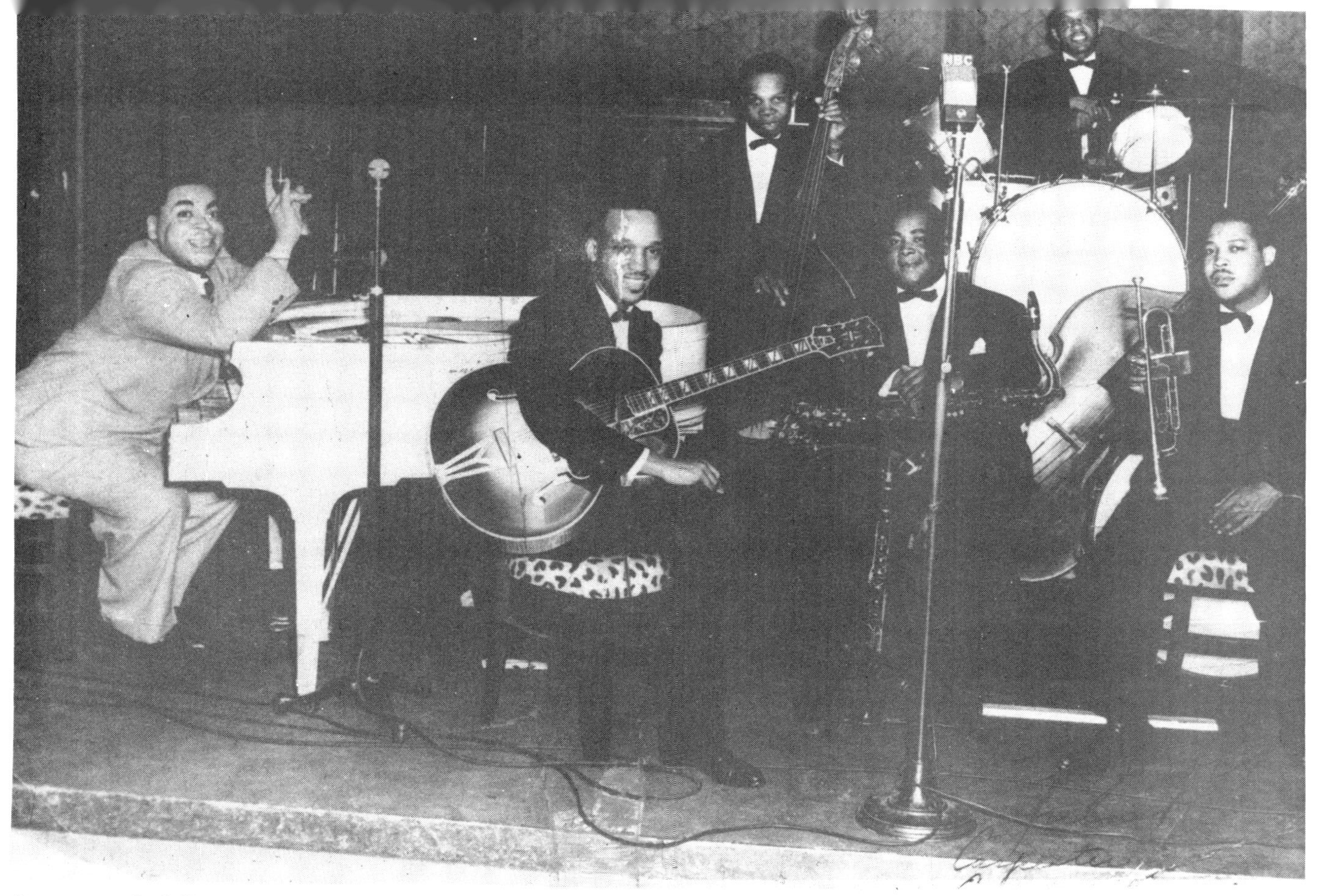

A personnel of Fats, Al Casey, Cedric Wallace, Gene Sedric, Arthur Trappier(?) and John Hamilton and the spotted seat covers suggest the Panther Room at the Hotel Sherman and this undated photograph may therefore date from early 1942.

appears that these events took place a little later in the year. The band was certainly back in New York early in March for they opened at the Apollo for a week on Friday, 6 March along with vocalist Myra Johnson, and Waller was said to be featuring his Hammond Organ as well as the piano. A note in the *Amsterdam News* of 21 March 1942 concerning the comedy and dance team of Harris, Burnham and Scott, mentions that they appeared at the Apollo with Fats Waller 'recently'. They were among the backing artists for the 6-12 March week.

*****

"Fats"/"fats" Waller, his Rhythm and his Orch. — Fox Trot or **Jive Waltz -3**
Vocal Refrain and Piano by "Fats" Waller -2
Hammond Organ by "Fats" Waller -3

John Hamilton, Joe Thomas, Courtney Williams, t; George Wilson, Herb Flemming, tb; George James, Lawrence Fields, as; Gene Sedric, cl-3/ts; Bob Carroll, ts; Fats Waller, p-1/v-2/o-3; Al Casey, g; Cedric Wallace, sb; Arthur Trappier, d.

Studio 2, New York City, New York — Monday, 16 March 1942

073440-1*	WE NEED A LITTLE LOVE (That's All) -1,-2 ("Fats" Waller-Ed Kirkeby)	BB B-11518-A
073441-1*	YOU MUST BE LOSING YOUR MIND -1,-2 (Ed Kirkeby-"Fats" Waller)	BB B-11539-A, *HMV/In B.D.1077,* RZAu G24989
073442-1*	TWO BITS -1 (Robert Hicks)	Victor unissued, no disposition noted. Issued on LP
073443-1*	THE JITTERBUG WALTZ -3 ("Fats" Waller)	BB B-11518-B, *Vi 20-2639-A, HMVSw HE2976,* HMVSc X8190

For the first time, a Victor recording sheet lists the entire Waller Big Band personnel, but makes no mention of Herman Autrey who has always been shown for this session. This is confirmed by Courtney Williams (see his piece elsewhere in this volume) who, despite the listing by Victor, avers that Fred Robinson rather than George Wilson was present and that the second alto player was named Jackie Fields rather than Lawrence. No dispositions are noted for any of the waxes, although an "A", usually signifying "accepted for issue" is shown against all eight. The first title was typed as *THAT'S ALL* with a note in manuscript above it "We Need A Little Love (per letter E. Kirkeby) 4/1/42". Similarly, the third title is typed as shown with a manuscript note "Really Fine (per C. Reddy 4/7)" added. It was later issued on LP under this amended title.

As noted after the 1 October 1941 session, HMV X8190 appears to be exclusively for Denmark rather than for general Scandinavian distribution.

*****

With this session over, Fats again took to the road with his big band, but a comment from reporter Roland Young in *Downbeat* for 15 April 1942 shows that the big band touring policy featured by Waller was not meeting with universal acclaim. Datelined Bridgeport, Conn., it says:

> *Although Fats Waller did fine business at the Lyric Theater here recently, when in for a 3-day stint, and almost broke house records (the management puts all bands in that bracket), the band and the show proved to be a big bring-down to all of Fats' friends who heard him. Fats used a big band that seemed lost about the entire affair. Why not, observers asked, have Waller use his own small crew on these theater dates? It's a shame to send him around like this, leaving a bad taste in everyone's mouth.*

*****

A number of other engagements may be dated from the columns of the *International Musician.* The issue of July 1942 shows that the Waller aggregation was at the Metropolitan, Rhode Island for the week ending 21 April 1942 where they followed Benny Goodman. Takings are reported as $6,000 for the week (Goodman took $7,000). They probably returned to New York after this, but two weeks later (week ending 7 May) they were at the Palace, Cleveland, Ohio, where they grossed $16,000, but this was eclipsed by the Gene Krupa orchestra which followed them and took $21,000. From there they went into Loew's Court Square Theatre, Springfield, Massachusetts for the week ending 13 May.

*****

One engagement by the small band is indicated by a report from Local 5, Detroit in the July, 1942 *International Musician.* It notes transfers are deposited for Fats Waller, John Hamilton, Eugene Sedric, Albert Casey, Cedric Wallace and Arthur Trappier, and probably relates to an engagement at the end of May or during June.

*****

For a few months prior to July 1942, when he joined Noble Sissle, Bill Coleman was a member of Waller's big band playing short theatre engagements in the *small towns of New York, Massachusetts, Connecticut, and New Jersey.* Thus he was probably in the band reported by Roland Young and the other engagements above, and his account helps to explain Young's adverse criticism:

> *Dave McRae, an alto player, was the one who engaged the musicians for the big band Fats was using. We were Jacques Butler, Johnny "Bugs Hamilton (Fats's regular trumpet man), and myself (trumpets), Herb Flemming (trombone), Cedric Wallace (bass), Al Casey (guitar), Arthur Trappier (drums), Bob Carroll (tenor sax), and there was another alto sax whose name I've forgotten.*
>
> *Fats was a natural hit everywhere we played. As Bugs Hamilton had been with Fats a long time, he was normally the leader of the trumpet section because he had parts that he played when Fats only used a small combo. He would give Jacques Butler and me the solos that he didn't care for. Sometimes when his lips were not feeling too strong, Bugs would ask me or Jacques to take one of the solos he enjoyed. If his lips were in good shape the next day, he would play the solos again. Jacques and I decided to have a discussion with him about that and he agreed that we should have our regular featured solos.*
>
> *These gigs were on a weekly basis and sometimes there would be periods of two or three weeks when Fats did not use a big band. Whenever he did, the same musicians were usually available. We had a few days once in upstate New York when Fats was suffering with the gout in one foot. His doctor had advised him not to drink any whisky but told him that he could drink a little wine. So Fats had a gallon jug of muscatel wine in his dressing room every day. He would invite the musicians to drink with him, but he drank most of the gallon.*

*****

Clyde Bernhardt also recalls a spell in the Waller big band:

> *After Edgar* [Hayes] *left for the coast, George Wilson, who was in Fats Waller's band, heard I was at liberty and got me to fill in when he went with Charlie Johnson to Atlantic City. Fats had Bob Williams, Eugene Sedric, Johnny "Bugs" Hamilton, George James,*

Hanc Duncan, Herman Autrey, Al Casey, Slick Jones and other good musicians. We did a week at the Royal in Baltimore and another at the Howard in Washington, D.C., around July.

Ed Kirkeby, Fats' manager, asked me to take a September tour, but I saw Fats only wanted his horns playing parts and that wasn't for me.

These engagements may have been prior to the next record session or immediately after it, although the inclusion of Slick Jones suggests a slightly earlier period.

*****

"Fats" Waller and his Rhythm — Fox Trot **Vocal refrain and piano by "Fats" Waller** or **Vocal refrain and piano by "Fats" Waller with the Deep River Boys -3**

John Hamilton, t; Gene Sedric, cl/ts-1; Fats Waller, p/v-2; Al Casey, g; Cedric Wallace, sb; Arthur Trappier, d; The Deep River Boys: Harry Douglas, Vernon Gardner, George Lawson and Edward Ware, v-3.

Studio 2, New York City, New York — Monday, 13 July 1942
1:30 to 5:00 p.m.

075423-1* BY THE LIGHT OF THE SILVERY MOON -2,-3 (Ed Madden-Gus Edwards) — BB B-11569-A, Vi 20-2448-A, *HMV B.10748*, HMVIt AV749, *HMVIn NE688*
075424-1* SWING OUT TO VICTORY -2 (Ed Kirkeby-Thos, "Fats" Waller) — BB B-11569-B, *HMVIn NE688*
075425-1* UP JUMPED YOU WITH LOVE -1,-2 (Ed Kirkeby-Thos, "Fats" Waller) — BB 30-0814-B, *HMV B.D.1045*
075426-1* ROMANCE A LA MODE -3 (Gannon-Altman) — *HMV B.D.1045, B.10748*
075426-2* ROMANCE A LA MODE -3 — Victor unissued, 'Hold'

According to the recording sheet the last two titles were originally selected for issue on Bluebird 30-0805-B/-A respectively, but this was withdrawn before issue. There is also a note in manuscript against 075426-2/-2A "Parts destroyed".

Hamilton and Sedric do not play on the issued take of the last title, although there is nothing on the recording sheet to indicate this.

The reverse of Italian HMV AV749 is *It Had To Be You* by **Orch. Earl Hines, con Green e le tre Varietes.**

This was the final session by the Rhythm and, although previous listings have stated that after this Fats disbanded it and had no intention of reforming, this was not so as will be seen Photographs taken at the session show him in a very happy mood and record the presence of his son Maurice in the studio.

*****

The Victor "First Nighter" Orchestra **Vocal refrain by "Fats" Waller and Men's Choruus**

Fats Waller, v; acc: Mannie Weinstock, Stephen Schultz, Del Staigers, t; Lloyd E. Turner, Chas. Butterfield, tb; Chet Hazlett, Fletcher Bereford, Eddie Stennard, Murray Cohen, saxes; Leo Kruczek, Harry Urbont, Joe Raymond, vn; John B. Giampietro, harp; Sam Mineo, p; Carl Kress, g; Edw. P. Brader, sb; Edw. C. Rubsam, d, and men's chorus.

Studio 2, New York City, New York — Thursday, 30 July 1942
Leonard Joy directing

075469-1 THAT'S WHAT THE WELL-DRESSED MAN IN HARLEM WILL WEAR (Irving Berlin) — Vi 27956-B

The reverse of Victor 27956 is by the same with Brad Reynolds replacing Waller. Both sides

Right: Fats in jovial mood at his final 'Rhythm' date for Victor

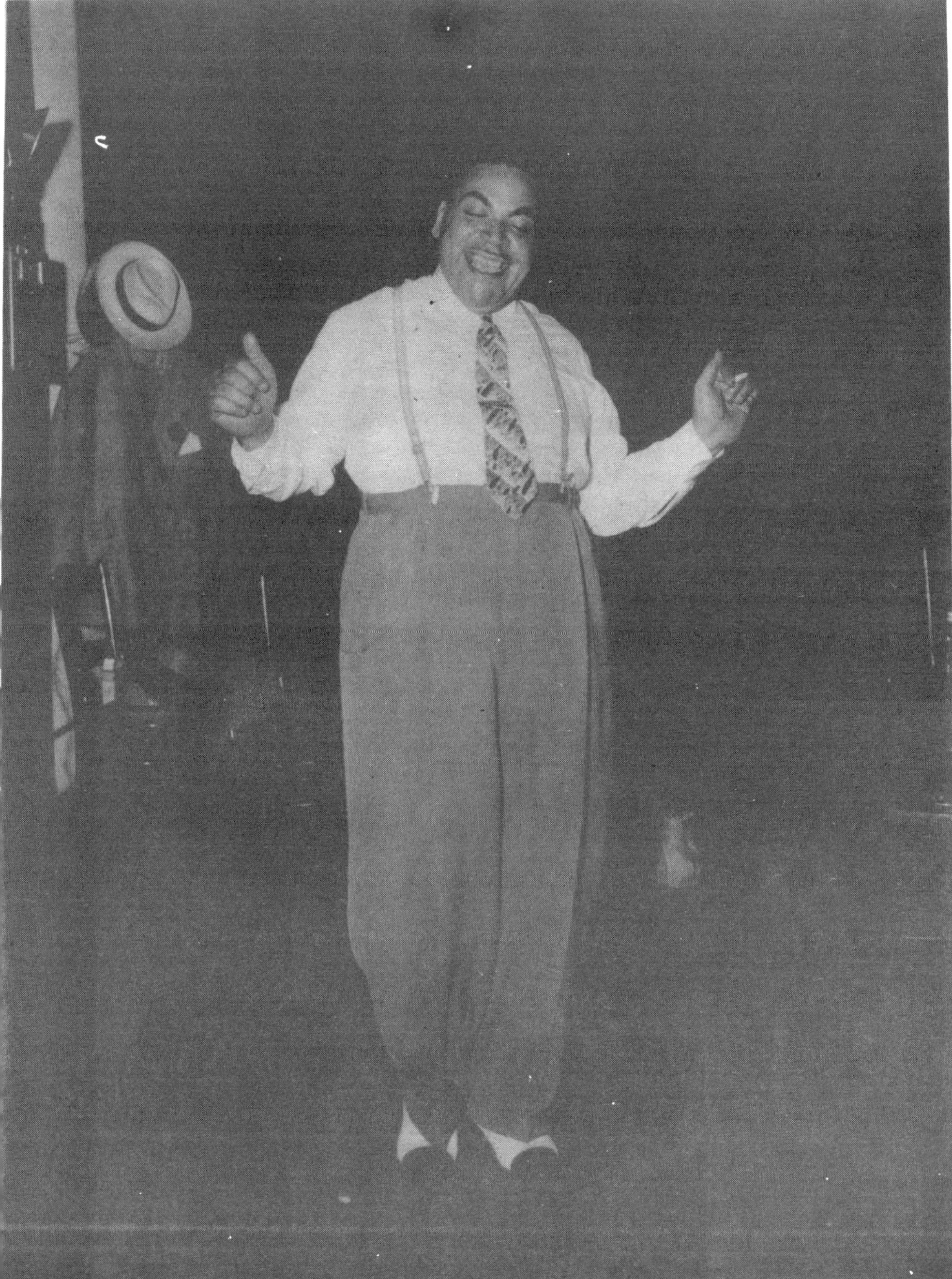

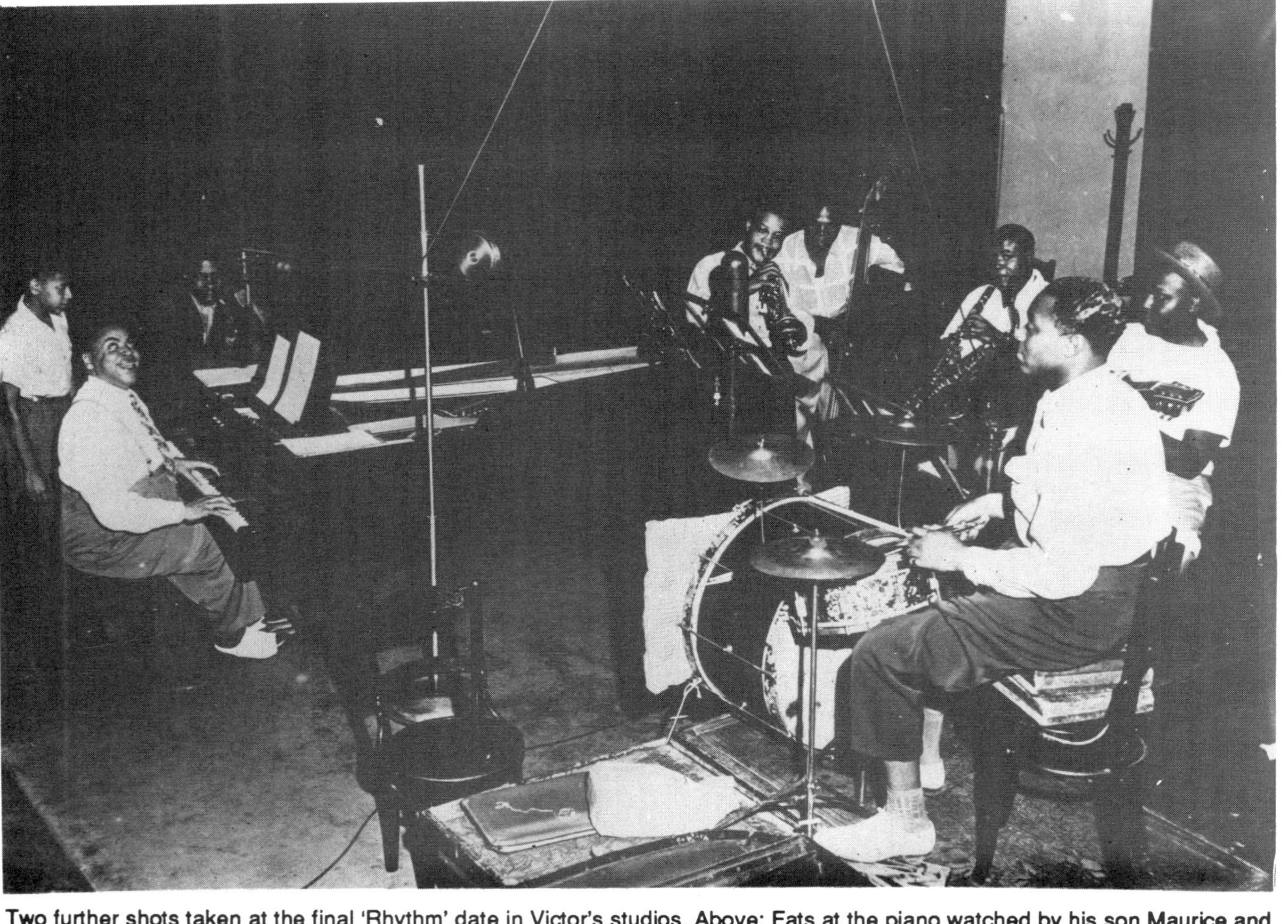

Two further shots taken at the final 'Rhythm' date in Victor's studios. Above: Fats at the piano watched by his son Maurice and

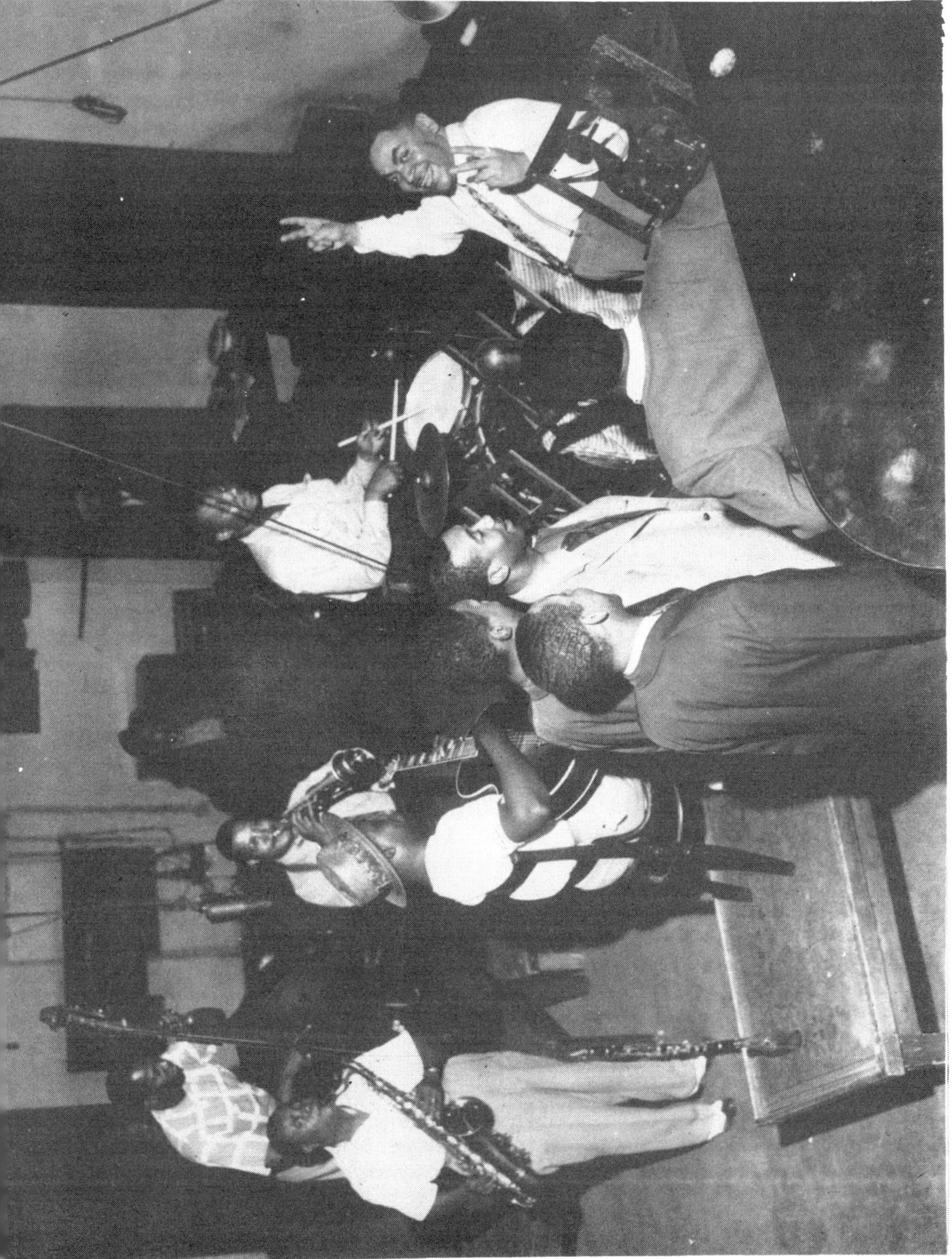

bear the additional credit **(From the All-Soldier Show "This Is the Army")**. Victor issued recordings from the show in Album P 131, and the Waller item is side 6 in this.

*****

This was Waller's final commercial recording, and the following day a recording ban on AFM musicians was called by James C. Petrillo, head of the union, effective from midnight 31 July 1942.

*****

An interesting sidelight appears in the *Pittsburgh Courier* of 29 August 1942 which reports that, according to a WW News Service release, Fats Waller had paid tax on an income of $72,000 'last year' — a sum equivalent to that paid to the President of the United States!

*****

Private Recordings

Fats Waller, p

Harry Smith Studios, New York City, New York — Thursday, 3 September 1942

You've Been Grand	Issued on LP
Pay-Off Double	Issued on LP
Untitled	Issued on LP

*****

Fats continued to tour for a time with his big band and assorted acts, making up a stage show of considerable proportions. There was obviously the tour in September which Clyde Bernhardt declined to make, and *Downbeat* of 1 October 1942 noted that, *Fats Waller opens at Club Top Hat [Toronto], October 5th, for a week.* It is possible that this report is in anticipation of the engagement confirmed below, but certainly during November Waller again went north into Canada with his small group. Art Pilkington has been able to date two of the events mentioned in the interview below and has established that he played the Civic Auditorium, Winnipeg on Thursday, 12 November. An unusually perceptive, enthusiastic and detailed review by Tony Allan in *The Winnipeg Tribune* of 13 November reveals that 5,000 people attended and that the band was comprised of "Bugs" Hamilton, Eugene Sedric, "Fats" Waller, Albert Casey, Cedric Wallace and Arthur Treacher (sic) on drums with vocalist Myra Johnson. Sedric was singled out for special praise, especially on ballad numbers like *Solitude* and *I Guess I'll Have To Dream The Rest.* Other numbers mentioned include *Someone's Rocking My Dream Boat* (Myra Johnson feature), *One O'Clock Jump, Jersey Bounce,* and *E Flat Blues* as well as the expected Waller perennials.

From Winnipeg, the group went on to Toronto where they appeared at the Club Top Hat from Monday 16 November until Saturday, 21 November. The Club Top Hat, formerly the Club Esquire, was situated at Lakeshore and Parkside Drive and also on the bill was Frank Bogart's Orchestra. Whilst there, Waller gave an interview to a reporter of the *Toronto Daily Star* in which he said he had had a session "last week" in Minneapolis with Dimitri Mitropoulos. He went on to explain that he'd had lunch with the famous conductor, and then the two men had played two and three-part Bach inventions and went on to do some fugues, after which "some of the boys got together and Dimitri conducted a jam session." If Kirkeby's recollection that this took place on a Sunday is correct and Waller's "last week" is also accepted at face value, then the lunch with Mitropoulos took place on Sunday, 8 November and the 'Happy Hour' engagement in Minneapolis probably on the previous day. However, this is somewhat

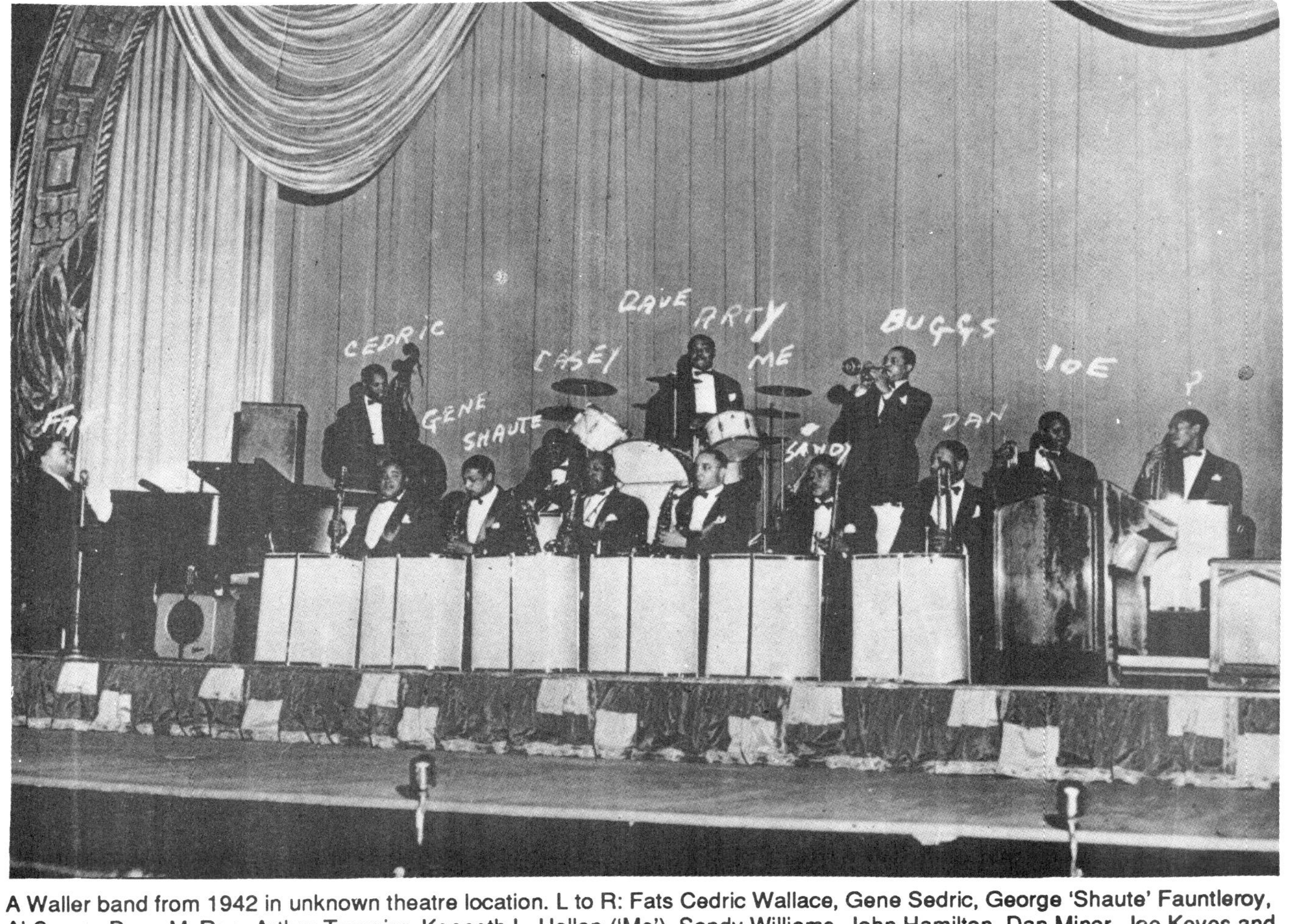

A Waller band from 1942 in unknown theatre location. L to R: Fats Cedric Wallace, Gene Sedric, George 'Shaute' Fauntleroy, Al Casey, Dave McRae, Arthur Trappier, Kenneth L. Hollon ('Me'), Sandy Williams, John Hamilton, Dan Minor, Joe Keyes and Henry Mason.

complicated by a report which had appeared in 'Band Briefs' column of the *Pittsburgh Courier* of 14 November:

> *Out Minneapolis way, Fats Waller is fronting a six-piece group at the Happy Hour Club there. So sensational has Fats been that the management has had to abolish dancing on the part of customers in order to accomodate additional persons and place tables on what was used as a dance floor. Between 600 and 700 patrons nightly hear the Waller music which is also featured at Friday, Saturday and Sunday matinees.*

Although Waller's own interviews and other reports imply that the 'Happy Hour' engagement was a one-off affair, the paper suggests otherwise and indicates that he was resident at least a week. Also if he played a Sunday matinee, he could hardly have had lunch with Mitropoulos unless he had been resident in excess of a week and had finished the engagement on Saturday night.

Continuing the interview above, Waller also revealed that the strain of constant travelling and one-night stands had caught up with him and he'd been in the hands of the doctors for three days. Fats also repeated his aversion to boogie woogie and told the reporter that he preferred working with a small band as it gave greater freedom and it was easier to improvise. He also added as a final comment against the use of a big band, "What's the use of having a lot of guys just sitting up there waiting for pay day?"

*****

Back home once more, he played New York's 125th Street Apollo for the week commencing Friday, 11 December 1942 with a number of acts that had been associated with him, including the Deep River Boys and Myra Johnson as well as a dance team and a troupe of acrobats. Whilst at the Apollo, Waller gave an unusually sober interview to *New York Age* reporter Dolores Calvin which appeared in the issue of 26 December. In it he told her that they had come to New York direct from Detroit and, after the Apollo stint would be leaving on the Friday morning for Philadelphia where they were to play the new Fays Theatre there *and then swing out to California and the Florentine Gardens. ... He gives 107 West 134th Street as his birthplace and said he even knew the exact situation of the room. ... In Canada the band did Winnepeg's Civic Auditorium and Toronto's Top Hat. In Minneapolis, Minn. they performed a jazz concert for the Happy Hour Club.*

*****

Waller's mention of the Fay's Theatre engagement is confirmed by a report in the January 1943 *International Musician,* which states that they played the Philadelphia theatre for the week ending Christmas Eve. No engagement has been traced for the next week and it is likely that Waller spent the holiday with his family.

Then a variation of the show opened at Chicago's Regal Theatre for a week commencing Friday, 8 January 1943 and the Chicago *Defender* of 9 January had this to say:

> *Fats Waller and his great orchestra come to the stage of the Regal the week starting Friday, Jan. 8, for 1943's first and biggest rhythm show. Fats distinguished gentleman of the hot piano and vocal chants brings with him a terrific stage show featuring, from out of the Southland that famous NBC radio quartet, the Deep River Boys.*
>
> *Harlem's head man of boogie woogie rhythm is really swinging like mad with his brilliant musicians and entertainers. They're coming direct to the Regal direct from a record-smashing road tour in which they have broken theatre, dance hall records from*

coast to coast and have entertained many thousands.

The Deep River Boys got their start over six years ago when they first sang together in the Hampton Glee club at Hampton Institute in Virginia. In New York they were discovered and named the Deep River Boys" by Rex Ingram, "De Lawd" of "Green Pastures".

Also in Fats Waller's great stage show will be Carl and Harryette, peppery dancing stylists, the Douglas Brothers, Harlem's favorite zany sons, and many others.

Note that despite Waller's disapproval of the form, the press couldn't get rid of the idea that he was a boogie-woogie pianist. An advert for the show, reproduced here, appeared on the same page.

*****

The 16 January 1943 issue of *The Billboard* ('Orchestra Routes' section) also reports Fats at the Regal Theatre, Chicago. It was to be the final performance, for Ed Kirkeby recalled that it was here that Fats disbanded his big band, sending them back to New York, and he and Waller travelled on to Hollywood, arriving there on [Wednesday] 20 January 1943 to film and record his contributions to the 20th Century Fox all-Black production *'Stormy Weather'.*

Under the heading *Fats Waller Leaves Piano Temporarily For Pictures,* and datelined Chicago, Ill. the *New York Age* of 28 January has:

Fats Waller has climed (sic)*off the piano stool temporarily after his successful week at the Regal Theatre here. Waller will concentrate on film work. He has been working with a six-piece unit in night clubs and cocktail lounges, filling in with theatre dates. Waller left for Hollywood last weekend with his magager Ed. Kirkeby, to begin work for Twentieth Century Fox on "Thanks Pal". His combine remains intact for bookings.*

The final comment was amplified in a similar report in the *Pittsburgh Courier* which said that Waller's 'leaving did not put the band in a quandary for it has been taken over by Eugene Sedric, saxophonist and Albert Casey, guitarist, who will keep it intact for future engagements until such time as Waller returns from the coast.'

Waller's part in the film is as the leader of 'The Beale Street Boys', a group assembled especially for the film by Irving Mills, an associate producer. This group recorded three items as follows:

Benny Carter, t; Alton Moore, tb; Gene Porter, cl/ts-1; Fats Waller, p/sp/v-2; Irving Ashby, g; 'Slam' Stewart, sb; Zutty Singleton, d; Ada Brown, v-3.

20th Century Fox Studios, Hollywood, California — Saturday, 23 January 1943

Ain't Misbehavin' -2	Time: 3:95
Moppin' And Boppin' -1	Time: 4:23
That Ain't Right -3	Time: 2:57

These timings are from Dr. Klaus Stratemann's book *Negro Bands on Film* and for a more detailed discussion of the musical aspects of the whole film, readers are referred to that. In the released print only two tiny portions of *Moppin' And Boppin'* were used. In the Beale Street Café sequence, *That Ain't Right* is used in its entirety, but *Ain't Misbehavin'* is edited. Waller's 32-bar introduction with rhythm is cut to 4 bars and Singleton's drum solo has the last 8 bars repeated. In the sequence which follows where a discussion takes place at the table between Ada Brown, Lena Horne and Emmet Wallace, the complete introduction is played as background music.

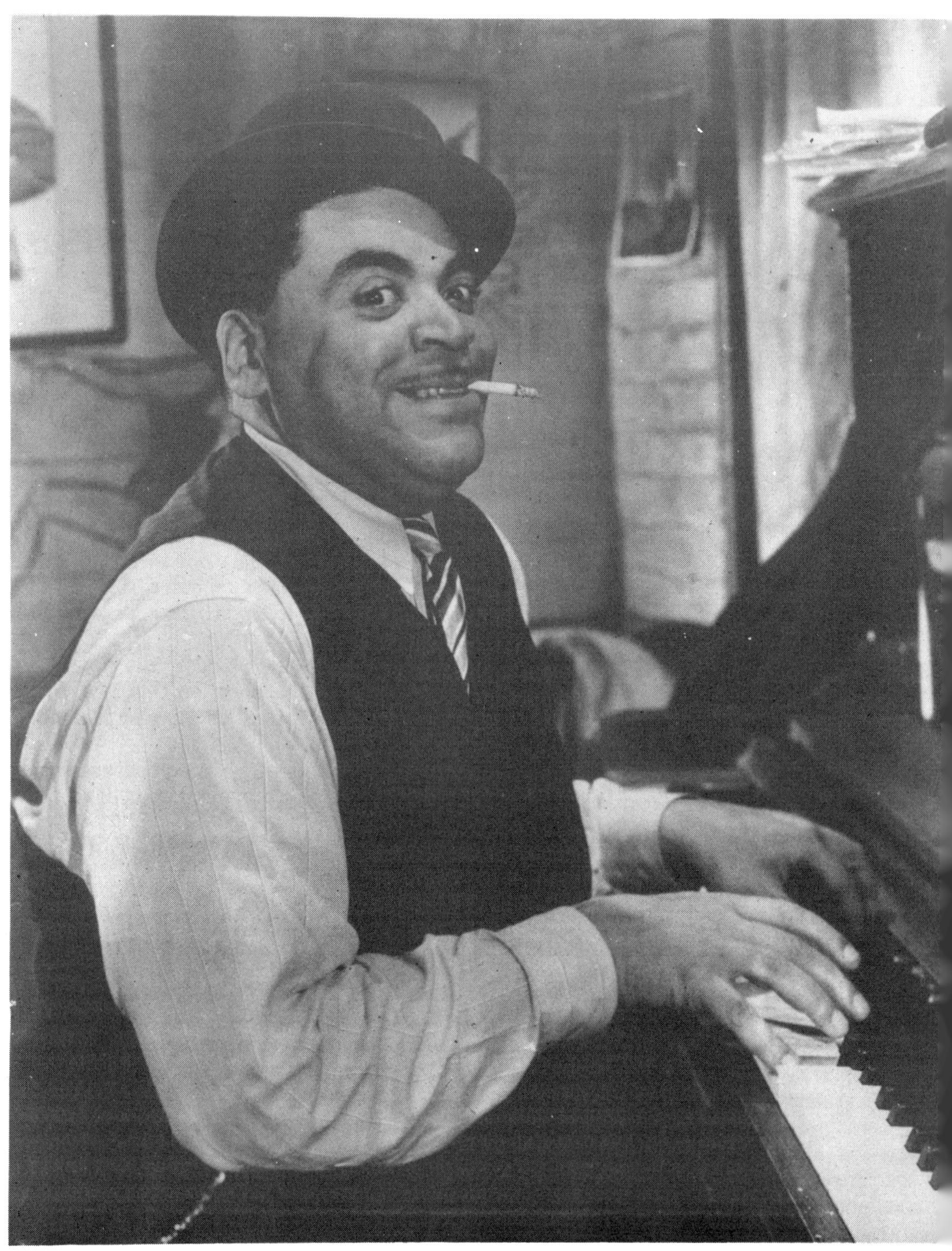

Two publicity stills from *'Stormy Weather'*. Above: At the piano. Right: With Lena Horne.

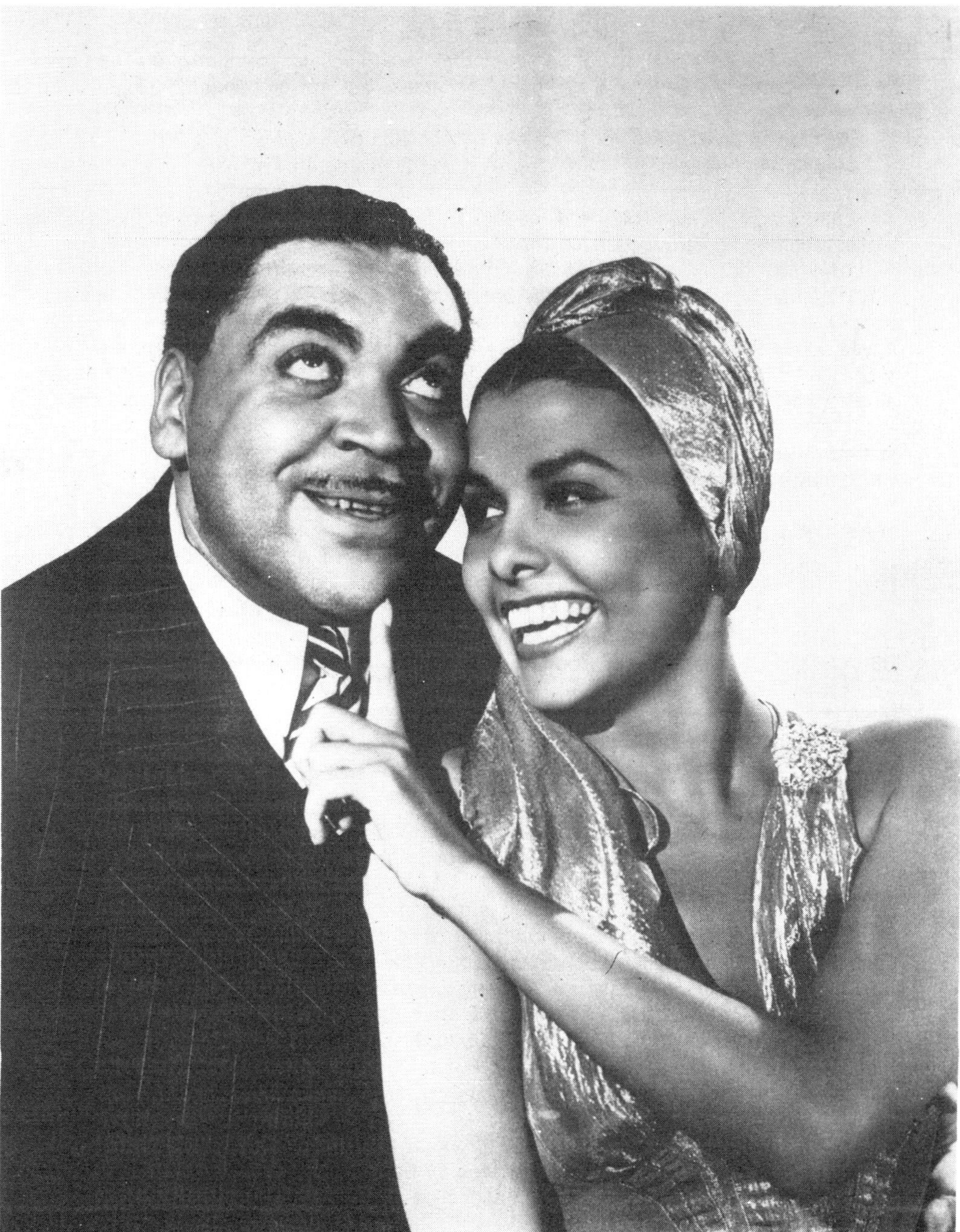

All three titles were made on "in-studio" recordings for company use and given the following numbers. They have not been inspected, but are probably 12" single-sided discs playing at 78 r.p.m.

Ain't Misbehavin'	20th Century Fox 103, 202
Moppin' And Boppin'	20th Century Fox 203
That Ain't Right	20th Century Fox 101, 201

Later that year, possibly on Tuesday, 16 September at the time of his V-Disc session, Waller recorded an introduction for *That Ain't Right* :

"Hey cats, it's four o'clock in the morning. I just left the V-Disc studios. Here we are in Harlem. Everybody's here but the police, and they'll be here any minute ... it's high time. So catch this song ... here 'tis."

It was added to the beginning of the tune, given matrix VP 471-D4TC 32 and was issued on *V-D 165-A.* Originally, the intention seems to have been to couple this with *Ain't Misbehavin'*, also from the film, but when issued in April 1944 the backing was by **Meade Lux Lewis**.

*****

In 1946, Victor's New York studios dubbed the first and second titles from 'an original lacquer' which may have been from the "in-studio" recordings noted above:

*****

"FATS" WALLER AND HIS RHTHM **(Piano by "Fats" Waller) -1**
(Vocal and Piano by "Fats" Waller) -2

Personnel as above - rerecording session "from a lacquer made from soundtrack of a film".

Studio 1, New York City, New York — Tuesday, 24 September 1946
1:30 to 2:00 p.m. S.H. Sholes directing

D6-VC-6215-1*	Moppin' And Boppin' -1 (Waller-Carter-Kirkeby)	*Vi 40-4003-B. HMV C.3737, HMVAu EB556, HMVSw FKX192, HMVIt S10611, HMVF SH.1*
D6-VB-6216-1*	AIN'T MISBEHAVIN' (I'm Savin' My Love For You) -2 (Razaf-Waller-Brooks)	*Vi 40-4003-A. HMV C.3737, HMVAu EB556, HMVSw FKX192, HMVIt S10611, HMVF SH.1*

Steven Sholes had been responsible for Waller's V-Disc recordings and, following his release from military service and return to RCA, had probably arranged for RCA/Victor to issue these.

*****

How long Waller remained in Hollywood is not known, but two items in the *Pittsburgh Courier* both datelined Hollywood, 11 February suggest that he was still there at that time. The first described how the presence of so many famous stars (Waller is among those mentioned) on the studio lot had caused the film company to install a grandstand to accomodate the huge number of would-be visitors. The second stated that plans were in hand for Fats and Zutty Singleton to 'combine their talents for an exclusive Hollywood nitery in the near future'. Singleton certainly did take a band into the Club Trinidad and was there until it closed early in August, but there is no indication that Waller ever worked there with him.

*****

With Waller now bent on a solo career, Ed Kirkeby was looking for ways to book his client and relates that whilst in Hollywood he negotiated for Fats to appear in a Broadway show. A phone call from producer Dick Kollmar, the prospective producer, had Waller and Kirkeby hurrying back to New York as soon as work on *'Stormy Weather'* was finished. There, they discovered that although everything for the forthcoming show had been arranged, no writer for the score had been found. Some fast talking by Kirkeby convinced Kollmar and his associates that Waller was the man and, with an advance of $1,000 in his pocket, Fats set about writing the music for each tune as the lyrics were presented to him. Eventually, the show, which was to be called *'Early To Bed'*, was completed, but before rehearsals were under way it was decided to release Fats from his stage role. During the time he was composing the music for the show, Fats paid two visits to a New York studio and made some private recordings which are probably try-outs for ideas he was working on. They were discovered in his effects after his death as mentioned in the note for April/May 1937 and, as far as they could be reconstructed, issued by John R.T. Davies in a special Ristic double album. Details are as follows:

*****

Private recordings: FATS WALLER piano solos

2, West 46th Street, New York City, New York — Tuesday, 2 March 1943

Smooth Velvet	Reconstructed from 11 pieces
Two Hands Fighting	Reconstructed from 11 pieces
Speak To Me	Reconstructed from 4 pieces
Martinique	Reconstructed from 4 pieces

Although 'Martinique' is not the generally known tune, the opening strain of that is introduced at the close of this.

Also made at the same sesssion, but not included in the set were:

Mirror Dust	Broken into well over 80 pieces with too many missing to
Walking Around	attempt reconstruction.

As above, but date unknown.

Early To Bed	Reconstructed from 10 pieces
Onion Time/Jump -1	Reconstructed from 10 pieces
That Does It/(Untitled)	Reconstructed from 6 pieces
Nylon	Reconstructed from 6 pieces
Long Time (No Song)	Reconstructed from over 20 pieces, with a large triangular
Short Time	piece missing (see note).

As with the earlier session the following were made but not included:

Horse An' Blue	Broken into well over 80 pieces with too many missing
Baby	to attempt reconstruction.

Although *Long Time* is listed on the insert accompanying the Ristic set (as above) it is not included on the label information and either it or *Short Time* is omitted unless the piece has a dual title.

*****

Two further recordings of unknown date and from an unknown source (Waller's private collection?) probably come from this period.

*****

FATS WALLER Piano Solos

New York City, New York — *March 1943*

Peekin' In Seek	Issued on LP
Onion Time	Issued on LP

*****

Howard Rye has uncovered an enigmatic report in *Variety* of 3 March 1943, which just states, *Myra Johnson at State, Hartford, with Fats Waller.* No date or further details are given. Possibly this is an assumption on the part of a writer, knowing of the association between Waller and Myra Johnson, but it merits further investigation in the local papers.

*****

With his writing for the show finished, Waller resumed his solo performing career with an engagement at New York's 125th Street Apollo Theatre which was to be the last there. He was the headliner for the week commencing Friday, 2 April and worked with Muggsy Spanier and his Band. The preview of the show in the *New York Age* of that week stated that Waller had recently completed a part in the film *'Stormy Weather'* and that he and the Spanier band were set to repeat the success they had enjoyed 'recently' in Chicago. The report also mentioned Waller's work on a Broadway Show and that his band was working without him in a Greenwich Village night club. This final statement may be explained by the fact that Una Mae Carlisle was working with a small group including Herman Autrey and Slick Jones and the press no doubt still associated these names with Waller, despite the fact that he had disbanded.

According to a report in the *Pittsburgh Courier* datelined 15 April, Muggsy Spanier had been 'knocked-out by the 'flu' and Waller had taken over leadership of his band for the Apollo engagement — the first time that Fats had fronted a white group.

Following this, the next known engagement was down to Philadelphia where he played the Celebrity Bar, as reported in the *New York Age* of 1 May. The following week the same paper reported him still there and commented, *Amazing thing is that Fats is taking down a salary of $750 a week and the bar doesn't accomodate more than 100 customers.* Then, into the State Theatre, New York, as noted in the 8 May 1943 issue of *The Billboard* ('Orchestra Routes' section). Probably on the return journey from Philadelphia to New York, he stopped off at Newark, New Jersey to attend the opening of the Sixth Stage Door Canteen of the American Theatre Wing on 20 May (*International Musician*). This was also reported in the *New York Age* of 18 June which added that among the other guests of honour was the State Governor, a keen record fan and that after playing a number of records, "Fats" asked for and got his autograph for Maurice and Ronald who were with him.

*****

With rehearsals completed, *'Early To Bed'* began its out-of-town try-out run at Boston's Shubert Theatre on Monday, 24 May 1943, and the Wallers and Ed Kirkeby travelled up from New York for the opening, where they encountered a rather nasty case of racial prejudice.

Saxophonist Joey Nash recalled this too in *Jazz*, and gave a slightly different version in considerably more detail. Fats had called him from New York to say he was on his way to Boston and for Nash (they were old friends) to meet him early next morning. Waller wanted to play his new music for him, but the Shubert Theatre piano was in use so they eventually found a bar which had a beat-up instrument in a back room and Fats proceed to play the entire score. The afternoon was spent with press interviews and the like concerned with the opening of the show. Late that night Nash got another call from a very depressed Waller asking him to come to his hotel, which proved to be a very dingy flop-joint. Apparently, Fats, whose name was above the Theatre and in all the local newspapers, had gone to the hotel where the cast of the show were staying and where he had reserved a room to be met with a blank refusal for accomodation. He then tried the hotel where he had been guest of honour at a cocktail party that afternoon, but they too were "full". Fats asked Nash if he could do anything for him. Nash knew all the top management in the 750 room hotel where he stayed and thought there would

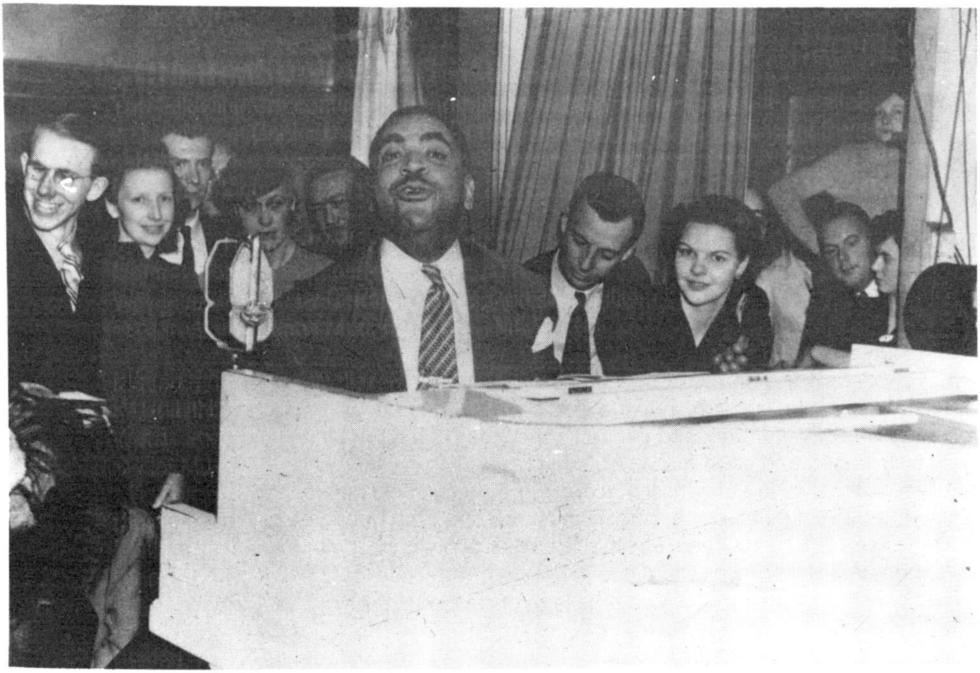

Two action shots of Fats from about this period, possibly during the Celebrity Bar engagement.

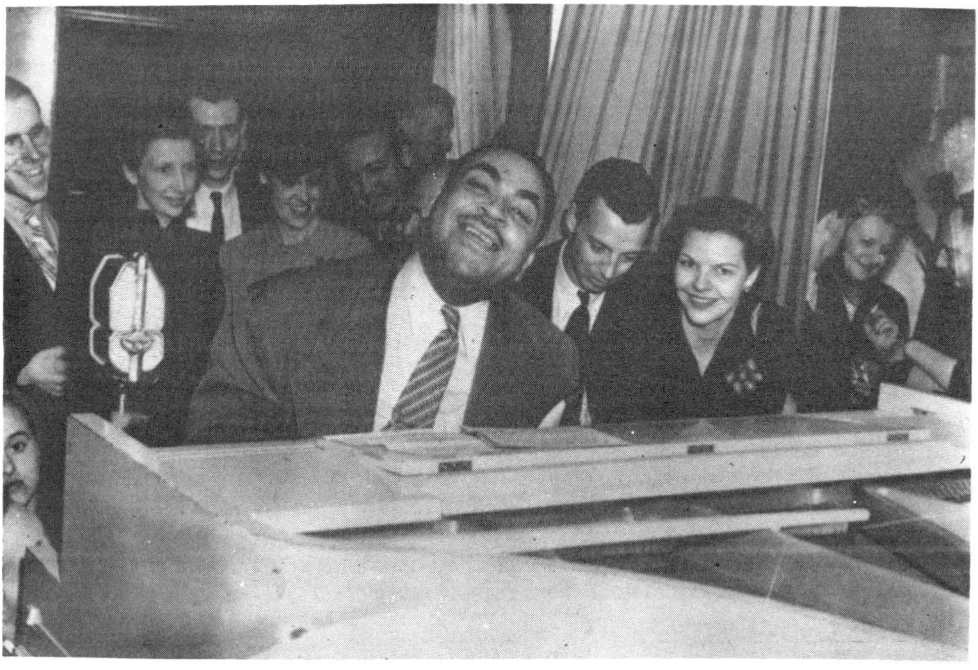

be no problem. But no, the manager couldn't help and when Nash suggested that Waller move in with him to share his own room (equipped with twin beds) the manager hit the roof and said if he tried "that trick" he'd throw him out! According to Nash, Waller left immediately for New York and home.

With the show safely under way, Waller travelled to Philadelphia for an engagement at the Cove Club. This is confirmed rather belatedly in 'Off The Cuff: Philadelphia' in *The Billboard* issue of 19 June 1943, which reports: *Fats Waller takes over the lead at The Cove with the Angie Bond Trio moving to Palumbo's, both spots under the same management.*

In fact, Waller left the Cove Club and was back in New York for the New York Premiere of *'Early To Bed'* which took place on Thursday, 17 June 1943 at the Broadhurst Theatre, 235 West 44th Street.

Reviews of the premiere of *'Early To Bed'* were generally lukewarm. Waller's music met with considerable acclaim, but the book was slammed as being weak and based on too obvious double entendres and general smuttiness, although all reviews admitted that the show was well staged and good to look at.

Probably thinking only of the score, Ed Kirkeby's *Ain't Misbehavin'* claimed that *'Early To Bed'* was a great success, and whilst in New York, Fats gave a Red Cross concert aboard the battleship *U.S.S. New Jersey* in the Brooklyn Navy Yard before heading for Boston and an engagement at the Tic Toc Club. However, this had to be cut short beause war-time restrictions meant that the place became over-heated in the very hot weather, making Fats feel ill and he returned home to New York.

*****

Back in New York there were appearances on NBC's "Music You Want" program on Friday, 9 July and NBC's "Lower Basin Street" show early in August.

*****

In between these two engagements, an offer came for him to appear for two weeks in the Sky Club of the Brant Inn, Burlington, Ontario, which he accepted and he journeyed there with Anita, his sons and Kirkeby and they were royally entertained during the day by the owner, Murray Anderson, and Fats entertained the customers at night. Art Pilkington has researched the local newpaper, the *Hamilton Spectator,* and from adverts in that it seems that Waller played with Gren Hobson and his Orchestra on Friday and Saturday nights 16 and 17 July and again the following weekend on 23 and 24 July.

*****

Broadcast — Chamber Music Society Of Lower Basin Street

Fats Waller, p/v; acc: "Lower Basin Street Orchestra.

NBC Studios, New York City, New York — Sunday, 1 August 1943

Honeysuckle Rose — Issued on LP

This show occupied a Sunday evening spot between Walter Winchell's news commentary and Jimmy Fiddler's Hollywood gossip programme, and presented a weekly offering by the top jazz and swing artists of the day. It was presented using a tongue-in-cheek format as a caricature of a programme of symphonic and light classical music. 'Dr. Gino Hamilton' (master of ceremonies Gene Hamilton) introduced Fats in this manner:

> *Serious students of the Harlem stride-school of piano stylings have long followed the cogent abilities of Professor Thomas Waller, both as a teacher, from whom much academic pianistic knowledge can be gleaned, and as a performer-without-peer, in the bringing forth of musical interpretations sometimes referred to as jam, jive and everything!*

> *Professor Waller, whose corpulent physical attributes have gained for him the nickname of Fats, will favour us tonight with a programme of distinctive interpretations of a series of his own compositions along with a number of compositions by some of the other 'masters of stride'.*

Despite this indication, only a single item has survived and been issued, even if others were played. A mention of the broadcast in *Time* of 9 August 1943 gives no indication of what titles were played, but does mention that Fats had just returned from Canada and "was cooking up some new tunes".

*****

Then down to Philadelphia again for a two week engagement at Palumbo's, the Italian restaurant mentioned in *The Billboard* report above. A report of this engagement in the *Pittsburgh Courier* on 18 September stated that Waller was impressed by the white swing quartet led by guitarist Freddie Baker and insisted that the unit worked with him during his residency and had arranged for them to accompany him when he left for Hollywood next month. Whilst at Frank Palumbo's, Fats made a quick return dash to New York on Saturday, 21 August to appear on the "Million Dollar Band" Show sponsored by Colgate-Palmolive Peet. All this time he was appearing in numerous War Bond Drives, Hospital Shows and concerts at military establishments and featuring his music from *'Early To Bed'* which was still enjoying a highly successful run at the Broadhurst.

On Friday, 10 September, Fats headed the show which re-opened the Greenwich Village Inn, 5 Sheridan Square after the summer shut-down, and was there for a three-week residency. Pee Wee Russell recalled strolling by one evening with his wife and, seeing Fats's name up outside, went in for a quiet drink. He was immediately spotted by Fats who press-ganged him into playing the blues on a borrowed clarinet. It was the last time Pee Wee saw Waller. Another visitor to the club was Art Tatum who was there at the same time as Waller's 'cousin' Henry Parker, as is shown from the snapshot below.

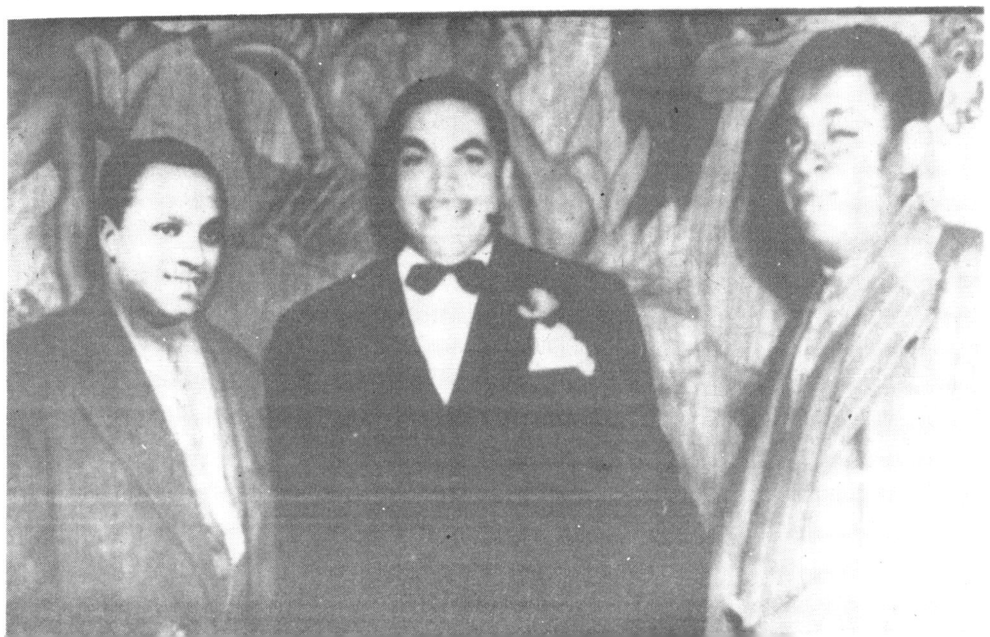

One evening Steven Sholes, who had known Fats when he was working for Victor came in. He had been drafted and was now working with the V-Disc Unit in Victor's studios and he invited Fats to come down and make a session "for the boys". Waller never refused a request to entertain the forces if it was humanly possible and this was a chance to get back into the studios and promote some of his new music.

*****

"Fats" Waller, Piano and Vocal — **Vocal** (32A, 32B, 133A, 133B)
"Fats" Waller — **Vocal** (74A)
"Fats" Waller, Piano and Vocal — **Swing** (145B)
"Fats" Waller — **Piano Solo** (74B)
"Fats" Waller — **Organ** (630A)
Fats Waller at the Organ — **Organ** (658A)
Fats Waller (at the Organ) — **Organ** (743A)

Fats Waller, p-1/sp/o-2
Victor Studios, 155 East 24th Street, New York City, New York 16 September 1943

VP154-D3-MC-193-1	AIN'T MISBEHAVIN' /TWO SLEEPY PEOPLE -1 Razaf-Waller-Brooks/Carmichael-Loesser	*V-D 33A, 133A* (Navy)
VP155 D3 MC 194-1E	SLIGHTLY LESS THAN WONDERFUL/ THERE'S A GAL IN MY LIFE -1 Waller-Marion/Waller-Marion	*V-D 33B, 133B* (Navy)
VP156 D3 MC 195	That's What The Bird Said To Me/ Hallelujah/Waller Jive -1	Unissued, test exists
No matrix number	There's Yes In The Air In Martinique -1	Unissued
VP157 D3-MC 196-1D	THIS IS SO NICE IT MUST BE ILLEGAL/ MARTINIQUE -1 Marion-Waller/Marion-Waller	*V-D 74A, 145B* (Navy)
VP 181 D3 MC 218	WALLER JIVE/HALLELUJAH -1 Waller/Youmans	*V-D 74B*
VP 414 D3 MC 480	You're A Viper (The Reefer Song) -1	Unissued
VP 419 D3 MC 485	That's What The Bird Said To Me/You're A Viper (The Reefer Song) -1	Unissued, test exists. Issued on LP
No matrix number	The Ladies Who Sing With The Band -1	Unissued
No matrix number	Medley: To A Wild Rose/Don't Get Around Much Anymore -piano only	Unissued

This completed the afternoon session, and Waller continued on Hammond Organ.

JDB 10 D6TC 5011	SOLITUDE -2 (Ellington-Mills-DeLange)	*V-D 658A*
JDB 11 D6TC 5012-1	BOUNCIN' ON A V-DISC -2 Waller	*V-D 630A*
JDB 12 D6TC 5013	SOMETIMES I FEEL LIKE A MOTHERLESS CHILD (Spiritual) -2	*V-D 743A*
No matrix number	St. Louis Blues -2 (no speech)	Unissued
No matrix number	By The Light Of The Silvery Moon -2	Unissued ? (see note)

The session, oiled by the consumption of several bottles of Cutty Sark whisky, started in the early afternoon with Waller on piano then, after a short break, he switched to Hammond Organ and continued until late evening, by which time Fats was feeling the effects of the whisky, and this almost certainly accounts for the rejection of the last two sides. Most sides have spoken introductions by Waller. Titles with the 'Marion-Waller' composer credit are from the show *'Early To Bed'. There's A Gal In My Life* was actually *There's A Man In My Life* as used in the show.

Although the final title is shown as 'unissued', it seems almost certain that it is a test of this that is the source for the version that has been tacked on to the George Jessel broadcast as reissued (see pages 200/201).

Because of the way in which V-Discs were prepared it is difficult to present them discographically, as the same segments might appear on more than one issue or test recording and, as an example, the material on VP 419 D3 MC 485 was also given the number J 609 USS 1039, but this and VP 414 D3 MC 480 were later cancelled and re-used for other performances. Usually army pressings omitted composer credits whilst navy pressings showed those given.

Reverses: V-D 145A is by **The Three Suns**; 630B and 658B by **Bunk Johnson and his Band**; 743B by **Buddy Weed and his Trio**.

Release dates: V-D 32, November 1943; V-D 74, December 1943; V-D 133, January 1945; V-D 145, February 1945; V-D 658, July 1946; V-D 743, March 1947.

*****

Tlhe following items from Fats Waller's personal collection were included in the Ristic double album (see note at April/May 1937).

FATS WALLER (p-1/v-2/o-3)

Victor Studios, 155 East 24th Street, New York City, New York *16 September 1943*

The Ladies Who Sing With A Band -1,- 2
To A Wild Rose - Don't Get Around Much Anymore -1
Martinique -1
Hallelujah! -1
St. Louis Blues -3
Organ Tests

The above version of 'Martinique' is the well known version. It is significant that these are the titles which were rejected at the V-Disc session and it seems reasonable to assume that Waller will have been provided with copies, hence the suggestion of location and date. However, unless tests survive of the V-Disc sides, this will remain pure speculation.

*****

Broadcast WABC "Off The Record

Fats Waller, p/v/sp; Hugh Conover, sp.

New York 23 September 1943

Ain't Misbehavin'	Issued on LP
There's A Girl In My Life	Issued on LP
Honeysuckle Rose	Issued on LP

The above broadcast has Waller telling the story of his life and playing and singing three numbers with background piano and talk with programme host Hugh Conover.

*****

According to Ed Kirkeby, Fats played a return engagement at Boston's Tic Toc club replacing the cancelled June one. This was apparently in the middle of October as he recalls that at the end of that engagement, they came back to New York for one day to pack for a trip to Omaha, Nebraska and on to the West Coast.

However, a paragraph in the *Pittsburgh Courier*, of 16 October 1943, datelined New York City and headed *Fats Waller Set At Beachcomber* has:

Fats Waller, who is currently appearing at the Greenwich Village Inn, has been signed for the Beachcomber, in Omaha, Neb. He will be there for two weeks beginning October 23. The former bandleader is the most expensive act to play the club to date since the Mills Brothers recent appearance.

Also, the *New York Age* of 13 November 1943 has a belated report under the heading *"Fats" Hollywood Bound* that gives the impression that Waller was still in New York and these two reports and Kirkeby's own account perhaps serve to illustrate some of the difficulties encountered in reconciling different accounts of the same event. It reads:

"Fats" Waller goes to Hollywood in two weeks for a short engagement at the Florentine Gardens nightery and for an appearance on RCA's radio program "What's New?". He will return to New York for a January return date at the Greenwich Village Inn.

At least this report indicates that the RCA broadcast was not a spontaneous affair and gives news of an engagement that he would be unable to keep.

By Kirkeby's account they left New York on Sunday, 24 October, travelling overnight and most of the following day, and arrived in time for the first show of the two weeks that were booked in the Omaha Beachcomber, finishing Sunday, 7 November. During this fortnight, Fats played a number of shows at local army bases during the day, and this was picked up by the *New York Age* on 20 November with:

"Fats" Waller, rotund ivory expert, took time from his engagement at the Beachcomber nightery in Omaha to entertain the boys at nearby Ft. Crook. Before his piano playing chores began, "Fats" was treated to a steak dinner at the Fort Commissary. With a steak so thick "he almost had to stand to see over it" and bread and real butter galore, "Fats" was ready to take the oath right then and there. "My, my," he whispered to manager Ed Kirkeby, "Let's play for Uncle Sam every day!".

This sounds like a press release from Kirkeby himself, but in gratitude, the army were instrumental in getting them on to a train to Los Angeles, travel at that time being very much geared to military needs.

They travelled overnight from Omaha and arrived in Hollywood on the morning of Monday, 8 November 1943 and Fats opened that evening, appearing in the floor-show at the Florentine Gardens as a featured artist and finishing out the evening as a soloist in the Zanzibar Room. This is confirmed by a report in the *Pittsburgh Courier* of 13 November which notes Fats at the Florentine Gardens and the Zanzibar Room. He became unwell on Wednesday (17 November) of the second week of the engagement and had to spend ten days in bed. Although far from fully recovered, he insisted on completing his engagement at the Florentine Gardens and also responded to calls to appear on a number of radio shows (in addition to his apparently contracted RCA date) during this second period. Among those he is known to have played are 'Colored USA', possibly on a Tuesday. There is an enigmatic note in Billy Rowe's column in the *Pittsburgh Courier* of 4 December which may refer to a broadcast: *On the all-sepia "Jubilee" program t'other night Fats Waller, Ernie Whitman, Ammons and Johnson, Joe Turner, Delta Rhythm Boys and Harlan Leonard and his orch.*

*****

Before listing the known broadcasts there is another brief note in Billy Rowe's column in the *Pittsburgh Courier* of 6 November 1943 which says *...for some unaccountable reason part of* *the lyrics of "When The Nylons Bloom Again" have been banned from the networks. It's a Fats Waller-George Marion tune from "Early To Bed".*

*****

The following week, on page 5, there was a large advert for Royal Crown Cola sponsored by Fats Waller.

*****

The following are broadcasts from which portions have survived. Exact dates for these have not been established, and they are thus not necessarily in the correct order.

*****

Broadcast "What's New" Radio Show

Fats Waller, p/v; Don Ameche, spoken introduction

RCA Studios, Los Angeles, California — December 1943

Medley: Tea For Two/Honeysuckle Rose — Issued on LP

*****

Broadcast "Command Performance" No. 95

Fats Waller, p/v, Dinah Shore, Abbott & Costello

CBS Studios, Los Angeles, California — December 1943

Your Feet's Too Big — Issued on LP

Handful Of Keys — Issued on LP

Abbott & Costello were in the show, but are not in any version heard on LP. Dinah Shore's voice is heard on some versions, whilst others utilise only the Waller performance. Harry Mackenzie suggests that this may have been mastered as early as September 1943 and distributed in October judging by its relationship with other "Command Performance" broadcasts. However, the presence of Abbott & Costello does suggest a West Coast recording location and therefore the approximate date given.

*****

Broadcast "Charlie McCarthy Show"

Fats Waller, p/v-1/sp-2; Edgar Bergen, sp-2; Ray Noble, sp-2

Los Angeles, California — ? Sunday, 5 December 1943

Interview -2

Ain't Misbehavin' — Issued on LP

Handful Of Keys — Issued on LP

Geoffrey Minish recalls hearing this show, he thinks on a Sunday, when a teenager in Toronto. He recalls that Fats played *Carolina Shout* during which he called out "It's easy when you know how!" after a virtuoso flourish which drew a laugh from the studio audience.

*****

Broadcast NBC "News From Home" (Sometimes reissued as the Nick Kenny Show)

Fats Waller, p/v; Spoken introduction by Nick Kenny

The Joint Is Jumpin' — Issued on LP

*****

Waller's health, despite appearances to the contrary, had given concern for some time. Ernie Anderson has recalled one bout of illness and other musicians have spoken to me of his disregard for his own well-being. In *Music On My Mind*, Willie 'The Lion' Smith had this to say:

> *But no matter what we said to Fats about taking care of himself, he wouldn't pay attention. Before he was forty, Fats's health was not at all good. He broke up his regular group in May 1943, and only took a few one-night engagements. The royalties on his songs were*

pouring in and he was riding around in a four-thousand-dollar Lincoln with a chauffeur at the wheel. But the years of running around all winter without an overcoat, eating like Richard the Lionhearted, and drinking like a fish were beginning to catch up. He should have tried to take off weight many years before and the last time I saw him, his ankles were swollen and he could hardly walk.

He had been getting attacks, like epileptic fits, for quite a while, and when he felt one coming on he would have to get up and walk around. These would act on him like a cramp, so he got one of his cousins to travel with him and whenever he felt an attack coming on, his cousin would turn him over on the other side and the cramp would disappear.

*****

On Saturday, 11 December, Fats was paid for his work and presented with a case of champagne by the management of the Florentine Gardens. Having finished that night, he went to an all-night party at Benny Carter's house. The following morning he was due to attend a Press Party given in his honour but, exhausted, fell asleep and was taken back to his hotel to rest in readiness for his final night's work. That completed, Fats caught the Santa Fé's Super Chief train at mid-day on Monday en route to New York to spend Christmas with his family. That night there was a party on the train and when he eventually got to bed, Fats slept all next day and died in the early hours of the next near Kansas City. Because of the sudden death, Ed Kirkeby relates that an autopsy had to be performed in Kansas City before the body could be released for the last rites.

*****

Although Waller had been well reported in the black press during his lifetime, *The New York Age* gave surprisingly sparse coverage to his passing and funeral, but in the obituary notice included the information that he had toured the country in a vaudeville act with Bessie Smith in 1925. The *Pittsburgh Courier,* on the other hand devoted almost a page to reports and tributes and, according to that paper, Waller's eldest son, Thomas Jr., then aged 21 and a corporal in the U.S. Army stationed at Coffeyville, Kansas was in Kansas City and was the first of the family to learn of the death. After the formalities were completed in Kansas City, the body was taken to New York where it lay in state at the Rodney Dade Funeral Parlor, 2332 Seventh Avenue. The funeral took place at 11 a.m. on Monday, 20 December 1943 at the Abyssinian Baptist Church, West 138th Street, the service conducted by the Rev. Adam Clayton Powell assisted by Rev. Ben Richardson. Pall bearers are listed as J.C. Johnson, J.P. Johnson, Bob Driver, Bob (Bud?) Allen, Perry Bradford, Claude Hopkins, Luckey Roberts, Clarence Williams, Andy Razar (sic), Count Basie and Duke Ellington. Huge crowds attended, blocking the streets near the church, and a special contingent of police was called in to control them. After the funeral service, the body was cremated at the Fresh Pond Crematory on Long Island and the ashes scattered from a plane piloted by 'The Black Ace', a World War I veteran, flying over Waller's beloved Harlem.

*****

At the time of his death, plans were being formulated for Fats to appear regularly on Television, which was then beginning to be established as *the* entertainment medium of the future. Having disbanded his 'Rhythm' and 'Big Band', he was planning to spend more time writing, and performing on radio as well as Television and to cut down drastically on travel and live appearances in clubs. He was also apparently to write music for a new Hollywood musical planned as a "follow-up" to the successful *Stormy Weather,* in which he would also have appeared.

*****

CODA

Ed Kirkeby mentions that he finally persuaded Fats to sit down and sign his will before setting out on what was to be his final tour. More than a year after his death, the Brooklyn Section of the *Amsterdam News* of 17 March 1945 had the following:

BATTLE OVER 'FATS' WALLER'S WILL

It was disclosed early last Wednesday before Surrogate Anthony P Savarese in Jamaica, that only $28,000 remains of the fortune earned by the late Thomas W. "Fats" Waller, boogie woogie piano king, and a fight was being waged over the will.

The fight over the will began when disclosed terms specified two-thirds of the estate to be invested and the income paid to Miss Anita Rutherford of 173-17 Sayres Ave., St. Albans, mother of Waller's two children, Maurice, 17, and Ronald, 16.

The other third, a dower right fixed by law, was to go to Waller's estranged wife, Edith, who lives in the Bronx. In the will, Waller indicated that he was cutting his estranged wife off with the minimum fixed by law "for reasons best known to her."

Mrs. Waller has begun an action against the estate for $65,000, representing $50 weekly alimony payments over her life expectancy of 25 years. That was the sum she received from the pianist-composer during his life.

Bernard Miller of Manhattan, executor and trustee, reporting that the gross estate totals only $28,000 is offering a compromise whereby Mrs. Waller, the legal widow, will accept one-third of the residuary estate, or $2500 plus $300 in accrued alimony, whichever is larger.

Surrogate Savarese will hear both sides on Tuesday, March 27.

Note that the "boogie-woogie" tag followed Waller even after his death. This report is revealing in several respects and an eloquent testimony to the fact that Fats *did* live life somewhat more than to the full.

*****

PIANO ROLLS

Because no actual recording dates are known for any of Waller's piano rolls, the known information is gathered here as a separate section but, before beginning the listing, some general comments and notes are in order.

Piano rolls were (and are) made by one of two basic methods, in both of which, variations will be found:

Hand played: In which the artist sits at a piano which has been suitably connected to a mechanism which produces a mark on a moving roll of paper for each note that is struck. These marks are then cut out with tools by a roll editor to produce the master roll from which commercial copies are produced. At this stage it is not uncommon for the roll editor to add embellishments of his own (these can usually be detected), and certainly, any errors detected in the original performance would be removed. A variation was the direct-punch method in which die punches actualy made the perforations in the master as the artist played. The resultant 'recording' still needed to be edited.

Arranged: In which the artist is dispensed with and an arranger works directly from a musical score, often that of a publisher, in cutting the roll. Some arrangers used a special master paper with pre-printed graphs and lines, and then cut out the markings they had made Others worked directly from the score through a machine to cut the roll. In the case of J. Lawrence Cook, he rigged a piano that could perforate (very slowly) as he held down the notes on the keyboard. The piano was activated by a foot pedal and Cook would decide how the next bar or two should sound, press down the appropriate notes and hit the foot pedal, and the piano would punch the notes in the master. Although this method came close in principle to a hand-played roll, it was still an arranged roll.

The terms 'hand-played' and 'arranged' are used in what follows. It might be observed, however, that many arranged rolls are considerably more spirited than some hand-played ones, and one must wonder if the mechanism used for the latter applied a dampening effect which detracted from an artist's performance. Rolls are either instrumental piano performances or performances to which words have been added to be sung by the player pianist. The words are printed in a narrow column on the right of the roll and are read from bottom to top as they pass behind a window in the player piano as the roll is played. Such rolls are known as 'word rolls' or 'song rolls' and, where known are indicated by (W) after the title in the listing. It should be noted that sometimes the same master was used to produce an instrumental and a song roll, with an appropriate increase in price to cover the extra work involved in producing the latter. For a further discussion of Q.R.S. rolls and their manufacture, please see *Storyville 114.*

Because of their very nature, it is very easy to 'doctor' piano rolls, by removing, adding or reversing sequences, and many of the Imperial rolls listed here fall into that category.

Although no recording dates are known for the Waller rolls, the release dates are known either from the box labels or advertising and, given a normal processing time of two months between recording and release, a rough estimate of the former can be arrived at. It was almost certainly James P. Johnson who introduced his protege to QRS and it was probably in December 1922, at the time he made his sides with Sara Martin, that Waller first went into the QRS Bronx studio.

CONFIRMED WALLER ROLLS

The following are confirmed hand played rolls by Waller, most, if not all, having been edited by J. Lawrence Cook. Date quoted is the release date. Additional information on composers, copyright, etc. appears beneath the title and is as given on the box labels* or as reported by correspondents. The QRS solo rolls bear a facsimile of Waller's signature on the roll leader.

Played by Thomas Waller, New York City — March 1923
Got to Cool My Doggies Now (W) Fox Trot — QRS 2149*
Words and Music by Schafer, Thompson and Williams
© Clarence Williams Mus. Pub. Co., MCMXXII

Played by Thomas Waller, New York City — May 1923
LAUGHIN' CRYIN' BLUES (W) Fox Trot — QRS 2213*, Q-137
Words and Music by Porter Grainger and Bob Ricketts
© Zipf Music, 1923

Played by Thomas Waller, New York City — May 1923
YOUR TIME NOW ('Twill be Mine After a While) Fox Trot — QRS 2245
Words and Music by Spencer Williams
© Leo Feist, Inc., 1923

Played by Thomas Waller, New York City — June 1923
SNAKES HIPS Fox Trot — QRS 2256, Q-108
Words and Music by Spencer Williams
© Leo Feist, 1923

Played by Thomas Waller, New York City — June 1923
'TAINT NOBODY'S BIZ-NESS IF I DO (W) Fox Trot — QRS 2270, XP-2270
Words and Music by Porter Grainger and Everett Robbins
© Clarence Williams, 1922

Played by Thomas Waller, New York City — July 1923
PAPA BETTER WATCH YOUR STEP (W) Fox Trot — QRS 2286*
Words and Music by Wells and Cooper
© Goodman & Rose, 1923

Played by Thomas Waller, New York City — August 1923
Haitian Blues (W) Fox Trot — QRS 2304*
Words and Music by Miles and Williams
© Joe Fishew (sic), MCMXXIII

Played by Thomas Waller, New York City — August 1923
MAMA'S GOT THE BLUES Fox Trot — QRS 2322
Words and Music by Sara Martin and Clarence Williams
© Clarence Williams, 1923

Played by Thomas Waller, New York City — August 1923
MIDNIGHT BLUES Fox Trot — QRS 2331
Words and Music by Babe Thompson and Spencer Williams
© Melody Music C., 1923

Played by Thomas Waller, New York City — September 1923
LAST GO ROUND BLUES (W) Fox Trot — QRS 2363*
Words and Music by Jimmy Cox
© Clarence Williams, 1923

Played by Thomas Waller, New York City — January 1924
YOU CAN'T DO WHAT MY LAST MAN DID (W) Fox Trot — QRS 2444*, Q-109
Words and Music by J.C. Johnson and Allie Moore
© Chateau Music Pub. Co., 1923

Played by Thomas Waller, New York City — June 1924
CLEARING HOUSE BLUES Fox Trot — QRS 2661, Q-138
Words and Music by Sadie Honesty and Harry Webb
© Joe Davis, 1924

Played by Thomas Waller, New York City — June 1924
JAIL HOUSE BLUES (W) Fox Trot — QRS 2670*
Words and Music by Bessie Smith and Clarence Williams
© Clarence Williams Pub. Co., 1924

Played by Thomas Waller, New York City — June 1924
Do It Mister So-and-So FOX TROT — QRS 2708*
Words and Music by Lukie Johnson and Myrtle Barger
© Spencer Williams, 1924

Played by Thomas Waller, New York City — June 1924
Don't Try To Take My Man Away (W) FOX TROT — QRS 2711*
Words and Music by Tausha A. Hammed
© Clarence Williams, 1924

Played by Thomas Waller, Orange, New Jersey — August 1924
A NEW KIND OF MAN WITH A NEW KIND OF LOVE FOR ME (W) Fox Trot — Standard Play-A-Roll 0677
Words and Music by Sidney Clare and Leon Flatow
© Jerome Remick Music Pub. Co., 1924

At this point it should be noted that a second roll for the Standard Music Roll Company is known only from a flyer listing new word rolls for August 1924 (along with the above). Mike Montgomery notes that such flyers were routinely mailed to music trade magazines which reprinted them as space permitted. In this instance, the reprint gave details of everything except the catalogue number as follows, but no copy of the roll itself has been found to date.

WEST INDIES BLUES — A Calipso Standard Play-A-Roll ???
Words and Music by Edgar Dowell, Spencer Williams & Clarence Williams
© Feb. 1, 1924 (sheet music shows 1923!)

Played by Thomas Waller, New York City February 1926
SQUEEZE ME (A Boy In a Boat) (W) Fox Trot QRS 3352*, XP-183,
© C. Williams Music Co. Inc., 1925 Imperial X5980

The Imperial issue is a 'doctored' version in which the introduction and coda are omitted and the sequence of verses/choruses reversed.

Played by Thomas Waller, New York City March 1926
18th Street Strut (W) Fox Trot QRS 3377*, Q-151
© Triangle Music Pub. Co. Inc., 1926

Played by Johnson & Waller, New York City February 1927
Cryin' For My Used To Be (W) Blues Fox Trot QRS 3800*
© Dreazen

Played by Johnson & Waller, New York City March 1927
IF I COULD BE WITH YOU (W) Fox Trot QRS 3818*, Q-152
Words and Music by Henry Creamer & Jimmy Johnson
© Jerome Remick, 1926

Played by Thomas Waller, New York City August 1927
Nobody But My Baby (Is Gettin' My Love) (W) Fox Trot QRS 3997*, Q-139
© Williams

Played by Thomas Waller, New York City November 1927
I'm Coming Virginia (W) Fox Trot QRS 4073*, Q-147
© Robbins

Played by Thomas Waller, New York City June 1931
I'm Crazy 'Bout My Baby (And My Baby's Crazy 'Bout Me) (W) QRS 5143*, Imperial 07787
Fox Trot © Davis

In a letter to Bill Bonner, J. Lawrence Cook stated:

> *Crazy 'Bout My Baby was indeed the last roll "Fats" Waller actually recorded for QRS ... "Fats" didn't have much time for this particular session and planned to come back the following day and finish the number, but he never showed up. So the arrangement turned out to be a combination of Waller and Cook, for it was I who had to make it into a complete production master.*

The Imperial issue, also released in June 1931, is a 'doctored' version of the QRS master. It is

understood that only 123 copies of this were sold.
Re-issue rolls in the 'Q' series bear labels inscribed 'From The celebrity vault', and Q-108 is as SNAKE HIPS.
QRS XP-183 is a long playing roll titled *Ain't Misbehavin'* issued to tie in with the Broadway show of the same name. It includes two original Waller rolls as noted in the listing above plus three other performances by J. Lawrence Cook; *Ain't Misbehavin', I Can't Give You Anything But Love* and *Honeysuckle Rose.* Note that a number of the above Waller rolls have been re-cut privately and (usually) issued in blank label editions, often cut to order. They are outside the scope of this listing.

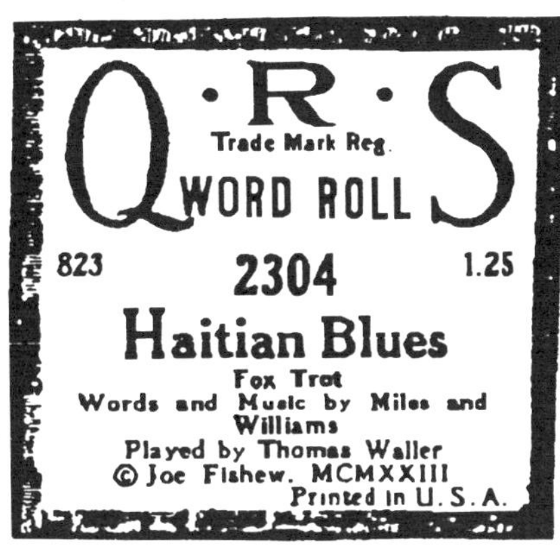

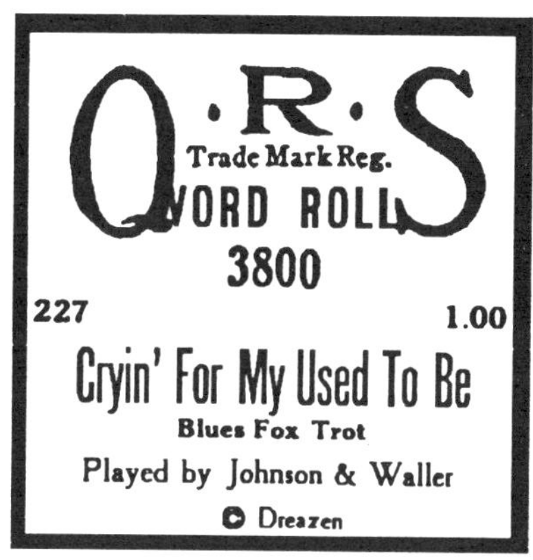

Q·R·S
Trade Mark Reg.
WORD ROLL
3800
227
1.00
Cryin' For My Used To Be
Blues Fox Trot
Played by Johnson & Waller
© Dreazen

POSSIBLE WALLER ROLLS

Played by Jack Clyde, — mid 1923
Cotton Belt Blues Fox Trot — Imperial X5313*
Words & Music by Spencer Williams
© Spencer Williams M. Co. Inc., 1923

Played by Jack Clyde, — August 1923
Low Down Papa Fox Trot — Imperial X5327
Words & Music by Spencer Williams
© Spencer Williams M. Co. Inc., 1923

Mike Montgomery believes that *Low Down Papa* is a "most probable" Waller roll and comments that the issue took place after the acquisition of Imperial by QRS. Apparently, this was not common knowledge and to the buying public the two companies were still separate and in competition. He feels that the explanation is that Clarence Johnson had also recorded the title for QRS and that his version (although not issued until October 1923) was preferred to that cut by Waller. The company then sent the Waller master to Chicago for issue on Imperial and, since Waller was a QRS artist, it was issued under the Jack Clyde pseudonym which was a blanket name used for many issues in the X5000 series. Something similar may have happened with *Cotton Belt Blues,* which was issued in a completely different version by Pete Wendling on QRS in December 1923.

THE J. LAWRENCE COOK/WALLER ROLLS

In 1935, the QRS Company began marketing rolls as **Played by "Fats" Waller**. These were ir fact played by J. Lawrence Cook, many in an excellent imitation of the Waller style. It appear that Fats was impressed with the way that Cook had been able to emulate his playing (possibl as a result of the latter's work on his final cut for the company and his fine editing) and ha given permission for his name to be used in marketing the rolls. This was, however, purely courtesy arrangement and after Waller's death, was withdrawn by the attorney acting for th estate. Thereafter those rolls which were still available either appeared with no artist credit, o credited to Cook himself. The following is a listing of all known Cook rolls which appeared a **Played by "Fats" Waller**, it does not pretend to be complete. Title, catalogue number an release date are given, along with other pertinent information.

AFTER YOU'VE GONE — QRS 561 (June 1936)

This catalogue number and title was originally issued in 1918, being played by Ted Baxter & Max Kortlander as a Cello-Rag. The above version was a reissue and a re-arrangement.

ST. LOUIS BLUES — QRS 1001

QRS1001 was originally used in 1919 for WHEN YOU'RE ALONE, a fox trot played by Victo Arden and Max Kortlander).

WHEN MY BABY SMILES AT ME — QRS1041

This catalogue number and title was originally released in 1920, being played by Pete Wendling.

I AIN'T GOT NOBODY — QRS 3293 (June 1936)

Again, this was originally issued in 1925 being played by Pete Wendling. The Cook/Walle version was a reissue and a re-arrangement. There is also a third version which was release in September 1944. It is a totally different arrangement described as "Blues Fox with Ja Chorus" issued as "Played by J. Lawrence Cook".

ROSETTA Fox Trot — QRS 6154 (April 1935), Imperial 08796

This catalogue number was originally the hymn TAKE ME AS I AM.

YOUR FEET'S TOO BIG — QRS 6155 (April 1935), Imperial 08797

QRS originally issued the hymn SAFELY THROUGH ANOTHER WEEK under this number.

NO SWINGIN' IN HERE — QRS 6156 (April 1935), Imperial 08798.

A second version was released by QRS in 1944 as "Played by J. Lawrence Cook". In som cases the dies used for labelling the rolls of the earlier version were also used for printing th rolls of the later version — hence while Cook's name appears on the box label, Waller's nam may still appear on the roll leader.

SWEET AND SLOW — QRS 6215 (August 1935), Imperial 08857

BASIN STREET BLUES — QRS 6233 (September 1935), Imperial 0887

I'M GONNA SIT RIGHT DOWN AND WRITE MYSELF A LETTER — QRS 6288 (December 1935), Imperial 0893

SING AN OLD FASHIONED SONG (to a young sophisticated lady) — QRS6321 (January 1936), Imperial 08963

SWING, MR. CHARLIE — QRS 6331 (February 1936), Imperial 08973

CHRISTOPHER COLUMBUS — QRS 6343 (March 1936), Q-223, Imperial 08985

HONEYSUCKLE ROSE — QRS 6419 (June 1936), Imperial 09061

QRS originally issued the hymn OLD HUNDRED under this number.

MR. GHOST GOES TO TOWN QRS 6531 (November 1936), Imperial 09173
I CAN'T BREAK THE HABIT OF YOU QRS 6589 (February 1937), Imperial 09231
BIG APPLE QRS 6746 (October 1937)
SHE'S TALL, SHE'S TAN, SHE'S TERRIFIC QRS 6760 (November 1937)
QUEEN ISABELLA QRS 6761 (November 1937)
THE DIPSY DOODLE QRS 6776 (December 1937)
SOPHISTICATED SWING QRS 6884 (June 1938)
THE FLAT FOOT FLOOGIE QRS 6885 (June 1938), Q-249
A-TISKET A-TASKET QRS 6896 (July 1938)
OL' MAN MOSE QRS 6904 (August 1938)
'TAIN'T WHAT YOU DO QRS 7044 (June 1939)
WELL ALL RIGHT, TONIGHT'S THE NIGHT QRS 7056 (June 1939)
THE JUMPIN' JIVE QRS 7090 (August 1939)
PEACH TREE STREET QRS 7138 (November 1939)
W.P.A. QRS 7233 (May 1940)
STOP PRETENDING QRS 7270 (July 1940)
CROSSTOWN QRS 7290 (August 1940)
RHUMBOOGIE QRS 7319 (October 1940)
BEAT ME DADDY, EIGHT TO THE BAR QRS 7324 (October 1940)
FIVE O'CLOCK WHISTLE QRS 7343 (1940)
SCRUB ME MAMA WITH A BOOGIE BEAT QRS 7368 (January 1941)
JAVA JIVE QRS 7383 (February 1941)
THERE'LL BE SOME CHANGES MADE QRS 7389 (February 1941)
BOOGLIE WOOGLIE PIGGY QRS 7483 (September 1941)
ALL THAT MEAT AND NO POTATOES QRS7489 (September 1941)
At least one copy is mislabelled ALL THAT MEAT NO AND POTATOES.
YEA MAN! QRS 7722 (August 1942)
FAT MEAT'S GOOD MEAT QRS 7729 (August 1942)
COW COW BOOGIE QRS7739 (September 1942?)
A shortened version was issued later
MAD ABOUT HIM, SAD WITHOUT HIM BLUES QRS7759 (November 1942)
MISTER FIVE BY FIVE QRS 7760 (November 1942)
DON'T GET AROUND MUCH ANY MORE QRS 7777 (December 1942)
JUKEBOX SATURDAY NIGHT QRS 7789 (December 1942)
THE CANTEEN BOUNCE QRS 7847 (June 1943)
DON'T STOP NOW QRS 7852 (June 1943)
THE FUDDY DUDDY WATCHMAKER QRS 7873 (June 1943)
SEE SEE RIDER QRS 7878 (June 1943)
THERE'S A MAN IN MY LIFE QRS 7893 (November 1943)
SHOO-SHOO BABY QRS 7899 (December 1943)

Note that several of the above may have been re-issued in shorter form after Waller's death, but these would then be credited either to Cook or be anonymous. Other rolls that have been claimed as Waller or Cook/Waller items in earlier listings may be disregarded and there seems no point in attempting to list them in full as information on them will be found in the standard reference sources. The number of 'Boogie Woogie' style pieces included in the Cook/Waller section together with a number of published music folios may have contributed to the impression held by the U.S. Press that Waller was a Boogie Woogie pianist, which he always denied himself.

WALLER ROLLS ON RECORD

Although all the known Waller rolls have appeared in LP format only the following 78 r.p.m. issues were made:

QRS 2213	Laughin' Cryin' Blues	Lon L.808, De BM 31059
QRS 2256	Snakes Hips	Pm 14027
QRS 2331	Midnight Blues	Ri 8, Les Amis de Fats (unnumbered)
QRS 3377	18th Street Strut	Ce 4001, JC L45, AFCDJ A.021

Paramount issue of *Snakes Hips* is played on a 65 note player and issued as *The Mess Around.* It has a reverse of *Jig Walk* by Duke Ellington (QRS 3565, released in August 1926 and actually played by J. Lawrence Cook). The reverse of London L.808 and Decca BM31059 is *Roumania* by James P. Johnson (QRS 1479, released June 1921), and that of all three issues of *18th Street Strut* is *Make Me A Pallet On The Floor* by James P. Johnson (QRS 3626, released in September 1926).

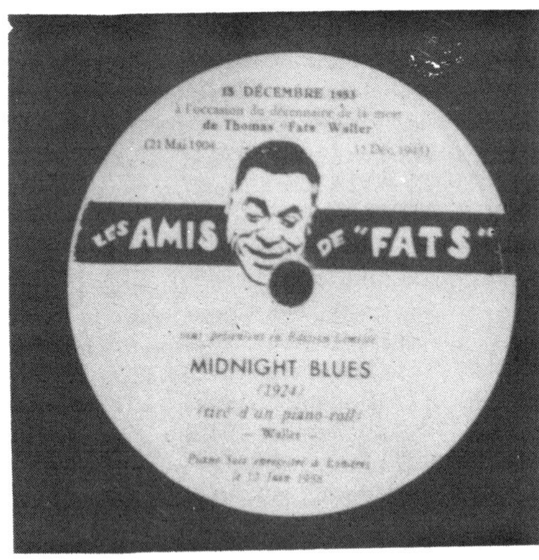

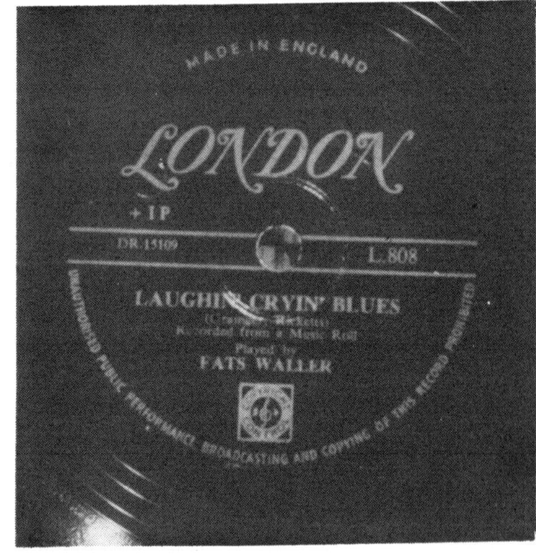

Acknowledgements

Grateful thanks are due to Ramsi P. Tick, the President of Q.R.S. and to Bill Bonner, John Farrell, George W. Kay, Tor Magnusson, Mike Meddings, and Mike Montgomery without whose assistance and enthusiasm, this listing of rolls would be much less complete.

THE MISCELLANEOUS FATS WALLER

In this section are listed those recordings which have been attributed to Waller in the past, as well as those which are recalled but for which no documentary evidence has been found. Also included here are references to Waller which, for various reasons, have not been included in the main listing, as well as other scraps of information. Dates are given where appropriate or known, but chronological order is not necessarily followed.

*****

First of all, a general note. A number of Victor executives have confirmed that Fats frequently used the Church organ in the Camden studio for his own purposes; playing new compositions and generally amusing himself, often with classical music. Such sessions were frequently recorded and played back for Waller's own interest. This immediately rendered the wax master unsuitable for processing and such masters were always destroyed. It is almost certainly from such sessions that rumours of the Bach sides, etc. stem and a number of diligent searches through the company files have revealed that no formal recording of this sort of material was ever undertaken.

*****

Walter C. Allen interviewed cellist Marion Cumbo at his home and he recalled that he had played the Roosevelt Theater in Harlem when Fats Waller was there on organ. No date is given for this.

*****

There are a number of references to Waller in Jack Schiffman's, book *Uptown: The Story of Harlem's Apollo Theatre* which should be noted:

Page 61:

> *Interestingly, before becoming a musical idol himself, Count Basie took every chance he found to drop over to the Lincoln Theatre, which Dad had run for a short while before getting involved in the Apollo, to sit at the feet of his idol, the same Fats Waller. Literally at his feet, too, for Fats' feet were as fast and unerring on the organ pedals as his hands were on the keyboard, and Basie was content merely to gaze for hours at his hero's footwork.*

Page 144:

> *The great Fats Waller was organist for my father at the Lafayette Theatre. One day, as Fats was playing a spirited accompaniment to the movie, a man started down the aisle. As soon as Fats spotted him coming, he deserted the organ and disappeared into the organ pit. The man was one of Fats's many creditors.*
>
> *Fats was one of a succession of organists hired to play at one of Dad's earliest ventures, the Verona Theatre. The Verona was located in the upper Eighties on Manhattan's East Side — the Yorkville district. Fats, like the organists who preceded him, quit the Verona after only one day on the job. When Dad asked for a reason, Fats clammed up. Finally, pressed for an explanation, he said:*

"I can't tell you why, but if you come down to the pit during the next show, you might be able to figure it out."

It didn't take much figuring. The reason for the mass resignations was obvious: guns. Dozens of revolvers, pistols, and automatics of every description, resting among the organ pedals. This was Yorkville — at the time, one of the centers of gangland activity. In New York, the Sullivan Law was strictly enforced, so the gangsters "checked" their weapons in the organ pit when they came to the movies.

*****

c. 30 April 1923
The Sara Martin/Clarence Williams duet of *Monkey Man Blues* on OKeh 8067 is often listed as a Waller accompaniment. The pianist, who is not named on the label [and the files no longer exist] plays certain figures that suggest Waller. However, this was one of a number of items considered for the final part of the listing which appeared in *Storyville* and at that listening session Ray Webb suggested that Clarence Johnson was responsible and comparison with the Edna Hicks Victor revealed a startling similarity of style and an almost identical coda.

*****

c. June 1923
In a letter dated 7 Dec. 1990 Bob Hilbert suggests that Kitty Brown's OKeh 8077 may have Waller as accompanist: "The pianist sounds like a cross between young Fats Waller and James P. I'm virtually certain it is not James P. It is certainly a first rate Harlem stride pianist." Having now heard the sides, I do not believe the pianist is Waller.

*****

2 November 1925
Perry Bradford's Vocalion 15156 coupling *Lucy Long/I Ain't Gonna PLay No Second Fiddle* has previously been shown as featuring first James P. Johnson *and* Fats Waller on pianos and, more recently as James P. Johnson *or* Fats Waller. Aurally it is Johnson.

*****

Little Mt. Zion Choir Piano Acc. **Negro Spritual**

X88	DIDN'T IT RAIN (Browne)	Ge 3334-A, Bu 8055
X89A	NO WAYS WEARY (Browne)	Ge 3334-B, Bu 8055

Despite rumours that the piano on these sides is by Waller, there is nothing to suggest his presence. Bob Kumm investigated the records of the Little Mount Zion Baptist Church of Harlem (whose choir this is) and could find nothing to indicate a recording association between it and Waller. Gennett 3334 was issued in September 1926.

*****

27 January 1927
Previous Waller listings have often included Fletcher Henderson's Brunswick recording of *Stockholm Stomp/Have It Ready.* However, the piano on this is unlike Waller and entirely consistent with Henderson's own work.

*****

4 November 1927
Crooning Andy Razaf: Columbia 14265-D has been listed previously as a Fats Waller accompaniment. This not so, and the piano on these sides is by J.C. Johnson plus Eddie King on organ on the second side per Columbia files.

*****

2 March 1928
Shilkret's Rhyth-Melodists Victor 21298 coupling *Chlo-e/When You're With Somebody Else* has been previously shown as featuring Waller on organ, mostly on the basis of an account related by Nat Shilkret himself to Brian Rust in 1963. In this, he said that things hadn't gone too well on the evening of 2 March 1928 when Waller walked in and started playing *Chlo-e* softly on the organ. Shilkret roughed out an arrangement which they recorded and then returned the following morning with additional musicians to make the second side.

Tor Magnusson contacted Milton Rettenberg (pianist on the record) in July 1976, who emphatically denied Waller's presence and said it was Sigmund Krumgold. The following year, in October, Tor was able to examine the Victor ledgers which reveal that the session of 2 March, with two organ pieces by Lambert Murphy following on, was completed by 4:35 p.m. — hardly "evening".

*****

19 December 1928
Clarence Williams's OK 8663 of *Watchin' The Clock/Freeze Out* has been suggested as a Waller item, possibly because Fats is composer of the second tune. Certainly, Waller was back in New York by the time this was made, but the playing, although not Williams himself, is not Waller either, lacking his firmness in the left hand and featuring some cross-handed work which is quite out of character.

Note that the suggestion in the VJM OKeh listing that 401467-D was also issued is now known to be erroneous as only three takes of each title were recorded.

*****

In 1973 Robert Brackney wrote to me stating that he'd had a letter from Paul Whiteman in 1961 in which Whiteman told him "that Waller had made organ records with the 'King of Jazz' Orchestra." No further details were given at the time, and Robert Brackney was unable to discover anything further prior to Whiteman's own passing.

*****

No doubt, because of Waller's known association with Gene Austin, the recordings of the latter have been subjected to the closest aural scrutiny in order to determine whether Fats might be present on sides other than those already listed in the main discography. Tor Magnusson has been particularly active in this respect and I am happy to draw upon his studies and references to Gene Austin below are based upon his conclusions.

30 July 1929
Peace Of Mind and *Ain't Misbehavin'* made on this date in New York by Gene Austin with an eight-piece accompanying group have excellent piano with a Waller flavour, but it is extremely doubtful if it is Waller.

24 October 1929 and 7 November 1929
Gene Austin made *All That I Ask Is Sympathy* and *Georgia Pines.* Only the former was issued and the pianist sounds unlike Waller.

*****

12 June 1931
The Vance Dixon session for Columbia has been suggested as a Waller session on the grounds that the pianist is addressed as "Fats" on one side. Aurally, it is not Fats Waller.

*****

17 August 1932
Old Yazoo by Baron Lee and his Blue Rhythm Boys has been suggested as a Waller item, but the pianist is clearly Edgar Hayes and, in any case Fats was out of the country. The source of the information was Billy Banks via Dave Carey who recalled:

> *When Billy Banks was over in this country I had the good fortune to meet him. Fats Waller's name happened to be mentioned, and suddenly Billy Banks turned to me and said, 'By the way, did you know Fats Waller played piano on OLD YAZOO with the Mills Blue Rhythm Band in 1932? I should know as I took the vocal, so I was there in the studio. Fats Waller took over the piano for that one number, and as you may already know, it is one of his compositions'.*

It may have been a rehearsal session that Banks recalled or a rejected version on another date.

*****

Mr. G. A. Wilmer copied out part of an article by James W. Poling which appeared in *Esquire* Magazine for June 1936. This stated that Fats Waller was a frequent visitor to staid Boston's *squalid, out-of-the-way Railroad Club.* No dates are given, but from the account, Waller appears to have been appearing in a solo capacity.

*****

3 March 1937
ARC recorded two titles in Chicago on this date as by 'Barrel House Annie' which were rejected. Matrix C-1837-2 *If It Don't Fit (Don't Force It),* appeared on a CBS CD in 1991 and has led to suggestions that the the pianist on the session may have been Fats Waller. The date falls between two 'Rhythm' sessions held in New York and, although Fats might have made a trip to Chicago at this time, there is no evidence either way. Aurally, there is a superficial resemblence to Waller on a first hearing, but I feel the left hand work is far too ponderous to be Fats.

*****

August 1938
Joe Daniels claims that Waller made four titles with him for the Parlophone label in August 1938. *Mood Indigo, Narcissus, Whispering* and *Limehouse Blues* are given as the titles cut. The first pair were cut by Daniels on 9 May 1939 (when Fats was back in Britain, but appearing in Brighton for the week) and the second pair on 31 August 1938 when Waller *was* in London doubling beween Holborn Empire and Finsbury Park Empire. There is no aural evidence on the issued versions of these titles to support Daniels's claim and Brian Rust has made a thorough search of the EMI files and could not locate any unissued session(s) which might fit this recollection.

*****

In a letter dated 3 December 1968, Joe Igo of Golden, Colorado mentions a tape of a Waller recording of *Singin' The Blues* with a vocal by a lady baritone named Mary Pearl. No other information is available, and I have never seen the item mentioned elsewhere.

*****

The story of Waller, Bubber Miley and Zutty Singleton recording jazz titles with a Scotsman playing the bagpipes in full regalia which is found in *Ain't Misbehavin',* has never been substantiated, although apparently all three musicians swore it happened and that it was not a leg-pull. Possibly, the appearance of this fuller account of the Waller life will enable researchers into the careers of Miley and Singleton to narrow down the field of research.

*****

Holmes "Daddy-O" Daylie in *An Autobiography Of Black Jazz,* page 265:

> *Floyd Smith and his trio furnished the music in the bar* [At the DuSable Hotel, Chicago]. *Floyd Smith was very famous at that time. He had written "Floyd's Guitar Blues" when he was with the Andy Kirk Band. In the lounge, a piano player named Wilbur Hobbs entertained the diners. Fats Waller, who was playing downtown at the Sherman Hotel, maintained a room at the DuSable. Some mornings Fats would come in from his Loop gig and literally take over Wilbur Hobb's piano duties. I remember that one morning Duke Ellington came down to the lounge. He and his band were working at the Regal, and Art Tatum came up from the Three Deuces downtown, and the three of them got into a piano jam session in the lounge that lasted from three a.m. until after one-thirty the next afternoon. I never went to bed that night. How could I with all that electrifying musical entertainment permeating the entire hotel?*

Page 266:

> *Most of the out-of-town artists stayed at the DuSable Hotel whenever they had a gig in Chicago. Remember, they played downtown but Jim Crow policies would not permit them to stay downtown.*
>
> *Fats Waller had a suite in the DuSable that was always available to him whenever he came to town. That was Suite 501 and 502. Eddie Flagg, the manager of the DuSable Hotel, would always have an organ in the suite for Fats Waller whenever he was in residence. Fats Waller loved flowers and when you entered the lobby downstairs, you could smell the fragrance from Suite 501 and 502. His fans, who were mostly white, knew that he loved flowers and they sent him forty or fifty bouquets of fresh flowers everyday. His suite was literally a bank of flowers.*
>
> *Many times Fats Waller would invite me up to his room just to listen to him play. He could entertain one or one thousand individuals. That was just the kind of person he was. As his bartender, I would pour him gin by the water glass, with no chasers. Fats would sometimes have me put a little ice and lemon in the glass to make it look like lemonade. He obviously had an elephantine capacity for gin, because I never saw him drunk, or even inebriated. With his glass of gin, he would sit at the organ and play, compose, create and entertain, and take several mouthfuls of gin between tunes. His organ music could be heard throughout the hotel in the wee hours of the morning, but no one ever complained. Who could? Would you stop a genius at work?*

*****

Fats Waller was a member of the Crescendo Club — an association of Negro song-writers of New York. — *Hendersonia,* page 382.

*****

In a letter to Roy Cooke dated 25 July 1972, Ed Kirkeby wrote as follows:

> *Fats loved to record and I am sad indeed when I think of the many session at the Victor that would have been done during the period of the AF of M strike. Consider this! Fats' last date for commercial records was on July 13, 1942. What a great pity. But how grateful I am that he left the many great things he did record.*

And speaking of "I Wonder what the Poor People are Doing", I don't know where Fats got that remark, but I do know he used it a lot, especially at the Panther Room in Chicago. That too was a time of "strike" when ASCAP and the Radio Staions were "having a go". Fats, who was ASCAP was unable to broadcast his tunes and grumbled about it on the air so much that I was called down to the front offices of the Hotel Sherman and warned by Ernie Byfield the General Manager that unless Fats stopped his chiding remarks about NBC they would pull out their lines. But Fats never quit, and the station was glad to have the greatest attraction it had ever booked stay around as long as he wished.

*****

Rumours persist of private recordings featuring Waller and Jack Teagarden, but no firm evidence has come to light.

*****

Storyville 63, page105
Account by Peter Stroud of *What's Your Name*, © 14 June 1938 written by Fats and J.C. Johnson

*****

Bob Kumm reported a broadcast by Waller on 3 July 1938, but no details of station, time or programme. In the absence of further information it has not been included in the main body of the text.

*****

MEMORIES OF FATS WALLER from ZAZA GELDRAY, formerly Scottish-born singer ZAZA PETERS (given name Sarah Prentice).

I met Thomas — everybody called him that — in 1939 when I was singing at the 'Palm Beach' then in Frith Street where Ronnie Scott's Club is now. As I was in the cabaret, I got to know everyone who came into the club. Thomas was at the Palladium and he'd come into the club and sit at the table with two bottles of gin: "that one's mine, and the other one is for everyone else." He used to drink a lot but I never saw him drunk.

I went out a few times with Fats and his girl-friend whose name, I think, was Paddy; funny name for a girl. She was a dancer at one time but not at the Palm Beach. He probably met her in one of the clubs.

But I was on my own the time he invited me a recording session. First we went to Denmark Street to get the sheet music and it was there that he said "Do you know who that is over there? That's one of your famous singers." It was Vera Lynn: she was probably getting her sheet-music too. It was free then, because they were plugging their own stuff and I used to get mine there as well. I think he only went to one place, on the left as you go down from Charing Cross Road. I've got a feeling that we were alone, and we went straight from there to the recording studio. We went by taxi, to Decca. We were in a little roorn, and it was all new to me. It was the first time I'd ever been in a studio. He and I were in tne same room together while he was recording, and you could see the other people — the engineers — through the glass in another room. I don't remember any other musicians being there, but I do remember him singing. He played piano and I remember when he made a mistake, he said "Break that one!" At the time, I didn't know what he meant, but he meant it was no good.

He was so down to earth. He said, "Come on, sing one with rne Zaza!" but I was shy and wouldn't. It was nice to know him, but I was never excited by any of it; I just took it for granted. He gave me his address to write to him in New York, but I never got round to it. I was too busy working, and going around all the clubs, living it up.

His girlfriend told me that they took a taxi to Scotland! Fancy that. And she said the door opened and he rolled out! Later she teamed up with Chris Gill, 'the Southern Gentleman', a dancer, and they went to live in Brighton.

Zaza Geldray in conversation with Val Wilmer, Highgate, London, 3 August 1991, and 9 September 1991.

Although Zaza Geldray's memories are no doubt a little confused and blurred with the passing of the years, she is almost certainly right in recalling the events as 1939 as Waller had his wife with him on his previous vist to the UK and would hardly have picked up a 'girl friend'. The recording session is intriguing. It is hardly the documented ones; that at Billy Higgs Studio featured all his own compositions and would not have entailed a visit to Denmark Street to collect music and the 13 June date at HMV can be ruled out for that and other reasons. However, there is circumstantial evidence for a private date the previous day at HMV (not Decca), and it may be this which Zaza Geldray attended.

*****

The *Pittsburgh Courier* of 28 September 1940 has a large photograph of Earl Hines in front of a bus being congratulated by Fats Waller and Erskine Hawkins. No date or location is given but the caption says that Hines was in Chicago 'last Sunday'.

*****

The *Pitsburgh Courier* of 30 November 1940 has a report datelined Columbus, O. Nov. 28 which is intriguing:

Waller's Ex-Drummer Hit With Own Band

Bill Tye's new band at the Roxy club is about the finest outfit the former Fats Waller drummer has ever fronted. It's an eight-piece ...

Who was Tye and when did he play with Waller?

*****

Al Casey recalled a broadcast done with the 'Rhythm' as a publicity stunt from an aircraft flying over New York City and said he played the guitar sitting on the arm of one of the seats. It's not clear whether the plane carried a piano or a Hammond organ for the occasion, but the latter seems more likely.

*****

Anita Waller died Jamaica, Long Island, New York, 12 March 1973 of heart attack. Aged 62.

*****

Andy Razaf died Hollywood, California on 3 February 1973 after long illness. Aged 77.

*****

Maurice Waller, died New York in October 1989.

*****

A NOTE FROM ERNIE ANDERSON

Lucie Barnicoat is a young girl who lives in Putney, a London village. She is a born musician, although both parents are painters. At six she entertained the family by playing a miniature violin. At eight somebody gave her one of those tiny electric keyboards, little more than a toy. She never had any formal instruction and she never practiced. It all began when the nuns noticed that the students tended to disappear from time to time. It turned out that they were congregating in an empty study room where there was a piano which little Lucie was playing. At ten Lucie told her mother that she wanted to be a professional musician. She began instruction on the violin and on the piano. Her mother got her a piano and put it the child's room. Lucie began to compose on it the same hour. Her advances in technique and expression were breathtaking. She decided she'd also like to play the viola and began lessons on that instrument as well. Her teachers all find her a most remarkable young musician. On summer vacation in a French Atlantic port she bought a harmonica which she plays effortlessly. She now is a regular member of three symphony orchestras in London and she also sings in two choruses. All this while continuing her usual grade school curriculum. Although all of her music is in the classical vein, she has always expressed an interest in the music of Fats Waller. Laurie Wright asked me to try to set down some of my memories of Fats. Strangely enough at the same moment little Lucie, who soon will turn fifteen, also asked me to tell her more about Fats Waller. This memoir is affectionately dedicated to both Lucie Barnicoat and Laurie Wright.

Ernie Anderson,
Palm Beach Shores,
Florida,
March 1990

AN ERNIE ANDERSON MEMOIR

Half a century ago, to a young white advertising man, Harlem was a secret happy place. By then it was already almost totally black. Today the legend is that it was a place of misery and oppression. In truth there were poor people all over New York City. The poor Irish of Bay Ridge in Brooklyn, and in Manhattan the poor Italians of Mulberry Street and the poor Jews of the lower East side, all lived in the same degree of poverty and squalor. But somehow black Harlem was really the happiest place in the entire city. Especially after dark and all night long. I was up there, and most welcome, too, almost every night.

Earlier still, at the turn of the century, Harlem had still been white. Rather palatial six and eight story apartment houses had been built. It was envisaged that a residential community of upscale whites would develop here. That ended when, in the wake of the first World War, in the twenties, blacks surged to the big cities from the rural south and Harlem became a lower income black community.

Those big apartment houses, like Twenty Forty Seventh Avenue, had to find another function, just to pay the rent. Twenty Forty became a vertical stack of what we called 'good time flats'. In a 'good time flat' there was always music. And there was always drink, even during Prohibition. To provide the music there was usually a piano. But there was always a phonograph, or possibly a juke box, known in the argot of the day as the 'piccolo'.

The collection of records inevitably reflected the taste of the proprietor. But from 1922 on, when 18-year-old Fats Waller's first blues records came out on the OKeh label, his music tended to be a staple in all of these establishments. Other favourites included Bessie Smith, Satchmo, and the early Duke, but the music of few white artists penetrated this particular after-hours culture until the more jazz-oriented big bands such as Benny Goodman came into vogue. Then their latest recordings were *de rigeur* in these places.

The fact that I was white in a black place didn't really seem to make the slightest difference. The first racial discrimination I ever encountered in the music trade was perhaps when George Brunies, a white trombonist originally from New Orleans, refused to go up on the bandstand with Eddie Condon at Nick's because Zutty Singleton was playing the drum. I must report that we were not irate at this overt display of naked racism. We all thought it was terribly funny, especially Zutty. Everybody knew George was crazy anyways. This was just another of his irrational eccentricities, like changing the spelling of his name, refusing to get into a plane and taking a slow train instead which often meant losing a date. "I wouldn't take a plane to my mother's funeral so I won't take one to no jam session!" he shouted.

We laughed so hard that George began to laugh, too. First thing you know he was up on the stand with Zutty and playing vigorously. The subject never came up again except as an excuse for further hilarity although I believe he lived out his life without ever getting into a plane.

The next time I ran into discrimination was in church. I remember that church so well. Some whites of my generation often used to venture into black churches to listen to the singing. There were even radio programmes you could tune in to that were just black congregations singing during their services.

In general Harlem was quite a religious community. There were store front churches all over the place. The church I'm remembering now was much more elaborate than that. That's what attracted me to it in the first place, that and its rather exotic name.

Deep in Harlem, just a few steps west of the community boulevard, Seventh Avenue, it was on the ground floor of what had been one of those nineteenth century brown stone front residences. The facade of the church was quite elaborately, and obviously lovingly, carved in wood that had been artfully painted in black with decorative borders of dark red and gold. Prominent was a plaque on which could be read in gilt gothic letters: Abysinnian Baptist Church. It had a very dignified and imposing look. But when I tried to enter, it was quickly made evident that no whites were welcome there. I was told that this was an extremely conservative black congregation that demanded segregation of the races as a simple courtesy to the dignity of their own colour during the practice of their religious rites.

Had I managed to get into the place, I might possibly have heard young Fats Waller play years earlier than I actually did. He played the organ here even when he was so little his feet could not reach the pedals. His father, the Reverend Edward Waller, often officiated as a deacon, preaching mighty sermons.

In the main whites were more than welcome in Harlem back then (they are not today). Evidently they were then also more than welcome in the black enclave on the South Side of Chicago. How else do we explain white teenagers such as Eddie Condon, Bud Freeman, Benny Goodman, George Wettling (who was still in short pants), Dave Tough, Gene Krupa and others of that ilk gaining free access to the black dance hall where Louis Armstrong was playing in King Oliver's band?

These youngsters circulated freely through all the places in the black ghetto where there was music, from the barbeque where Pinetop Smith played his boogie woogie piano to the big silent movie house where Erskine Tate conducted his Vendome Orchestra.

Mezz was one of those white teenagers who discovered Louis Armstrong in Chicago's black ghetto. He was the one who did not become a great jazz virtuoso. He shared their fanatical enthusiasm for the music but, unlike most of the others, he just didn't have enough musical talent to respond to the inspiration. He was trying to play the clarinet. But in that same little high school gang were such clarinetists as Frank Teschemacher and Benny Goodman. Still, back in those days, he was always trying to make up for this deficiency. If you looked him over closely you might feel that he was the villain of the lot. There was always something sinister about Mezz.

His young pals were all broke but Mezz usually had money and a car. He had five older brothers, all pharmacists. In their drug stores he managed somehow to get quantities of illicit alcohol, prohibition was still the law of the land, and before he was old enough to vote Mezz was an affluent bootlegger. What he lacked in musical skills he made up for in three categories. He always had a car so he could provide transportation, out to the Southside to catch Louis, or even up to Lake Delavan to hear Bix playing in a resort dancehall. He also had booze which these younsters otherwise couldn't have afforded. He also usually had some cash which none of the others ever had. Thus he became an almost accepted member of the musical gang centering around young Condon, those other two clarinetists, McPartland, Freeman, Tough, Wettling, Krupa et al.

Then, during these musical adventures, Mezz, through an extraordinary accident, stumbled into the source of the finest marihuana ever seen anywhere. He tied up the source, then distributed the stuff nationwide on the wave of interest in jazz that began to sweep the country. In a very short time wherever jazz was played there were some musicians smoking 'Mezz', as his stuff was known everywhere.

He now drove a huge Pierce Arrow and had his monogrammed shirts handmade by Sulka. He still posed as a clarinet player and this may have misled a law officer or two but never a musician. He was the top dealer in marihuana anyplace in this world for years.

Louis Armstrong was an habitual and grateful user and he let everybody know it which only made the product known as Mezz more in demand than ever. Louis's rigidly observed routine was to smoke the stuff only after work. He never touched it until he had played the last note of the day.

Louis was now getting quite famous. He was regularly broadcasting on network radio from the various dancehalls he played. It is a fact that he often sent signals over the air to Mezz. "Those fine arrangements from Mezz arrived today," he'd announce, which merely meant that he had just safely received a new shipment. Mezz never wrote an arrangement in his life, although after those Satchmo announcements he often clained he had.

Back in the early twenties Eddie Condon was particularly energetic in searching out the best jazz music wherever it might be found. As he moved around South Side Chicago he made a friend of every jazz player of quality. It was such a friend, Earl Hines, who first spoke Thomas Waller's name to him. There was no question at all but that Earl was the best piano player in Chicago and he was suggesting that this Tom Waller was his peer.

In the middle twenties Tom Waller had played in Chicago. Once in Erskine Tate's band at the Vendome where he first played with Louis Armstrong, a featured artist in that orchestra. And again as intermission organist at the Regal Theater which was the other black movie house. On these occasions Earl had prowled the South Side 'after hours' joints with Fats. They had even played duets together at the Sunset Cafe where Louis was the bandleader. Now Eddie was about to leave Chicago, making his first visit to Manhattan, to play a vaudeville stand with a band including Jimmy McPartland and Bud Freeman. Earl was urging him to look up Fats when he got to the Big City. This was a powerful endorsement and Eddie recognized that fact.

The McKenzie-Condon Chicago record date had just been a minor sensation and Eddie was under the misaprehension that the New York record studios would be paved with gold. They were not. Times for a jazz musician in Manhattan were even tougher than they had been in the Windy City.

Although as usual he somehow managed to hear the best jazz in town, even hitting the Harlem 'after hours' joints, it was months before he heard that name Earl Hines had confided to him.

The record business was by now a huge industry but the jazz segment of it was not only minuscule, it was frowned on by most record executives. There were a number of disturbing elements in it and one of the principal ones was race. Blacks bought lots of records but they were usually made by black blues shouters and black musicians, singing and playing for blacks. The record companies made a different sort of record for the white trade and the artists on those records were all white. Many white sophisticates, however, found they liked those black records. Moreover, it became obvious that some black musicians were influenced by some of the white players, arrangers and song writers featured on the recordings made for the whites. Eddie wanted to make some records in which some of the players were white and others black. This was firmly rejected by everyone to whom the proposal was presented. There was, however, one exception.

This was the mysterious Ralph Peer, head of the Southern Music Company. He had powerful influence with the Victor label and, in fact, sometimes operated as an Artists & Repertoire director for it. Peer told Eddie that he couldn't see how the colour of the players mattered in the least because you couldn't see it on the record and if you could hear it - why good luck to you. The record was always going to be black in any case. So, under Peer's sponsorship, Eddie made the record, which was of Peck Kelley's tune *I'm Gonna Stomp Mr. Henry Lee*.

Back in those days Eddie's instrument was still the tenor banjo. Two of his musicians on the date were Happy Caldwell, black, and Jack Teagarden, white, and born in Texas to boot.

Both Peer and Condon felt that they were making the first record to break the colour bar. (It was six years later that Benny Goodman made his first trio sides with Gene Krupa and Teddy Wilson and still a year after that when in a concert in Chicago he first publicly presented the mixed trio with his black piano player.)

During that first mixed session, Mr. Peer unburdened himself to Mr. Condon. Publisher Peer was pleased with the authoritative way Eddie was handling his little orchestra. How he ever got the idea that Eddie was a stern disciplinarian who could rehearse a band and keep all the players sober is a mystery that can never now be solved. The publisher declared that he was having desperate trouble with a Harlem piano player. He wondered if Eddie knew Fats Waller? "I don't know him, but my information is that he's a master!" declared Condon. "Oh, he's talented enough," admitted the publisher, "But when he shows up for his date he's always drunk and unprepared." Thus Peer arranged to hire Eddie to rehearse Fats Waller and a small band for a record session at which four sides were to be made on an afternoon just three weeks away. Perhaps he judged that this white had a special rapport with blacks.

Eddie's black and white mixture on *Mr. Henry Lee* didn't cause any race riots and was a mild success in jazz circles. Eddie went to the OKeh label, then famous for their many all-black releases which they frankly billed as 'Race Records', a category in which young Fats had been happy to be included.

He suggested to them that they might like to make a mixed band date, too. He thought he got a favourable reaction. More likely they were seeming to agree with his proposal just to get him out of the office. They had some big recording attractions under contract, artists who sold tens of thousands of copies. Eddie's small band jazz dates caused a lot of talk but didn't produce too many sales. The consensus was that he was some kind of a nut. Louis Armstrong, one of their premier artists was due in town for a session and this guy was actually proposing that Louis play in one of Condon's little combinations.

The date Ralph Peer had set for the Fats Waller session was noon of March 1st, 1929. Fats hadn't made any recordings since 1927, a year during which he had five record sessions in which he had recorded two dozen titles.

It was February 28th before Eddie made the slightest move about the Waller date. He didn't even have the remotest idea how to find Fats Waller whom he had never even met. He took his pork chop and caught a subway uptown.

In Harlem he moved around the various speakeasies frequented by musicians he did know. In Small's Paradise he learned that Tom Waller usually hung out at Connie's Inn.

Connie Immerman had been the proprietor of a very successful Harlem delicatessen. With prohibition he had added bootleg booze to the commodities he sold and he prospered mightily.

Fats Waller was a particular friend of the management. As a boy of fourteen Fats had an angelic face but he was a very big kid. He wore a blue serge suit with enormous knickerbockers. He could stow a couple of quart bottles of bathtub gin in these oversize pantaloons with nobody the wiser and then deliver them to whichever address the bootlegger indicated even if it meant walking right through a cordon of revenue agents. Fats's youth and beatific smile dissipated all possible suspicion.

Now, with prohibition still raging, Connie Immerman had opened a speakeasy cabaret adjacent to his deli where you could drink your booze on the spot while you saw a show. Connie loved Fats and put him in charge of the music. Fats made sure there was a good piano in the place, which together with the gin, was all he needed to pass the time happily.

Nobody at Connie's would ever think of handing Fats a tab. Naturally Fats was here every evening. He was there on the evening of February 28th, 1929 when Eddie passed him regards from Earl Hines.

Within minutes they discovered that they were kindred spirits. This is where Eddie first heard Fats Waller play the piano. In subsequent conversations with me he ranked this occasion with the night he first heard Louis at the Lincoln Gardens in Chicago and the afternoon he first heard Bix on a day coach en route to Syracuse.

There is no question but that Eddie sat in with Fats that night. His instrument was right there with him. He would have been out of character if he hadn't played it. They were almost exact contemporaries, both aged 24, but already both seasoned and thirsty veterans of the speakeasy generation.

We know that Leonard Harper staged the show at Connie's and that Fats wrote the music for it. He did this without effort, sometimes writing a whole new show with as many as eight new songs every week. Fats could improvise new melodies instantly. When he was cheated of the rights to his songs he never minded because he found it so easy to compose new ones.

Of course Fats was a Harlem man. He knew every inch of that black community. In his early post-adolescent years the only other place they knew his name at all was in the cluster of run down buildings a block or so north of Times Square that was known as Tin Pan Alley. Every flyblown office here had some kind of a piano that was more or less in tune and that fact in itself made the place irresistible to the young Fats Waller. He was a legend among the song publishers before anybody else in show business had ever heard of him.

Hard up and with no prospects of any kind in sight, young Fats would hop a subway four miles downtown to Times Square. In those days the fare was only a thin dime. Arriving, he'd walk into, let us say, the Brill Building at Forty-ninth and Broadway. He'd get off the elevator at any floor and walk into the first office in sight. There he'd sit down at the piano.

Instantly the word would race through the building like a brush fire, "Fats Waller is here." Somebody would get a bottle. There always seemed to be a lot more booze around during Prohibition than there ever was after Repeal. Life in a publisher's office was usually a pretty drab affair but that all changed when Fats hove into view. He turned a dull day at the office into a party.

Fats would sit at the piano and play. He was always most entertaining. Especially when the gin was flowing freely. His audience was just these men whose whole business was music. Sitting at the keyboard, playing continuously. he was forever pouring out new melodies, new themes, brand new songs. They were all in the song business and he would offer to sell them anything they heard that they liked. He didn't charge much either. Twenty-five dollars was the usual suggestion.

All the publishers, and the songwriters who frequented their offices, loved these exhibitions by Fats. They sensed the quality of the music he was producing. Sometimes a publisher would buy a song from Fats, put it on the shelf and forget he had it. Sometimes a song writer would buy a melody and put his own name on it as composer. Fats didn't mind as long as they gave him his twenty-five. They appreciated his performance and sometimes they bought a song just to pay for the show.

When Fats had scored with a sale he'd make his adieus and get back in the elevator and get off at another floor and walk into some other office, sit at some other piano. Somebody would open another flagon of gin and the whole fandango would begin again.

Everybody loved Fats's music but nobody loved it quite as much as Fats.

He'd be mad about some new theme and it would keep creeping into whatever he was playing. Some publisher would be fascinated by it and insist on buying it. The office copyist would be summoned to write down the new melody Fats was playing, Fats would sign a form contract for the tune and take his twenty-five.

You might never believe it but Fats was only human. Sometimes something he'd sold on the eighth floor he sold all over again on the fifth. That was part of the legend. Another part was that there were songwriters with their names on hits they never wrote, melodies they'd bought on an alcoholic afternoon from Fats. No one will ever know how many of these there were.

Fats's profligacy was so extraordinary that while they were arguing in Tin Pan Alley about whether it was his song or someone else's he was playing half a dozen completely new songs. As long as the piano worked and the gin held out he just didn't care.

He displayed the same attribute uptown at Connie's. The entertainment at Connie's Inn that night when Eddie Condon first turned up was titled *'Hot Chocolates'* and it became so popular that a few months later they doubled it into the Hudson Theater downtown on Broadway.

With Fats in the pit and Louis Armstrong on stage it quickly became a box office smash. One of those songs that Fats threw off so casually for the cabaret at Connie's became a world hit under another title and with another name listed as composer. Fats sold it to the man for a quick cash touch. With new lyrics it became *I Can't Give You Anything But Love.* But Eddie Condon always sang the melody with the completely different original lyric which had been written for Fats by his pal, Andy Razaf, and which was sung at Connie's for weeks before the big time songwriter bought the tune alone from Fats.

The truth is that this was only one of a number of Fats Waller melodies that came to have other composers's names on them. But whether Fats's name was on them, or someone else's, it didn't seom to matter to Fats. One night, later that same year he first met Eddie, Fats sold all rights to his entire *'Hot Chocolates'* hit score plus thirteen other Fats Waller songs to Irving Mills for five hundred dollars in cash. He put the money in his pocket and walked away with a smile.

Among the titles he handed away that night were: *Ain't Misbehavin'; Can't We Get Together;* and *What Did I Do To Be So Black And Blue.* He never earned another penny from any of them. Never within my hearing did he ever make the slightest complaint about this.

News of this shabby transaction echoed through the corridors of Tin Pan Alley and in some barroom came to the ear of Eddie Condon. If Fats didn't complain, Eddie did and to anyone within hearing. He thought the deal outrageous. Bud Freeman tried to calm him. He said, "Eddie, you must remember that Duke also sold eighteen compositions to Irving Mills. They were all supposed to be Duke's original tunes. Irving put his own name on them immediately. But If you listen to them carefully you can see that they are all versions of Gershwin's *I Got Rhythm.*" Eddie laughed at Bud's exaggeration. But there is a modicum of truth in Bud's canard. *Cottontail* is surely a variation on the Gershwin classic and *Stompy Jones* is surely *The Sheik of Araby.*

About the night when Eddie first met Fats at Connie's inn we have scant detail. Neither Eddie nor Fats were ever able to say much about what actually transpired that evening at Connie's Inn.

Charlie Gaines who played trumpet in the little show band at Connie's Inn recalled that Fats did mention to him a record date planned for the following noon. "He said he'd speak to me about it later. But by the time I went home at four in the morning he hadn't mentioned it again. He and Eddie were drinking up a storm. They were both in a wild state and roaring with laughter. So I split and left them there. I had no idea whether the date was on or off."

Charlie Gaines was a solid professional and a record studio veteran. He had made many sides accompanying blues singers and was a regular in Clarence Williams's pick-up combos. But this was his first record date with Fats.

All Eddie or Fats could ever tell me about that night at Connie's Inn was that the gin rickeys were flying thick and fast and that ultimately both parties drew blanks. Which is to say that although they carried on in their usual ways, all memory of the night vanished. Their first signs of life returned the following morning at ten.

They came to out of black unconciousness, both rigidly prostrate on the banquettes of a booth in the nightclub. According to Eddie this is when they actually first seriously discussed Mr. Peer's imminent record session.

"Holy Mackerel!" Eddie exclaimed, "It's ten Ayem and we're due at the record studio at noon!" There was a pause while both reflected upon this hard fact. Then Eddie added, "With a band!"

"With a band?" asked Fats. When he saw if not pure terror at least real concern in his new friend's eyes, he took a small address book out of his pocket and added, "Don't worry, we'll make it. Have you got any nickels?" Back in those days you could still make a phone call with a nickel.

Within seconds he was talking about players Eddie had never even heard of and making call after call from a pay phone on the men's room wall. Eddie attempted some simple matutinal ablutions while Fats called rooming houses and other pigeonholes where out of work musicians might be lurking and most of the time he was getting no result at all. But now and then he hit a lucky number and got someone. He was telling them to drop everything and come to Connie's Inn right away.

By eleven-thirty that morning he had again found Charlie Gaines to play trumpet, and also saxophonist Arville Harris who had been a regular in King Oliver's New York recording band, and Charlie Irvis who had been Duke Ellington's first trombone player when Duke started his career in New York at the Kentucky Club.

Eddie had been expecting a few more musicians. These three were all who showed up. They gathered at the entrance to Connie's.

"Well, look at it this way, Eddie" said Fats with a grin. "We'll only need one cab." The five musicians crammed in, and the hack took off for midtown Manhattan. Eddie noted in some alarm that Fats had not managed to turn up a bass player or a drummer. But Fats didn't seem in the least perturbed by this and, in the cab as it raced down through Central Park, he began to sing a strain to the musicians and call out keys for a brand new melody.

Those who managed to live through the Prohibition Era can attest that there were various species of hangover. Rarely encountered was the one in which, although the nerves are shattered, the reflexes are quicker than usual and ideas by the million proliferate in the head. This happily was the state in which Fats and Eddie now found themselves.

The studio which Victor had booked for the session was the old wooden walled beer garden which in pre-prohibition days had been called the Liederkranz Hall. It was spacious and the walls and ceilings were all of ornately gilded, carved wood. For many years it was the best acoustical premises in New York City. Then a decade or two later André Kostelanetz and his symphony sized orchestra demanded it for a CBS radio series sponsored by Coca-Cola. CBS took a permament lease on the place, at hideous expense installed radio control rooms, mostly of aluminium and glass, and a few tons of recording gear and the magical acoustical properties of the Liederkranz Hall just floated away.

Eddie and Fats and their three sidemen arrived at the studio at ten minutes to twelve. Ralph Peer greeted them with a grin, he noted that for one thing they were actually on time. He had no way of knowing that this group hardly knew each other.

Here I must interpolate that Eddie Condon often recounted this adventure in considerable detail. I have even heard him tell the story in the presence of Fats, who nodded solemnly in confirmation. But in fact the times were all wrong. It is a fact that in those less than prosperous days neither Eddie nor Fats sported a wrist watch. Still, I was quite surprised to learn that the indefatigable Laurie Wright, prowling through the ledgers of the Victor Record Company, has discovered that, in fact, the record date was scheduled for one-thirty in the afternoon. But Eddie and Fats, and their three musicians did not arrive until ten minutes to three. That is the fact of the matter.

Instantly on arrival at Liederkranz Fats gravitated to the big piano. He warmed up by playing a fantastic piano solo. It was such a clever composition and so brilliantly played that Ralph Peer asked Fats to start the date by recording it as a solo. Thus the world first came to hear Fats's *Handful of Keys.* Almost eight years later Benny Goodman was to make it one of his quartet classics with Gene Krupa, Lionel Hampton and Teddy Wilson.

Now Fats gathered his little combination around him and ran his hands over the keyboard. New aspects of the strain he had been singing in the taxi began to emerge. The little band set up and began to romp. Eddie's banjo and Fats's walloping left hand provided the only percussion. Within minutes they had the first take.

As Fats huddled with his horn players on a new melody, Ralph Peer took Eddie aside and congratulated him on having so carefully prepared the little band for the date. "I've made half a dozen record dates with this man and this is the very first time he's been properly prepared to record. I congratulate you!" and he squeezed Eddie's right hand and gave it a vigorous shake.

The date proceeded so rapidly that the technicians in the control room were caught off guard. As a take was approved the control room would ask for the title over the speaker system. Actually, these particular technicians had no experience whatever with jazz. They didn't have an inkling that the titles were references to the tempos of the compositions, Thus they managed to mix up the titles Fats had assigned to the two band instrumentals and what Fats created as *Harlem Fuss* will thus be known forever as *The Minor Drag.* And vice versa.

Once the two instrumentals were in the can, Fats went to the piano and cut another piano solo that has now also become a standard, *Numb Fumblin'.*

Victor distributed the two 78s across the country. Despite rave reviews they were not smash hits but sales were nevertheless encouraging. Within an hour of first hearing *The Minor Drag* in Chicago, Gene Krupa called Eddie Condon in New York. "Who's on drums on that record?" he wanted to know. He found it hard to believe that there were no drums. "It swings like crazy!" he insisted. Over the years it has been accepted as one of the greatest pure jazz sides ever recorded. The gin-crazed rout that produced it evaporated away. When you listen to that music there is no trace of it. But those alcoholic furies pursued Fats Waller and Eddie Condon all their short lives.

It was only four days after that *Minor Drag* record date that Eddie sparked off another famous session. Louis Armstrong arrived in Manhattan and when

Eddie found him, Louis enthusiastically agreed to participate in his mixed black and white record date for OKeh. "I'm making two sides for OKeh myself the night of March fifth anyway," he explained to Eddie. "You just bring your cats along and we'll slip it in as part of the same session."

In those days a Louis Armstrong record session in New York was almost a social occasion. Music pluggers and musicians not connected with the date tended to drop in, sit on the floor and observe the proceedings. Everybody knew that Louis didn't mind in the least.

Once more Eddie overshot the mark. He arrived three sheets to the wind with his banjo and also a quart of gin, which he generously offered to all hands. For his mixed band Eddie had brought along Joe Sullivan, Jack Teagarden, Happy Caldwell and Kaiser Marshall. Unlike Fats, Louis never drank when he was making records, but others in the company did. None more so than Eddie himself.

Luis Russell had assembled the band for Louis's own sides. The group rejoiced in the name 'The Savoy Ballroom Five'. This was despite the fact that not one of the musicians had been in the group when Louis Armstrong made his original and only other Savoy Five date, the previous year in Chicago. In fact Louis Armstrong and his Savoy Ballroom Five on this occasion numbered nine players which number became ten when Louis insisted that Eddie and his banjo sit in, although Lonnie Johnson was already playing guitar.

They cut that New Orleans bordello classic, *Mahogany Hall Stomp.* And then with Louis singing the vocal, they made *I Can't Give You Anything But Love,* the song that Fats had written and, with other lyrics, casually sold for a pittance. Louis's own date was complete. Now he signalled that he was ready to make the mixed band recording.

They looked around for Eddie, who was the originator of this project. Unfortunately Eddie had by now overdosed. He had passed out cold, deeply asleep on a chair. But Louis was resolute. He had Eddie's little black and white group set up to record, with Eddie Lang on guitar substituting for Eddie Condon on banjo. Louis led the little group in a classic blues as Eddie Condon slept. He named the pure improvisation *Knockin' A Jug* in tribute to Eddie's alcoholic ways. He was, nevertheless, a bit upset by Eddie's behaviour.

A decade later he was still berating his friend about getting drunk on that particular job. "You should have waited until you got off," he cautioned. These admonishments caused Eddie particular hurt because they came from Louis, the man he habitually referred to as 'Mr. Strong'. They did not, however, seem to curtail his habit in the least.

Now, more than half a century later, you could hardly make any list of jazz classics without including *The Minor Drag* and *Knockin' a Jug,* two recordings made with totally different personnels only four days apart. A good deal of illicit alcohol went into the production of both of them, yet there is no sign of it in the music nor in it's execution.

Like most midtown Manhattan blocks, West 52nd Street between Fifth Avenue and Sixth, was two rows of nineteenth century brownstone residences. Each had a stone stoop, under which had been a service entrance. The kitchen had been on this floor. Now, more often than not, there was a small iron grating in this door.

When you rang the bell, someone appeared behind this grating to identify you. For now many of these brownstone residences housed speakeasies which operated as private clubs, but which could in any event be raided for selling liquor in any form.

A block to the east was CBS and very near to the west was NBC. These were the two national radio networks, then in their most prosperous period. The musicians's union, Local 802, was also only a block away. In those halcyon days some good jazz musicians who could read music could earn big money. All the big radio shows of the era featured big orchestras. A job playing a radio show required the musician to play a rehearsal, usually in the morning or early afternoon. Then he was off until show time which was usually at eight or nine in the evening.

These shows, sponsored by important advertisers, earned big money for the networks and the musicians's union knew it. They saw to it that the pay for a rehearsal plus the evening show paid very well. The big trouble with these jobs was killing the time between the rehearsal and the show. Thus that block on 52nd Street became a musicians's mecca.

Thus 'The Famous Door' was a speak in that block where a musician member of the club could come in and pass the hiatus comfortably. The club took phone messages for you and cashed your cheques. They could keep your instrument safe for you while you might walk a couple of blocks west to the Times Square area to catch a movie or shoot some pool. Or, alternatively, you could stay right there and play cards or read the papers and, incidentally, drink some of the forbidden stuff.

It was supposed to be like a gentlemen's club, a preserve where one might be shielded from the outside world for a while. Benny Goodman didn't get the idea. He was a member in good standing. One day outside the entrance there was a summons server trying to get in. Of course no member in his right mind would vouch for the man so he was refused access. Until Benny Goodman, fresh from a rehearsal for the Lucky Strike Hit Parade, came by.

Benny, despite his unquestioned musical talent, had a warped sense of humour. He thought it was funny that one of his fellow musicians was in trouble with the law. He passed the man in and the summons was served on a well-known trombonist who was in arrears on the alimony payments. Benny laughed, fit to kill. The trombone player and everybody else in the place save the server stared at Benny in contemptuous wonder. Of course Benny never did have close friends especially among his fellow union members.

When Prohibition ended 'The Famous Door' ceased being a speakeasy and became a night club. Across the street another speak became 'The Onyx Club'. And a few steps to the east, at number 21, 'The 21 Club became the most luxurious café restaurant in town and still is today.

One block further west was a chop house called 'The Hickory House'. The owner of the place, a very masculine, bulky, cigar-smoking type, loved the jazz music as accompaniment to the fare he featured which was mostly steaks and whisky.

The premises were a high ceilinged cavernous joint with an oval-shaped bar, in the centre of which he gave his friend, former Chicago truck driver and now clarinetist, Joe Marsala, unfettered reign to turn out some small band jazz every night.

In this little band we saw for the first time young Joey Bushkin and also teenager Buddy Rich whose father and mother used to come in early to set up his drums. On Sunday afternoons Joe put on a bit of a jam session. You never quite knew who might be there but you could always count on seeing Joe's great friend, Eddie Condon.

Those Sunday afternoons in the thirties everybody dropped in at 'The Hickory House'. It was here that I had first met Eddie Condon. I used to see him there every Sunday. One Sunday he took me to the back of the place and introduced me to Fats Waller.

Fats, neatly dressed in a brown business suit, seemed smaller than I had imagined him. There was nothing jolly about him at all that day. In fact he was quiet and, so it seemed to me at least, he emanated a mood of deep melancholy. The three of us sat together in the booth. I ordered a drink. Eddie and I had our usual scotch and sodas but Fats took nothing. It is the only time I ever remember seeing Fats without a drink or on his way to one, in a saloon or out of one.

In retrospect I now surmise that Fats had just come out after a spell of illness caused by over-indulgence in the drink. Eddie understood this but I did not. In those days I lived in an apartment in the Beaux-Arts on East 44th Street, just a block west of the East River slaughterhouses that provided the steaks for the whole city. By an ironical twist a few years later they razed the slaughterhouses and put up Le Corbusier's United Nations building instead.

At five that Sunday afternoon the music stopped as usual in 'The Hickory House'. The musicians and the crowd left, scooting off in all direction. Eddie and I had planned to take a taxi to my place. I had just scored with a small stash of Mezz and Eddie was anxious to see if it was up to Mesirow's usual high standard. The law was being particularly brutal at the time and such matters had to be dealt with in extreme secrecy. Fats seemed to be at a loose end so we took him with us.

In the taxi going crosstown, Eddie turned to me and said, "Would you look at the dukes on this guy!" At this Fats held up his hands, thumb to thumb, and spread them out palms forward. It was a formidable display. They were perfectly shaped hands, but they were enormous. You could scarcely imagine hands more suited to the keyboard of a grand piano.

I had no piano in my place but Fats came anyway. Once at home I poured a drink but Fats declined it. Then I got out the tea which I had hidden in my Atwater Kent radio console. Eddie took his Zig Zags out of his pocket and rolled up a couple of joints. At this point Fats surprised Eddie by indicating that he would like to partake too. In a few minutes the three of us were laughing like crazy. It was very powerful jive. Fats's participation was unique. In the succeeding years when I came to know Fats really well I never even heard of him indulging in the stuff again, although people all around him including the members of his own band were smoking it nightly.

Then suddenly Fats made a phone call, summoned a taxi, and was gone. A couple of weeks later early one morning I was in an after hours joint in Harlem doing my weekend Rest & Recreation when I was grasped from behind in a bear hug. My first impulse was to be terrified. I thought I was being mugged. Instead it was Fats in ebullient mood. There was nothing melancholy about him now.

He greeted me as though we had been cellmates for years. I was surprised he even remembered me but he called me by the diminutive of my first name and led me to the little upright piano where he proceeded to give me a solo concert. He was drinking all right that morning. There was a little blue-mirrored bar on wheels near the piano with a comely barkeep whose only duty seemed to be replenishing the piano player's oversized gin and Seven Up which sat on the piano directly in front of him.

I would say that Fats played for about two hours or so without stop on that occasion. It was beautiful music. There were no comic interludes, no clowning. In fact he didn't sing at all. His playing was effortless, his enormous hands stroking the keys delicately, then crashing down with thunderous harmony. It was all virgin improvisation, new untitled melodies and fresh variations on old tunes.

The playing was impeccable although the gin was flowing very freely indeed.

Fats's easy virtuosity was breathtaking. No musician could ever resist his graceful flowing improvisation. It was hard to believe that such talent could have evolved without the customary academic training. He insisted that he learned the rudiments by studying the movement of the keys of a player piano as James P. Johnson's piano roll of *Carolina Shout* turned. His ambition to play like that inspired a relentless determination. No one will ever know how many days, nights, weeks, months, he sat in study at that keyboard as that roll revolved. In the end he played it exquisitely and he played it that night as I listened. The fact is he continued to play it as long as he lived. It became one of his show stoppers.

I don't know how much he might have consumed that night before I ran into him but I saw that he had consumed an entire fifth just while I listened and watched him at the keyboard. Now his private bartender was setting up another fifth for his exclusive use. Under this flood of alcohol other musicians would have at least faltered a bit. But not Fats. He was unperturbed, playing beautifully and still thirsty. I gazed at the man in wonder. He was a phenomenon on two fronts. He was the most gifted piano player around. And he could drink more than anybody on earth! There was a something a bit frightening about it. I thanked him, made my excuses and split for home downtown. I felt guilty about it but it was all too much for me.

It was now that I discovered another impressive element in Fats's makeup. He had an oversize libido. In these oases there was often passing feminine company that came and went. These girls were not hustlers, at least in my own experience. They were co-workers in show business or on the periphery of it. They worked erratic tours of duty and after work they were looking for company as I was myself.

As far as I could see they found Fats irresistible. You might think that his obesity might put him out of the running. If you did you were wrong. First of all, from the keyboard he was capable of hypnotising a girl. Then his sly humour would take over and you would hear her laughing. She was done for, plain and simple.

Up until that night I had thought Eddie Condon was a top flight toper. In fact I thought I was a pretty good hand at the bar myself. But the simple fact was that Fats left us both in the starting stalls. He could polish off bottles and it didn't seem to faze him in the least. That was where the fright lay. Because you knew in your heart that no human frame could stand it forever.

Of course alcohol must be recognized as the jazz musicians's chief occupational hazard. He only works where booze is sold. Naturally when he steps away from the bandstand his delighted fans offer him a drink. The better he is the more they pour. Usually the fan is just there for the night. The musician is there every night.

Some musicians recognize this menace early on. Louis Armstrong was one such. He described for me the place where he first started. "It was a dirt floor saloon in the district; I mean Storyville. There were no hours — it was open day and night. The pimps and whores played cards and drank, killing time between tricks.

Whisky was five cents for a big glass. It was poured from a spigot in a barrel. There was a tin can under the glass to catch any of the droppings. Every once in a while they'd pass up that tin can to the musicians who sat in the back of the joint on the band stand which was some planks across two sawhorses. No uniforms, nothing like that. Just an undershirt and a towel around your neck.

I was the youngest so when the tin can came up I was the last to get any. By the time the can got to me it was usually empty. But I didn't mind because almost from the first night I saw that if you dipped too heavy into that can, you lost control of your chops. Cats who got drunk played sloppy. And that isn't the only thing. A lot of those hard drinking cats in New Orleans were able to cope with it physically. But they ended up going crazy." I interpreted this as an oblique reference to Buddy Bolden. When I mentioned this to Louis he did not deny it, he just nodded and added, "a whole lot of cats!"

Throughout his career Louis rarely drank, and then only after hours. Fats regarded Louis's abstention from alcohol as an amiable eccentricity. Louis, while full of praise for Fats's extraordinary musical talent, had misgivings about his life-style. You seldom saw them together in their off duty time even when they were co-starred at the Hudson Theatre downtown on Broadway in Connie Immerman's *'Hot Chocolates'*. Louis tended to avoid all lushes. He hung with the vipers. You usually found Mesirow in Louis's dressing room and no fifths of Gordon's Dry Gin ever.

Whiskey sometimes harmed musicians viciously. Marihuana was somehow more benign. At one point the use of it was so prevalent that some of those Harlem good time flats became known as tea pads. Tea merchants regularly made the rounds of these establishments.

Their big conversational ploy was discussing the provenance of the variety being offered. This one came from Yucatan, this other from Northern California. The most colourful of these purveyors was a dynamic young black who featured a species packed in two quart mason jars. "A railroad brakeman cultivates it", he proclaimed. "He grows it way out in the Michigan countryside, in the rich soil on the sides of an embankment alongside a railroad siding for freight cars." We called this fellow Detroit Red. He later went on to write a page in the history of the times as Malcolm X.

For some years Mezz had the greatest. He didn't do the rounds of the 'good time flats', he had emissaries to do that for him. Mezz's tea came from some place near Pueblo, Colorado. It was celebrated in song and story. "Dream about a reefer five feet long. The mighty Mezz but not too strong."

Mezz grew rich with it for some years. He had runners in Los Angeles, Chicago and Boston, that I know of, distributing his product. He also had a steward on the French line, carrying the stuff over to supply entertainers touring Europe. It was this Mezz, six sticks for a buck, that Louis Armstrong passed to the Prince of Wales when he played a private engagement at Fort Belvedere.

Mezz rode around Harlem in his deluxe limo. He wore his monogrammed shirts. But even at the zenith of his affluence he invariably posed as a working musician. When he delivered his merchandise, he always carried his clarinet in its small black case. Should he happen to be picked up and arrested, he would protest that the drug was only for his own personal use. It was Mezz's private fantasy that he, was black although he came from a good jewish famly on the north side. He spoke the patois of the south side ghetto, rich in black idiom. Most of his customers were black.

When Dave Tough cabled Mezz from Europe in 1929 asking him to come over for a job and to be sure to "bring music and records", what he meant was to bring plenty of Mezz. Dave hardly wanted Mezz to play the clarinet. He was well aware of his severe limitations in that department. But there was no superior marihuana in Europe and Dave wanted some. He couldn't wait and left before Mezz even arrived.

Mezz, now always in funds, had taken a stateroom on the French line, and on his way over lined up the steward who became his courier, carrying batches of Mezz to European destinations for years.

It was on this 1929 excursion that Mezz first encountered a rich-kid jazz fan, aged 17, named Hugues Panassié. He introduced the lad to the powerful drug and saw that he, too, had an unbroken supply. Thus he seduced the man who from that point on never missed an opportunity to propagandise Mezz as a great jazz player, although how the youthful critic could come to this conclusion is baffling. In fact I have heard him insist to anyone who would listen that Milton Mesirow was the greatest of all white jazz players. Even Mezz knew that was so much bosh.

Panassié knew that Louis himself and Mezz were very close friends and that the drug was their bond. It could hardly have been Mezz's clarinet playing because Louis, a prolific recording artist, in those days used a variety of clarinet players, such as Johnny Dodds, Boyd Atkins, Jimmy Strong, Don Redman and

Albert Nicholas on his dates, but never Mezz. Although Mezz is credited with ringing the train bells on Louis's *Hobo You Can't Ride This Train*, it always seemed to me that Mezz just happened to be in that studio to deliver his latest batch.

Eddie Condon, a chronic Mezz smoker, actually did cast Mezz on some record dates in his early Chicago days. Eddie, a kind man, tried to excuse himself for this in later years. He said to me, "Sometimes Mezz wasn't really too bad on some of those blues choruses." But, as a matter of pure fact, Eddie never had Mezz play any of his Friday Club gigs, his Town Hall concerts, or his Blue Network Broadcasts.

In 1938 when Hugues Panassié first came to America I was unaware of his connection with Mezz. I approved of Panassié. He wrote that jazz music was high art and I agreed with him, although that was by no means a popular assumption in those days. Thus I arranged a little welcoming party for him. We staged it in the luxurious apartment of Minerva Pious.

Min was a great fan of our music. She was the comedienne of the day, costarred with Fred Allen every week on the biggest network radio program of those times. Her constant companion was Bernie Hanighan, a fine jazz violinist whose student band had been a sensation at Harvard. Now Bernie was in Manhattan writing songs with Johnny Mercer, and Billie Holiday was recording them; such record classics as *When a Woman Loves a Man*.

Min's pad was in an elegant East 54th Street apartment complex called the Southgate. Eddie Condon always called it the Gatemouth. In addition to Eddie we had such as Maxie Kaminsky, Bud Freeman, Lips Page, Peewee Russell and George Wettling among others that I can recall. Naturally I had invited Fats who was playing at the Onyx Club on West 52nd Street, just a half a dozen blocks away. Fats had enthusiastically accepted. But in the end something had come up and he never showed.

Panassié's book, *'Le Jazz Hot'*, had been published in Paris in 1934. Two years later an English version, entitled *Hot Jazz* came out in New York. To most Americans at the time hot jazz was still something to be avoided at all costs and the book was never in the best-seller charts. Very few of us had actually read it but there had been many newspaper stories about it. Evidently Hugues Panassié adored Louis Armstrong and that was what was usually quoted. That was enough for us. Satchmo was our religion.

None of us yet realized Hugues Panassié's peculiar obsession with Milton Mezzrow.

At our little cocktail do Eddie studied the Frenchman for a considerable time. There wasn't much conversation between them. Eddie had zero French and

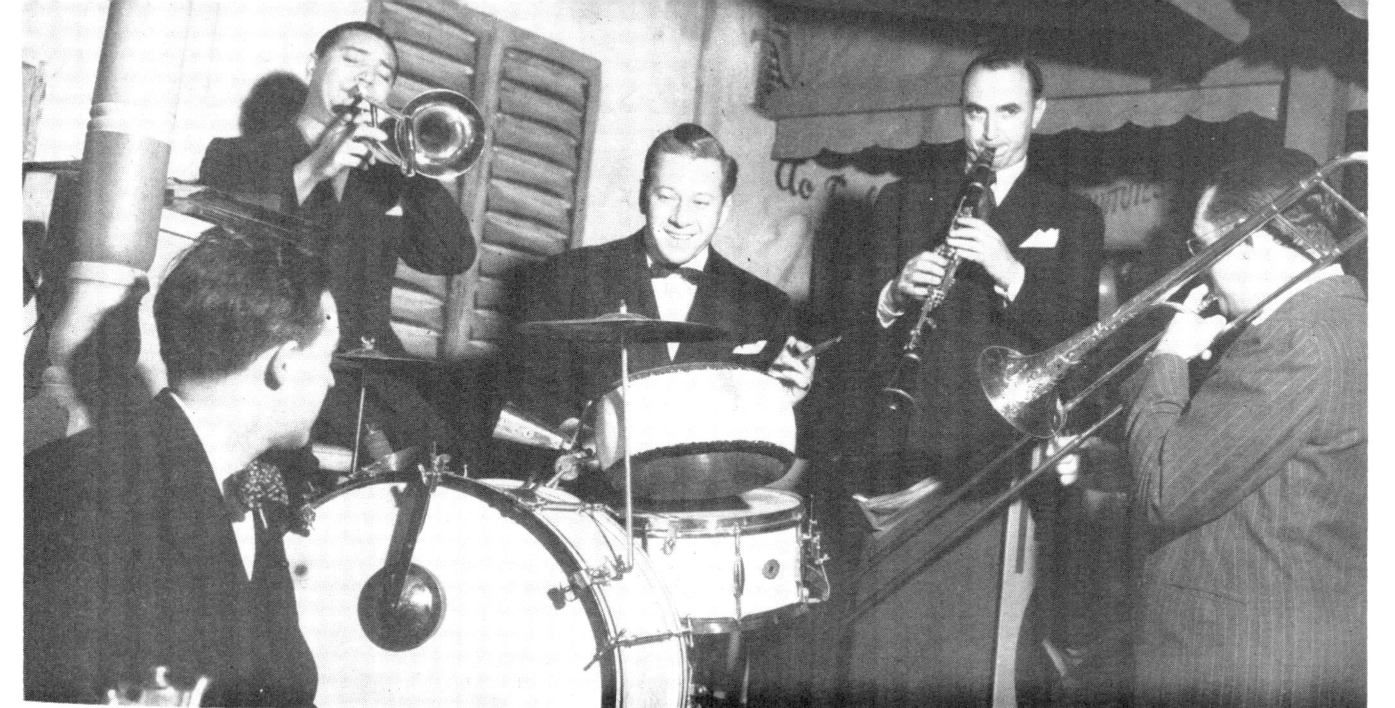

Mezz had two fantasies. One was that inside his white persona he was actually black. The other was that he could play the jazz clarinet. He was wrong on both counts, but somehow he convinced Panassié that these illusions were true. In France, years earlier, Mezz had introduced him to his excellent marijuana. When the French critic came to New York in 1938 Mezz towed him around town, introducing him to the greatest players. Here, he has organised an unlikely jam session. In the left foreground the bow tied Panassié watches Mezz as he plays with trombonist Jack Teagarden (who never used marijuana), drummer George Wettling (who was an enthusiastic user of Mezz's product, but who never played with him if he could get out of it — his preferred clarinettists were Frank Teschmacher, Pee Wee Russell or Edmond Hall) and finally, the most unlikely participant of all, trombonist bandleader Tommy Dorsey, who reviled marijuana in all of its forms and especially reviled Mezzrow himself, not only as a bad clarinettist, but also a drug pushing criminal outside the law. Tommy, however, was partial to publicity. He could not resist the opportunity to be in the same frame with the author of *Le Jazz Hot* in a photo taken by his musical pal, Charles Peterson.

Panassié wasn't really speaking a whole lot of English. Then as we left, Eddie turned to Bob Sylvester, who had a gossip column in the *New York Daily News*, the biggest paper in town, and said, "This French guy comes over here and tries to tell us how to play our native music. Would I go over there and tell him how to jump on a grape?" It was very deliberately stated and I listened as Eddie repeated it so that Bob could copy it down. It was at the top of his column the next morning. In the succeeding weeks there were numerous Panassié stories and interviews in the American press. The recording execs, seeing all the publicity, even had him make some sides. But I noticed that Mezz was in total charge at every date. On piano they wanted Fats but had to settle for James P. Johnson. James P. showed up drunker than I've ever seen him before or since.

I was curious enough to look in on both dates. Despite the presence of Panassié, and the high calibre of the other players, (such musicians as Tommy Ladnier, Teddy Bunn, Pops Foster and Zutty), I found the mood more of a undiscipled rout than a serious musical occasion. Mezz, who dominated the proceedings, was at his abysmal worst, according to one critic.

On previous occasions Mezz had managed to snag a record date or two by producing some high quality players. One side he made he titled *Swinging With Mezz*. One interpretation might have been that under the influence of smoked Mezz you swing. Bud Freeman, who had known Mezz since their short pants schoolboy days, was particularly offended by this. He didn't approve of Mezz's musicianship and he didn't approve of marihuana either. So he made a trio recording for Milt Gabler on the Commodore label which he entitled *Swinging Without Mezz*. With Bud, Jess Stacy and George Wettling, it swung like mad. If you look at the label you will see that he put my wife's name down as the composer which, of course, for such an improvisation she could not possibly have been.

Then one day some years later Mezz's marihuana connection, a character known only as 'Mootah Bill', was shot to death in a Pueblo back street. Wherever it had come from around Pueblo, that superior product was never seen again. Mezz tried to keep his trade intact but the only tea he could come up with was inferior. Mezz's affluence waned and never did recover.

Ultimately he was arrested, marihuana, clarinet and all. In open court a Manhattan police official pointed out to the presiding judge that Mezz was largely responsible for the spread of the use of the drug in the Metropolitan area. They gave him a jail term and, despite extensive legal manoeuvering and the application of a good deal of political pressure, Mezz actually did 18 months in the pokey.

Eddie Condon had used Mezz in 1927 in Chicago when he made those famous sides, *Nobody's Sweetheart* and *Lisa*. But Frank Teschmacher played the clarinet. Mezz is credited with playing the cymbals. Gene Krupa was the drummer. I can only imagine that Mezz had delivered a batch of his stuff and Eddie gave him the date in return. The cymbals would have normally been Gene Krupa's responsibility but he was a viper, too, and Mezz had the best stuff after all.

Fats, who, as I have already explained, was not an habitual user of marihuana, liked Mezz. Mezz never quite learned how to tell the truth and he was apt to steal anything not nailed down. Still there was something about this white Chicagoan who wanted to be black that appealed to Fats.

In 1932 when his usual clarinetist, Gene Sedric, had the flu, Fats slipped Mezz in on clarinet for the session and that day his little band made six classic sides including: *How Can You Face Me?; You're Not the Only Oyster in the Stew; Mandy;* and *Serenade for a Wealthy Widow.* Mezz did not disgrace himself but Fats never did use him again.

In time Mezz became so famous that a publisher commissioned an autobiography and a ghost writer to write it. Mezz fought to have his book entitled *Passing For Black.* But the publisher wouldn't take that title, finally deciding to call it *Really the Blues,* which Eddie Condon translated to 'Really the Booze'.

In one of his more spectacular adventures, Mezz actually put together and led a twelve piece thoroughly mixed band for a night club called The Downtown Uproar House. Players included Max Kaminsky, Frankie Newton, Floyd O'Brien, Al Casey, Benny Carter, J. C. Higginbotham, Chick Webb and other famous vipers. He tried to get Fats for the piano chair but Fats, although interested, was busy and Mezz had to settle for Willie 'The Lion' Smith. The band caused a sensation and Mezz got some record dates. On one date he titled an adlib blues *Dissonance.* Bud Freeman, who was his tenor player that day, questioned his choice of title. He said, "Mezz you know Webster defines dissonance as 'a mingling of discordant sounds'". Mezz replied, "Webster doesn't understand the negro."

The National Biscuit Company had plans for a major radio show to be called Let's Dance. Three orchestras were to be featured: a sweet band, a Latin band, and a swing band. In the end Benny Goodman won the competition for the swing band. Benny's triumphant success as the King of Swing followed.

But at one point they were mulling over giving Benny's spot to Mezz Mezzrow's Downtown Uproar House Band. They asked Mezz to play an audition. It was a full dress affair in the major network's main studio, Studio 8H. Mezz beefed up his usual group with a few more hot names. The sponsor's booth was crowded with network executives and big shots from McCann-Erickson, the biscuit company's ad agency. The trouble with such a jazz ensemble, and the great attraction of it too, is that everything is impromptu. Rehearsals don't do much good. Mezz tried to beat off his orchestra but the players couldn't seem to grasp the tempo. No sound issued forth. Mezz turned to the sponsor's booth and said, in explanation, "Man! Am I high!" The execs fled out and the audition was over.

On my usual weekend forays into Harlem I continued to encounter Fats and now he presented to me one more extraordinary attribute. He never seemed to sleep. I managed to stay with him on several long nights but, believe me, it took prodigious stamina. On other occasions it was just impossible to keep up with the man.

Every 'good time flat' operated around the clock, seven days a week, year in year out. Prohibition was on and even when it was lifted new licencing regulations were imposed. But no such rules were observed in these places. You could always get a drink there day or night. In Prohibition days it might be the finest imported spirits, Bacardi from Havana or Haig Dimple from Glasgow, smuggled in from Rum Row, where all during the Volstead Era the fleet of booze freighters rode at anchor just off the three mile limit.

Back then, however, more likely it was simple bootleg hooch, Gordon's Gin or William Penn Rye Whiskey. When you drank it you already knew it was counterfeit and made in somebody's bathtub out of distilled water, medicinal alcohol and Arpeako flavoring. After all you could buy Arpeako on any drug store counter. There was nothing illegal about that. You were often more complimentary about the quality of the labels than you were of the product itself.

For the big bulk of his trade these were the products that Connie Immerman sold and that young Fats Waller had delivered. But there were other places that served you home distilled corn whiskey, said to have the kick of a Georgia mule, and even lower on the scale, some places you got only something known as King Kong which tasted vile but which was wickedly effective.

Teenage Fats had known all these spots. They were scattered all through Harlem. He knew which had pianos and which had not. He practiced on these keyboards whenever and wherever the opportunity presented itself. His poor father would have been grievously shocked had he known where young Fats's delicatessen delivery errands were taking the boy every afternoon after school.

Fats was always keenly devoted to his mother. His relationship with his father was more of a problem. He never spoke of these matters in my presence but the people around him were always whispering about them. His father was a fiercely dedicated religious man. Perhaps it would not be too strong a term to label him a fanatic. He was a fire and brimstone fundmentalist. His religious beliefs were his whole life.

He believed that music should only be heard in church. He was convinced that the theatre, the movies, popular songs and records, and everything pertaining to these things, were instruments of the devil. According to well founded rumour, the day that Fats got the job of playing the organ at the Lincoln Theater, the news provoked a serious family crisis. Such an occupation for his son was strictly against his father's religious principles.

Despite all this Fats did not decline the job, as his father surely prayed that he would. It was said that this caused his father to fall ill. Some said it marked the beginning of a decline in his father's health which ended, some years later, in his death.

I remember when Fats played the Apollo. The Apollo was Harlem's own theatre. Headlining at the Apollo meant that you were the biggest attraction in town. Fats got there through some records that became juke box hits. He'd take a little pickup band into the studio and record whatever they wanted. Sometimes it was his own songs, that was what he seemed to like best, and sometimes it was songs that a publisher had talked, or even bribed, the record company man into waxing.

Then, months later, one of the songs would hit and Fats would be in demand for theatres and dance hall one nighters. By this time he'd completely forgotten the song and they'd have to play his record for him so he could learn it all over again. This time it had been a really big hit so they had booked him into the Apollo where he was doing smash business.

That meant he had to be in the theatre ready to work at ten thirty in the morning. They sometimes did as many as seven shows a day, particularly on Wednesday when they staged their famous midnight amateur show that produced such stars as Sarah Vaughan and Ella Fitzgerald. When Fats conducted this performance it was a spectacle indeed.

Ordinary mortals were exhausted by such bookings. Some famous names folded under the strain. Not Fats! He sailed through it, staying up day after day while drinking vast amounts of hard liquor and brightening all the while. It really was beyond belief. Only those who actually saw it can understand.

You must appreciate that, offstage, there was nothing flamboyant about Fats. He was always well groomed and well tailored in a conservative manner. There was never anything flashy about his off-stage attire nor his demeanour either. When he was on-stage or making a movie, you might see him with a derby hat cocked at an arrogant angle. But that was just a comic prop he picked up from Willie 'The Lion' Smith. Then in later years Jonah Jones picked it up from

Fats. But off-stage I don't think Fats ever even owned a derby.

I particularly recall late one night, after the last show at the Apollo, I was with him as he strolled out of the stage door onto the broad sidewalk of 126th Street and moved west with stately elegance towards Eighth Avenue. In those days whoever was the headliner at the Apollo was the reigning monarch of the Harlem community even if it was only for that one short week.

I drifted along beside Fats and behind us there was a whole entourage moving at the same slow pace. A few inches from the curb Buster Shepherd, a cousin of Anita and Fats's driver and constant companion, drove Fats's gleaming green Lincoln at the same leisurely glide. It all looked like a religious procession in an Italian village on the patron saint's day.

At the corner of Eighth Avenue stood the Braddock Hotel which for more years than anyone can remember has served as the dormitory for the acts, the musicians, the dancers and the showgirls playing the Apollo. When he got to the corner Fats turned left onto Eighth Avenue and his retinue followed, including the Lincoln.

I felt the big car must be there to take Fats home whenever he decided it was time to go. Meanwhile it was a sort of totem, registering the importance of its owner. The fact that it was a Lincoln was in itself symbolic. After all Lincoln was the President who freed the slaves.

Fats had played four vigorous shows that day, signed several hundred programmes, autograph books, record sleeves and photographs, did an interview with Dan Burley of the *Amsterdam News,* whose column everybody in Harlem read, had a dressing room fling with a lusty young dancer, even found a half hour to go on the radio from his dressing room with Fred Robbins, who was then the hottest disc jockey in Greater New York.

Halfway down the block, now we all turned into the main entrance of the Braddock Bar & Grill on the ground floor of the hotel. This was almost the official oasis for the Apollo Theater. It was a long, dark tunnel of a room. In the gloom you could make out a long, long bar that ran along the left hand side of the deep room.

Fats gravitated to the deepest recesses of this bar, where, at almost the end, stood his favourite barkeep, Foster. Foster always attended to the Apollo headliner and the headliner's friends. He was a headliner himself. Fats immortalised him in his hit record *The Joint Is Jumpin'.*

It was now one o'clock in the morning. Quite naturally I assumed that Fats, after an exhausting day, was going to have a drink or two and then go home. I was quite wrong. Fats was chatting affably in the centre of a group of half a dozen, sipping, sipping, sipping, as time slid by.

In those days they closed the Braddock Bar at four in the morning. As they turned out the last lights, Fats and I, all that was left now of the retinue save Buster, sauntered out of the place and turned left on Eighth Avenue. Buster was once again back in the Lincoln, piloting it along beside us at curb's edge. Now we turned left again on 126th Street where a score of steps in slow time later we found the wide entrance to the Apollo Theater with its marquee proclaiming the week's attraction 'Fats Waller & His Rhythm'.

We had been chatting for hours but Fats had never mentioned this destination. Perhaps he just wants to check his billing, I thought. Well, you couldn't blame him for feeling proud of it. But then suddenly he turned sharply and went through the lobby. I followed him as he moved into the dark and empty theater. Fats was now going down an aisle towards the bare stage. I remained at the back of the auditorium. Buster, who had now parked the car directly in front of the theatre, joined me there.

As my eyes became accustomed to the gloom I now noticed that, on stage, actually there was some dim illumination. A naked light bulb hung down from the flies. Directly beneath it stood a bulky shape which I gradually made out to be a Hammond Organ. This was confirmed when a huge chord filled the theatre. I realised that whoever put that light there had done so in the expectation that Fats would be by.

By now Fats was improvising lovely Bach-like music. Perhaps it was Bach. It was four-thirty in the morning and I was now quite tired. My stamina was at its lowest ebb. I turned to Buster standing beside me in the back of the hall. "He never mentioned to me that he was coming over here," I said. "I wonder how long he'll be?"

Buster grinned. "He comes here every night when they shut down the Braddock. He loves to play that organ!" A great crescendo filled the house. "Nobody knows how long he'll play. Not even Fats," Buster went on." He might even keep right on playing until the first show." That was coming up in a little less than six hours, I guessed, after looking at my watch.

"What about sleep?" I asked. "Oh, at the Apollo Fats doesn't bother too much about that," Buster replied. "He might catch a little nap between shows."

The rich music was pouring through the theatre as, in some desperation, I made an excuse that I was expected at home, then turned and fled out of the theatre towards home and bed. I remember feeling quite guilty about leaving while Fats was playing so magnificently but I was too beat to appreciate it.

It was some months before I saw him again. This time I was feeling great. I resolved to outstay him tonight no matter what. I found him in Harlem and we rambled around the whole place together from piano to piano. He sat down and played in night clubs, bars and finally after hours joints. In the end we ran out of pianos. So he took me to his home. That was the only piano left.

At that time he was living on an upper floor of an old tenement on Morningside Heights. It must have been about five when Fats took out a key and opened the front door. Everything was very quiet, no one was stirring. No one at all.

It was a railroad flat with a deep, narrow airshaft running through the whole building from top to bottom. We came into the living room which was almost filled by a beautiful Steinway Grand.

Even before Fats's name was known to the general public, he had been discovered by Fritz Steinway, heir to that fine piano company. Whenever Fats needed a piano he had this man's personal attention. Fats would go down to The Steinway Company, which was on West 57th Street almost across from Carnegie Hall, and Fritz would show him all the grands on hand. Fats would play them and pick out those, the actions and tones of which, he particularly liked. Then, when he went on tour, playing theatres and night clubs, they reserved two of these grands for him: one to be where he was working; the other to be in transit to his next stand.

It was plain that the piano in his living room was a special instrument. He sat at it now, and despite the hour, he now began playing it at full volume. "Don't worry," he explained, "I can play here at any time. Why the old man who lives just below sometimes calls out requests and I am always delighted to oblige."

In Fats's own special way he was playing exquisitely; things I'd never heard before, as well as new variations on more familiar themes. As he sat at the keyboard his only view was through a window facing directly at that airshaft. Some housewife had rigged up a line the whole length of the airshaft on a set of pulleys. Clothespins held several dozens of brilliant white diapers to that line and they were all fluttering in the early morning breeze. It was easy to see where the inspiration for that classic composition, *Clothesline Ballet,* had come from.

This impromptu concert went on for some time. A hall opened into the living room. I knew that this corridor, like that clothesline, ran the whole length of the apartment and all the bedrooms opened off of it. Now I began to hear some sounds from this direction.

Fats had never introduced me to his wife or to any members of his family. They were bound to think that I was the one who had been keeping him out all night. I might be suspected also of encouraging him to drink so much. There was also one more question. In our midnight rambles through Harlem, I had often seen Fats dallying with a pretty girl or two. I knew all about this. The question was; did his wife know. It seemed to me time to take it on the lam. I made my adieus to Fats and scarpered.

Fats loved all piano players. He showered them all with compliments whenever he heard them. I must believe that in his innermost heart he knew absolutely that he was the best. But he was always most gracious in the presence of his peers.

He expressed open-mouthed astonishment at whatever Joey Bushkin might be playing. He had a special reverence for Earl Hines. Whenever he encountered Lee Wiley he inevitably made a point of expressing admiration for the playing of Jess Stacy, knowing that she was enamoured of Jess. He was forever congratulating Eddie Condon on the musicianship of Joe Sullivan, or Alex Hill, or Dave Bowman or Gene Shroeder, or whoever sat in Eddie's piano chair at the moment.

Fats always kept track of such things. He even had some Harlem piano players close to him who determinedly attempted to play like him, an impossible feat on the face of it. His great friend, Hank Duncan, accomplished this better than anyone else. In fact Hank did it so well that Eddie Condon got him hired as the intermission pianist at Nick's down in the Village.

When told the Art Tatum was in the audience, Fats proclaimed, "We have God in the house tonight." Of course we must realise that Art Tatum had actually come to hear Fats Waller play and this announcement underlined this otherwise salient fact. Teddy Wilson was another of Fats's special favourites. It is a fact that one afternoon in Milt Gabler's Commodore Record Shop I actually overheard Teddy Wilson, helping one of his piano students make a selection of recorded piano solos for study, suggest that she take the set of Fats Waller solos rather than the set of Art Tatums.

Of all jazz piano players, however, Fats reserved a special place for Mary Lou Williams. One day, reminiscing about the Connie's Inn days, Fats said to me, "She came down there one afternoon while we were rehearsing a new cabaret and she played for me. Right then I like to have adopted that child." Instead he had Connie Immerman hire her as his substitute.

She was a keen student and she regarded him as The Master, the perfect virtuoso of the jazz piano. "He'd slip away from Connie's for an hour or so to play a turn at the Lafayette Theatre down the street," Mary Lou recalled to me. "While he was gone I'd play for him and I was lucky to get the work. But more than that I was thrilled to bits to get a compliment from Fats because, without any doubt, he was the greatest. I will never forget watching him whenever they rehearsed a new show for next week at Connie's.

More often than not he hadn't really prepared anything. Leonard Harper, who was staging the shows, would be out on the floor with all the chorus girls. 'In this spot the girls do a dance number at about this tempo,' and Leonard would snap his fingers in time. Instantly Fats began to play something at that tempo, something brand new, and Leonard would begin working out a routine. What Fats had played was something he had composed on the spot.

What always amazed me," Mary Lou went on, "was how much Fats enjoyed doing it. It was no work for him at all. The music just came out of him like a fountain. I've actually watched him as he composed all eight melodies for the next week's show while accompanying the rehearsal and without losing a minute of time. He was an extraordinarily gifted composer. There was never anybody else like him.

Unfortunately, it seemed to come so easy that the music business underrated him. I put the musical quality, and the originality of his composition, right up there with the best of George Gershwin, Vincent Youmans and Irving Berlin."

Late one afternoon, just as I was about to leave my office, I had a phone call from Fats. He was in midtown, he told me. He'd just had a meeting with his new man, Ed Kirkeby, and the Victor people. And if I wanted to go uptown with him he'd pick me up. I went down into Madison Avenue, saw the big green Lincoln and jumped into the back seat with Fats. This was the first time I had heard Ed Kirkeby's name. No further explanation was offered.

Fats then took me to somebody's apartment in Harlem where there was a nice upright and a parlour bar. Thus the evening began. We made another stop. And then another. It was now sometime after nine oclock in the evening and we were moving along 125th Street in the Lincoln. It looked to me that we were going to the Apollo and so we were. It was Thursday, and in those days the new show at the Apollo always opened on a Thursday. I now saw that Fats had timed this arrival perfectly.

Count Basie was playing in Kansas City when he was discovered by John Hammond. Perhaps you'll recall that Hammond was listening to a Basie broadcast on a radio in a car parked outside the Sherman Hotel in Chicago. Benny Goodman was sitting beside John Hammond and the two of them decided that this band was so good that it deserved a wider audience.

John Hammond then turned agent Willard Alexander loose on Count Basie who got him a Decca record deal, added half a dozen players to the band, and started booking him. This headline week at the Apollo was the band's first exposure in New York.

All the publicity was about Kansas City. But the truth was that Bill Basie was a special protegé of Fats Waller in Harlem. When young Fats Waller played the intermission organ in the Lincoln Theater in Harlem, young Bill Basie used to sit in the front row right behind him. He was Fats Waller's earliest dedicated fan. Fats had given him lessons on the organ.

When Count Basie had just got his big band contract with Decca, the very first side he recorded was Fats's most famous melody, then and still today, *Honeysuckle Rose.* That Thursday evening we got to the Apollo and the place was packed. Basie, resplendant in his first ever set of white tie and tails on his opening night, was overjoyed to see Fats coming down the aisle. I assure you he wept with joy, I could clearly see the tears running down his face.

By this time Fats was on the stage and, as the crowd recognised him, the whole place exploded with applause. Fats played with the band and there was a standing ovation. Then Bill Basie sat at the piano and the band stomped out that new band's first recording, *Honeysuckle Rose*, which everyone in the theatre knew was Fats Waller's song.

Basie played it just as Fats might have played it. Just for that moment he abandoned his usual economic style and played the full keyboard with both hands. It really sounded like Fats to me for a moment. The audience stomped and shouted. No one who was there that night will ever be able to forget it. There were no announcements. Nothing was said. But all knew that this was a unique musical occasion. I thanked Fats from the bottom of my heart for arranging that I was there to see and hear it.

I sometimes called Fats Tom or even Thomas. I thought it more dignified, especially when we were alone together. Fats realised my intention and smiled in appreciation. But I soon came to appreciate that he really preferred to be called Fats. Fats was the name the public recognised and it was his billing. He liked it. Once you knew that you could call him by no other name.

Even in those days everybody knew that too much drink was bad for the health. Yet many jazz artists couldn't seem to escape from drinking heavily. The music was only played in places that sold the stuff. They were always organising a benefit for some jazz player.

Fats was the heaviest boozer I ever encountered anyplace. In 1934 I lived for a year in Paris with Malcolm Lowry as a roommate. He was a jazz fanatic, too. He particularly loved Joe Venuti and Eddie Lang's Blue Five with Jimmy Dorsey and Adrian Rollini playing *Pink Elephants On The Ceiling,* which in itself was a comment on Delirium Tremens. He had a cardboard wind-up phonograph and that one record. We didn't have any other records. We must have played that one ten thousand times.

Then in the 1950s I hung out in Dublin and New York with Brendan Behan. Both Malcom Lowry and Brendan Behan were heavy drinkers, too, but nowhere near Fats in the consistency of the drinking and in the amounts consumed.

Fats's palliative against boredom was the gin. The only alternative according to Fats was, "Step out the window and turn right. Cement!" He often uttered that line. It made him laugh. It made me sad.

Dave Tough died at forty on a bender. Bob Zurke died in his cups at thirty-two. The gifted Beiderbecke only lasted twenty-eight short years. Some of the greatest players died of drink. But nobody I ever personally saw drank as much as Fats. His closest contender was Eddie Condon.

Eddie drank every night, until the last place closed. That was his policy. He was working at the Famous Door on Fifty-second Street. Eddie was working in Bunny Berigan's little band. Young Joey Bushkin, just out of short pants was the piano player, Forrest Crawford was playing tenor, Cozy Cole was playing the drums and Mort Stuhlmaker played bass. It was a great little band and musicians used to come by to sit in. One of these was a fine clarinetist who just happened to be a medical intern. "We called him Doc Slovak and he could really play that thing," Joey Bushkin remembers.

Just across the street was the Onyx Club. Eddie always made it a point to have an intermission retreat. This was his alternative bar close to where he worked. When he worked at Nick's this was Julius's. But now at the Famous Door, it was the Onyx.

Johnny Meagher was the bartender at the Famous Door and he loved Eddie. Joe Helbock was the barkeep at the Onyx and he was also a keen admirer of Eddie. Between the two of these advocates Eddie sailed through the nights in an alcoholic haze. As a result he ultimately encountered a particularly brutal hangover. In those days Eddie lived in a decrepit deadfall called the Elk's Hotel, under the El on West Fifty-third Street. When he checked in there they asked him for a name and number to call in case there was any trouble.

"I guess I was the only guy he knew who had a phone," Joey Bushkin recalls. "Anyway, he put down my number. I only had a phone because I was still living at home with my father and mother, uptown on One Hundred and Fourth Street."

The hangover was so bad Eddie decided to go on the wagon. Of course Eddie's idea of going on the wagon was unorthodox. He decided to drink nothing but beer. There was some very powerful home brew going on at the time and Eddie told Johnny Meagher to chill up a case of twenty-four bottles for his exclusive use that night. Eddie drank the lot before the place closed.

He managed to get home to his cell at the Elk's all right. It was only a few blocks away. But the next morning he didn't wake up. In alarm, the hotel called the number Eddie had written down when he registered.

Joey Bushkin recalls, "They called me. I grabbed a cab immediately and dashed downtown to the Elk's. Eddie wasn't unconscious by this time but he was doubled over in extreme pain. Of course I didn't know what was wrong. He was just in very bad shape. The place he was living in was a real crumb joint, he even had a broken window in his room. The hotel thought he should go right to a hospital and they suggested the Polyclinic which was a few blocks further west.

Suddenly I remembered that clarinet player. The Polyclinic was where he worked. I said, 'Wait a minute,' and I ran over to the hospital and found our brother musician, Doc Slovak. I told him what was up and he dashed back with me to the Elk's.

When Doc saw Eddie he was really alarmed. He said, 'There's no point in taking him to the Polyclinic now. The wrong head surgeon is on. He'll just say, This patient is inoperable. It's a case of acute pancreatitis.' He regards the mortality for that condition as one hundred per cent. He'll just say, 'Try to make him as comfortable as possible until he expires.' Then he gave Eddie an injection to ease the tremendous pain.

Finally he said, 'Let's take a chance and keep him here in the hotel for another day because Dr. McGrath, the great stomach surgeon is coming on duty tomorrow. If anybody can save him, he can.' So I stayed with Eddie and Doc dropped in every few hours and gave Eddie another shot. I went home, put on my dinner jacket, which was the band uniform, and came right back to the Elk's. Then I went to the job. That night between Johnny Meagher and Joe Helbock every musician on Fifty-second Street knew that it was touch-and-go with Eddie. After work I came right back to Eddie at the Elk's. I was in touch with Doc all the time and every once in a while he'd dash in and give Eddie another shot. Eventually Doc told me it was time to take Eddie over to the Polyclinic.

I got Eddie into a cab and we took off for the hospital. But the cab, bouncing around, threw Eddie into paroxysms of pain. So we got out and tried to make it on foot. Eddie was walking like a monkey but we eventually got there. A couple of male nurses with a table on wheels were waiting just outside. They laid Eddie out and wheeled him up to the operating theater and Dr. McGrath took over.

The operation went on for a very long time. I was beat. I had been up for most of two days. I fell asleep on a chair in the corridor. After some hours Doc Slovak came out and woke me up. He said, 'There's no use waiting around. He's not going to make it.' I went home very depressed. The next day I went straight to the hospital. Eddie was still alive but only just. They needed transfusions of blood.

They decided that they couldn't use mine because I wasn't twenty-one yet. My father and my brother went to the hospital and volunteered. Then all the guys in the band came, Bunny, Forrest, Cozy, Morty. Within a few hours half the musicians from Fifty-second Street were there offering their blood. Even the bartenders came. It just depended on what type you were. Johnny Meagher, for one, turned out to have the right kind and he gave a pint or two. They didn't want any from Joe Helbock and he was disappointed."

The transfusions continued for some days as Eddie lapsed in and out of consciousness.

In the middle of one of these Eddie came to and demanded to know what was going on. The doctor explained that he was giving him blood. Condon responded instantly, "It must be Fats Waller's 'cause I'm swingin'!" That night this line ran up and down Fifty-second Street like a breeze, cheering up the musicians who had all but given up Eddie for good. Pee Wee Russell said, "Eddie talked the Reaper out of his dues!"

In time, a matter of some weeks, Eddie managed to get out of the Polyclinic and reported back on the bandstand at the Onyx. Dr. Joe Slovak turned out to be a very fine hot clarinetist indeed and in later years Eddie featured him in a number of his concerts at Town Hall and other places. In fact the day came when the doctor had to decide whether he wanted to switch careers, give up medicine for good and play the clarinet professionally. He declined to do this and now has his own clinic in Schenectady, New York.

It would be wonderful to be able to say that Eddie tapered off his drinking and modulated down to moderation. I'm afraid that wouldn't be true. He always insisted to the end of his days that it wasn't the alcohol that put him in the Polyclinic. "That beer was just too cold!" he reasoned. Knowing Eddie as well as I did I had to think he actually meant it.

I remember years later when Eddie worked at Nick's and spent his intermissions across the street in the bar at Julius's, he often took a day's hiatus from his steady scotch and soda diet and, just for the day, mind you, went on the beer wagon. Only at Julius's he didn't drink beer on these occasions. He drank Guinness from St. James Gate, Dublin.

Harold Fitzimmons, the head barkeep at Julius's, would put aside a twenty-four bottle case of Guinness behind the bar just for Eddie. Eddie claimed he didn't really like the taste of Guinness. "That first one is so bitter," he was inclined to protest, "but the twenty-fourth one tastes like French pastry!"

I remember one evening, it must have been about seven, I ran uptown looking for Fats. I looked into the Braddock Bar. It was half empty. I decided I'd walk back and ask Foster if he had any idea where I might find him. As I walked down into the room towards Foster's station I noticed just at that moment that I was the only white in the place.

As I looked in that direction I could see that he was busy with a cluster of dignified looking black men just past middle age. They were well groomed and richly attired but they surely were not in show business. I guessed they might be well paid butlers and chauffeurs from some of those millionaires's mansions down along Fifth Avenue where they still prefer blacks for such jobs.

As I came to this conclusion I noted that although they had just been served their drinks they had turned and were all staring at me, the only white face in the saloon. When they realized that I was heading for Foster, they turned as one man, tossed off their drinks, then moved straight out of the Braddock.

I realised that, as at the Abysinnian Baptist Church so long ago, I was being given a signal that I was invading the privacy of blacks. These men, who had probably been working for whites all day, now objected to my presence here in the evening in their private black place. The signal was clear and unmistakable. I turned on my heel and left the Braddock and returned downtown.

Usually, however, when I went up town I found him, and without troubling anyone. I would drift around to his various waterholes until I ran into him. He always seemed glad to see me, so the search seemed to be worthwhile. Of course sometimes he was on the road. Or in Hollywood. A musician in a bar would give me the news.

One day the news was unhappy. Gene Sedric, who could be spotted a block away by the sharp camel's hair wraparound overcoat he featured back then, passed me the word that Fats was sick in bed. 'The alcohol has caught up with him!' was my first thought. Gene's report seemed to confirm it.

Gene had been to see him at home in the Morningside Heights apartment. He was evidently very, very ill. "He won't let a doctor in and his wife is terribly worried," said Gene. Apparently the booze had caused some sort of rheumatic reaction. "He hurts all over, man" said Gene.

He then described in detail how Fats's arms and legs and torso were wrapped in wet bandages. "Wet bandages?" I had never heard of such a thing. "Yes, he's all wrapped in cotton that has been soaked in some medication," Gene was now giving me a visual explanation in pantomime. "They even wrapped his fingers and his hands! They have to put new stuff on every few hours. Man, poor Fats is really suffering!"

According to Gene, Fats was lying flat out with his arms akimbo and he'd been in this state for some days. He had no idea what the medication was but since no doctor was on hand I guessed it must have been some homeopathic remedy. Whatever it was it seemed to work and Fats was soon up and around again.

Jack Robbins, the publisher, knew I was a special friend of Fats. I had mentioned my anxiety about his illness. One afternoon Jack called me at my office. "Your boy's downtown," he said, "He just came into the building. He must be making a record date in one of the studios upstairs."

I beatled across town to 799 Seventh Avenue where Jack's office was and in a studio on the fourth floor here was Fats, quietly sitting at a piano. He gave me a big smile but he didn't seem to have much to say. The usual gin bottle wasn't on the piano so I said, trying to make conversation, "Are you on the wagon?" He thought this was very funny and he nodded affirmatively. So far he hadn't said a word.

Directly across the street was Charlie's Tavern, a refuge for musicians for many years. They used to sell you a quart of cold draft beer, to go, in a buff coloured cardboard tube about a foot long and four inches in diameter. I now saw Buster, in a great hurry, rushing one of these cylinders out of the elevator and through the studio door. He put it on the piano.

Buster and I both went into the control room as they were just about to record. I looked through the control room window and saw Fats in the studio taking a huge draft out of the Charlie's Tavern tube. I said to Buster, "Look at him! He does love that beer!"

Buster, startled, turned and stared at me. "That's not beer," he said, "That's a fifth of Madeira Wine, some cracked ice and a little Coca-Cola." Whatever it was Fats was enjoying it and soon he was his usual talkative and laughing self again. I never sampled this curious mixture myself, but it was plain to see that as a restorative for Fats in his present condition it worked wonders. The next time I saw him he was back on the gin, buckets of it.

Despite the insurance that Fritz Steinway's patronage offered Fats, he was always running into bad pianos. One night he came down to Nick's to see Eddie Condon. Nick Rongetti who owned the place considered himself a master ragtime pianist. He was not. He knew some of the tunes, by ear, it should be added, but he had a touch like Primo Carnera.

He had two small uprights on the night club floor just in front of the raised bandstand with a small grand up there for the orchestra. He employed some of the greatest jazz players of the day and expected them to permit him to play with them once in a while. This expectation met with stiff resistance.

When Fats came into the place that night the band was playing. Fats rushed directly to the nearest piano, which was one of the uprights on the floor. He sat down and started to play but it sounded like a busted zither. He instantly got up as the band still played on and he moved to the second upright. After a chord or two he rejected this one as well and then climbed up on the bandstand where Dave Bowman was playing the small grand.

Dave with a grin, rose from the piano bench and Fats sat down and started to play with the band. Eddie, who was vigorously playing his guitar, looked over and asked, "Is that one all right, Fats?"

Fats replied, "It's pine but I'm the master of it!" You had to love Fats. Even when the deck was stacked against him, he smiled and made the best of it.

One Sunday evening Eddie and I were walking on First Avenue in the Fifties. We had just come From a cocktail party in that neighborhood. Suddenly here's Fats. Whatever brought him to that part of town I have no idea.

The three of us were standing there chatting when a tall blond teenager came up to us. Eddie and I knew him slightly. He was Hotch Ely, a rich kid from Old Lyme, Connecticut, who used to hang around the bandstand wherever the best musicians played. He knew it was bad form to crowd in on us like that, but he just couldn't resist the urge to meet Fats Waller and he was trying to make the most of it.

"Would you like to meet Agatha Christie?" he asked right out of the blue. He was addressing himself to Eddie and Fats. I must confess I rather doubted that either Eddie or Fats had ever read that particular author. But Eddie surprised me. He asked, "English writer, isn't she?" Fats said nothing. He was going to let Eddie do all the talking.

Now that young Hotch had their attention he was so eager he looked like he was about to boil over. He leaned back his considerable height and pointed sharply up towards the sky. "My mother's got a condominium up in that building," he was indicating a skyscraper that began only a few steps away and went straight up for a long ways. "Agatha Christie's my mother's guest up there on the thirty-eighth floor", he went on. Eddie looked at Fats, Fats looked at me, nobody said anything. I suppose we could have said, "We're busy, get lost!" But nobody did, he was a nice kid loaded with enthusiasm.

Instead Eddie said, quite calmly, "Is there a piano up there?" This was an eminently sensible query. "Oh, yes! A wonderful grand. My mother's had it for years," was Hotch Ely's instant reply. Fats was smiling. Now Eddie asked the only question left, "Is it in tune?" And Hotch replied, "Of course! Do you think my mother would allow an out of tune piano in her house?"

In a very few minutes we were getting out of an elevator on the thirty-eighth floor, a luxurious apartment overlooking not only the East River but also all of Queens and a good deal of Brooklyn. There were about a dozen very pleasant older ladies and gentlemen and the celebrated author. A butler was pouring Johnny Walker Black Label which served to break the ice most efficiently.

As the introductions were made it was clear that these nice people didn't quite know who in the world Eddie and Fats might be but they were more than pleased to meet anyone of whom young Hotch was so fond. They smiled and nodded.

There was the piano, a highly-polished, shining, mahogany instrument. Fats was already sitting at the piano, a butler placed the Waterford crystal tumbler holding a generous measure of the scotch on a coaster. Now Fats was trying to open the cover above the keyboard. It seemed to be stuck and then suddenly it sprang open, bringing with it several little dusty clouds. It hadn't been opened in some time.

Then Fats began an arpeggio and we knew the awful truth. The piano was a half a tone out. This is the moment that I expected Fats to rise and make his way to the door. But he showed no sign at all of any dismay. Instead he smiled as he played The *St. Louis Blues,* covering the entire keyboard, and as he did so that unique mind of his was operating like a computer, discovering which notes were fit to play and which keys would finesse the notes which were not.

Then he played for about an hour, non-stop, and you might have thought that the piano was practically in tune. It was a remarkable demonstration. Agatha Christie, a grey-haired lady in a frock from the school of Mother Hubbard, shook Fats's hand warmly and said she had never in her entire days ever heard anything quite like it. We left and as we thanked our hostess at the door I heard Eddie whisper to her that she must have that instrument tuned as soon as possible. She assured him that this would be done, but I am afraid that she was innocently under the impression that Fats had put it out of tune.

Sometimes when I came up to look for Fats he was away on tour. Often this turned out to be an engagement or two in Chicago, the town where Eddie had first heard of him.

By this time Fats was very well connected in Chicago. One of the biggest wheels in town was Ernie Byfield who, among other things, owned some of the best hotels in the city, including the Ambassador East and the Sherman.

Ernie Byfield loved the jazz music. He particularly loved Fats and he often paid an extravagant fee to bring Fats out his way for a private party or two. But although Mr. Byfield often hospitably assigned a room to Fats at his Sherman, I never knew Fats to stay there. Instead he swung out to the South Side, the Harlem of Chicago, where he took a suite at the DuSable.

I don't know exactly how he arranged it, but somehow just before Fats checked in, a Hammond Organ was always installed in that suite. There was a bar cum night club on the ground floor of the DuSable. But for those in the know, whenever Fats was in town the action was up in Suite 506. You could hardly miss it because you could hear that organ all over the hotel. And nobody ever even thought of complaining.

In those days big bands were the fashion. But Fats travelled with his little five piece group. One week the Regal Theater decided to put two small band combos on instead of one big band.

They booked Fats & His Rhythm. And they booked Muggsy Spanier's Ragtime Band. They set them up on the big stage with the two grand pianos end to end. Fats sat on the right. And on the left, almost back to back, was little Joey Bushkin.

In the centre of the proscenium arch they had rigged up two huge thermometers with a series of legends in between and, when Fats played, a red line, simulating the mercury, would rise higher and higher. Then Muggsy's band would play and their thermometer would go up and up. Then the two bands would play together and both thermometers would seem to go through the roof.

The show was a smash hit. The day after the opening the theatre announced it was holding the whole show over for a second week. Then as word spread about the sensational show at the Regal, The State Lake Theater, the big white theatre in the Loop downtown, anounced that they would headline the same two band show for two weeks. This meant that Fats Waller & his Rhythm and Muggsy Spanier's Ragtime Band had a run of four straight weeks in Chicago.

Joey often has spoken to me about that experience of working with Fats. "It was one of the great lessons of my young life," he explains. "I don't mean the piano, although there will always be plenty to learn there. For all time, Fats must be recognized as just about the greatest all around piano player and with no serious contenders. I mean what I found to learn, from Fats's way of life. Fats insisted on having fun at all times.

If you're having fun, it isn't work. And Fats managed to have fun all during every show, between shows, all day and all night long. His policy was; if it isn't fun, why do it?

I can remember moments during those shows when Fats, just by the simple beauty of his playing, would reduce that noisy house to total silence. Then, as he delicately trilled in the treble, he would turn to the audience and say softly, 'It's so easy when you know how!' Then the place always errupted in a roar. Of course he did hit the booze pretty hard. But at the time I just reasoned that he had the frame to stand it. I tried to follow him with the booze but I just couldn't make it. But I did resolve to enjoy whatever work I took on or walk away from it. That was a powerful lesson Fats taught me and I have profited richly from it ever since.

The other thing was that Fats never got tired. When there was a wild good time going on I could stay up for a couple of days and nights but then I'd have to fold. It looked like Fats could go on all month. I tried to go along with him but I pulled up short. One night I just retreated to my hotel and slept. The next day I showed up at the State Lake at eleven fifteen for the first show which was at noon and the stage doorman had word that Fats wanted to see me urgently in his dressing room.

I went up to his dressing room and Fats said, 'Where were you last night?' I knew he hadn't been to bed at all and he was staring me straight in the eye. Then he took a bottle of that Gordon's Gin he was featuring and poured out a half a glassful into a water tumbler. He handed it to me and said, 'We have to start even.'

I looked at him and he looked at me. Well I drank it down. What else was there to do? We started laughing and we laughed all day. We did five shows that day and both bands swung like mad. I could never understand when he ever found time to sack out. The only possibility was that he fell out for a big sleep between engagements, the way a bear hibernates."

Today Bushkin is in rude good health, playing better than ever as he moves into his seventh decade, although he looks about half that. He sat in with Ruby Braff and Jack Lesberg the other day in a Manhattan night club and he swung that club right into a standing ovation. As far as I can see he always seems to have a smile on his face. Fats was never short on smiles either.

I remember visiting Fats at the DuSable and eventually leaving his suite at about four in the morning. As I got into the elevator on the fifth floor the full harmonies from Fats's organ filled the place. There was a new elevator boy on duty and his eyes were wide with curiosity. He knew I had just come out of Fats's quarters.

"Did Mr. Waller play over at the Regal all day today?" he asked. I replied that he had, that he'd been playing there all week. "Well I love that music," said the elevator boy. "But what I can't understand is; how can Mr. Waller play at the theatre all day and then come home here to the DuSable and play all night?" I explained that nobody had any answer to that question, least of all me.

At just about that time Eddie Condon formed up a band of eight superb musicians. In the fashion of the time it was decided that it would be a cooperative band, all members of it owning equal shares and getting equal pay. In fact there were nine shareholders to that eight piece band. I was the ninth.

Eddie was going with Paul Smith's sister, Phyllis, who was writing ad copy for Gimbel's department store. She suggested that we call the new band 'The Summa Cum Laude'. We all agreed that was a splendid idea. We had a contract drawn up and all nine of us shareholders signed it. Who would be the band

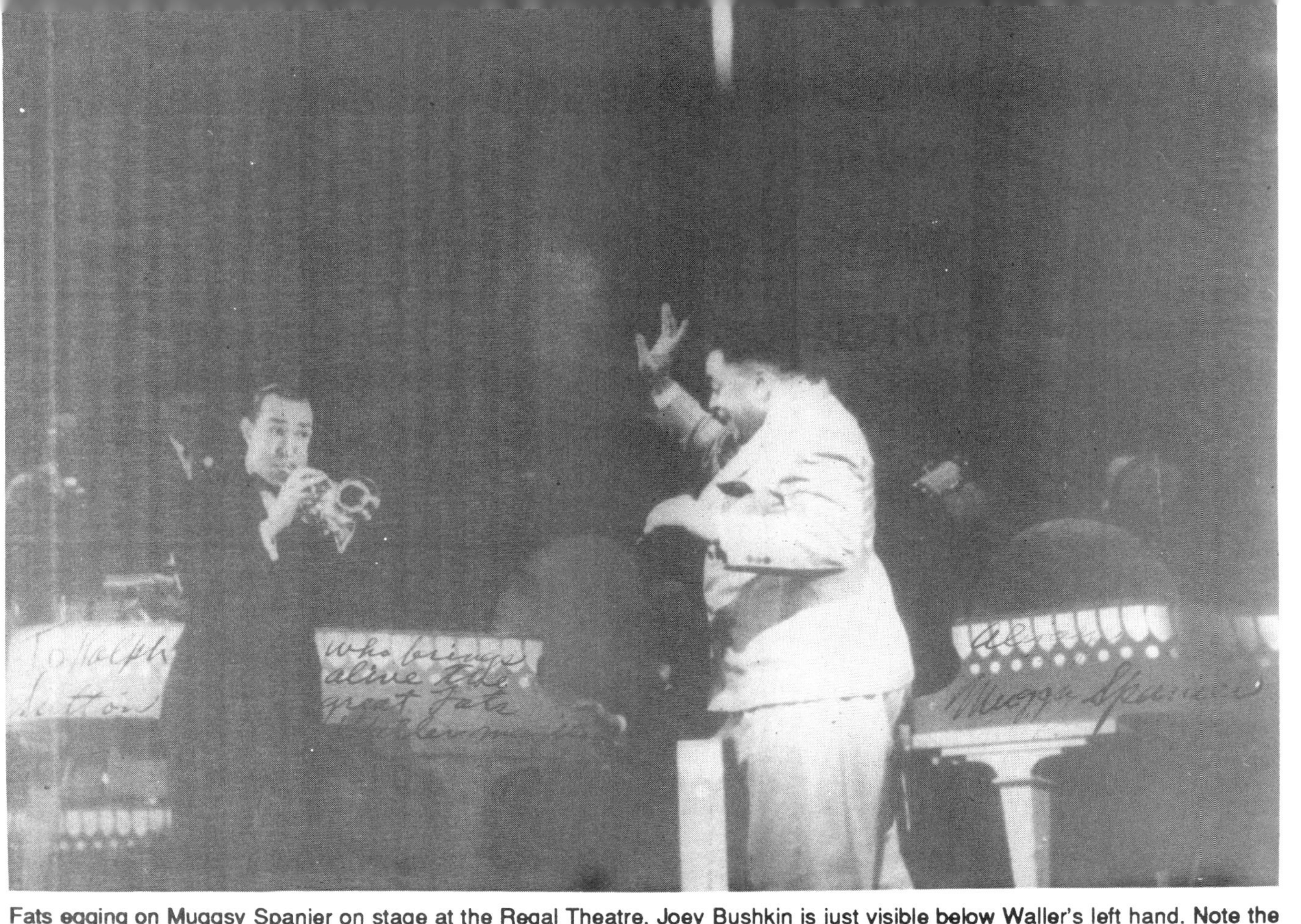

Fats egging on Muggsy Spanier on stage at the Regal Theatre. Joey Bushkin is just visible below Waller's left hand. Note the dedication from Muggsy: "Ralph Sutton who brings alive the great Fats Waller music. Always, Muggsy."

leader? Well, when the band played Eddie was always sitting down playing his guitar.

Bud Freeman stood up, playing his saxophone. Eddie was quite nervous about making any announcements and that sort of thing anyway. Bud Freeman, on the other hand, had histrionic ambitions. He loved to make announcements and talk to the audience. So we all voted to have Bud be in front of the band. This didn't mean he got a dime more than any of us. We all got the same, down to the last penny.

At that time we were the house band at Nick's but we had ambitions for higher things. It looked like we were on our way when we were selected to be featured in a big deluxe Broadway musical called *'Swingin' The Dream'*. Louis Armstrong was in it and so was Benny Goodman's Sextette.

Despite these attractions the show laid an egg. It folded in two weeks and we had no job at all. Nick was mad because we'd taken that show job in the first place. Now he wouldn't let us go back to work at his place. 'The Summa Cum Laude' was in grave danger of curling right up and expiring.

Lips Page had been working in a sleazy night spot called 'The Brick Club'. He got a job on the road, so he recommended us to this joint and they offered us the job. We didn't have any other work in sight so we took it. Our nine shares of the net income from this engagement meant that we each got eighteen dollars a week. It was a lifesaver because it kept the band together. How we squared it with the musicians union I have no idea but they let us go ahead with it.

'The Brick Club' was on the ground floor of a notorious Mafia hotel on Forty-seventh Street between Sixth and Seventh Avenues. Lucky Luciano had run this place and in an effort to clean it up they named it the Hotel America and a huge electric sign outside proclaimed this fact. The club was run by the toughest gangster I ever saw and his name was Harry Brock.

The place was empty almost all the time. There had been so many arrests on that block over the years for drug busts that the newspaper guys all called it Dream Street. The band was playing beautifully. We all wanted to stay together: Maxie Kaminsky, Pee Wee Russell, Brad Gowans and Davie Tough. So we put up with all the unpleasantness of the job.

I remember one evening the band was just great. Harry Brock came up to the bandstand. There were very few people in the place. Harry Brock made Bronco Nagurski look like a choir boy. He stood right in front of Bud and requested that the band play *Melancholy Baby*. He was dead serious. Bud had a very funny line of patter and he started laying it on this gangster.

What he was implying was that 'The Summa Cum Laude' would not be playing *Melancholy Baby*, but it was all well laced with Bud's humour. Harry

Brock listened to all this with no change of expression. Then he unbuttoned his jacket and his coat fell open and plain to see was a big old stained leather holster with a great big pistol in it. He didn't say anything. He just stared at Bud.

There was a pause and then Bud turned around and just said, "Two beats - *Melancholy Baby*" and they just went right into it. They played it for about ten minutes and, I must say, that group played it pretty good. Fortunately a few nights later we got a new job.

Out in Chicago, that jazz lover, Ernie Byfield, had started a new policy at his Panther Room in the Hotel Sherman. Just like at the Regal Theater out on the South Side, here in the Loop instead of featuring a big band he was putting in two small bands. We went in opposite Stuff Smith with Jonah Jones and Cozy Cole. We were thrilled. Stuff's band loved our band and we loved theirs. There was a pop song of the time called *With The Wind And The Rain In Your Hair*. Stuff was a particular fan of Bud Freeman's playing. He used to say, "Bud, play that *Wind And the Rain In Your Moss.*" Then Bud would play the ballad beautifully, Of course, Bud didn't have a speck of hair himself.

The night we opened we discovered that Fats Waller & His Rhythm and some other small combination had just closed. Ernie Byfield loved Fats. He discovered that Fats was particularly fond of a very special scotch called Old Rarity. As an extra bonus to Fats, on the last night of his engagement, he had sent up to Fats's bandstand a whole case of Old Rarity.

All I can say with any certainty is that when Fats left the bandstand that night there was none left. Now Gene Sedric and Herman Autrey hardly drank. Al Casey drank to a certain extent. Bassist Cedric Wallace was no drinker and neither was drummer Slick Jones. Let's say the five of them accounted for three bottles although, honestly, I can't believe it.

What happened to the other nine bottles? Herman Autrey told me that when they packed up their instruments that night there was no Old Rarity left at all. I asked Gene Cedric. He said, "Fats drank it, all of it." This story raced around jazz circles. Dr. Joe Slovak refused to believe it. He said firmly, "Two or three bottles should be a lethal dose." I said, "Doc, you'd better revise that because I've actually seen Fats drink more gin than that myself."

I asked Fats, when I next saw him back in Manhattan. "What about that case of old Rarity at the Panther Room?" "Oh, Man," he exclaimed. "That's very good stuff." I said, "I know that but tell me on your closing night how much of that case Ernie Byfield sent up did you drink?" Fats stared at me in silence. Then, "How many bottles, you mean?" he inquired. When I nodded. He broke into a broad grin and answered, "Man, I don't know but they was delicious."

I began to notice Ed Kirkeby, who now had the official title of Fats Waller's manager. Actually I seldom saw him. He was never around after hours with Fats. It looked to me that he really did not have a whole lot of social contact with Fats. But he was always there when there was money to be transacted, as on the closing night of a theatre engagement.

He did travel with Fats, however, sharing his quarters on the train whenever Fats hit the road. Ed was a dapper little fellow, a caucasian, who had performed as a singer in vaudeville as long as vaudeville lasted. He was slim and well pressed, usually in sharp gray sharkskin, which went well with his small and pointy, waxed moustache. He had a quick smile and a ready line of inoffensive patter.

Since 1916 he had been making phonograph records with one variety turn or another. That date was not only the beginning of his recording career, it was the beginning of the entire record industry. He knew absolutely everybody of any account in that business.

He was especially well connected with the people at the Victor label. It was through Victor that he became Fats's manager. On various labels he had been a featured vocalist with such turns as The California Ramblers and the Goofus Five, just to name two. Sometimes he had taken over the duties of band manager, especially to set up record dates.

His last show business adventure had been to launch a new career as a singing bandleader. In this effort he had recorded a whole batch of sides. The label for this venture was Bluebird, a subsidiary of Victor. Perhaps it is significant that on his very first side of this batch Ed Kirkeby sang *I'm Gonna Sit Right Down And Write Myself A Letter*.

He made this record just seven months after Fats had first originated the song on Victor. Fats's recording had been a hit. His was not. His career as a singing bandleader went out the window.

He was a strange choice to take over Fats's affairs and I got the impression that it suited Victor more than it suited Fats. It reminded me of Ralph Peer's selection of Eddie Condon as the proper choice to bring Fats to his record dates, on time, properly rehearsed and cold sober.

By the time he first encountered Ed Kirkeby, Fats had already been making records for fifteen years. He had developed his own way of going about it and he continued to operate according to the same unorthodox routine. When Duke Ellington, or Benny Goodman, or even Eddie Condon made records in those days, they'd make four sides and the date was over. But at his dates Fats would sit at his piano surrounded by his little band. There would be a bottle of gin with a glass and some ice just above the keyboard and Fats would knock off as many as thirteen sides at a crack. If he ran out of gin, Buster was always there to run in another fifth.

Fats could have given them thirteen originals every time. But the publishing contacts of the record people were always pressing new songs on him. Fats was always an amiable man. He'd knock out practically anything they gave him and then he'd go back to doing his own stuff.

I'm Gonna Sit Right Down And Write Myself A Letter was such a song that some publisher had brought to Victor. They handed it cold to Fats. He worked out a little routine for it with his players and made it and then went on to something else. It became the biggest hit he ever had and will be associated with him forever.

The melody of the song had been written by one of the Tin Pan Alley greats, Fred Ahlert. Among his other songs were pop classics, *I'll Get By* and *Mean To Me*. The lyric was written by Joe Young. Other artists made recordings of the song, including, curiously enough, Spooky Dickinson with Red McKenzie's Mound City Blue Blowers, Chick Bullock, Slim Green and also Wingy Manone. But only Fats Waller's version became a solid hit.

The other day I asked another gifted pianist, Dick Hyman, if he had any idea why Fats record of *I'm Gonna Sit Right Down And Write Myself A Letter* was so successful. Dick replied, "Actually I have studied that particular record and tried to analyze its appeal. I believe that the main factor was tempo. Fats established a light tempo with a lot of swing, and that is what caught the public's ear."

At the time it turned out to be one of the sides that he had to learn all over again after it had become a hit and was playing on juke boxes all across the land and spinning on radio disc jockey turntables everywhere. It brought him a whole rack of theatre and dance hall engagements.

On all these sides Fats was invariably accompanied by his little five piece band. They were always billed as 'Fats Waller & His Rhythm'. The virtues of this ensemble didn't appeal to Ed Kirkeby. He thought Fats should have a big band like so many other attractions at the time, attractions such as, say, Jan Savitt and his Orchestra.

At first Fats resisted this proposal because he felt that he now had his little band swinging just the way he liked. Then a compromise was effected. Victor made a date in which the little combination was expanded by another half a dozen players. On the label the billing now was 'Fats Waller, His Rhythm And His Orchestra'.

Unhappily the box-office explosion that Ed Kirkeby had been predicting never turned up. The new big band proved to be a much less of a draw than the small band so it was quickly abandoned, to Fats's relief. Ed Kirkeby's next move was to book him in Europe with no band .

The musicians's union in England was run by a militant communist named Hardie Ratcliffe. He was anti-American to the core. Before he came to power in the union there were American bands, such as Hal Kemp, playing very successfully in the West End of London. He put an end to that.

Fats, however, as an entertainer without an orchestra, came in under the auspices of another union which covered variety artists. It was the summer of 1938. Back then you went to Europe by boat. On arrival, Fats was wonderfully received by the musicians and jazz fans of England. They were always keener about jazz there than they ever were in America, the home of the music. The English still are.

Fats had a wonderful tour of the music halls, always performing as a single. Ed Kirkeby also managed to arrange to have him record there for His Master's Voice which was an associate of Victor. He made a half a dozen sides with a small band of British players including George Chisholm and Edmundo Ross. Those labels read 'Fats Waller & His Continental Rhythm' and the British Musicians's Union permitted the date as that of an American Variety Artist accompanied by British musicians.

Then he made eight more sides on organ, practically all spirituals, with Adelaide Hall singing on two popular song sides including *I Can't Give You Anything But Love,* the melody which he wrote, then sold to another songwriter. Adelaide Hall had come to England with *'The Blackbirds of 1928'* and stayed. The last time I looked she was still there, and still stopping shows in concert halls and night clubs at the majestic age of eighty-one.

In Paris, on a previous visit, Fats had been greeted by Marcel Dupré, the master organist who recorded for Victor's Red Seal classical label. One afternoon he took Fats to a cathedral which Marcel Dupré said had the finest organ in Europe. Fats always assumed that this was Notre Dame cathedral, the only cathedral he had ever heard of in Paris. Actually it was not Notre Dame. It was another great cathedral, a hundred yards south of St. Germain des Pres, along the rue Bonaparte. This is St. Sulpice. The Cathedral is noted for a pair of huge murals painted in 1856 by Eugene Delacroix the artist, whose studio in the Place de Furstemberg a few blocks away is still maintained as a museum. But when he painted them the church had already been famous for its superb organ for almost a hundred years. Since the organ was first commissioned in 1776, the greatest organists of the day have been appointed to the cathedral staff. Marcel Dupré had been rated the outstanding organist and in consequence had the appointment when Fats came to Paris. All of those Red Seal records Marcel Dupré made for Victor were made with this instrument.

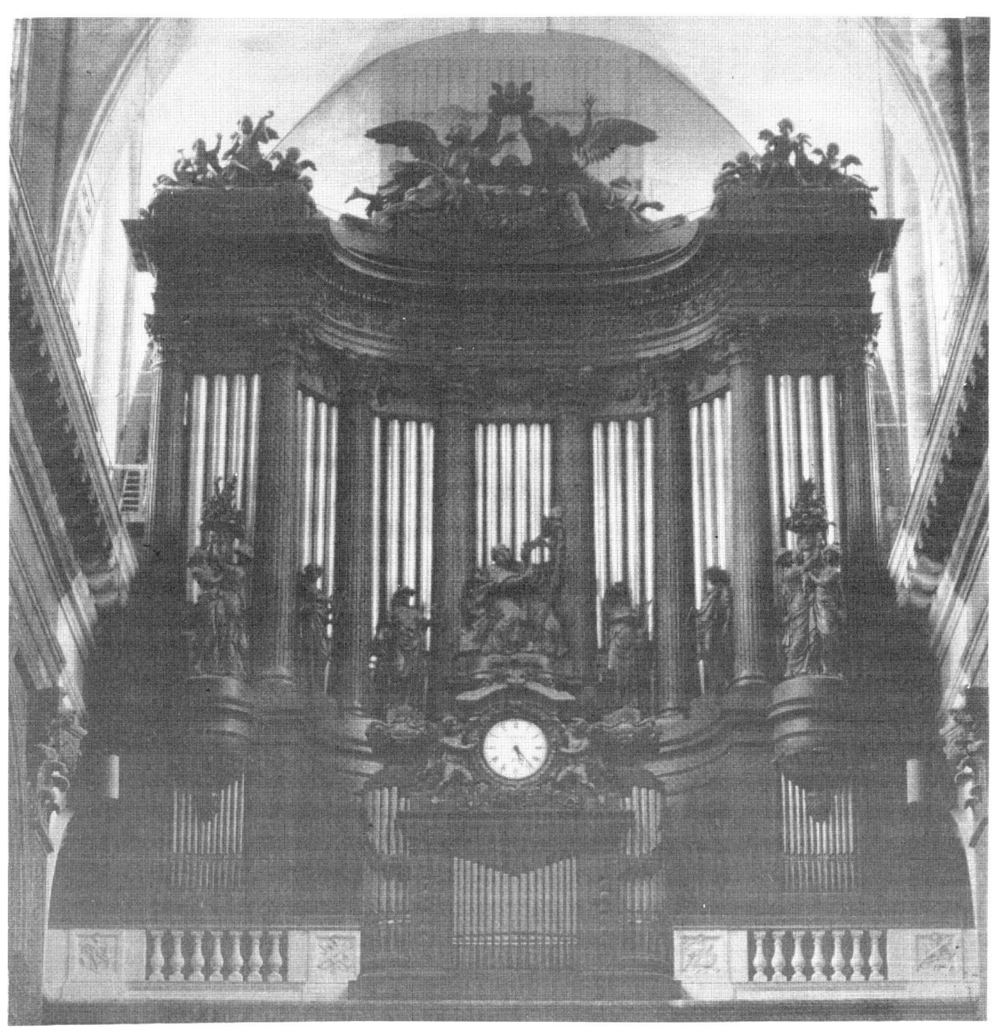

Above: A general view of the Grand Organ Aristide Cavaillé-Coll of Saint Sulpice. It is situated over the main entrance to the cathedral. In the summer of 1991, French newspapers carried an announcement that it was to be renovated and restored by master craftsman Jean Renaud and a team of workers and it was estimated that 15,000 hours of work would be required. No starting date was given for this undertaking and the organ was still in use in the autumn when a Festival of Sacred Music was held in the cathedral in October and November.

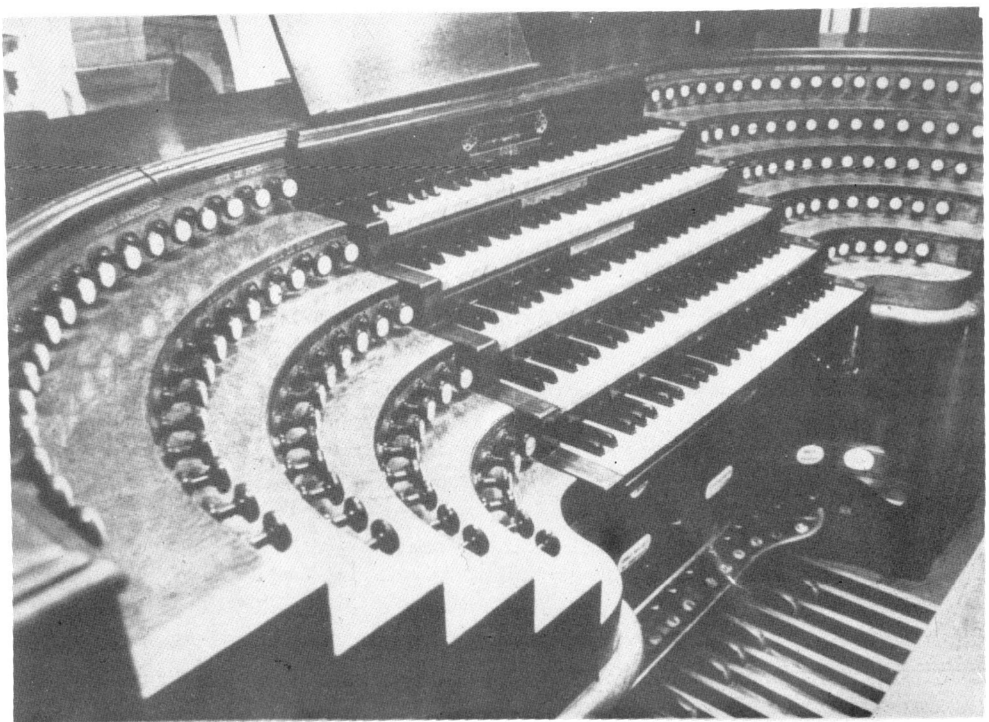

Above: A view of the console of the organ.

Most authorities still consider the St. Sulpice organ the finest in the world. It comprises five manuals, one pedal-board, twenty composition-pedals, one hundred and eighteen tone-qualities, one hundred and two stops, six thousand seven hundred and six pipes and six air-pumps. "It is those air-pumps," Marcel Dupré assured Fats, "that give such a glorious quality of softness to the keyboards."

Fats always told me that the afternoon he spent there playing that grand organ was one of the great musical experiences of his life. At the end of his trip, Fats caught the *Ile de France,* then the most luxurious liner afloat, and came back to Manhattan.

Ed Kirkeby was disappointed in the bookings in America that were available to Fats. He had been impressed by the huge success Fats had scored in England. He became convinced that Fats would do much better there than in America. So six short months after his return to America, he was back in London.

It was too soon. In the music halls Fats was no longer the draw he had been on his first go-round. This was completely unexpected and very bad news indeed.

Old habits die hard. In London Fats Waller discovered the British version of Tin Pan Alley in Denmark Street. Bob Musel came to England as a distinguished War Correspondent attached to General Eisenhower. Bob combined his newspapering career with writing popular songs. He recalls the day Fats Waller walked into the offices of the Peter Maurice Music Company and started moving towards the piano.

"Jimmy Phillips was in charge of the office and he was delighted to see Fats come in," Bob told me. "In the British tradition of hospitality, he offered his distinguished visitor a drink. Fats said he'd love to have a drink." By this time Jimmy was starting to open a brand new bottle of Bell's Whiskey. Fats had begun to play the piano.

"Then Fats told Jimmy that if he'd put the whole bottle on the piano, he might compose some music that his company might wish to publish. Jimmy was a bit discomfited by this remark. He had been rather planning to have a social drink with his famous guest. But then, wishing to be welcoming, he did as Fats requested.

"That was the afternoon that Fats, in a sudden creative burst, composed the six movements of his The London Suite: *Bond Street; Piccadilly; Whitechapel; Chelsea; Soho* and *Limehouse.* The Peter Maurice Company published the suite and Fats recorded it as piano solos for His Master's Voice a week later. Without that bottle of Bell's that music might never have happened." The new melodies were Fats's rather sentimental reaction to his love for the city. Subsequently the publisher, Lou Levy of Leeds Music in New York, had Bob Musel write a lyric for the Chelsea sketch.

But this trip things had cooled down considerably for Fats. His Master's Voice didn't even release the new recordings. In the music halls Fats was playing to half empty houses. The bookings collapsed. The unforseeable happened. Fats was stranded in England. His manager couldn't raise the boat fare to get him home. Fats, himself, was stony broke and there was no cash reserve available from any quarter.

Ed Kirkeby tried everything. Victor wouldn't advance another penny, Fats was already badly overdrawn on advances against royalties. If Ed Kirkeby had any spare funds he did not declare them. He shot off a few panicky cables but there was no response. Then Fats remembered a man who had often bailed out jazz artists in desperate trouble. This was John Hammond, discoverer of Count Basie and many others.

Once, just seven years earlier, Eddie Condon had brought Fats up to Westchester County to play in a little band- with Frankie Newton, Pee Wee Russell, Benny Carter, Zutty Singleton and Artie Bernstein. It was John

Hammond who had asked for this band for a country club dance. He always spoke of how much he had enjoyed Fats's performance that night. "I put a big jug of gin on the piano for Fats and he played *Bugle Call Rag* for twenty-two minutes."

Fats dictated the text of a cable to Ed Kirkeby. He sent it off to John Hammond and the next day they were in funds again. Fats never forgot this completely generous, but life-saving, move to rescue a musician in dire straights, that was so typical of John Hammond. On arrival back in the States after three months abroad, there was a bit of a surge in bookings and Fats hit the road with his little band.

Fats arranged that their very first takings be dispatched to John Hammond in repayment, together with his own grateful thanks. John Hammond never mentioned the incident to anyone and this too was typical of the man.

Lee Wiley was born and raised in Muskogee, Oklahoma. Her mother, who I met in her later years, was pure white Anglo Saxon Protestant, looking for all the world like a Grant Wood portrait. Of all possible things, she had fallen in love with and married a full-blood Oklahoma Indian and this beautiful girl was the result.

Lee had a brother and he looked Indian all the way. I met him on several occasions and I can report that he resembled exactly the Indian on the Buffalo nickel. When Lee was a school child she was told by her mother exactly which streets to take for her walk home. This was to circumvent the section of town that was called Niggertown. Fortunately Lee didn't pay too much attention to these instructions. Her route home took her right through the forbidden territory and specifically past a music store where, more often than not, they were playing recordings by Ethel Waters on the Black Swan label. Back then she never managed to own one of these records, for her just hearing them was enough.

In time she grew up and got to Chicago where a musical renaissance, black and white, was in progress. Lee, as a young singer, became an integral part of it, and the musicians she performed with were as often black as white. Then she came on to New York where she was instantly accepted as a singer of rare quality. I remember Lee telling me about one of the early French explorers in America. "In his anthropological report he wrote, 'All Mohawks sing.'"

Lee already had dedicated fans. One of them named Norma Deloris Egstrom changed her name to Peggy Lee in tribute. I visited this young lady with Lee. She was on the porch of a low rent flat, rocking her new baby. Her husband was guitarist Dave Barbour.

Now it was the time of the big radio programmes on coast-to-coast networks. Lee Wiley became the star of the top musical show, The Kraft Music

Hall, where she was billed as 'The Girl with the Blue Velvet Voice'. She was highly paid for this weekly programme and she prepared for it meticulously. She had many big-money offers to appear in cabaret and in theatres but she turned them all down on the grounds that there could never be anything routine about her performance.

Her show drew high ratings. She was always absolutely correct musically and there was always a high sexual quotient in her voice. Musicians were all mad about her and, Stanley Resor, the Vice-president of J. Walter Thompson the ad agency in charge of the show, was madly in love with her, too.

Fats Waller told me, "When Lee was on, all the musicians were all tuned in. I'd never think of missing one of her programmes." Lee loved the musicians, too. Sometimes too deeply for her own good.

At this moment she was secretly in thrall to Victor Young, violinist, composer and conductor. Stanley Resor thought she was in love with him. He wanted to further upgrade her programme so he proposed that for her new season, for which she was supposed to sign new contracts at an even higher boost in salary, he wanted her to be accompanied by Paul Whiteman's Concert Orchestra, which was then the most successful musical attraction in the land.

Lee Wiley rejected this suggestion and told Stanley Resor that she would only sign new contracts if Victor Young became her conductor. Resor had heard a whisper that Victor Young was her lover and now her new demand seemed to him to confirm this. Burning with jealousy, he went to the Board of Directors of the Kraft Cheese Company and told them that it was time to drop Lee Wiley and begin a new programme series with Paul Whiteman. Very reluctantly they accepted his recommendation.

That season Paul Whiteman and His Concert Orchestra made up the programmes and a voice, which up until now had only been identified on the labels of the Paul Whiteman records as 'With Vocal Refrain', began to sing the song hits of the day on the Kraft Music Hall. This voice was that of Bing Crosby. In the course of time Bing Crosby took over the programme.

The public forgot about Lee Wiley but the jazz musicians did not. A new bit of gossip about Lee was always being passed along wherever musicians gathered. She was off on a desert idyll with Artie Shaw. A torturous attachment to Bunny Berrigan went on for some years. But always it seemed she came back to Victor Young.

One day Eddie Condon had a brand new item. "Poor old Lee," he told me between sets at Nick's. "She called Jack Kapp 'a Jew' to his face and he told her that he'll see that she never makes a record in this country again." We all found the details of this new item quite funny.

It seems that Victor Young had been directing the house orchestra for the Decca label for some years. He thought he was due for a raise. Jack Kapp, who was the great record tycoon of the day and totally in charge of the Decca Company, didn't want to give him a raise. This made Lee very mad indeed.

The next time Victor Young had a meeting with Jack Kapp he took Lee along. This time when Kapp vetoed the raise, Lee flew into a furious tirade. She called Jack Kapp many things but it was only when she uttered the two syllables 'a Jew' that she got his full attention. He rose angrily from his desk and said, "You'll never make another record in this country again!"

You must realise that, like Jack Kapp, Victor Young was also a Jew and very proud of it. Just as Lee was proud of her own Indian blood. You must also realise that it was 1938, Hitler was already on the move in Europe, and racism was rampant. But Lee Wiley was never at any time a racist. The remark was unfortunate, ill-timed, and even as she uttered it Lee regretted it. It wasn't what she meant at all. Her hot Indian temper was to blame.

In those days three men ran the entire record industry: Eli Oberstein at Victor; Manny Sachs at Columbia; and Jack Kapp at Decca. Jack Kapp called his two confrères and all agreed never to record Lee Wiley again. He made the calls alright and he didn't give Victor Young his raise. But he didn't fire him either. Victor Young remained director of the Decca house orchestra until his death two decades later.

Now can you possibly understand how it was that Eddie, myself, Maxie Kaminsky, Bud Freeman, Joey Bushkin and others, found it regrettable, but nevertheless funny? If Jack Kapp said she'd never make another record, well that was it. Lee Wiley, the very finest jazz singer of the day, would be silent.

In those days there weren't a lot of fly-by-night labels. Records had to be cut in wax. It was quite an expensive job. It looked like the boycott would stand. Everybody knew she had done wrong. But wasn't it a shame we'd never hear her again, not on radio, and now not on records?

Everybody in our set was talking about it. Johnny DeVries was the most talented young man I ever ran into. He was always wildly funny. He could draw and paint like an angel. And he was a gifted lyricist. Among other songs he wrote with Joey Bushkin was *Oh, Look At Me Now* .

He had a job as art director of an advertising agency and due to his undisciplined ways they had given him a wonderful big office in a nice old building overlooking Union Square. I used to go over and meet with Eddie Condon every day when he got up, which was about three. He lived down in the Village. Then we'd usually stroll over to Johnny's office.

The repartee exchanged between Johnny and Eddie was classic. The Kapp vs. Wiley controversy produced some irresistible humour up in Johnny's place. We decided, among ourselves, to put Lee back in the record business, Jack Kapp or no Jack Kapp.

The Manhattan social set on the upper East Side bought all their records and phonographs at the Liberty Music Shop. Johnny was acquainted with a young salesman named Billy Hill who just happened to be the son of the owner. Johnny and I called on Billy. We actually just wanted some advice. But I guess it was a dull day and Billy got so interested in our idea that we ended up promoting him.

We told him all about Lee Wiley and Jack Kapp. We told him we wanted to make an album with Lee. We told him we wanted to use all the great jazz musicians. That's when we found out that Billy Hill was a jazz fan himself. This was long before LPs so we were going to make an album of four ten inch 78s.

We told him we were going to do eight George Gershwin songs. Nobody had ever made a George Gershwin album yet, nobody. This would be the very first. He loved the idea. Suddenly he exclaimed, "Let's do it." There was a silent pause. Then he quickly said, "Well, I'll talk to my father about it." He did and his father was so impressed by his son taking such an active interest in the family business that he approved the project at once.

There was a kind of conspiratorial atmosphere. We operated as discreetly as possible. The truth is we were scared to death of Jack Kapp. We were afraid he'd try to sink us if he ever heard about it. I took Lee up to Harms Music Company, who published most of George Gershwin's songs and we went over everything. Five of the eight songs we selected had never been recorded before. These songs were *I've Got A Crush On You, My One And Only, How Long Has This Been Going On, Sampson And Delilah* and, finally a song that Claude Thornhill suggested, *But Not For Me.*

Joey Bushkin rehearsed Lee at her home, where there was a good piano, every day. I booked the Liederkranz Hall because Eddie and Lee and Joey Bushkin were all convinced that it was the most acoustically perfect studio in town.

Eddie was the contractor and we filed union contracts at Musicians Union Local 802 without mentioning the name of the singer. The day before we were to go into the studio, Eddie ran into Fats Waller and told him all about it. Fats asked if he could play on one of the dates. This was an enormous thrill for all of us, especially Lee.

He was under contract to Victor at the time and this would be a violation of his contract. He didn't care. He just wanted to be sure Ed Kirkeby didn't know about it. Fats said, "Put Maurice Waller on the label. That's my little son. I can always say I taught him the chords."

Fats had never raised the subject of money. According to the union rule, the sidemen all had to get thirty dollars for recording four sides within three hours. The contractor got double that, sixty dollars for a date. So we paid Fats sixty dollars and he was very pleased. Fats never bothered much about money anyway as far as I could see. He could just walk in anyplace and sit down at the piano. Once he started to play they'd give him anything he needed. Food, drink, - even girls found it hard to resist his easy charm at the keyboard. Money was something he never quite seemed to get the hang of. That's what Ed Kirkeby was supposed to remedy.

We went to the Liederkranz Hall two afternoons running and the records almost made themselves. Lee had prepared herself immaculately and was in her best voice ever. We had brought Brad Gowans along in case there might be a difficult key someplace and some little sketch might need to be written. It turned out that didn't happen so Brad just sat, watched, listened, and marvelled.

Joey Bushkin played the piano on all four sides on the first date, with Bud Freeman and Maxie Kaminsky playing the horns. Then on the second date, Fats took over at the piano as we laid down the first recordings ever made of *I've Got A Crush On You, How Long Has This Been Going On* And *But Not For Me,* all three of which went on to become favorite Gershwin standards.

For his fourth side Fats dismissed the orchestra and moved to the organ. He then made with Lee what has become the definitive version of the classic ballad, *Someone To Watch Over Me.*

We had Pee Wee Russell on the second date and Eddie Condon sat in on guitar as well. On both dates George Wettling was the drummer and Artie Shapiro the bassist

Johnny DeVries designed a masterpiece of an album cover. These recordings have continued to be always current in the shops for half a century plus two years as I write these lines. Like all fine art they remain completely undated and will continue to be so forever. They sound as fresh today as they did the minute they were recorded.

My only quarrel with that is that somewhere along the line some inartistic reissue executive abandoned Johnny's album cover, perhaps to make it look like a brand new recording which is what it always sounds like. This was a grave error and it should be corrected no matter how difficult that may prove to be.

I never took a penny for all my effort on this project and neither did Lee. I was making a decent wage writing ads for somebody or other and I was happy to participate in such a worthy venture. I didn't even put my name on it as the producer. The truth is, it was my very first recording and I didn't know I was supposed to do that.

When it came time to put down the copy for the label I had to make a decision. Whose band would it be? I put down 'Max Kaminsky and His Orchestra' on three sides, and 'Joe Bushkin and His Orchestra' on four sides. On the eighth side I wrote that "Maurice" played the organ. Over the years they have changed this to Fats Waller.

This marks the very first occasion that Maxie and Joey ever had bandleader credit and they thanked me profusely. Everybody had assumed that it would be 'Eddie Condon and His Orchestra' for everything. But, although Eddie was the official contractor as far as the union was concerned, he missed the first date for some reason or other, although he got paid sixty dollars for it. On the second date he also got sixty dollars. So Eddie's hundred and twenty dollars was the biggest payoff of all.

Poor Lee was just in love with music. Whenever some fine musician appeared on her horizon, she crumpled at his feet. She was happily married to Jess Stacy, the great jazz pianist, for five mostly happy years. He had a big band at the time and Lee sang with it. But she insisted on top equal billing. This caused difficulties until an ingenious ad man devised a poster diagonally split in two. Each took half of the display and they alternated which would be first. She loved Jess and his music but she was never quite satisfied with the billing.

She had great highs but also some fearsome lows. She was finally permanently rescued from the depths of the latter by an unglamorous, unmusical pharmacist she came to trust and ultimately to love. He had the drug store in the lobby of the Astor Hotel in Times Square. When Victor Young died she married the pharmacist and when she died at the age of sixty she was Mrs. Nat Tischenkel.

Like myself, Paul Smith was another advertising man who loved the jazz music. He was the art director for Kenyon & Eckhardt. He worked a few blocks away from me. We used to meet for lunch, and sometimes just for a quick drink.

When they built the Grand Central Station in midtown Manhattan, the New York Central Railroad had to run its trains under a number of buildings. Sometimes it was difficult to get permission to do this so they just bought the building. That's what happened to the Park Lane Hotel, a deluxe establishment at the north east corner of Park Avenue and East forty-eighth Street. They let the existing management run the place but, since the railroad wasn't in the hotel business under usual circumstances, they didn't exercise any supervision at all. Consequently the luxurious Park Lane Hotel just went to sleep.

There was a lovely big bar just off the avenue and there was hardly ever anybody in it. Paul's office was a block or two to the south and I worked a couple of blocks to the north. We used to slip over there now and then for a quiet drink and a chat.

At the Park Lane everything was first class. All the servants were in livery. They were always glad to see us and I can't remember a time then when there was anybody else in that bar but us. We got to know the head barman very well. One day he took us through an archway beside the bar and we found ourselves in a large stunning ballroom set up for a banquet. It was all white napery and two story crystal chandeliers. Without any doubt it was the most beautiful room of its kind in New York City. But hardly anybody ever used it anymore.

Paul and I had an idea. We wondered if we could get the use of this room every Friday afternoon from five until eight? Our friend the head barman said, "Why ever not?" Within a few minutes he had summoned the manager of the hotel. This was a very gracious gent in striped trousers and swallowtailed coat.

My proposition was that we would fill the big room every Friday at five and for three hours this crowd would be ordering drinks which the bar would serve. If they'd give us the room free, we'd take no commission at all on the drinks. The hotel manager and the head barman quickly approved this deal.

Thus 'The Friday Club' was born, one of the most colourful of all jazz venues and one which produced some of the best music ever performed in the thirties. We instantly put Eddie Condon in charge of the music. Paul's sister, Phyllis, was writing ad copy for Gimbel's, a New York department store, and she wrote this little brochure, which we circulated to all of our friends in the advertising fraternity, all of whom, I hasten to point out, were through for the week at five p.m. on Friday and looking for any excuse at all to have a party.

Here's what she wrote below her byline:

True jazz music has a cult of its own. Its followers are as frigid to popular current "arranged" swing as they are to Guy Lombardo, Johannes Brahms. Hard, fast and faithful to the rigid, intellectualized [but hot] style known as "Chicago" or "Dixieland", these musicians and music lovers have still found no prophet to out-trumpet the late Bix Beiderbecke no leader to out-clarinet the great and simple Teschmaker. Among a small group of living artists, however, the style they look for still exists.

Not in one single band. Not in any band. But in the living styles of a scattered group of musicians [most of them now playing in large commercial bands]. These men, with their backgrounds of improvisation, easy knowledge of the great jazz tradition - are now in demand by highly paid organizations, for their spontaneity, solid tempo. They are employed by Whiteman, Dorsey, Shaw, Berigan, some have their own bands.

In The Friday Club cultists and musicians have gotten together. Have done something about preserving the great tradition that Bix and Tesch so far advanced.

Here such names as Fats Waller, Bud Freeman, Pee Wee Russell, Jimmy Dorsey, Eddie Condon, Artie Shaw, Bobby Hackett, Jess Stacy, Arthur Schutt, George Wettling will come, play, or just attend.

The mid-town office crowds, music lovers - many who work in the busy forties and fifties - have accepted this idea enthusiastically. Here they start their week-ends. Here the scattered Mid-West boys with their music followers will again pick up, accumulate, add to that strange phenomenal store of blues, jazz, musical ideas - that flashed out so unaccountably during the late twenties. Here once again can be heard that unmatchable, stomp-down, free-style music which started in Chicago dance-halls; little, cold, one-night-stand towns along Lake Michigan - just ten short years ago.

Below this screed was my name and office telephone number, and Paul's name and his office number, and then the words *The Friday Club, five to eight PM on Fridays. Park Lane Hotel, Forty-eighth Street and Park Avenue.*

I thought Phyllis had written a fine précis, evocatively capturing our enterprise. I hoped she'd write a novel about jazz, but she died last year before she got around to it. Word of 'The Friday Club' spread through town like wildfire. We opened as a solid hit. The place was packed with a wonderful crowd. We charged them all five dollars a head as they came in. They ordered rafts of drinks and the Park Lane waiters coped as best they could. Eddie took the entry money and spread it among the players.

We had twenty two musicians on that stand the first afternoon and they were all special. There were fantastic surprises, I particularly remember wonderful duets between Buck Clayton and Willie 'The Lion' Smith that you could never in the world have anticipated.

Everybody played 'The Friday Club'. Fats Waller showed up about the second Friday and tied up the place in knots. He never sang or did any of his comedy routines on such occasions, he just sat in with the band and took choruses. Nobody ever got on that bandstand unless they had been specifically invited by Eddie Condon.

At this stage of his career Eddie hated the microphone. He delegated all announcements to Joe Marsala who made them very professionally. But Eddie was always in total charge of the music and all the musicians knew that. He programmed the event in a very disciplined manner, yet, in his usual Chicago way, everything was quite impromptu.

Eddie usually opened up with a rhythm section and three horns. Then he might put on a piano player with a drummer, such as he did with Fats with Dave

Tough at the drums. Then Dr. Joe Slovak stepped in with his clarinet and it was a trio, with Fats amazed at the medico's proficiency, and Doc amazed that Fats could drink more than the pharmacopoeia proscribed. Other pianists who did such shots on 'The Friday Club' were Arthur Schutt, Jess Stacy, Joey Bushkin, Dave Bowman and even Meade Lux Lewis and Albert Ammons who came uptown from the Café Society. Then Eddie'd usually put on a soloist like Jack Teagarden or Pee Wee Russell or even Sydney Bechet with a rhythm section. Everybody was there.

We had a wonderful choice of rhythm. George Wettling dropped in from the Paul Whiteman band. Zutty came by almost every week. We had brilliant bassists, Artie Shapiro, Pete Peterson, Mort Stuhlmaker and others. Teddy Bunn played the guitar. And of course we had horns galore. Lips Page stopped the show every week and we also had Maxie Kaminsky, Bobby Hackett, Marty Marsala, Frankie Newton, just to mention a few.

Then Eddie might put on a singer, with whatever accompaniment he thought most suitable, selected from whomever was on hand. We had Billie Holiday, I remember, and we had Lee Wiley. We also had Leo Watson, scatting like mad. Bud Freeman and Ernie Caceres were regulars and on a couple of occasions we had Jimmy Dorsey and sometimes Happy Caldwell.

A little after seven a piano duet would set up, sometimes with two drums, a couple of basses and a guitar or two, and Eddie would start them up on the blues in a bright tempo. Then he'd bring the horns on one at a time, each taking an open four bar break and then playing it out with the full ensemble. Ultimately he went into *Bugle Call Rag* or W. C. Handy's *Ole Miss* and then we'd all go home.

I remember those afternoons so well. Isn't it a shame there wasn't yet any such thing as a tape machine back then? We never advertised or looked for any press publicity. We didn't tell any disc jockeys. But we did get some attention from music critics and jazz writers who just happened to find out about what we were doing.

When Duke Ellington was in town some of his guys came by. Ralph Gleason wrote about it when he saw Barney Bigard, Johnny Hodges and Harry Carney putting up some sheet music, to play their little trio in *Mood Indigo.* It was the only sheet music we ever saw at 'The Friday Club'. Week after week the shows were wonderful but things were often hectic and there were two occasions when things got a bit out of hand and I found myself in a panic. My first sign of panic was when I saw that the old waiters were stuffing cotton into their ears. When I could get the attention of one of these characters I asked, "Why?"

"Well we only have five waiters here," he tried to explain. "We really need at least a dozen. When I take an order to a table and start back to the bar, people

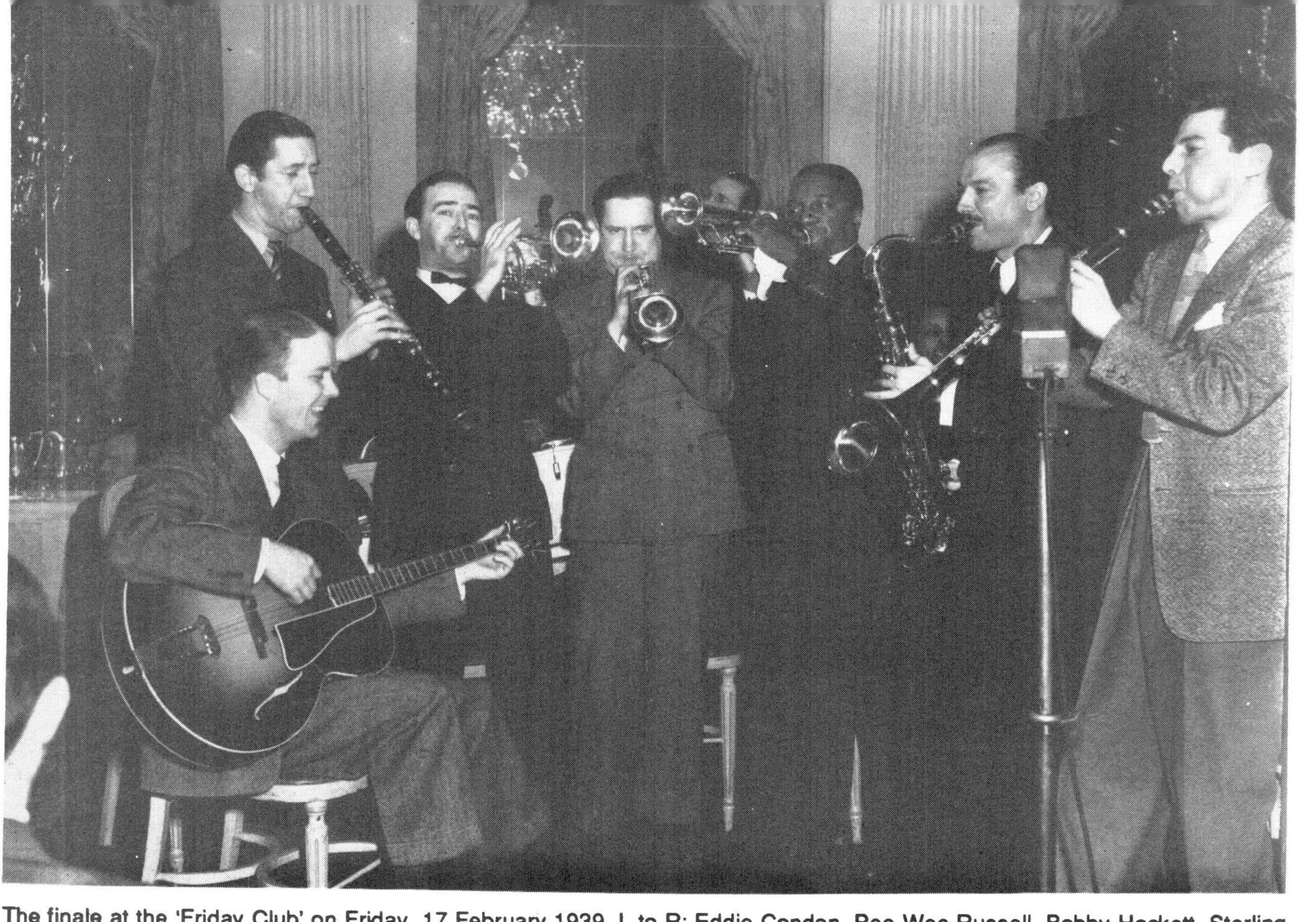

The finale at the 'Friday Club' on Friday, 17 February 1939. L to R: Eddie Condon, Pee Wee Russell, Bobby Hackett, Sterling Bose, Mort Stuhlmaker, Hot Lips Page, unidentified pianist, Bud Freeman and Joe Marsala.

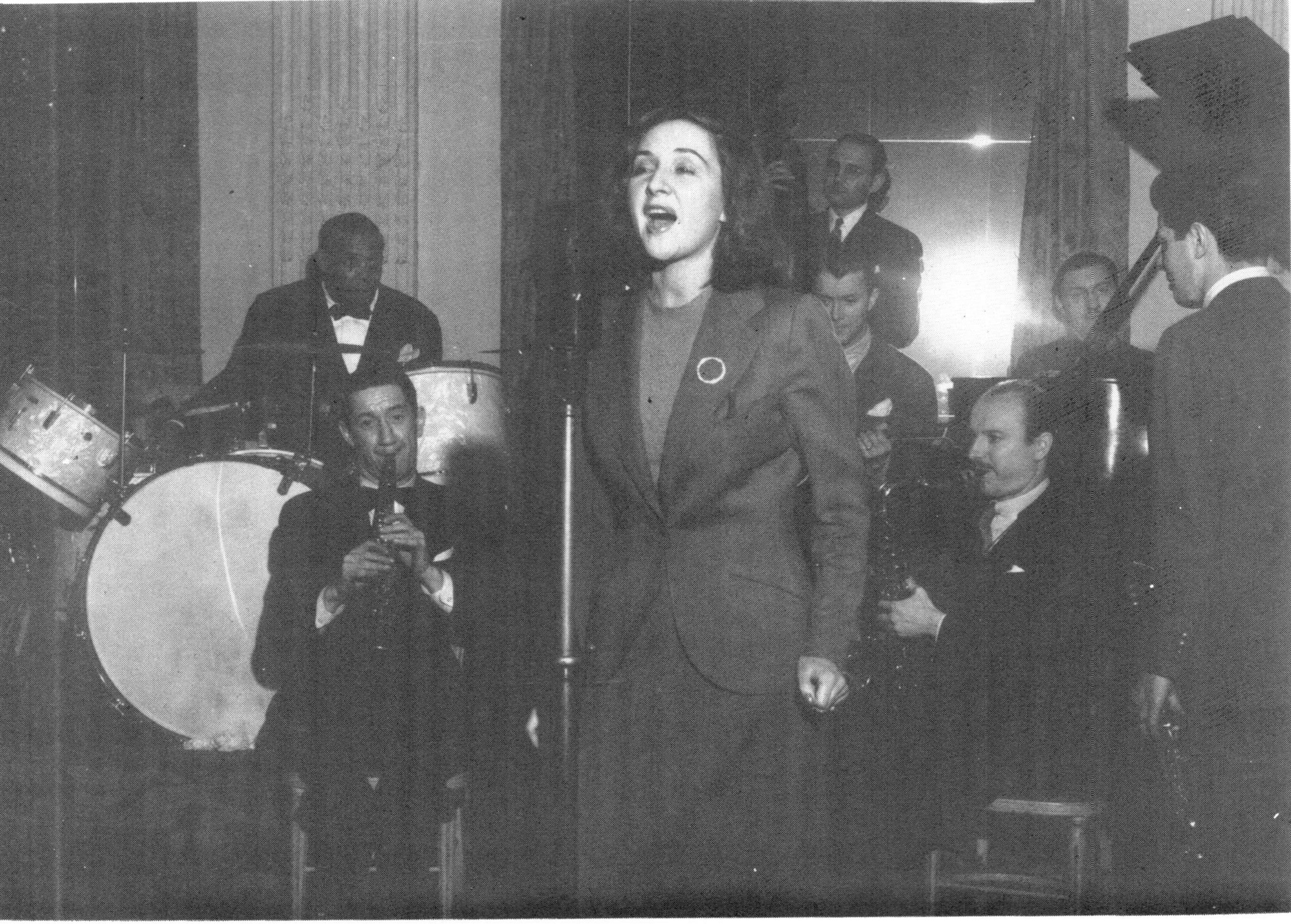

shout at me and start pulling at my sleeve and ordering more drinks than I can possibly handle. With the cotton I can get back to the bar and fill the order I already have."

My second sign of panic came at about six with two more hours to go when the head barman told me that for the first time in its long history the Park Lane Hotel had run out of scotch. The amazing thing was that the customers didn't seem to mind and switched to gin, rum, and other things.

That first 'Friday Club' we had twenty-two famous jazz players performing on the bandstand. Within a few weeks every jazz artist of any consequence in the Manhattan area had appeared. I think it was on our second Friday that Fats Waller came.

It must have been about the fourth session that we particularly looked forward to Fats coming again to our 'Friday Club' session. He wasn't there when the band took the stand at five. Jimmy Dorsey had come by with his alto. He had run over between shows at the Paramount Theater in Times Square where his big band was headlining. I had hoped Fats would be here early to accompany him and so had Jimmy.

I made a trip to the entrance. Here I learned that there had just been a brief fracas. "What happened?," I wanted to know. "A big black guy was trying to get in," said a waiter, not one of our old timers but a new recruit who obviously didn't know the ropes yet. There were at least a dozen black musicians already in the place. But this new man had refused Fats admission, I was told. I rushed into the street but there was no sign of Fats. I knew that Fats, at the first speck of any sign of race trouble, would vanish.

Much later that night Eddie and I made the rounds in Harlem until we found him. At the end we were in one of his favorite gin mills, The Colored Actors & Performers Club on West 126th Street, almost directly across the street from the stage door of the Apollo. We had gone there in desperation and had all but given up trying to find him.

This place was unique. You entered from under the stoop of a brownstone residence in the usual speakeasy way although Prohibition had already been repealed. You were supposed to be a member, or the guest of a member. This regulation was not strictly observed, you may note, because neither Eddie nor myself qualified for membership. Once inside you continued on right through the whole ground floor.

Then you came to what would in ordinary circumstances be the back yard. Only at the CA&P, as the establishment was known, the entire back yard was the floor of an oversize saloon.

I don't imagine anybody ever bothered to get building permission for this unique structure. The roof had been extended all the way to the end of the yard. The whole place was paved and enclosed. There was a nice carpet and many tables with white tablecloths. The back facade of the brownstone was clearly visible, its windows indicating the rooms of all the upstairs floors.

It was open twenty-four hours a day and it was a hard drinking establishment. I remember they served spirits, gin, rum, whisky, in quite a big tumbler that was called a shortie. I estimated that it must hold something like at least five ounces or, more likely, a half a pint. It was without doubt the biggest drink I have ever run into in a saloon. With it came another glass with ice and whatever mixer you preferred. But this second glass was hardly as large as the first.

It must have been about three in the morning. We were both beat from the afternoon session at the Park Lane and from the many stops we had made in Harlem in pursuit of Fats. We had decided that after this drink we'd catch a cab and go back downtown. Just as this decision was agreed upon, one of those upstairs windows was flung open and Fats leaned out, arms flung wide apart, and he grinned at us as he shouted, "Don't anybody give their right name!"

Fats came down and joined us and we ordered still another round of scotch shorties with soda on the side. Eddie and I both tried to apologise for the incident earlier in the day at the Park Lane but Fats brushed these pleas aside, insisting that no afront had ever been made.

Eddie had been particularly mortified by the incident and pressed Fats to excuse it on the grounds of the ignorance of a moronic waiter. Fats laughed and managed to change the subject. We had no doubt but that Fats had been hurt by the rejection at the door but we also felt that he had a certain degree of gratification from our coming uptown to apologise even as he smilingly protested that there was really nothing to apologise for.

There really wasn't much more that we could do about it. By the time Eddie and I left to take a taxi back downtown Fats was saying that he would definitely see us at the Park Lane Hotel on Park Avenue at East Forty-eighth Street next Friday at five. But he never did come. Not that Friday. Nor any other Friday either.

Eddie was most articulate about Fats's talent. He felt that the records Victor was making and which were now playing on every juke box and on every radio station were vulgar exploitations of a great musical virtuoso. "After all these years they know that Fats Waller is capable of producing very important music. Listen to what they have him doing! *Your Socks Don't Match!*", which was his current pop hit. "He's not a clown!," protested Eddie. "He's a great artist!"

Eddie was also quite emphatic that Fats should not be heard playing with the musicians he had assembled for his little touring band. He didn't specifically criticise any one of them. He just said, "They are inferior to him. He should only be presented playing with his musical peers."

Why did Fats Waller drink so intemperately? The time and place of his adolescence were undoubtedly factors. He was moving through a network of Harlem speakeasies before he was out of his teens, while others of his age enjoyed more sedate environments. He was also almost pathologically shy and he found early on that a little alcohol seemed to bolster his confidence. It made him bolder, happier and consequently, more entertaining.

I asked his great friend, Maxie Kaminsky, now eighty-one, if he had observed any relationship between Fats's heavy drinking and his remarkable creative powers. Maxie replied, "I don't think anybody knows just yet how it all works, but just from watching some musicians over the years, I have no doubt at all but that there is some kind of a powerful connection.

I remember once I ran into Beiderbecke in Sudbury, Massachusetts. We knew each other and he wanted to know if there was anyplace he could get some whisky. Between sets I went outside the dance hall and asked around. I was told I could get something at a certain drug store. The pharmacist gave me a pint bottle of a colourless liquid, saying that it was one hundred and eighty proof alcohol.

I took it to Bix. 'I couldn't get any whisky', I said. 'But I did get this'. I gave him the bottle. He took a bottle of ginger ale, emptied half of it out on the ground. Then he refilled the bottle with the alcohol. It was a murderous mixture, I thought. But then he put the ginger ale bottle up to his mouth and drank it, the whole thing. I thought 'after that he won't be able to play'.

By now the intermission was over and we went back up on the bandstand. All I can say is that Bix started playing like an angel. Whatever the psychologists might say, I assure you that that powerful infusion of alcohol definitely enhanced his playing that night.

I think it was the same thing with Fats. He drank constantly while he was playing. Somehow the alcohol provided the energy that fuelled his creative talents. There is no other possible explanation.

I first met Fats when Eddie Condon took me up to his flat in Morningside Heights. I had a job and Eddie didn't. He was living with me at the Lismore Hotel on West 73rd Street. You can figure out when this was when I tell you that Babe Ruth was living just down the street at the Ansonia. I didn't have one job, I had two jobs. They were network radio shows. I was playing with Leo Reisman's Orchestra. Originally he had a society band in Boston. He liked to feature jazz musicians. At times he had Bubber Miley and Adrian Rollini and Lee Wiley sang a vocal or two for him. On Tuesdays I did the Phillip Morris cigarette programme and on Fridays I did a programme for some mince meat company. I got eighty-seven dollars a week which was a huge salary at the time and quite enough for Eddie and me.

Eddie wanted some whisky. So we went up to see Fats and he got us some corn whisky that only cost fifty cents a pint. It was terribly hard to get that first drink down but after that it was all right.

Fats used to call me to play rent parties with him. We'd get ten dollars apiece for the gig. Plus, of course, all you could drink. In Fats's case that was a lot. He liked the way I played. Later on when he became really successful, he tried to put me in his little band. But Ed Kirkeby, the manager, wouldn't stand for it. He only wanted Fats to have black musicians even though Kirkeby, himself, was white.

I remember once I was in Jack Marshard's band, another society orchestra in Boston and we were scheduled to play this big ball for all the socialites. It was an annual affair called 'The Snowball'. Fats just happened to be playing in a local theatre with his little band. Jack knew I was a friend of Fats. Jack said, 'I'm going to invite Fats to play a number for us at the big ball.'

I said, 'Jack, that's not the way you do it.' He asked, 'What should I do?' I said, 'Well first you send Fats a case of good wine at the theatre.' So he went out and bought a real good case of French wine and sent it to the theatre. I was backstage with Fats and Fats said, 'What's this wine for?' I said, 'Oh, Jack wonders if you'd come over to this big society ball and play a number or two.' Fats, who was delighted with the wine, said, 'Maxie, anything you want.'

That night I was up on the bandstand and they had a big Steinway concert grand on the dance floor just below us for Fats. Fats came in and he was all dressed up in formal gear. He sat down at the piano, then he looked up at me sitting up in the brass section and waved at me to come down. I didn't move. Then Fats got up from the piano and walked over to the bandleader, Jack, and said, 'I'm not going to play unless I have Maxie with me.'

Well Jack told me to come down and I stood in the well of the piano with my horn and a mute and we played some duets together. That society audience didn't quite know who Fats Waller was but they liked our act. We stopped the show cold. The same routines we played for the poor blacks at the rent parties went over very big with these rich white society folk. These people didn't even know what a rent party was."

Creative powers are believed to emanate from the subconcious. Some artists seem to be able to motivate this genie naturally. Picasso was mostly abstemious during his most productive years and never even used drugs either except for a few youthful experiments with hashish. Yet he poured out paintings in an unending stream most of the time. He was frank to confess that the works were all the product of his unconscious and, as far as he was concerned, they were so mysteriously produced that he never ascribed a title to a single work in his long lifetime. Nor did he ever explain a painting of his, even in the most cursory way. The titles that exist for his various works were all invented by his dealers.

On the other hand, all critics agree that Jackson Pollock's art was somehow produced as a result of his self-destructive drinking. It is also a known fact that Jackson Pollock produced those celebrated drip canvasses to the accompaniment of his collection of Eddie Condon, Louis Armstrong and Fats Waller records.

We know that all of Samuel Taylor Coleridge's *Kubla Khan* that exists came to him verbatim under the influence of laudanum. Eugene O'Neill and even Graham Greene, among others, have admitted to the use of opium in pursuit of their literary muse. The legendary jazz pianist, Peck Kelley, was said to be on opium also. Despite bids to join the touring orchestras of Jack Teagarden, Jimmy Dorsey and even Paul Whiteman, always at excellent salaries, Peck preferred to remain in San Antonio where he was the resident pianist at the Rice Hotel. His reason was that he feared breaking his connection for the drug.

Around the turn of the century the use of opium was widely accepted. Irving Berlin used it. So did Ned Washington, whose ballad, *Midnight On The Street Of Dreams,* sung by Lee Wiley among others, was actually a paean to the drug.

It is not generally known that when Louis Armstrong played the Dreamland Cafe on the Chicago South Side, Joe Glazer, whose mother owned the premises, ran a hop joint upstairs. Eddie Condon, who was there at the time, told me, "The white swells from the North Side would come down to the black South Side ostensibly to hear Louis's hot jazz. Actually that was just a front. As soon as they got inside they'd go upstairs and hit the pipe."

Perhaps his immoderate use of alcohol spurred Fats Waller's own unconscious to pour out so many musical compositions, rich in melody and harmony. No one else in our time has produced anything like as much fine music in such a brief span.

Doctors and psychiatrists have been talking about these matters for a couple of centuries, yet today nobody knows much about them with any degree of certitude. I must feel, however, myself, that Fats's heavy and deliberate use of alcohol must have played a large part in the creation of the complex and, at the same time, delicate, torrent of music that poured out of him as long as he lived.

His substantial build and sturdy constitution, as well as his endless stamina and energy, must have been responsible for his remarkable ability to withstand the ravages of alcohol to the extent that he did.

Many of our finest creative artists habitually over-indulged in alcohol. Among writers we might mention Ernest Hemingway, Scott Fitzgerald and William Faulkner. We must include in this list the great Irish writer, Brian O'Nolan, who usually signed his works Myles na gCopaleen. He explained, "In life one has to choose between drinking and being bored to death. You're in danger all the time, not only from death, but also from boredom." Then speaking of his great friend, Brendan Behan, who had just passed over at an early age due to drink, he added, "Brendan made the choice." Shortly after delivering this theory O'Nolan went to his own premature grave as well.

A century ago cocaine was prescribed by Dr. Sigmund Freud 'as a tonic'. It was generally considered to be an exotic pharmaceutical with no harmful side effects. There were no laws against it and it was used in many products. There was even a panacea manufactured in Atlanta, Georgia, by a pharmacist named Chandler. It didn't cost much and it made you feel very good. It became wildly popular. The principal active ingredient was cocaine from the cocoa leaf imported from South America. It also contained elements from the cola nut imported from India.

Very soon Mr. Chandler had a chain of drug stores, then a big company and finally a whole network of big companies. His panacea was called Coca-Cola. It was sold then only as a cheap medication to cure whatever might ail you, particularly anything causing pain. It was famous for relieving hurt of any sort. This panacea aspect of Coca-Cola ended in 1906 when the Congress of the United States enacted into law The Pure Food and Drug Act which specifically prohibited, for the very first time, the manufacture and sale of such drug-laden products.

A clever advertising man from St. Louis named Bill D'Arcy rescued Coca-Cola. He had chemists work out a formula using the cocoa leaf and the cola nut to retain the exact taste of the panacea but, at the same time, removing the active chemicals of the drugs. Then he advertised and sold the product as a refreshing soft drink. Part of his strategy was to insist that any retailer who wanted to stock the product had to agree to sell it only when it had been chilled. The new variation of Coca-Cola caught on, as you know, and its flavour today remains that of the panacea. Bill D'Arcy always stayed within the law. Part of the new law stated that any product containing any active particle of these drugs must state so clearly on the label of the bottle. First he eliminated any active ingredient of the drugs, then he eliminated the label. Can you think of any liquid product sold that carries no label? Coca-Cola is the only one I ever encountered.

That was Bill D'Arcy for you.

In the thirties when I was writing ads for that famous soft drink, they were still getting its flavor directly from the cocoa leaf. I was actually present when four and a half kilograms of cocaine, extracted from the leaf during the manufacture of the essence for the soft drink, was burned in a laboratory in Fort Lee, New Jersey, in the presence of U.S. Federal Marshalls.

Up until the end of the twenties, some theatricals continued to use raw cocaine, sniffing it as a brightener in the wings just before going on stage. John Barrymore delighted hipsters among his matinee audiences on Broadway and in the West End of London, with mannerisms with his hands and nostrils, indicating that he had just turned on with it.

Tallulah Bankhead was an habitual user, her only problem was getting it. "I know just where to get it in London," she told me, "But here on Broadway it's more difficult. You have to deal with such unsavoury types. I can't imagine why. It's good for you and it is definitely not habit-forming!"

Tallulah loved jazz and I made some records with her, in which she was accompanied by Joey Bushkin and a small group. Joey used to sign off his nightly radio broadcasts with a blues he entitled Portrait of Tallulah. She adored this little tribute. She spoke of the 'underlying quality of sadness' in Louis Armstrong's work and compared his music to that of Mozart.

Louis Armstrong had his own way of summoning his unconscious. He believed he was a medium. If he kept himself immaculately in shape, healthy, rested and sober, with a fine instrument and with his embouchure properly salved, that miracle would happen again every night. He took no personal credit for his performance at all.

He had an austere routine he religiously went through every evening before hitting his first note. He awoke, bathed, dressed, ate, in total silence. Then got into the car and was taken to the job. No one was ever to talk to him during all this time, not even Lucille, his wife, nor Dr. Pugh, his valet. If by any chance someone innocent of this routine did happen to interrupt Louis's contemplative mood, steps were taken instantly to ensure that it never happened again, which usually meant removing that person, whomever he might be, from the Satchmo coterie.

Louis was a constant user of the best marihuana since his earliest Chicago days. He spent large sums to be sure always that he had the finest available, and that he would never run out. But he never smoked any before playing. Like drink, that was for after the job. He seldom broke this self-imposed rule until his very last years. He nevertheless was convinced that his use of the drug was associated in some mystical way with his creative accomplishments.

Fats knew all about Louis's intense association with marihuana. As I have mentioned, Fats sometimes was a casual user himself. He chose not to use it to the extent that Louis did, much as Louis chose not to hit the bottle the way Fats did. But Fats did not disapprove. In fact he involved it in his music. His beautiful piano composition, Viper's Drag, is a direct reference to the drug.

Fats also made two recordings of *If You're A Viper,* even singing the lyric on one. In the argot of that day, the word viper had but one meaning, someone who smoked marihuana. The general public may not have been aware, but all Harlem surely knew it. Don Redman wrote, and with his orchestra played, a smokily atmospheric piece called *The Chant Of The Weed.*

It captured the public imagination. The weed, of course, had to be marihuana. What other weed could he have been talking about? If you had any doubt, the music set up a weirdly mysterious mood. Even André Kostelanetz had his version of it orchestrated for his symphony sized combination and broadcast it from the Liederkranz Hall studios over the CBS network for Coca-Cola on at least one Sunday afternoon broadcast that I can remember.

Fats never made a recording of Don Redman's composition but under the influence of it he did improvise and record something called *The Chant Of The Groove* which cannot be too distantly related.

When Fats and I sat and talked together in some Harlem after-hours joint, I found he was really more than just interested in serious music. I was actually quite shocked when he told me that he used to go to Carnegie Hall to hear Vladimir Horowitz. "I would always get a single ticket in the Second Balcony for two dollars and seventy-five cents", he told me. Attending those concerts seemed to be terribly important occasions for him. As he spoke of them, which he did frequently, I was surprised to detect that he had a curious reverence for Carnegie Hall. He spoke of the place in hushed tones as though it was some sort of a religious temple.

Probing this unexpected mood, I asked, "You'd really like to play there some day?" This provoked an instant reaction. A warm grin came over Fats's features as he answered, "Oh, how I'd love to!" He was positively ecstatic at such a prospect.

Until that moment in all my young life I had hardly ever paid any real attention to Carnegie Hall at all. A girl friend had once towed me over there to hear some classical thing or other but we left before the intermission. The place that meant so much to Fats meant nothing to me at all. I remembered that Paul Whiteman and his big orchestra, with young George Gershwin playing his *Rhapsody In Blue,* had played Aeolian Hall in 1924 and that Benny Goodman had played Carnegie in 1938. The finest concert venue in Paris was the Salle

Pleyel and in 1934 I had watched and listened as Louis Armstrong and a five piece pick-up band played four great concerts there. They do these things much better in Europe, I decided.

Why shouldn't Fats play Carnegie Hall? I decided to look into it. After work in the ad agency late one afternoon, it must have been about six, I walked over to Carnegie at West Fifty-seventh Street and Seventh Avenue. It certainly was not very preposessing from an architectural standpoint, a big nineteenth century brick edifice with a rather ugly decorative cast iron canopy over the entrance. There were some posters there advertising some coming attractions, symphonies and operatic recitals mostly. A dull lot, I thought.

I walked around the building along Seventh Avenue and turned in at Fifty-sixth. There was a big German bierstube on that corner which advertised beer from Munich on draft. Alongside this place I discerned the stage door. I walked on through it and on my left espied a large business office full of desks and filing cabinets. Except for one man, the room was empty. The office staff had long since gone home.

The man was in the far corner. He stood before the biggest desk in the room. He was well tailored and he was smoking a Havana cigar. He also kept his hat on. It was a stylish brown trilby set at just the proper angle. A real showman, I thought.

"Good evening," I ventured. "I was wondering how much it would cost to rent this place some evening for a concert." He took the cigar out of his mouth, smiled and said, "I'm Mr. Totten. I've been the manager here for thirty two years."

He pointed to a table on which was a large volume. We both walked to it and he began turning the pages. This was the booking ledger. It was early in November in 1941. He turned to the upcoming January and scanning the bookings said, "We have an opening here for the evening of January fourteenth," he said, pointing with his index finger to an open space on the page. I knew that date would suit Fats beautifully, he was wide open on the fourteenth.

"How much will that cost me?" I asked. He instantly replied, "Six hundred dollars." I couldn't help but note that he never even asked who I was proposing to put on that so highly revered stage that evening. As long as I paid the six hundred it didn't matter in the least. This further reinforced my lack of respect for the place.

"It's payable in advance," he added, not to waste any time. I wrote a cheque on the spot. It was a bit of bravado on my part. At that precise moment I wasn't absolutely sure it would clear. I felt I had to build a little character with Mr. Totten. He didn't know me at all. I was just someone who had, literally, just walked in off the street.

As a matter of fact my cheque did clear. I was making a good wage for a young fellow, three hundred clams a week. But I never was one for putting much aside.

He now got some forms out of a desk, filled in the date, signed them and then asked me to do the same. I looked them over in what I considered to be a professional manner, but the fact was that they were full of fine print and also some archaic and unintelligble text. I signed them anyhow, put one copy in my pocket, shook hands with Mr. Totten, who was grinning broadly, and walked into the auditorium on my way out to West Fifty-seventh Street.

The hall was empty and the huge uncurtained stage was bare except for about a hundred chairs and music racks for the symphony concert scheduled for later that evening. I waited for the deep spiritual feeling that Fats talked about but it never came. The place was just empty and drab. The boxes and the proscenium arch had some carved decorative elements but the walls were painted in a lifeless brown about the same hue as a Hershey Bar. I found it all depressing.

I walked up the steeply raked aisle to the entrance lobby. There on the extreme right was the highly secure box-office, also painted that same dreadful shade of brown. Here the six Heck brothers had their sinecure. They controlled every penny that came in to Carnegie Hall.

They not only sold the seats, they also sold many seats that were not ever on the floor plans. They ordered the tickets. They reported to you on those that they sold that were on the floor plan. The receipts from the ones that were not was just so much velvet for the Hecks. In years to come they were unmasked in some of their illicit enterprises and the law stepped in. But in my time I was inclined to treat them like the Bank of England. They probably took even more advantage of a tyro like me than they did with their regular clients.

You can see that there was absolutely nothing sacred about Carnegie Hall. I gave one of the Mr. Hecks the copy for the tickets, worked out the price scale, and signed something else I couldn't make head or tail of. Not one of the six Hecks had ever even heard of Fats Waller. They told me how many poster spaces I could have outside and they told me to get my programme copy ready for the printer.

My inclination had always been to bill the attraction as Thomas Waller. This is what I felt Eddie would have liked and he was going to be the Musical Director of the affair. The Heck brothers frightened me into billing it as Fats Waller's concert, but I softened the blow by putting the sobriquet in quotation marks, thus 'Fats'.

A Mr. Heck then asked, "And would I be having a programme note?" I really didn't know the first thing about staging a Carnegie concert and the Hecks all knew it.

The best seats in the house for our concert were priced at two dollars and twenty cents, ten per cent of that being tax. The cheapest seats in our house were seventy five cents, including tax. There were almost three thousand seats to try to fill in that place.

It was now just about seven oclock in the evening. I knew enough about the New York *Times* to know that they were just about putting the paper to bed. This would be the ideal time to make the first announcement of the concert. And the *Times* would be the ideal place to plant it, the most important and the most serious paper in town. Unfortunately I didn't know anybody I could call at the *Times*. I found a pay station and called the paper, asking for the music department. It took a considerable time for anyone to respond. While waiting, the operator came on the line asking me to insert another coin. Just at this moment someone from the paper asked "Yes?" I said that I'd like to tell them about a concert Fats Waller was giving at Carnegie Hall.

"Who?" asked the obviously puzzled music reporter. I said, "Fats Waller, the great jazz piano virtuoso." "Jazz? In Carnegie Hall?" were the next two questions. The operator now came on, asking for yet another coin. Of course the *Times* man heard this, as he had heard her previous request.

The *Times* now wanted to know who was I and where was I. I explained that I had just signed a lease for the hall for the concert and I wanted the *Times* to be the first to know about it. Quite reasonably I was told that perhaps it would be better if I sent them something in writing. I thanked the man and hung up.

I called Fats's house. He had moved from Morningside Heights to a house of his own in St. Albans, a residential community in Queens. A lady answered, presumably Mrs. Waller. She said Fats wasn't there but could I leave a message. So I told her about the January fourteenth date at Carnegie Hall. She took it all down.

Now I dashed downtown to see my Musical Director, Eddie Condon. I found him, as usual, in Julius's, a corner saloon in the Village, just down the street from Nick's. Julius's was operated by Pete Pesci, a foot soldier in the ranks of the Mafia, a position he was given because of a strange facility he had with figures. He could look at a sheet of numbers for an instant or two and then reproduce it like a Xerox machine.

Pete had a home with a wife and child someplace in town, but he also had a little flat upstairs at the saloon where he had installed Slats, his girl friend, a leggy beauty who danced in the chorus of a show on Broadway.

Julius's was a classic New York City sawdust joint. It was mostly a long bar. There were a few tables which seemed to have been cut down from barrels in a rustic style. The sawdust on the floor was about an inch deep. Pete had accentuated the homely ambiance of his establishment by finding someone with a machine that could spray out plastic counterfeits of spider webs. The whole place was festooned with these dusty and tangled skeins.

Eddie sat in a corner, nursing a scotch and soda, waiting for nine o'clock when he would hit the bandstand at Nick's. I told Eddie the momentous news about Wednesday night January fourteenth at eight thirty when Fats Waller would be at Carnegie Hall. He did not jump up, shake my hand and say 'Hurrah' as I had hoped. Instead he frowned and gave me two ultimatums. "One," said my Musical Director, "He cannot have that dogass band with him, and two, absolutely no singing, and none of those allegedly comic songs either."

I agreed to this and said that I'd have a serious talk with Fats about it. Then Eddie and I began to work out a programme. We decided that he should open with a piano recital of improvisations of Fats's own compositions. Then he'd go to the organ and play some Negro Spirituals.

At some point we should see that he played something more serious at the piano, then perhaps he should return to the organ. Then we'd also have a small all-star orchestra to improvise with him as a sort of finale. We decided to beef up this group with some box-office names who were, nevertheless, fine jazz players.

Gene Krupa would fit in beautifully and he was going to be in town playing at the New York Paramount with his new big band on that date.

Then we thought of Artie Shaw who was in town, living in an apartment in Central Park South. I got Krupa on the phone and he agreed to participate instantly. Then I called Artie and his reply was ambiguous. He'd love to play but he wasn't sure he could make it. It sounded more like 'Yes' than 'No'.

The next day I managed to find Fats and I went over all this with him. He acquiesced in every detail. I tried to get him to make some suggestions but he said what we were proposing was exactly what he had in mind. I was quite surprised that he never asked us to use his little band. Perhaps mentioning Gene Krupa and Artie Shaw took that idea out of his head for the moment.

I never went near Ed Kirkeby, and I also made a wide detour around Victor Records. I thought they might not agree to the idea of Fats Waller playing in Carnegie and try to get Fats to cancel the deal. Then I'd lose the six hundred dollars I'd laid out so far. But I really believed that Fats in Carnegie would turn out to be a very important musical event. And so did Eddie Condon.

I had a session with Paul Smith and he designed a knockout poster for the concert. His poster design was where that little round silhouette of Fats playing a miniature grand originated. On his design Paul had lettered, "The Girth of the Blues".

Now I got the maquette of the poster, a photographer and Eddie, and we took a long taxi ride all the way out to Fats's new home in St. Albans. It was a great improvement over the Harlem railroad flat. In his big living room stood a Steinway concert grand. And just a yard away from that keyboard was the keyboard of a full size Hammond organ. Fats would play the piano, then the organ.

The photographer took a photo of Fats and Eddie with the poster between them. It turned out to be a great photo. I sent it out to all the papers, in those days there must have been a dozen in New York City. Nobody printed it.

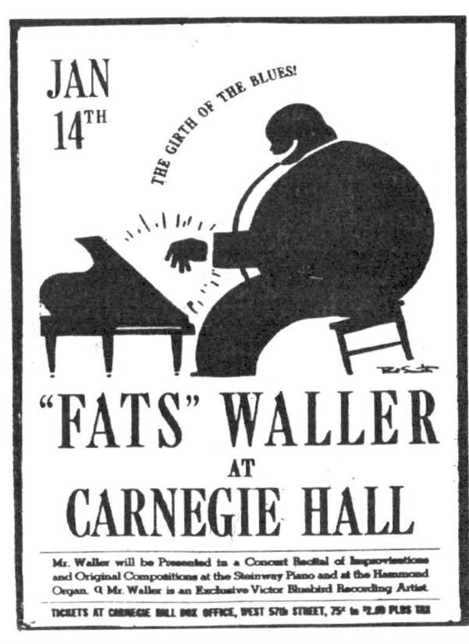

Right: The original poster design.

Below: The photo of Eddie and Fats in Waller's apartment.

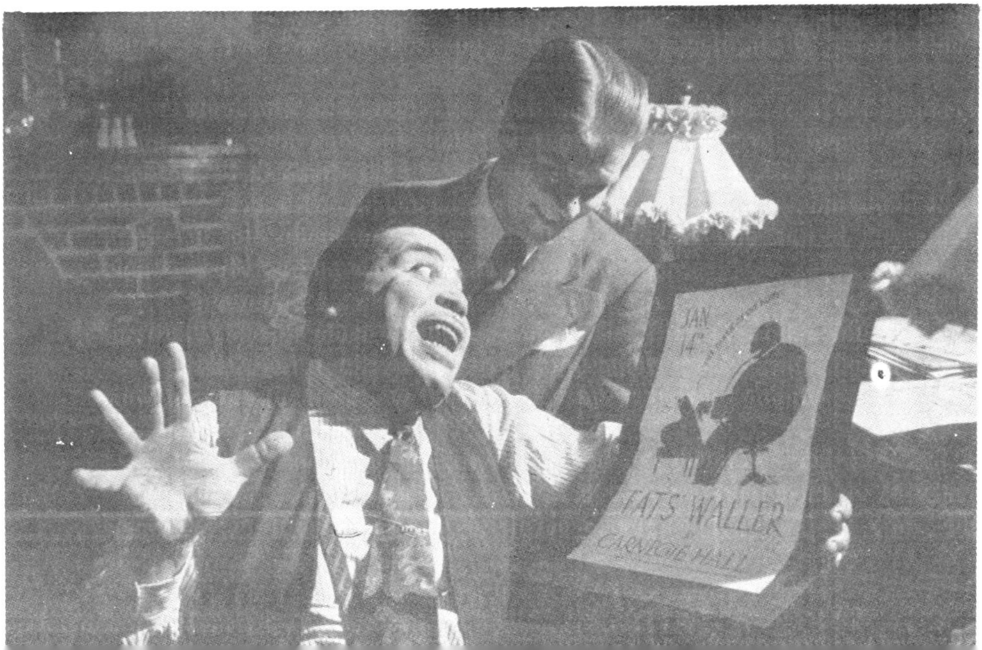

I prepared a press release, detailing exactly who Fats was. I sent that out to everything in print, too. That wasn't picked up either. Then the New York *Times* printed three lines at the bottom of a column. It only said that Fats Waller would give a concert in Carnegie Hall on January fourteenth. I then put a very small paid advertisement in the New York *Times* and also in the New York *Daily News,* the tabloid with the largest circulation in the country. These little ads cost a bundle and that was very worrying.

Every day I'd call on the Heck brothers in their high security bunker at Carnegie. I wanted to know how many seats we had sold. The sale was very discouraging. That box-office was selling about fifty events at a time. The tickets for each event was kept in a separate rack. The tickets for each event were of a different colour. The Fats Waller concert had white tickets. Finally I knew just where to look through a brass grill to see the Fats Waller rack. From day to day it didn't seem to change at all. If, by any chance, we sold out, the Heck brothers would tell me that our rack 'had gone clean'.

There didn't seem to be too much danger of that happening.

Newspaper advertising was fiendishly expensive. I decided to try direct mail. I got Phyllis Reay to write the text of a letter. She used Paul's little round silhouette of Fats as the letterhead with the numerals '88' just below it. (As we all know, there are eighty-eight keys on a piano keyboard.)

Then she wrote this text:

I'm gonna sit right down and write yourself a letter...

About a gr8 d8 that's definitely on the sl8, for about half past 8 on January 14th.

You see, on this d8, there's going to be a deb8, (well, a sort of t8-a-t8,) between this humble advoc8 of the piano laure8, and a few intim8 sk8s. (Friends, by the way, of the L8 Sister K8.)

It'll be at Carnegie Hall.

I'd like to prognostic8 - it's going to be some conglomer8 of that brand of vertebr8 that loves to gravit8 around a musical cr8 and a str8-bar-8 and start to cre8...good music.

Most of the evening I'll be playing a Steinway grand and a Hammond organ. But some of the time Artie Shaw and Gene Krupa and Eddie Condon and some other marvellous musicians will be helping out by sitting in.

*Don't forget the d8, 75 cents to two dollars plus tax pays the fr8. By the way, don't be L8. See you at the g8, (signed) Fats Fats Waller, 88**

**The first 88 keys are the hardest.*

Once again Phyllis Reay came through with a little masterpiece. No wonder Eddie Condon later on took her hand in marriage. We printed this up on especially nice stationery and we mailed it out to all of our friends and then to everyone we could think of.

In the Heck brothers rack at Carnegie, I was just beginning to see some small sale starting, when we were hit by a devastating blow. The Japs bombed Pearl Harbour and the entire United States of America went to war.

Ticket sales for everything froze up. The papers were chockablock with grim news. Nobody wanted to know about jazz concerts. Everywhere you went they were playing the national anthem. Somebody instituted an ordinance and from now on you had to close every public gathering of any kind with the *Star Spangled Banner,* at best an awkward composition. We'd have to play it to close our concert. I decided that Fats could probably make something special of this on the organ. I discussed it with him and he agreed.

I called up John Hammond. "Would he like to write the programme note for the Fats Waller concert?" "Oh, yes, he'd be delighted," was his instant reply. A few days later, when I called on him to pick up the copy, he apologised, he hadn't had time, would I please write something and sign his name to it?

There were a hundred things going on at once. Eddie and I decided we had to get a more definite commitment from Artie Shaw. Eddie and I had both known Artie, a superb musician, for years. He had struggled to get his band started and for a long time it looked as though he was never going to make it. I remember when he was so broke he had to bunk up with Maxie Kaminsky in Maxie's mother's place in Dorchester, Massachusetts.

When he finally hit, he hit very big. I remember when he played a one-nighter in Hartford, Connecticut, and he and the band were staying in the annex of the Bond Hotel. Lana Turner was a very big movie star. She came all the way from Hollywood to Hartford to see him. He wouldn't see her. So she sat in the lobby of this rather crummy establishment on the off-chance of catching him. Oh, he was a big shot.

At the very top of his career he had just taken a breather and he was padded down in these luxurious quarters overlooking Central Park. Eddie and I phoned and he said come on up. At this period he was in the upper reaches of his high intellectual phase.

Now Artie knew that Eddie and I were just a couple of saloon bums, but for some reason he couldn't help trying to lay some of his intellectual jive on us. We rang and he came to the door in a smashing silk dressing gown that would have made Noel Coward blush. He was carefully holding an open book so that we could dig the title. I remember it to this day. It was *The Varieties of Religious Experience* by William James. The author was the latest hot psychologist-psychiatrist.

Artie, however, was cold. He loved Fats and all that but he just couldn't be sure he'd be free between ten and eleven on Wednesday evening, January fourteenth. We'd have to call later and he'd let us know.

Eddie and I left and as we went down in the elevator, Ed said, "He seems to think it's some kind of a clambake and he'll drop in for a few minutes if he can get away from his shrink.' I said, "Let's scratch Artie Shaw." And so we did. I called Chicago and got Bud Freeman on the phone. Bud said he'd come if we paid his fare and if we put him up someplace in New York while he was here. I paid the fare and I put him up in my flat, much to my wife's objections. She claimed he always left the bathroom looking like the Battle of the Marne.

"But we must have a clarinet," Eddie said. I asked, "How about Pee Wee?" Eddie said, "Nick will never stand for it. He has been raising absolute hell about my taking off Wednesday evening up until eleven-thirty. He'll explode if we take Pee Wee too."

Nevertheless, I went down to Nick's that evening and talked to Pee Wee about it. When he heard the details he insisted on playing with Fats. "I don't care if Nick fires me," said Pee Wee, "I'll play the date."

I was sending all sorts of things to the newspapers and now and then they printed something. When they printed that Pee Wee Russell would be playing on the Carnegie stage with Fats Waller, Nick got mad. He told Pee Wee, "You play that job and you're fired."

Just as I got this news I was writing a programme note which was to be signed by John Hammond. I could not resist including a few lines of scurrilous comment about Nick Rongetti and the way he continually exploited an artist like Pee Wee Russell.

Of course Maxie Kaminsky would play the trumpet. He was always Eddie's first choice. "What a tone," he would exclaim. John Kirby and his little outfit with Maxine Sullivan was the big noise on Fifty-second Street. We set Kirby to play bass in our little group. Although every musician in this little band knew every other musician, they had never played together as a band and of course there would be no rehearsal.

The concert was assuming a definite shape. It would begin with Fats playing at the piano improvisations on the tunes associated with him. Then he'd play the organ. we'd close with Fats at the Steinway jamming with the jazz band we had put together. Then he'd walk to the organ and play *The Star Spangled Banner*.

There was only the intermission to worry about. We needed something very strong just before the intermission. And we needed something very special right after it, to open the second half. I suggested to Eddie that in the first of these two spots we might use Lips Page. Eddie thought this over for a minute or two and then said, "Fats is at the piano. He plays some blues, say in A. Then Lips comes on, with his trumpet. You turn those two loose on the blues in the key of B flat and they'll wreck any joint, including Carnegie Hall."

Fats agreed to this with real enthusiasm. "Yes," he said the next afternoon, "Have Lips come on and sing a few choruses of the blues, just whatever he wants to make up. Then he starts playing his horn and we swing it on out."

Everything about the concert sounded great to me. I used to walk over to the Hall in the evening and look in on Mr. Totten. Noting my enthusiasm, he casually mentioned that there was a way of getting an especially good souvenir of the concert. It seems that there was a little privately owned recording studio on one of the upper stories of the hall. They had a microphone hanging down, way up above the centre of the stage.

"They'll make an acetate copy of whatever happens on the stage that night for fifty bucks," he informed me. "But don't tell the Musicians's Union or they'll charge you a wopping amount." I couldn't imagine that a single mike hanging forty feet above the Carnegie stage could produce a very good recording but I thought it would make a nice souvenir of the occasion.

I went up and found the little studio that had rented an office in the Carnegie Hall building and gave the man a hundred dollars and ordered two sets of acetates, one for Fats, the other for me. I never mentioned the fact to anyone. I had a contract with the union for the concert but it did not include the right to record.

I was frantically searching for little items to send the papers in hopes of stimulating our turgid ticket sales. Just after Fats had returned from Europe after his second tour there, he happened to include on a Victor record date a little instrumental he had named *Bond Street.*

Now I learned that this was just one item of a series of six pieces he had composed and recorded on the piano in London. Each of these was named for a London locale and Fats called the whole set 'The London Suite'. Victor in the States had not been too enthusiastic about his *Bond Street* so they hadn't bothered to have him record his *Piccadilly, Chelsea, Soho, Limehouse,* or *Whitechapel.* They hadn't come out in London either.

I took the long taxi ride out to Fats's house in St. Albans. As usual he was in the living room alternately playing his Steinway and his Hammond. I never saw a drink in that house. I guess Mrs. Waller must have laid down the law. Fats was in wonderful shape and playing brilliantly as always. I discovered that he loved his little musical impressions of London.

I went back to Manhattan and wrote a little release that at the Carnegie concert he would play the premiere performance of his 'The London Suite'. It turned out to be the most successful release of all. It even got prominent display in the New York *Times*. I decided that Fats's playing 'The London Suite' would be the perfect way to open the second half, after the intermission.

A few days later the Heck brothers professed themselves as being very pleased with the sale. They reported that the house was almost half sold. Half sold? What about the other half? I wasn't very pleased at all. There was hardly any time left.

Fats, Eddie and I had arranged to meet at Carnegie at five o'clock on the day of the concert. We were going to be sure that the piano and the organ were in the proper positions and we were going to decide where to set up Gene Krupa's drums and other such details. We expected this might take us a quarter of an hour or so. Then the plan was for Fats to be driven home where he would get into his tails and report back to Carnegie at eight o'clock, half an hour before showtime.

As I came into the hall that day through the backstage entrance, I saw a long line of people, a kind of raggedy looking bunch, all blacks. There must have been about a hundred of them and they were lined up right around the corner and down the street. They were just standing there waiting, patiently. I couldn't imagine who they were. If it had been a line for tickets it would have been at the front of the house, where the box-office was. There still wasn't any line out there.

Mr. Totten was standing there in the doorway to his office, with his hat on, smoking a cigar, smiling. I said, "Hello. What's all this?" He said, "These are fans for your Mr. Waller. I know all music fans are a little crazy but I never saw them this crazy before. Your concert doesn't even go on until," he looked at his pocket watch, "three hours and forty minutes from now." Typical jazz crowd, I thought. We were doing better at the stage door than we were at the box-office.

Now Eddie Condon arrived. He walked past the long line waiting at the stage door and came up the steps into the building. "That's Fats's second line," he remarked, referring to the mob that followed the New Orleans street bands.

"You know what they're all carrying?" he asked. "No," I answered. "Well, they all know Fats, and they all want to bring him something he'd like," Condon went on. "You mean drink?" I asked. "There's enough booze in that line to stock Julius's for a month," was Eddie's response.

"Fats is really amazing," I put in. "It's a scientific marvel how he manages to drink all that stuff without impairing his faculties. It would kill anybody else." "Amen," declared Eddie. Then we went up to the star dressing room, the one that Toscannini used when he played here. We didn't find Toscannini there, however. In this luxurious suite there was a mahogany Steinway upright and Fats was sitting at it.

Fats greeted us by indicating a change in schedule. "Instead of going home to St. Albans to dress," he informed us. "I think I'll stay right here. I'll send Buster home to pick up my tails, and I'll shower and dress right here. Did you see all those people out there? I can't shut them out.

They've got a porter here and he's going to let them in, one or two at a time and I'll talk to them. It may take half an hour or so, but we've got plenty of time." While he spoke he was playing the piano so beautifully you could hardly argue with him.

Eddie and I checked the stage. The piano and organ were in position. We marked a spot on the stage floor with white chalk, where Gene Krupa's man could set up his drums. I had a million things to do and so did Eddie. We left Carnegie. Fats stayed.

I dashed home, changed and was back in the front lobby at seven forty-five. I was cheered to see a definite line at the box-office. One of the junior Hecks spotted me and said, "You're going to be all right. You've got a nice sale here. You sent passes to a lot of press and you also had quite a free list. All together, I'd estimate that you'll have about eighty per cent of a house."

This was thrilling news. I had dreaded seeing a half-empty house. I rushed backstage to tell Fats. When I walked in, it looked to me as though there was a big party going on in the star dressing room. The stage door fans had left but now there were a dozen of Fats's close friends there, laughing and carrying on. Fats was not dressed and he didn't seem to be in any hurry either.

Buster came up to me and whispered, "He's terribly nervous. I never saw him this nervous about a job before." I walked over to Fats and said, "Come on, Fats. Let's get moving. You've got to get into your gear. This show hits at eight-thirty sharp. You cannot be late in Carnegie Hall."

In retrospect I think this was a mistake. I shouldn't have mentioned Carnegie Hall. That just made him more nervous and he was as nervous as a cat already. I was getting pretty nervous myself. Buster told me not to worry, he'd have him ready on time. I went back downstairs to the stage and tried to find something else to be nervous about.

Eddie had been worried about Nick Rongetti. He didn't want Nick to start any trouble at the last minute. So Eddie decided to work on the bandstand for the first set at Nick's which began at nine and ended at nine-thirty. Then he and Pee Wee would take a cab up to Carnegie. They'd surely be there by ten. They were already in their tuxedos, which was then the uniform at Nick's.

I had John Kirby braced to be there at ten with his bass. I knew I didn't have to worry about Gene Krupa. He had just that very week broken the house record for an orchestra at the New York Paramount. *Variety* said he did something over a hundred and ten thousand dollars for the week. He had a man with a full drum kit for him already backstage at Carnegie. And Gene had arranged with the Paramount management to be through for the day there by ten-fifteen. It would only take him a few minutes run up Seventh Avenue from Forty-fifth Street to Fifty-sixth Street. I knew I didn't have to worry about him.

As usual Mr. Totten stood in the doorway of his office. His trilby cocked at a saucy angle, he smoked his fine Havana cigar, and watched the excitement brewing up all around him. I came up to him and said, "I'm told we'll have an eighty per cent house." Instantly sensing my anxiety, he said, "You haven't got a thing to worry about. The Hecks are consummate professionals. They'll dress your house so it looks like a sell out. It's all in the way they distribute the seats sold around the auditorium."

'The Dutch Treat Club' was a very chic dining society. Mostly illustrators for the magazines of the time, they met every now and then at an elaborate luncheon at which they honoured somebody in show business. The honoured guest would perform. Being invited to perform for 'The Dutch Treat Club' had almost the cachet of getting an Oscar in the movies. They had written to me that day inviting Fats Waller to their next session. I hadn't told Fats about it yet.

I dashed back up the stairs to the Toscannini Suite, which was a floor above the Carnegie stage level. I came in to a scene of total confusion. There were the remnants of a party still going on and Buster was trying to get Fats dressed in his elegant set of tails. Fats didn't seem to be fully cooperating. He seemed to be lagging a bit. I said, "Come on, Fats, you've absolutely got to hit that deck on time."

I then told him about the invitation from 'The Dutch Treat Club'. He stared at me for a moment and then he broke into a big grin. "Wonderful," he almost shouted, "Tell them I'll be there!" Fats shouting in that tone wasn't really in character. I had the distinct impression that right at this momment he would be happy to talk about anything but Carnegie Hall. I looked at my watch. It was eight-twenty and he wasn't nearly ready to go on.

I managed to get a quick word in with Buster. He said, "The man is terrified! It's this place Carnegie. I never saw him like this before."

Well, there really wasn't anything much more I could do. Fats knew what time it was and he knew it was past time when he should have been on stage. Finally I was told, "He's ready."

I opened the door and the two of us went down the stairs towards the huge Carnegie stage. I noted that Fats was not moving as sprightly as when he had come in some hours earlier. But he looked marvelous. I don't know who Fats's tailor was but he certainly made him some fine clothes. In the wings Fats tried to stop again. I refused to let him. I said, "Go on out there Fats," I looked at my wrist watch, "We're eighteen minutes late right now."

At this he stepped out, and as he was seen by the audience for the first time after that long delay, there was a great burst of delighted applause. I was mentally measuring it and I thought it was the beginning of an ovation. At that instant I had not even a small shadow of a doubt that Fats Waller was going to have the triumph of his life this night.

As the house applauded, and a handful of enthusiasts even stood up as they clapped, Fats made his way to the keyboard of the big Steinway. It was a distance of only about twenty feet but Fats was not moving with his usual grace. I didn't worry. I knew that once he got to the piano everything would be all right.

There was a piano stool there in front of the keyboard. Fats had picked it out days ago. It was already raised to just the right height. Buster had attended to that. Fats bent forward and lifted up his tails to sit down on it. My heart fell as he almost missed the stool. But he didn't tumble to the stage as it seemed he must. He just managed to get part of one cheek on it and then awkwardly sidled over and until he was properly seated. There was just the tiniest ripple of laughter as though some thought Fats was opening his show with a bit of comedy.

Then his hands hit the keyboard and he ran a complex keyboard length arpeggio full of mighty chords with both hands. As he got up into the treble, at full volume, he hit a clinker. It was the first and only clinker I ever heard from Fats Waller.

I dimly began to realize that Fats was hopelessly smashed. I was deeply shocked at this realisation. All my experience with him heretofore had indicated that by some freak of constitution, Fats was impervious to the effects of alcohol. Now, this was proven to be untrue. Although somehow he was able to continue to play he had lost all powers of concentration. His mind was wandering.

Fats and I had gone over the printed programme a dozen times. I thought perhaps I had better place the routine on the piano so he could refer to it. He vetoed this suggestion, insisting that he knew the whole sequence by heart. But now he had lost all memory of it completely.

He was playing *I'm Gonna Sit Right Down And Write Myself A Letter* and some might even think that he was playing it quite competently. But I heard none of Fats Waller's brilliance there. In fact he was not supposed to be playing that number at that point in the concert at all. Although it was his most popular recording, he had not written it. He had decided that the first item on our programme would be a selection of the songs he had written himself.

According to the programme, the first item was: *The Songs of Fats Waller.* This was qualified with a short statement, to wit:

> *In order to give Mr. Waller all possible liberty in selecting his material and in order to retain a maximum of spontaneity for his performance, no formal program has been arranged. In this, his first group of selections at the piano, he will play some of his own popular compositions. A list of the best known of them follows. He may be expected to play several of these items. Some of the best of Mr. Waller's popular songs (which are not included in this list) are not credited to him simply because he sold all rights to them to unscrupulous Tin Pan Alley authors.*

Then followed a carefully compiled list of the titles of 91 Fats Waller compositions together with the dates of composition, beginning with his 1919 *Squeeze Me* and ending with his 1941 *Blue Velvet.* Of course *I'm Gonna Sit Right Down And Write Myself A Letter* was not on this list, since Fats had not written it. Some song plugger had passed it to Victor and Fats had recorded it for them on demand. It had become, however, his most popular number.

The audience listened listlessly. They had no way of knowing what was wrong, or even if anything was wrong. The dynamic reaction I had been praying for never came. I am sure he would have had it had he been right. Naturally I was terribly disturbed but of course there was nothing I could do about it now. He had moved into some of his own things and suddenly he was playing *Honeysuckle Rose.* This stirred the audience into a burst of applause. But I could see that Fats was not himself, he was on automatic.

Stirred by the applause, Fats now got up from the piano and made his way to the organ. Here he began to play spirituals.

The programme read:

> *SPIRITUALS. Among the spirituals Mr. Waller may play are the following: Go Down Moses, Swing Low, Sweet Chariot, Deep River, All God's Chillun Got Wings, Water Boy, Sometimes I Feel Like a Motherless Child and Lonesome Road.*

He began playing one of these and it sounded pretty good. The house was silent and attentive. I had hoped there would be such periods during this concert. It was now going along beautifully and I was just beginning to recover my composure when suddenly he lurched into *All That Meat And No Potatoes,* one of his recent big popular comedy hits. He didn't sing it. But just playing it on the organ in the middle of a batch of religious hymns brought the house down.

Then he was back playing the spirituals. Or was it a spiritual? As I listened to the sound swelling through the auditorium I thought to myself, 'That's no spiritual! That's *Summertime* from Gershwin's opera, Porgy and Bess!' Then he seemed to drift out of *Summertime* and back into a spiritual.

In the printed programme we had scheduled a little after piece to the spirituals medley. This was something based on a classical theme that Fats had been playing in his sessions at home. The programme read:

> *This selection, says Mr. Waller, was inspired by eight bars of Sir Edward Elgar's Pomp and Circumstance.*

I had heard Fats playing with this melody on his Hammond in his St. Albans living room. There he had done such extraordinary things with it that I had asked him to include it on our programme and he had agreed.

Now at Carnegie he started it all right, but then he seemed to forget what he was doing, then he started up again and went off in a completely different direction. It was most erratic. He just couldn't seem to get it going in the way he had played it so easily at home. He got a bit of mild applause for this.

Then he left the organ and returned to the Steinway. Here, just as programmed, he played some Blues. Drunk or sober he could always play the Blues. Then Lips Page came on and began singing about Fats Waller having a ball in Carnegie Hall. Then he picked up his trumpet and, alternately growling with his plunger and screaming with his open horn, he shook Carnegie to the rafters. Fats and Lips got an ovation after this. Then they left the stage for it was intermission.

I asked Mr. Totten how long an intermission should be. He said "Ten minutes." I met Fats and Lips in the wings as they came off. Fats's elegant set of tails was soaked with perspiration. I knew he had to shower and get dressed again. He'd never be able to do it in ten minutes. I said, "Fats this is very important. You must be back on stage in fifteen minutes. Buster, look sharp. That's all you got, fifteen minutes, Come on. You can do it."

A party was already starting in his dressing room. I tried to clear it out but I was afraid of hurting somebody's feelings so I desisted. I raced back into the auditorium and up to the best box, which I had reserved for Mrs. Waller and the family and guests. I had put a couple of bottles of chilled champagne in the box, together with glasses. I suppose young Maurice was there. They all seemed pleased with the concert and unaware that anything might be wrong.

I could only stay a minute, then dashed back to Fats in the star dressing room. The quarter of an hour was up but he wasn't dressed yet. Finally Buster got him organised and out the door. I walked down the stairs with him and headed for the wings. Suddenly he stopped and I could see that he was terrified again. He just did not want to go out on that Carnegie stage. I said, "Fats, there's nothing to worry about. You're just going to play your *London Suite*." I tried to move him towards the stage. Then he said, "Just one more cigarette."

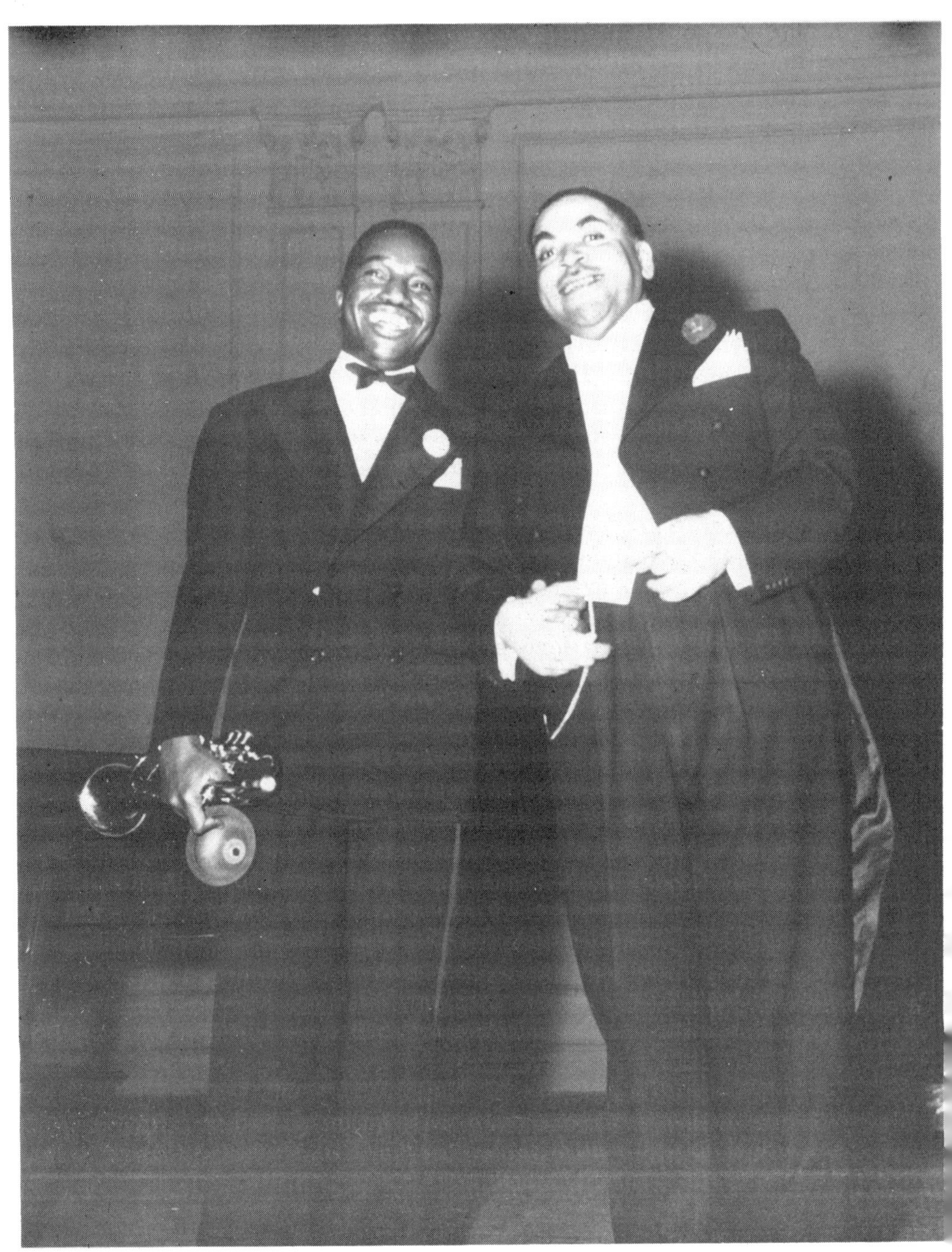

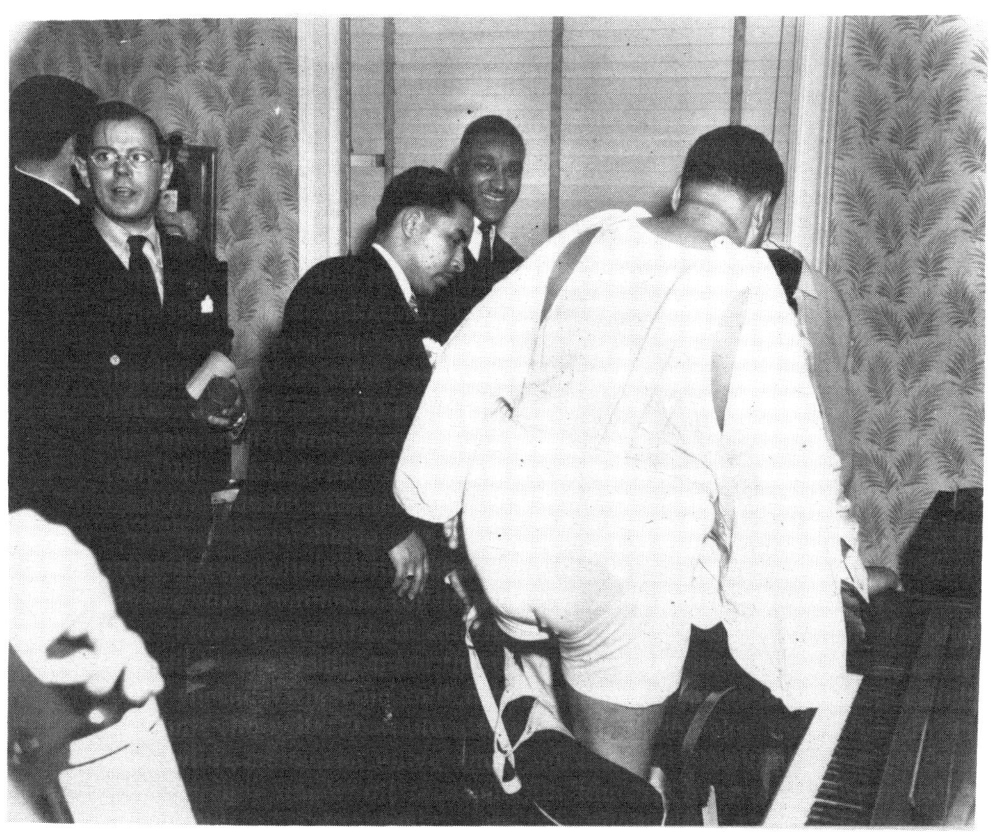

Above: The dressing room scene in the interval with Fats changing into his second half gear. A distraught-looking Ernie Anderson is on the left and Al Casey claims to be in the centre looking at the camera. Note the bottle in left foreground and another held by the man behind Ernie.

Left: Lips and Fats respond to the ovation after their blues duet.
The only truly triumphant moment of Fats Waller's concert happened when he brought on Oran Thaddeus 'Hot Lips' Page and the two of them playing some impromptu blues brought the house down. Lips began his career as a kazoo entertainer in a Texas hotel men's room. By the time he hit New York he was the 'leader' (cum Master of Ceremonies) of the Count Basie orchestra. He was such a sensation when the band first played the Apollo Theater in Harlem that Joe Glaser went backstage and signed him to an unbreakable term contract. Then he cynically kept Lips out of work. Glaser believed he was throttling any competition to Louis Armstrong. Armstrong, of course, never knew about this. Despite such obstacles, Lips's unique talent as a blues shouter, and his wicked style of growling the blues through a plunger in the bell of his horn, were recognised as exceptionally moving throughout the jazz world. All musicians loved Lips. He played hard and lived hard. So hard, in fact, that he only lasted halfway through his forties.

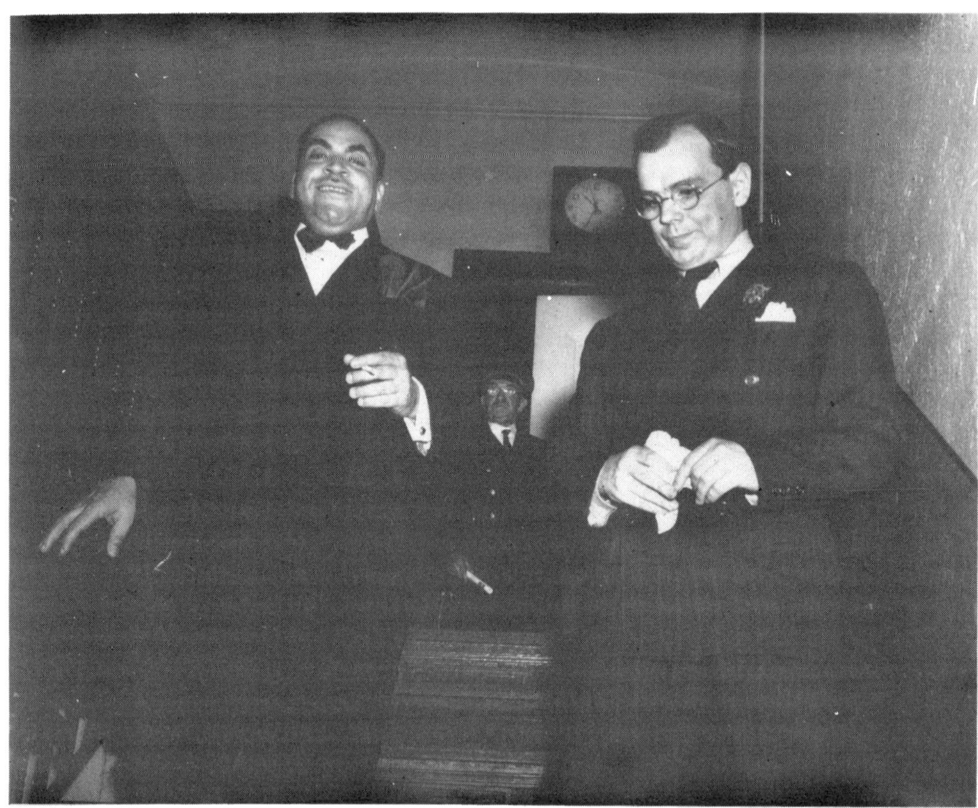

It was 10:34 p.m. and the intermission should have long been over. But Fats was so nervous about performing in Carnegie Hall that he had to fortify himself. Unfortunately he over fortified. The first half had been a disaster and it was only with great difficulty that I finally got him out of his dressing room and down the stairs to the stage. He kept insisting, "Please, just one more cigarette!" We were half way down the steps when he spotted Charlie Peterson and broke into a beam for his camera. I managed to get him past the photographer and down into the wings. He had finished his cigarettes by this time, but said he absolutely had to have one more. He finally walked on to an ovation. But in the next morning's paper one critic wrote that he had returned from his intermission 23 minutes late.

I really felt dreadfully sorry for poor Fats. I lit his cigarette for him and waited while he smoked it. Then he went out to the Steinway. He got a pretty good hand as he entered. Then he started to play *Bond Street* and I thought everything was going to be all right. But all this stress, the immoderate dose of alcohol, the terror of playing Carnegie, were too much for him. He could not concentrate. Once more he drifted into *Summertime,* then I couldn't make out what he was playing.

Naturally enough, I was distressed. The dream I had of showing Fats's extraordinary talent had turned into a nightmare. Just to put a new highlight on it I clearly spotted Gene Sedric holding his naked saxophone in the backstage shadows. This could only mean that Fats was going to sneak his little band on for an unprogrammed item or two. I didn't mind. In fact if Fats had asked for it I'd have been delighted to include the little group. Eddie had always been against it but I could certainly have talked him round once we had lined up our all star group. They would surely make his point.

I turned and made for the lobby and the box-office. I had accounts to settle. The Heck brothers admitted me to their inner sanctum and we began to settle up. First I got my six hundred dollars back. Then we got a cheque for seventy-five dollars for Eddie Condon and another for the same amount for Bud Freeman. Then there were cheques for fifty dollars each for Gene Krupa, Max Kaminsky, Pee Wee Russell and John Kirby. There was a cheque for Bud Freeman's round trip train fare from Chicago, one to cover the champagne for Mrs. Waller's box, and another to cover the cost of newspaper advertising and our direct mail letter. Phyllis had asked for nothing.

The net after all that was something just a little over three hundred dollars and I had a Mr. Heck give me a cheque for that amount made out to Thomas Waller. As usual there was nothing for me. They made up a very business-like statement of accounts on a Carnegie Hall bill heading and I took that with the cheques and headed backstage.

Timing is everything in show business. The instant I got backstage I saw the smiling face of Ed Kirkeby. I hadn't seen him in months but here he was again at payoff time. He greeted me with a compliment. "I don't know how you did it," he began, "that's a nice looking house and you got them all out for him!" He shook my hand in congratulation and, before he had a chance to ask for it, I handed him the box-office statement and the Waller cheque. He studied the statement for a long moment while smiling broadly but he had nothing more to say. A minute later I looked around again for him but he had gone already.

Whatever had been going on on-stage, Fats now came off and there was some desultory applause. He was drenched in perspiration. I could see he was

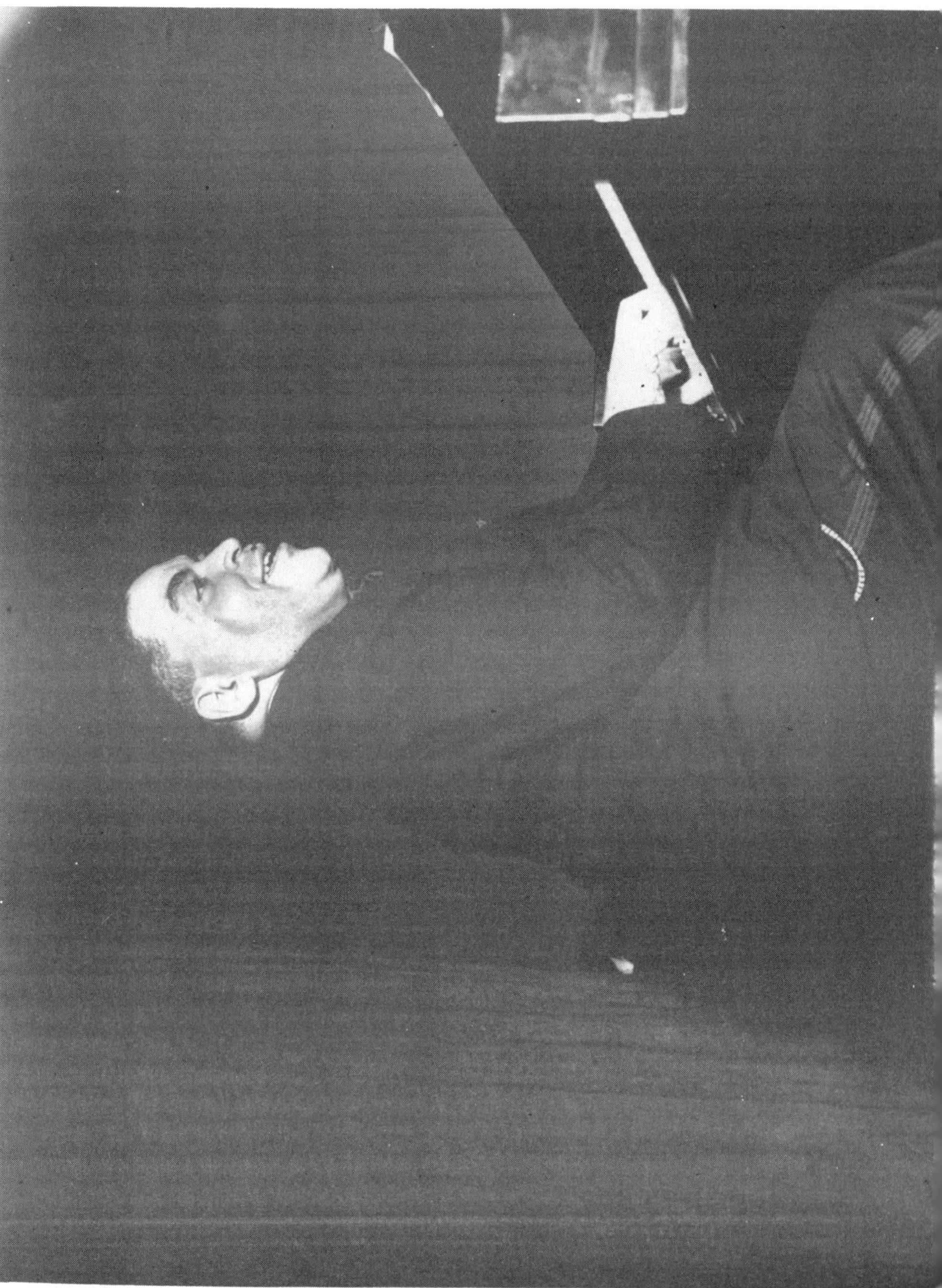

very tired. But, it looked to me, that he was coming around at last. His eyes were alert and he grinned reassuringly when Gene Krupa came bounding up the steps from the stage door. Gene's man was already on the Carnegie stage setting up his drums. Kirby came in through the stage door bearing his bass.

As Eddie got them all together in the wings before shepherding them on stage, I handed each of them their cheque. Each slipped it into a dinner jacket pocket. Except for Gene. He opened his cheque up and read it carefully then, with his characteristic grin, he came up close to me, shook my hand, put the cheque in my outer pocket and said in my ear, "Not for me, Ernie. I'm just honoured to be here." Then suddenly they were all on stage and there was a roar of applause from the audience.

They were supposed to take off on Gershwin's *I Got Rhythm*. Gene realised that this item was for his benefit. At the very last moment he said, "We should play something by Fats. How about *Honeysuckle Rose?*" and suddenly they were playing it.

I thought Fats had almost regained his usual command. But he was terribly tired and with Krupa and Kirby and Condon swinging away, the little band was on fire. They were moving at a rather bright tempo. Freeman took a flock of dynamic choruses, Fats took another batch while Kaminsky, Russell and Freeman riffed behind him, then Gene took off on a solo flight for a few minutes and then they played ensemble for some more choruses as the excitement mounted. The audience was aroused to its highest pitch of the evening.

It was getting late and we were into overtime, which could easily prove very expensive. Fats was supposed to get up and walk to the Hammond now and play the national anthem. He was too tired to move. He began to play it at the piano. This meant that the little band had to play it with him. You must remember that the whole nation had now embarked on the greatest war in history. It had only begun a little over a month earlier.

Actually as I remember that evening now, they sounded pretty good. Gene was rolling away on the snare drum in top military style. But these fellows, including Fats, hadn't played, or even listened to, the *Star Spangled Banner* since childhood. They didn't really know it. As they approached the release the thought began to dawn on them that nobody knew the sequence of notes for the middle part at all.

Then at the very last moment Pee Wee Russell squeaked it out and they all fell in with him. It sounded like it had been planned. As the audience poured out of the hall I went to the front lobby and listened to whatever I could hear. There was Oscar Levant, one of Fats's strongest supporters. He had actually bought a ticket although I'd have given him a pass in a minute. After all he was the man

Left: Fats at the Steinway in the second half of the Carnegie Hall Concert.

who first referred to Fats as 'the black Horowitz'.

Someone was asking his professional opinion of Mr. Waller's *The London Suite* which had just had its world premiere performance. Oscar Levant said, "It shows the strong influence of Gershwin." I wanted to tell him that he hadn't heard *Piccadilly* at all. What he heard was *Summertime.* But I was too depressed. The miraculous thing was that nobody seemed to have twigged to the fact that Fats had been blind drunk all night.

I went back to the star dressing room. Fats was quite bright now. After showering and dressing in another new outfit he had revived. He had already sent Mrs. Waller and the family home. Now he was waiting for Buster to come back to pick him up. But he wasn't going home. Oh no. "I had a hard night tonight," he declared. "Now I'm going out and have a little fun." He was heading for Harlem. I declined his invitation to go along.

He was back in shape. But I was a wreck. As far as I was concerned the whole night had been a disaster, a smashed dream. I regretted it all. I didn't blame Fats. I blamed myself. I could have kept him from the whisky. I had just been convinced that it never bothered him. I had been wrong. It had been my own fault.

I went home to my apartment and I didn't come out for three days. I couldn't bear to see anybody. When people called I said I was very busy. I did get all the papers and read all the notices. The critics all knew something was wrong but they couldn't figure out what it was. This didn't make me feel much better. Never at any time in my life have I felt as low as I did in the days immediately after that concert, which was, you may remember, my first.

The consensus of the critics was that Carnegie Hall was not the proper place for Fats Waller. The New York *Times,* among other things, said:

> *There is undoubtedly a large field for Mr. Waller's talents, as was shown by the size of last night's audience. But why his specialized abilities were exposed to the rigors of Carnegie Hall is an issue that lies beyond the reviewer. Mr. Waller would most likely offer pleasant entertainment in a cafe, but his extended improvisations at this concert were overlong and shapeless.*

The New York *Herald Tribune,* long famous for its music criticisms, was also interesting. Their review included these words:

> *The news is bad. The program according to a note by John Hammond,* [and you know who wrote that], *was dedicated to Fat's artistry as a musician and composer, and the pianist apparently took this seriously. Instead of being his buoyant, rhythm-pounding self, he improvised soulfully, for long stretches at a time, first on the piano and then on the Hammond electric*

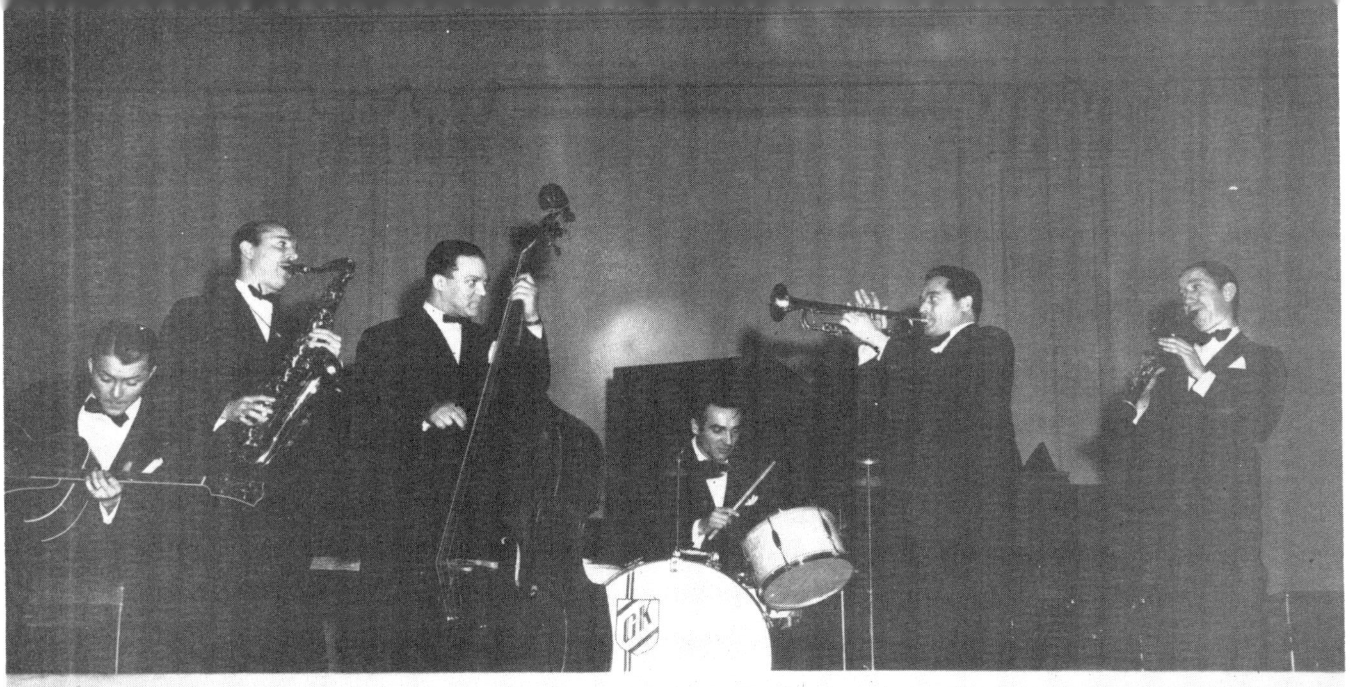

A CARNEGIE CONCERT WITHOUT SHEET MUSIC

L to R: Eddie Condon, who taxied up to Carnegie from Nick's in Greenwich Village where he was supposed to be leading the band; Bud Freeman, who flew in from Chicago just to play this show; John Kirby, who dashed over from Fifty-Second Street where his band was then the premiere attraction; Gene Krupa, who with his big new band had just this week set the house box-office record of $110,00 in the Paramount Theater, thirteen blocks south in Times Square; Maxie Kaminsky, who Fats tried to hire permanently, but Fats's manager, Ed Kirkeby, blocked by insisting that Fats's black band could not have a white trumpeter; and the immortal Pee Wee Russell, who alone of all these famous musicians knew the middle part of the *Star Spangled Banner* which, of course, the band had to play at the end of the concert because the country was at war.

> *organ. Long pauses between his groups did not help matters.*
>
> *The audience responded when Fats started his improvisation on eight bars from Elgar's Pomp and Circumstance on the organ. But Fats stopped playing with a swinging rhythmic bass, and went off into fancy ornamental figures again and the audience relapsed.*
>
> *After a twenty-three minute intermission the audience just sat numbly through a long London Suite and the succeeding variations on a Tchaikovsky theme which was undistinguishable from the suite. The combined talents of Gene Krupa, Eddie Condon, Bud Freeman, Pee Wee Russell and John Kirby could not save the evening.*

Robert Bagar wrote in the New York *World-Telegram:*

> *Where we might have expected real, untrammeled, soaring individuality in a group of improvisations the massive maestro let us down. All the improvising he did came briefly between lines of melody in simple and fragmentary chord formations.*
>
> *A lift was given proceedings with the appearance of the noted Negro trumpet player, Hot Lips Page. He and Sir Fats contrived a really neat bit of extemporaneous stuff.*

You could hardly blame the critics. The poor critic could not be expected to realize that he was not hearing the true Fats Waller. After all, he saw the musician sitting up there at the Steinway. He was impeccably attired. His posture at the instrument was correct. His hands rambled easily over the keyboard.

This in itself was remarkable for what the critic could not see, in fact what no critic even guessed, was that Fats's entire mental facility was stupefied from drink. He was operating entirely by rote. It was all mechanics with no intellect. What the critic heard was the palest of simulations, a cramped and crippled version of the talent Fats truly possessed when in his right mind.

I had a full recording of the whole concert on a set of acetate discs, all paid for and just waiting for me to pick it up upstairs at Carnegie Hall. Perhaps you can gauge my disappointment in the whole event when I tell you that now, half a century later, I still haven't picked it up.

The concert was on a Wednesday evening and Buster had picked up the duplicate set for Fats on Thursday morning the minute the little recording studio opened.

It was Sunday before I came out of purdah. I was quite surprised to observe that everybody knew about the concert and everybody thought it had been a triumph. New York was a city of something over ten million souls. Only twenty six hundred had been in Carnegie Hall that night. The rest just assumed Fats had had a triumph. This was a reasonable assumption in itself.

"What about the music critics?", I asked a friend who I considered knowledgeable in such matters. The reply was, "First of all, nobody much reads the music critics. Those that do are interested in classical music. When they see it's a notice about a jazz concert, they skip it. As far as the true jazz aficionados are concerned, they won't pay any attention to what a longhair music critic writes. 'What does he know about it anyway!'"

This was all reassuring and I began to heal up rapidly. Of course I knew exactly what had transpired at that concert and I was embarrassed even to bring it to mind. But, obviously, hardly anybody else did. In the vast public consciousness, Fats's appearance at Carnegie had been a hit.

Monday just before noon I went out to St. Albans, to pick up Fats for his appearance at 'The Dutch Treat Club'. He was sitting in the dining room eating a solitary late breakfast. He was all dressed and ready to go to the date. Up high on a wall a small record player played. I could hear a solo pianist. "What's that?" I asked. Fats replied, "That's the concert." It was one of the acetates. Fats went on, "It's beautiful, man."

'Well', I thought, 'there's one person who was at the concert who liked it.' Fats and I never had any further discussion about the concert. I took him to 'The Dutch Treat Club' where he was received like an emperor. Everybody there was convinced that his Carnegie appearance had been a triumph.

That Monday lunchtime he then sat down at the Steinway and played the concert he had been unable to play at Carnegie Hall on the previous Wednesday evening. He was brilliant. He got standing ovation after standing ovation. What I should have done was book him right back into Carnegie Hall as quickly as I could get an open date. But I was too badly bruised.

That year Fats toured more than usual. The Carnegie shot, which was mentioned in papers across the country, produced more bookings for Ed Kirkeby. I didn't see Fats so much. Then I heard he was in Hollywood. He had told me what happened out there.

Ivie Anderson, Duke Ellington's great vocalist, had a kind of hostelry for black theatricals called to work in Hollywood. It was out in Central Avenue, the black ghetto of Los Angeles and you might be forgiven for thinking it was just a rooming house. But what rooming house has a grand piano in the living room with a nice bar beside it? Fats had told me that when in Hollywood, the minute he arrived, the party started and it didn't stop until he caught the train back to Manhattan.

Then came the flash news bulletin:

Fats Waller is dead!

A great chord sounded through me, painfully reverberating, on and on. It had happened in Kansas City. He had died of pneumonia in the berth of his drawing room on the Santa Fé Chief on his way to New York.

It was in the depths of a very cold winter, one day less than a week before Christmas. Eddie and I talked about it. We could visualise Fats partying at Ivie's until the last minute, then, soaked to the skin with perspiration, dashing to the Los Angeles train terminal and getting on his train just as it was about to pull out from the station. Exhausted and full of whisky, he piled into the berth of his drawing room and sacked out, probably still in his wet clothes. He would have been very tired you can be sure. His perspiration evaporated and, according to the laws of physics, his temperature fell sharply and he died in his sleep.

I don't really know the actual details yet, only what various people had said they thought were the details. Evidently after leaving Hollywood there had been a party in the club car which continued in his drawing room. Ed Kirkeby had slept in the same drawing room. When I saw Kirkeby in New York I got an account directly from him which ended with, "And then at four in the morning I heard a sound from Fats, It was his death rattle."

That's the only time in my life so far that I have heard those two grim words used in a sentence. I'll be quite content if I never hear them again. In the course of time it developed that some of those financial arrangements Ed Kirkeby had been making for Fats had some subsidiary and under the table financial benefits for Ed Kirkeby.

I really don't believe this would have been any surprise to Fats. If he didn't know about them he would surely have guessed that they existed. He was quite cynical about the business side of music. He had no real respect for money in any case.

On that dread day in December of 1943, Thomas Waller, Jr., had been in the U.S. Army and stationed in a camp not too far from Kansas City. He had arranged to get leave, so that he could go to the Kansas City train terminal early in the morning, in order to have a few minutes with his Dad during the brief scheduled stop.

He met the train only to learn that his father was dead. Half a century later, that sad chord still sounds in my head. I mourn him still and I know I will continue to do so as long as I live. And so will every other human who was ever touched by the musical genius of Fats Waller.

That Irish philosopher Brian O'Nolan suggested that alcohol is an anodyne for boredom. That may be true, but whether it is or not, I honestly do not think that Fats often allowed himself to be bored. He had a happy life, albeit a short one and he died in his sleep, death rattle or no death rattle.

The whole truth of the matter can be stated very simply. Fats was killed by scotch and soda just as surely as if he had been submerged until drowned in a vat of the stuff. We must assume he was willing to settle for that in exchange for being permitted to live his short life in the free and joyous spirit of a party.

All parties have to end sometime.

MY DAYS WITH THE FATS WALLER BIG BAND

by Courtney Williams
(as told to Nigel Haslewood)

The opportunity for me to join Fats Waller's band was provided by my friend George Robinson, the trombone player. George and I had been members of Tommy "Steve" Stevenson's very fine but short lived orchestra. "Steve" left the Jimmy Lunceford band, with which he had been the high note trumpet specialist, and had formed his own band with the advice of Harold Oxley, who had continued to be Lunceford's booking agent.

George Robinson, having heard that Fats was about to rehearse a big band in preparation for a road trip, wanted to be in it and suggested that we attend the rehearsal and try out for the job. We were both hired, as we showed that we could read and play suitably. I remember the rehearsals at the Haven Studio on 54th Street in Manhattan. Fats was so genial and made everybody comfortable by remarking jokingly that the music should be played "M— F—" and then adding innocently that in case we didn't realise, this meant "Mit Feeling".

On my first road trip with Fats Waller the personnel was Herman Autrey, Johnny 'Bugs' Hamilton and me trumpets, I played lead; George Robinson and John 'Shorty' Haughton, trombones; Jimmie Powell and William Alsop alto saxes (Powell playing lead); Gene 'Baby Bear' Sedric, Al Cobb, tenor saxes and Freddie Skerritt, baritone sax. Fats was on piano and organ, Al Casey on guitar, Cedric 'Bass' Wallace on bass and Wilmore 'Slick' Jones, on drums. Don Donaldson went along as musical director, arranger and alternative piano player and Myra Johnson handled the vocals.

On the road trips, we played theatres (booked mostly by the Theatre Owners Bookers Association, or TOBA and known as 'Tough On Black Asses'), segregated hotel ballrooms, tobacco warehouses set up for concert-dances, and town auditoriums where 'coloured' audiences in remote balconies listened to the band concert that preceded the dancing in which only the 'white' audience could participate. I remember particularly a theatre date in a southern town when the State Governor was in the audience and Fats finished off with one of his fun acts. As he left the stage he wrapped his very large backside in the curtain at the side of stage and wiggled it at the audience. We made a hasty exit to the bus waiting to take us out of town just in case there was some reaction from those southerners who might not have considered it funny.

I also remember Fats's fabulous appetite for both food and Old Grandad whiskey. When the bus stopped at a hot dog stand or a pastrami sandwich place, he would order seven or eight just for himself. Fats also had a Lincoln Continental automobile which he used to use when he didn't travel in the bus. This was driven by the band's valet, Bobby Driver. His brother Lawrence, often accompanied Fats on such trips and also helped as band valet. Some of the journeys between jobs were long, and directions on how to get there often vague. However, Fats could always make a joke out of the situation, and when asked about directions would often reply, "Keep straight ahead 'til you hear glass breaking".

On jobs we played stock arrangements of some popular tunes, along with special arrangements recorded by, associated with, or favoured by Fats. Don Donaldson was the primary arranger and musical director, but I also contributed a number of arrangements along with playing lead trumpet. We also had arrangements by others, and I always enjoyed playing Fletcher Henderson's arrangement on *Sometime I'm Happy.* Head (blue book) arrangements were usually worked out in rehearsals where someone (often the section leader) would come up with a riff or phrase to play behind a solo or vocal and the other section members would improvise the harmony or play unison. Sometimes the bandleader or musical director might distribute notes to be played by each player. The given notes might be played from memory or might later be transformed into written parts by an arranger or copyist. I believe Duke Ellington was known to practise developing arrangements in that fashion.

The records that I played on with the 1938 band came out on the Victor label, and back in those days there weren't too many 'coloured' bands recorded on the major labels. Mostly the companies had some sort of secondary or auxiliary label which they distributed to certain parts of the country (mostly the south) and they featured what was then called 'Race' records or rhythm and blues. We were pleased to find that we were going to be one of the first 'coloured' bands to be recorded on the Victor label, and not to be considered just a 'rhythm and blues' band. I recall that there was some urgency because we had to prepare quickly for the upcoming date and Fats wanted to include some current tunes. Listeners to the records today will notice that the first tunes we recorded were not blues, but popular tunes of the day.

In the Fats Waller discographies, my name is listed as Nathaniel. I suppose that's an additional listing which matches one that appeared on a French issue of an album by Benny Carter. Apparently the researcher must have got an original record from Local 802 of the Musicians Union, which I joined in 1934. At that time I gave my full name as Nathaniel Courtney Williams, and although I never used the name 'Nathaniel', that's the name that appears on the Benny Carter album and in the listings of Fats Waller. But that's me!

The other personnel from the road trip were almost the same as in the band that made the recordings. The one exception was the tenor player, Al Cobb. I had not known him before that time and I never heard about him after he left the band. He was a tall, dark, carefully groomed fellow from Texas who most of the time kept himself to himself. He had very little to say unless spoken to, but was very polite in company and stood straight as a soldier whenever he had to play a solo. He did not seem to be one of Fats's favourites, and did not stay with the band too long. He managed to beat Fats a number of times in the intermission crap games and, it was said, was somtimes an unwelcome interloper in some of Fats's other social activities. Certainly, some of us felt that Fats was sometimes annoyed when Cobb tended to win out in both the crap games and social competition. The tenor sax player on the 1938 record session was 'Lonnie' Simmons. Lonnie was a young fellow with whom I worked on several local gigs with 'Lips' Page and others before he returned to Chicago.

I have provided a listing of the numbers we recorded of which I still have copies, together with my comments and identifications. These are based on my best recollections and recognition of the players's styles and sounds.

(Courtney Williams's notes will be found at the foot of the session of 12 April 1938 — LW)

The personnel of Fats's band often changed in the lay-offs between road trips. During my second stint with the orchestra in March 1942, we played the Apollo Theatre. However, I didn't stay with the band long after this second occasion because by this time I had decided not to go on the road any more. I soon left to join Snub Mosley's small group and played local gigs during 1942-43. At this time we had Johnny 'Buggs', Joe Thomas and me on trumpets. I don't recall Herman Autrey being there at that time. Herb Flemming and Fred Robinson were the trombone players, not George Wilson whose name I have seen listed. First alto player was George James and the other was Jackie Fields, not Lawrence Fields as some people have suggested. We had two tenors, Gene Sedric and Bob Carroll, but there was no baritone sax in that band. With Fats in the rhythm section were Al Casey and Cedric Wallace as before, but the drummer was now Arthur Trappier. Myra Johnson still handled the other vocals and Don Donaldson was still the musical director.

It was this band that recorded *The Jitterbug Waltz* which was written with the organ in mind. Gene Sedric played the clarinet part. Fats liked to carry an organ with him on tour with the band and he loved to play it. Often after the last

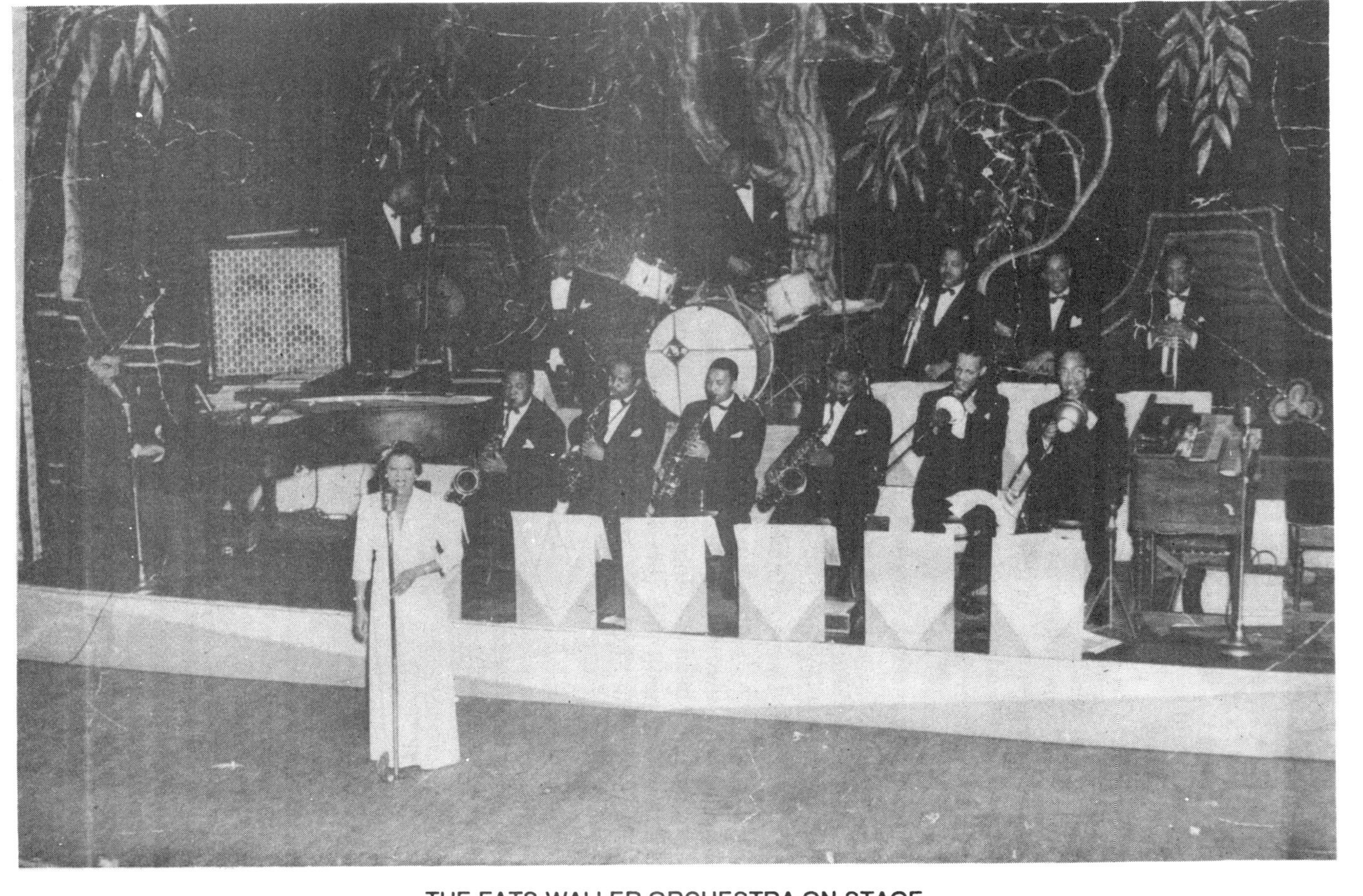

THE FATS WALLER ORCHESTRA ON STAGE

L to R, back: Cedric Wallace, Al Casey, Arthur Trappier, Johnny 'Bugs' Hamilton, Courtney Williams, Joe Thomas. Front: Fats, Myra Johnson, Gene Sedric, Jackie Fields, George James, Bob Carroll, Herb Flemming, Fred Robinson. Note organ at right.

show at a theatre, he would have us stay on stage as an audience while he played the organ for us. He always said that one of his fondest memories was having played the great organ in the Cathedral of Notre Dame in Paris. When he spoke of that he always did so with great pride and joy

I never knew who arranged *The Jitterbug Waltz*. In later years some of the fellows believed it to be my arrangement, but that's not true. I always loved this number and I do remember a meeting at Fats's Morningside Avenue apartment in New York where he, songwriter Andy Razaf and I talked about the proposal that I write an arrangement of it for André Kostelanetz who wanted it for his big concert-type orchestra on a popular radio show. That idea was never carried out. However, I do have another reason for remembering the tune well. When we recorded the number I was entertaining a royal fever blister on my lip and enjoyed the playful concern of my section mates, Joe Thomas and Johnny 'Buggs'.

I don't recall anything about *We Need A Little Love* which was issued on the back of *The Jitterbug Waltz* and my copy has been cracked for years, so I've been unable to play it. However it was issued as the 'A' side of the record, so presumably that was the side that Victor thought was going to sell. Hearing it again recently, I think it may have been a stock arrangement as it's not Don Donaldson's style. I have no recollection of recording the other two titles, but I suppose I must have been playing lead trumpet as usual because the records do sound like the 1942 band and the soloists sound like Johnny 'Buggs', Al Casey, Gene Sedric and Jackie Fields on alto sax.

MUSICAL ATTRIBUTES OF FATS WALLER, THE PIANIST

by Henry A Francis 18 March 1991

Thomas "Fats" Waller (1904-1943) has been renowned continuously since the middle 1930's as one of the greatest jazz pianists, an equally great organist, a prolific songwriter, an ebullient singer and entertainer, and a gifted, subtle comedian. He was the most famous, and one of the best, exponents of a unique style of piano playing known as stride piano, which evolved directly from ragtime music, but is firmly anchored in the mainstream of jazz. To set the scene for an analysis of Waller the pianist, therefore, it will be useful first to define and discuss the musical idiom of stride piano.

The Stride Piano Idiom

A list of those who played authentic stride piano must include James P Johnson, Fats Waller, Willie "The Lion" Smith, Joe Turner, Donald Lambert, Cliff Jackson, Luckey Roberts, and, early in their careers, Art Tatum, Duke Ellington, and Count Basie. To further define the boundaries of the idiom, a list of great jazz pianists who did not play stride piano would include Jelly Roll Morton, Earl Hines, Teddy Wilson, and Joe Sullivan.

The Stride Piano School of American Music dictates that both hands earn a living. The most obvious attribute of this style is that the left hand occupies itself principally with striking a bass note, octave, or tenth on beats 1 and 3 of the 4/4 measure, and a dense chord near middle C on beats 2 and 4. The left arm is therefore continuously engaged in reciprocating motion (hence the name "stride"), and this athletic activity provides a very strong rhythmic and harmonic foundation. The even-beat chords usually contain four notes and are closed voicings (as tightly bunched as possible) which gives them a percussive striking power comparable to the odd-beat bass notes. Thus all four beats are more or less equally accented, which enhances the "swing" of the rhythm. [F1]

However, this oom-pah-oom-pah left hand is merely necessary, not sufficient; its presence does not guarantee the real thing, the genuine article. The unique characteristics of stride piano are subtle — readily detected aurally, but not easily described verbally. Suffice it to say here that the idiom is distinguished by a particular rhythmic and contrapuntal feel produced by the combined effect of the sturdy striding left hand and various playful right-hand figures which, as is usual in swinging jazz, are phrased in a meter close to 12/8. [F2]

Above all, stride is a truly solo idiom; it is entirely self-sufficient and requires no rhythmic or harmonic assistance. In fact, the addition of rhythm instruments usually obscures the impish strut of solo stride piano. The style generates a very full, orchestral sound, as the oscillating left hand activates simultaneously both the low and middle registers, while the right hand operates in the upper registers. The bass notes often comprise a line or voice which moves in proper (i.e., 19th-century European) counterpoint to the melody and harmony above, further solidifying the edifice. At fast-to-medium tempos, stride is played without using the damper pedal, to achieve a crisp rhythmic drive, while at medium-to-slow tempos, the pedal is customarily used to enable the left hand to produce legato [F3] full-value quarter notes which emphasise the harmony.

Stride piano evolved from classic American ragtime piano music of the period 1895-1910, adding harmonic and rhythmic complexity and subtlety, and attained its mature form by the middle 1920's. It was developed in the Northeast (mostly in New York; in fact it is often labelled "Harlem stride piano") by a fraternity of black musicians as a frolicsome, flashy, swaggering, aggressive solo piano style able to forcibly entertain and command attention, to be audible in a room full of raucous people, and to provide strong enough rhythm for dancing — all for the price of one piano player. Paradoxically, this robust music created by blacks originally for blacks is currently performed and appreciated almost exclusively by whites. The style is applicable not only to the formal pieces written by the stride pianists to display their wares, but is also admirably suited to theme-and-variations presentation of all types of American popular songs and jazz compositions.

Fats Waller, the Pianist

Having elucidated the definitive characteristics of stride piano, we can now proceed to the particular attributes of Fats Waller that ensure his greatness and distinguish him from other pianists.

To most listeners, Waller's dominant quality is his remarkable hypnotic beat and rhythm — powerful, yet also calm, smooth, and totally under control. Like Louis Armstrong and all the other great jazz voices of the classic era, it was simply impossible for Waller not to swing. Every note and chord was chosen, placed, struck, and held in such a way as to optimise the rhythmic drive and to generate intense swing. And, like Lionel Hampton, he was a catalytic rhythm machine, who instantly and infallibly supercharged both his fellow performers and his audience with energy and well-being.

Waller was also an outstanding melodist, evidenced not only by the hundreds of high-quality songs he composed, but also by the graceful and well-structured melodic lines created in the course of his day-to-day improvisations and embellishments.

Most music can be assessed completely in terms of three categories of attributes:

1. The notes that are played; these can be specified, at least approximately, on paper by conventional staff-and-note notation.

2. The exact time-placement and duration of the notes, as they are played by the performer.
3. The quality of the sound — both the sound of the "attack" or beginning of the note (or chord), and the sound of the "ringing" or body of the note.

In the analysis and aesthetics of European "concert" music, the type-1 attributes, the notes of a musical piece as an intellectually abstracted system, receive the most emphasis — indeed, a work of music is often considered to be completely defined in the form of a printed score. In jazz, however, the performer's "voice" is at least as important as the notes he plays (hence recordings, not scores, are the principal archival material), and attributes 2 and 3 must be considered carefully. Most importantly, these two attributes determine the delicate balance of rhythmic tension that provides the essential swing and momentum, without which the music falls flat and ceases to be jazz.

Applying this classification of musical attributes to the piano music of Fats Waller, we will consider first some general characteristics of the actual notes he chose to play, which can be described in musical notation. We will then discuss the distinctive ways in which he executed his chosen notes on the piano, most of which are too subtle and rhythmically complex to be indicated conveniently by conventional notation.

His Choice of Notes

A stride pianist's voice and personal style depends at least as much on the nature of his rhythm section, the left hand, as on the sound of his "horns", the right hand. On beats 1 and 3, Waller's left hand employed equally both tenths and single notes, in distinction to the other great stride pianists who favoured single notes or octaves. He typically played a middle-register tenth on beat 1 and a low single note on beat 3. The tenths contributed considerably to the overall fullness of his sound. Waller had three different ways of phrasing his stride tenths: Usually the two notes were hit simultaneously, but often, for rhythmic and textural variety, he played the lower note before the beat and the upper note on the beat, thus "rolling" or "breaking" the tenth chord. [R1,R2,R3] Occasionally, he played downward-broken tenths, the upper note before the beat and the lower note on the beat; this produced an exhilarating rhythmic effect. [R4,R5] Whenever possible, usually at slower tempos, he used open three-note chords instead of "empty" tenths, either on beats 1 and 3 when striding, or in "walking" parallel motion on all four beats, as illustrated in Example 1.

The nature of Waller's right hand is best introduced by a short catalogue of his most often-used or typical right-hand stride figures. In these examples presented in musical notation, the usual convention in notating jazz applies — namely, that notated 8th notes represent a rhythm close to 12/8 meter. [F2] The chord symbols below the staff indicate the nominal harmony played by the striding left hand.

Most of the music Waller played (and indeed most of American popular music and jazz) consists structurally of 8-measure (bar) or 16-measure units which are usually terminated by a 2-measure cadence marking the return of the harmony to the tonic chord. Four favourite Waller cadences are illustrated in Examples 2-5. In Ex. 2, the vital rhythmic and harmonic punch is provided by the first right-hand chord which is not the tonic chord C but the subdominant F, thus creating tension by delaying the return to the tonic until beat 3. Ex. 4 illustrates a very characteristic Waller use of triplets at the beginning of each measure. Ex. 5 shows a general note pattern Waller used somewhere in practically all of his solos. The 12/8 "shuffle" rhythm of this figure is emphasised by the accented 2-note chords on the second half of beats 1 and 3.

Examples 6 and 7 are representative figures Waller used on a dominant 7th chord. Ex. 6 exhibits the same note pattern and rhythmic feel as the cadence in Ex. 5, and Ex. 7 is similar with a rising overall line in contrast to the falling lines of Exs. 5 and 6.

Examples 8 and 9, although harmonically different, both illustrate the same characteristic rhythmic structure over the 2-measure phrase, with one strong syncopated (off-the-beat) accent in measure 1 and two in measure 2.

Many of Waller's right-hand figures can be categorised as "riff-type" [F4], where a short group of notes is played repeatly. Examples 10 and 11 (both of which are as instantly recognisable as his face) are strict repetitions of length 1 beat and 3 beats, respectively. In Exs. 12-15, the repeated figures are identical rhythmically but are successively altered melodically. Exs. 12 and 13 repeat each beat, while Exs. 14 and 15 repeat every 2 beats. The descending triplets of Ex. 14 are a common feature in Waller's melodic landscapes, particularly in his early career.

As with human personality, the flavour of a jazz pianist's musical personality is determined as much by his various personal embellishment and ornamentation of the principal musical theme as by the theme itself. Waller had his own arsenal of right-hand runs used to punctuate the interstices between melodic phrases, and ornaments used to decorate chords or a melodic line.

Some typical runs are illustrated in Examples 16-18. Ex. 16 is a pentatonic run [F5] used over the tonic major chord, while Ex. 17 is essentially the same run slightly altered to go with the dominant 7th chord. At slower tempos, these two runs were usually played faster than 16th notes. The pentatonic run of Ex. 18 was often used as a "break" at the end of an 8-measure unit. The arpeggio-type run of Ex. 19 is, along with Ex. 17, representative of the fast runs Waller frequently employed to sprinkle his slow-tempo melodic excursions with "stardust".

Example 20 shows a typical ornamental figure Waller used to fill space and sustain rhythmic momentum between melodic phrases — a short downward run covering two octaves, starting with a fast triplet at the top. Ex. 21 illustrates his characteristic use of a triplet turn to decorate an unchorded line of melody.

Waller often embellished and strengthened a note in a melodic line by playing it as an octave with either upward or downward grace notes to give it a "ringing" attack. These were white-key octaves executed by sliding off the adjacent black keys with both fingers. [R6] He also ornamented octaves with an upward grace note applied to the top note only.

The piano is technically a percussion instrument in that once a note is struck, its loudness will steadily diminish, its tone cannot be controlled, and vibrato is impossible. Pianists have always been concerned with devices for producing the effect of "singing", to approach the emotional intensity of the sustained tone of the voice and wind instruments. Earl Hines, Jess Stacy, and many other jazz pianists used the octave tremolo to maintain note loudness and to simulate vibrato. Waller, however, made unique use of the trill to sustain long notes in a melodic line. [R7,R8] The trilled interval was usually either a whole tone or a minor third.

Finally, we should mention the role Waller's harmonic style played in his overall musical voice. His harmony was unusually rich in that he employed very full chords containing as many notes as feasible. His chord voicings and harmonic sequences were always tasteful and musically correct (that is, by classical European standards), and his voice-leading [F6] was impeccable. His use of harmony was never "advanced" in the sense that Tatum's and Ellington's were. Waller rarely used altered chord functions such as the flatted fifth, flatted ninth, or sharped ninth degrees of the dominant 7th chord, which constituted a major component of the pianistic voices of Tatum, Ellington, and others in the 1930's. Even Waller's original mentor, James P Johnson, employed these harmonic devices in his later career.

The Way He Played His Notes

What were the nature and sources of Waller's distinctive sound? Hugues Panassié wrote, in his account of Waller's 1932 visit to Paris: [F7]

> *He hardly raises his hands from the keyboard. So the unbelievable power of his playing comes not so much from the speed of his attack as from his weight. His strength is not at all nervous but muscular. Instead of taking his impetus from above to strike the keys heavily, Fats attacks them rather from quite near, and would appear to be trying to push the keys into the piano. That is surely why his playing, in spite of its terrific force, appears so much more placid than that of other pianists.*

Panassié was right on target here, both in his description of what he heard, and in his interpretation of how Waller achieved this sonority. Waller's striding left hand produced relatively long note duration (without using the damper pedal) and exceptionally smooth attack, even at fast tempos, and this was accomplished primarily by arm muscle control. A note or chord lasts only as long as the keys are held down, and so to attain a more legato stride sound, the fingers must remain in contact with the keys for a longer fraction of the beat interval, which shortens the time left for moving the arm to the next note or chord. In addition, to avoid a harsh, strident, banging, clanging sound, the keys must be depressed without too much velocity; to accomplish this, the arm must decelerate and stop moving before the fingers contact the keys. These two requirements make extreme demands on left-arm strength, speed, and control, and Waller was a supreme athlete in this respect. The feat was not merely moving the arm laterally from bass note to chord and back at fast tempo, but to be capable of such rapid and accurate acceleration and deceleration that the keys were always depressed with controlled speed and held down for a large portion of the beat length. Panassié's observation that Waller kept his hands close to the keys indicates that he moved the keys using finger action and/or a short wrist stroke, but without appreciable vertical arm motion. The low trajectory of his striding left hand can be plainly seen during his solo chorus of *I've Got My Fingers Crossed* in the 1935 movie *'King of Burlesque'*. Lesser pianists can duplicate the smooth sound of Waller's striding left hand only by "vamping" with both hands (using the left for the bass notes and the right for the chords), for then no lateral arm motion is required. It should be added that when striding with his usual rhythm section of drums, bass, and guitar, particularly in his later career, he usually played his left-hand notes more staccato (shorter duration) than when playing unaccompanied, to give the collective rhythm a lighter, more relaxed sound. However, his two-handed "vamp" accompaniments were usually of comparatively long note duration. [R9]

In addition to his exceptional arm, wrist, and finger control, Waller was blessed with enormous hands. He did not flaunt this gift by using his abnormally large finger spread to play unusually wide intervals. However, his large hands enabled him to play moderately large, dense chords (usually a tenth wide and containing three or four notes) very cleanly, without strain, at all tempos — see Examples 1 and 15. At fast tempos, he played even the widest left-hand tenths (such as Db-F) firmly, securely, and with both notes struck simultaneously. In addition, his large hand size allowed him to execute cleanly and smoothly certain characteristic "Fats" right-hand figures that would have been awkward or impossible for smaller-handed pianists — see Examples 2 and 22.

Much of Waller's elegant, smooth, legato sound and rhythmic feel at slow and medium tempos is attributable to his superb right-ankle control on the damper pedal. The damper pedal, when depressed, lifts all the string dampers, and its mastery is one of the keys to a legato, "singing" sonority on the piano (the other key is finger control). It must be rapidly and deftly lifted and depressed at the junctions between notes so that there is neither dead space nor overlap between successive notes. Waller used it principally to extend the note duration of the striding left hand, ideally achieving exact quarter notes. Thus, the pedal is lifted just before each beat, to terminate the notes of the preceding beat, and is then depressed just after the beat, and held down, to sustain the new notes until the next beat. To use this technique successfully at medium tempos, as Waller was able to [R10,11], requires fine ankle speed, timing, and control.

Waller's incomparable overall piano technique, touch, and sonority is well illustrated by his "classical" version of *Honeysuckle Rose.* [R12] In the third chorus in particular, he achieves a very full-bodied sound, with the different simultaneous activities all clearly audible. From the same session, *Ring Dem Bells* [R13] similarly demonstrates his rich sound. Finally, Waller's general pianistic sure-footedness is pointed up by his well-documented ability to play with undiminished control, accuracy, and sensitivity when drunk.

Miscellaneous Attributes

Waller's basic style essentially changed very little throughout the 15 years (1929-1943) of his mature career. Perhaps the most notable change, during the later 1930's, was that his slow-tempo ballads were decorated with increasing amounts of baroque filigree, such as illustrated in Examples 17 and 19. Also, as jazz steadily evolved and the Swing Era began (ca. 1935), the prevailing rhythmic feel in jazz became generally more understated and subtle. In keeping with this trend, Waller, when playing with his band, tended to play his striding left hand more staccato, to emphasise the overall lighter feel of his rhythm section.

Most great musical performers have the ability to control simultaneously several different neuromuscular activities, and Waller's multifunction mind was exceptionally well-developed. On hundreds of records he demonstrated this aptitude when he accompanied his own entertaining and swinging singing with brilliant stride piano (not just two-handed "vamping"), consisting of intricate, demanding right-hand figures, perfectly chosen and impeccably executed. Since in the recording studio he was usually presented with unfamiliar sheet music to record, part of his mind was necessarily focused on reading the lyrics and melody, altering or embellishing them to suit his musical and dramatic temperament, and finally delivering the vocal, often with jiving asides inserted in the interstices. Yet in addition to all this mental activity, the remaining portion of his mind was able simultaneously to produce a stride piano accompaniment worthy of standing on its own as a solo. [R14,R15,R16]

Waller was a very exciting, inspiring, and catalytic ensemble pianist, whether striding or merely "vamping". When striding as part of the rhythm section behind an instrumental soloist or ensemble, a steady stream of notes usually flowed from his right hand (the antithesis of the space and economy of Count Basie's pithy accompaniments), yet the end result was never obtrusive. His right hand purveyed brilliantly conceived rhythmic figures and airy riffs which never obstructed the soloist or muddied the background (in contrast to Art Tatum's accompaniments), and often spurred the horn-men to perform above their usual artistic levels. With his striding left hand firmly and gracefully defining the beat, he was a rhythm factory which energised and drove the entire band without being loud or overbearing. [R17,R18]

As with many other great jazz performers in the 1930's, particularly the more popular and commercially successful ones, Waller was often given trite, banal songs to record. These were usually foisted upon him sight-unseen in the studio by the recording authorities. It is to his credit, and for posterity's gain, that he was able single-handedly to transform this hack material into musically valuable performances, often by merely playing the melody unaltered but exquisitely phrased and ornamented, and firmly supported and propelled by his striding left hand. [R19,R20,R21] This is what Waller had in mind when he said: "Regardless of how sweet the line, how fast or slow, the good old left hand can always swing it out" [F8].

FOOTNOTES

F1. The term "swing" refers to a rhythmic feel in jazz which simultaneously has both strength and buoyancy, both tension and relaxation, plus a relentless bouncing momentum. Swing is a subjective property and cannot be defined in musical terms. A performance that does not swing, however, is like a car with a flat tyre — it is immediately apparent when one drives off that something is very wrong.

F2. Thus, if a measure of melody consists nominally of eight 8th notes, when phrased in "swinging 12/8" the odd-numbered notes will have approximately twice the duration of the even-numbered notes.

F3. Legato means phrasing a melodic line so that there is no silence and no overlap between successive notes.

F4. A riff is a short melodic figure (generally 1 or 2 measures long) which is repeated, unaltered or slightly altered, over an extended section of changing harmony.

F5. A pentatonic melody uses only the five notes of the pentatonic scale; the C pentatonic scale is C, D, E, G, A.

F6. Voice-leading refers to the relationship between the notes of successive chords, treated as being made up of two or more melodic lines or "voices". Voice-leading is part of the academic discipline of Harmony.

F7. *Storyville 40;* April, May, 1972; translated from the French by Roy M Cooke.

F8. *Hear Me Talkin' To Ya,* Nat Shapiro & Nat Hentoff, eds., Rinehart & Co. (1955) p. 266.

MUSICAL EXAMPLES

The matrix number and date of the recording are given in parentheses.

Ex. 1. *Sweet Savannah Sue* (49493-2, 2 August 1929) Chorus 2 (after verse).
Numb Fumbling (49762-2, 1 Mar 1929) Chorus 2.

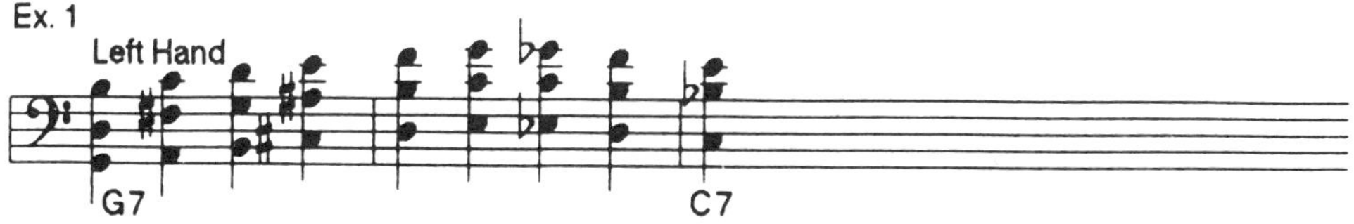

Ex. 2. *Smashing Thirds* (56710-2, 24 Sepember 1929)

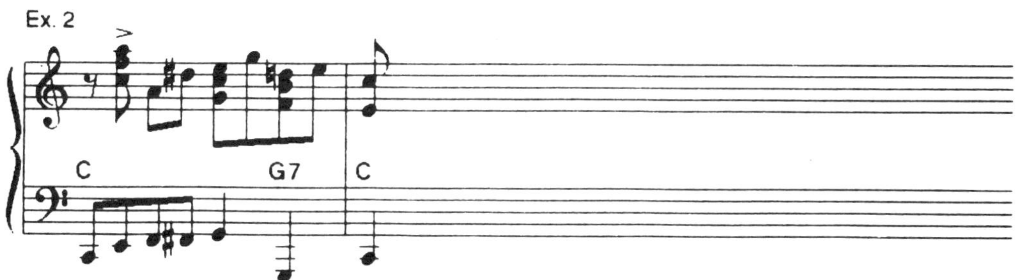

Ex. 3. *Bach Up To Me* (102017-1, 8 June 1936) Chorus 2.
Lounging At The Waldorf (102020-1, 8 June 1936) Chorus 1.

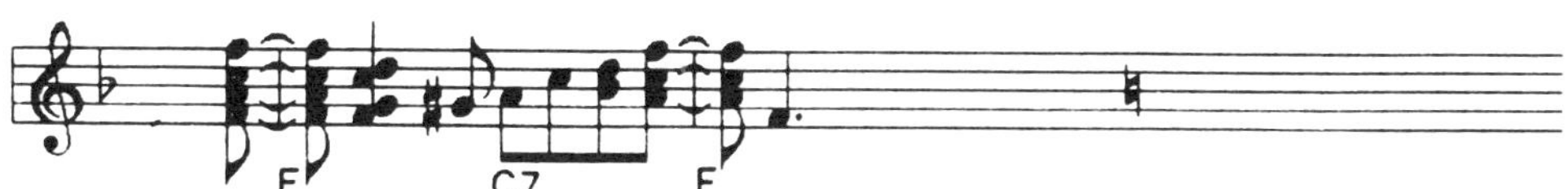

Ex. 4. *Fractious Fingering* (102018-1, 8 June 1936) End of chorus 4.

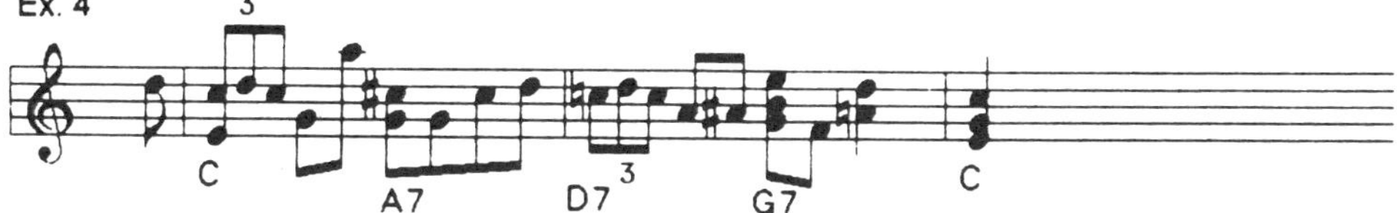

Ex. 5. *Handful Of Keys* (49759-1, 1 March 1929) End of strain B (key of Bb).

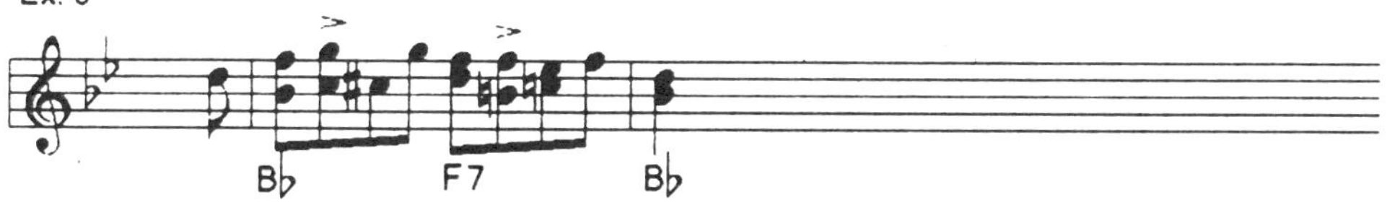

Ex. 6. *Sheik Of Araby* (ZZ-2143, 7 August 1939) Choruses 2 and 4.

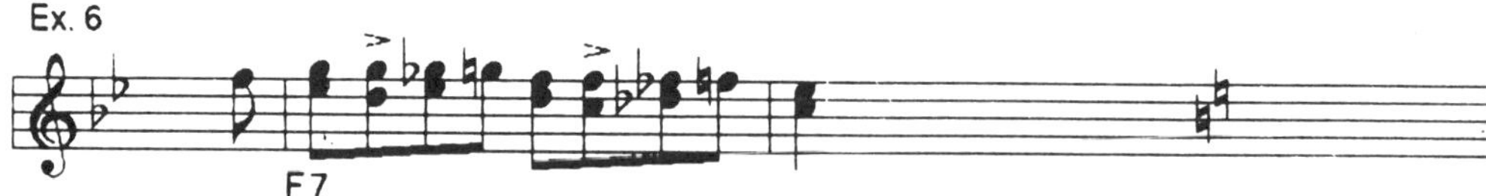

Ex. 7. *California Here I Come* (A-272, 11 March 1935) Choruses 2 and 3, measure 23.

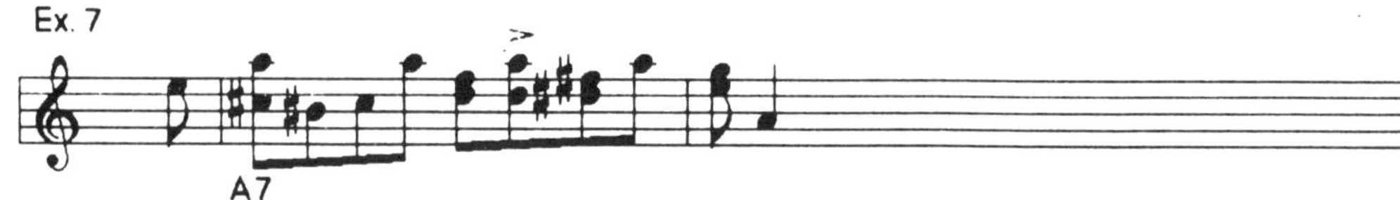

Ex. 8. *I Got Rhythm* (98198-1, 4 December 1935) Waller's solo.

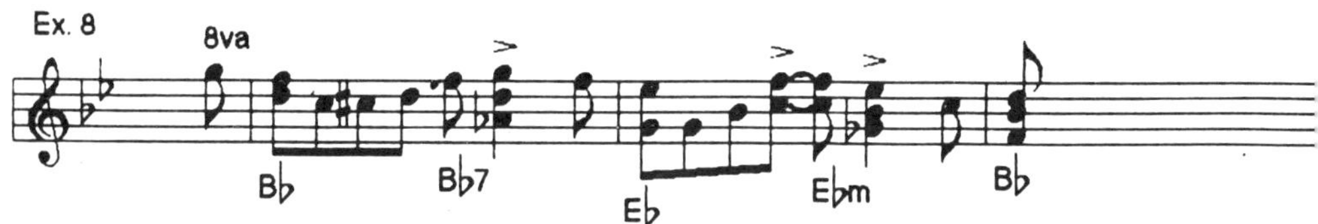

Ex. 9. *Black Raspberry Jam* (102016-2, 8 June 1936) Chorus 1.

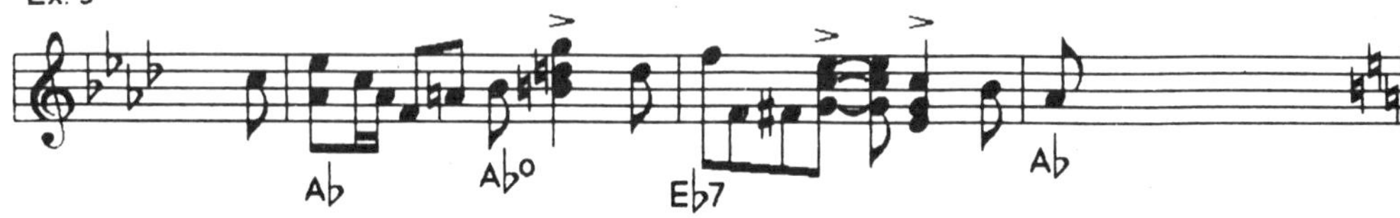

Ex. 10. *On The Sunny Side Of The Street* (19 October 1938, Martin Block broadcast withArmstrong) Waller's solo.
I'm Gonna Salt Away Some Sugar (057084-1, 6 November 1940) Chorus 3.

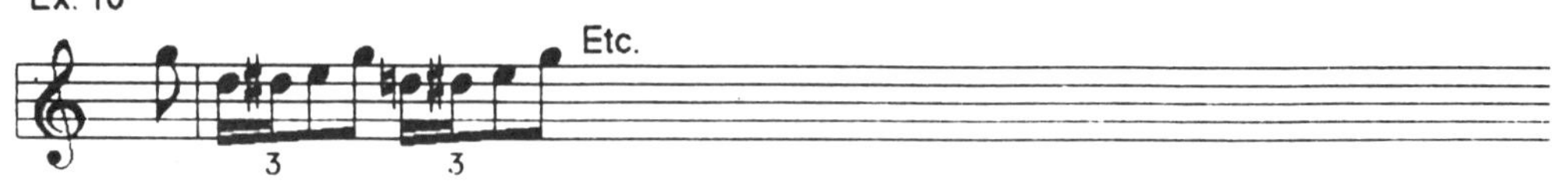

Ex. 11. *Christopher Columbus* (101190-1, 8 April 1936) Waller's solo.

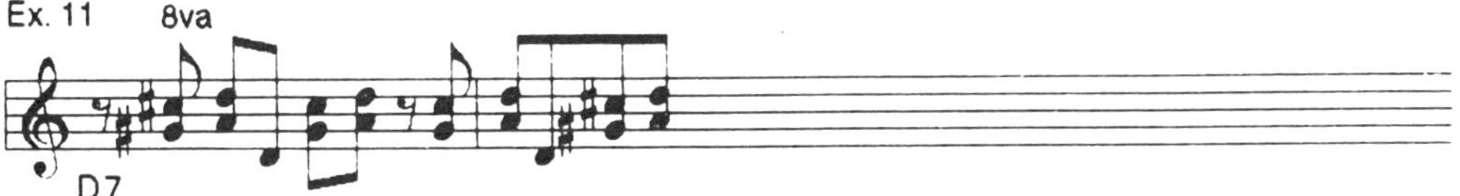

Ex. 12. *Do Me A Favor* (82529-1, 16 May 1934) Chorus 1.

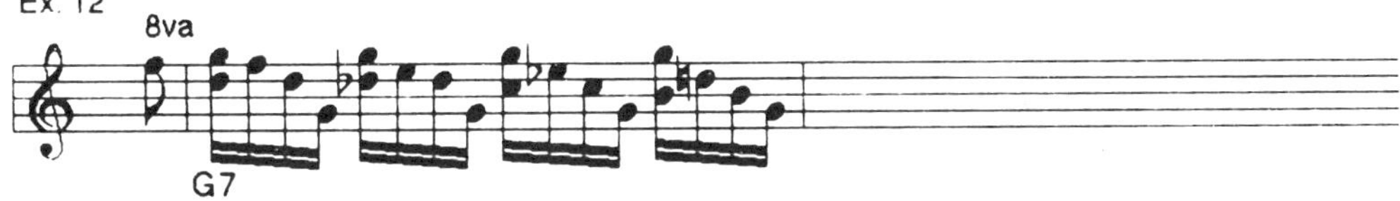

Ex. 13. *We The People* (023765-1, 1 July 1938) Chorus 1.

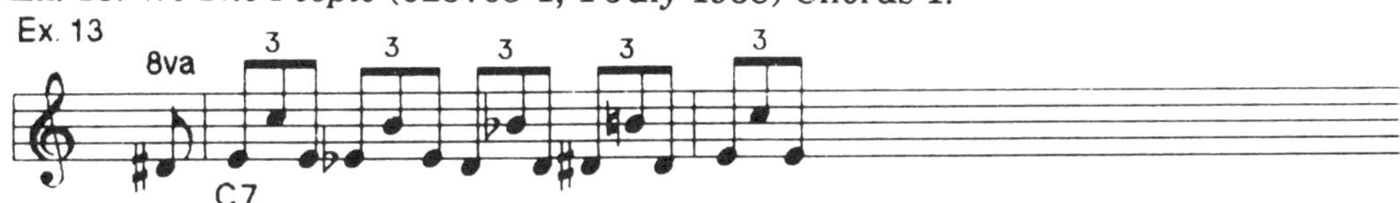

Ex. 14. *Valentine Stomp* (49497-1,2, 2 August 1929) Strain A.

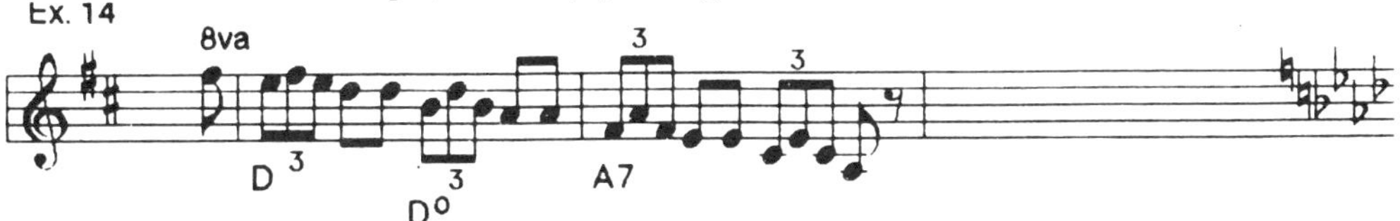

Ex. 15. *Black Raspberry Jam* (102016-2, 8 June 1936) Chorus 1.

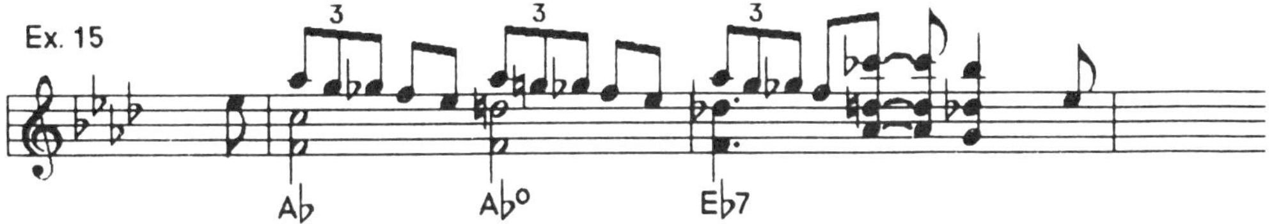

Ex. 16. *Numb Fumbling* (49762-2, 1 March 1929) Last chorus.

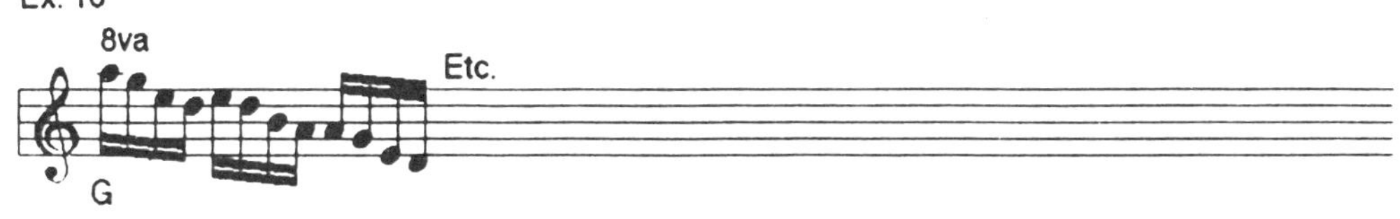

Ex. 17. *I Ain't Got Nobody* (with vocal, 88777-1, 6 March 1935) Chorus 1.
Lounging At The Waldorf (102020-1, 8 June 1936) Chorus 1, measure 23.

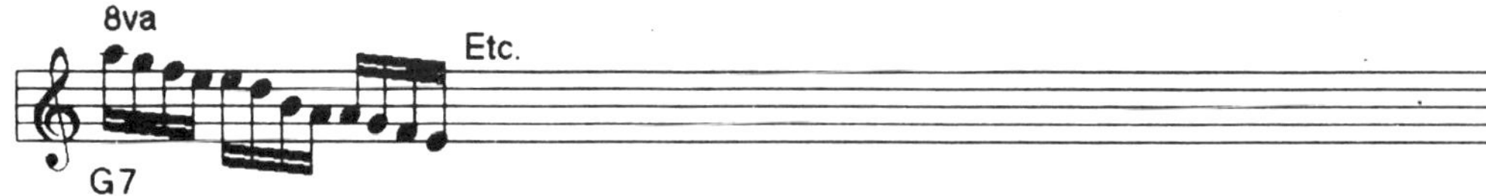

Ex. 18. *I Ain't Got Nobody* (with vocal, 88777-1, 6 Mach 1935) Chorus 1.

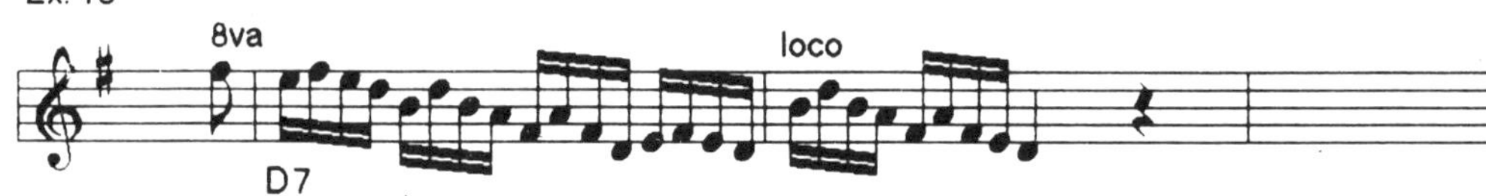

Ex. 19. *We Need A Little Love* (073440-1, 16 Mach 1942) Chorus 1, measure 5.

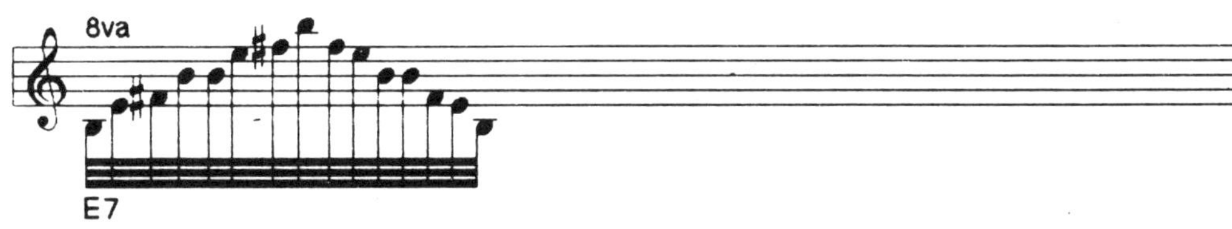

Ex. 20. *How Can You Face Me* (A-265, 11 March 1935) Chorus 1, measure 4.

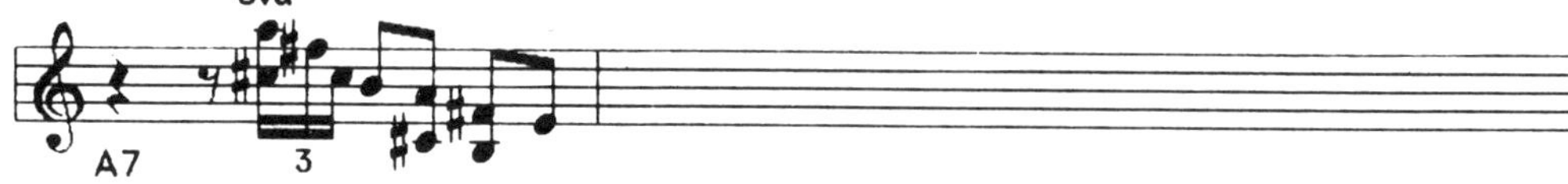

Ex. 21. *Ain't Misbehaving* (23 January 1943) Chorus 1.

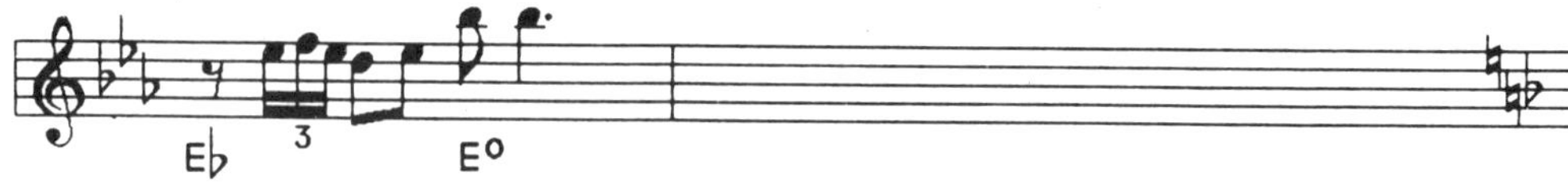

Ex. 22. *Honeysuckle Rose* (84921-1, 7 November 1934) Chorus 1, measures 12, 14.

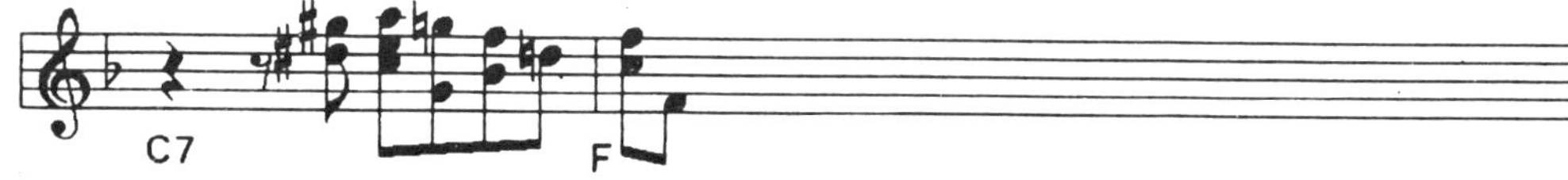

ILLUSTRATIVE RECORDINGS

The matrix number and date of the recording are given in parentheses.

Upward-broken tenths.
R1. *I Ain't Got Nobody* (with vocal, 88777-1, 6 March 1935) Chorus 1.
R2. *Do Me A Favor* (A-272, 11 March 1935) Chorus 1.
R3. *Rhythm And Romance* (92994-1, 20 August 1935) Chorus 1.

Downward-broken tenths.
R4. *Gladyse* (both takes, 49496-1,2, 2 August 1929) Strain B (key of G), statement 2.
R5. *Sweet Sue* (ZZ-2145, 7 August 1939) Waller's solo.

Octave grace notes.
R6. *Who's Afraid of Love* (03842-1, 24 December 1936) Chorus 1.

Trill as note sustainer.
R7. *Because Of Once Upon A Time* (A-269, 11 March 1935)
R8. *Last Night A Miracle Happened* (031532-1, 19 January 1939) Chorus 1.

Two-handed vamp.
R9. *The Joint Is Jumping* (014646-1, 7 October 1937)

Medium-tempo pedalling.
R10. *You Fit Into The Picture* (87087-1, 5 January 1935) Last chorus, measures 1-8.
R11. *I'm Sorry I Made You Cry* (03841-1, 24 December 1936) Chorus 1.

Harmony and voicing.
R12. *Honeysuckle Rose* (063890-1, 13 May 1941)
R13. *Ring Dem Bells* (063891-1, 13 May 1941)

Playing and singing.
R14. *I'm Crazy 'Bout My Baby* (151417-3, 13 March 1931) Chorus 2, measures 17-24.
R15. *Believe It Beloved* (A-267, 11 March 1935) Last chorus.
R16. *Do Me A Favor* (A-272, 11 March 1935) Chorus 2.

Ensemble accompaniment.
R17. *Patty Cake Patty Cake* (030369-1, 7 December 1938) Last 2 choruses.
R18. *I'm Gonna Salt Away Some Sugar* (057084-1, 6 November 1940) Last 2 choruses.

Hack-song melody played straight over striding left hand.
R19. *Don't Let It Bother You* (84107-1, 17 August 1934)
R20. *I Wish I Had You* (030364-1, 7 December 1938)
R21. *You're Gonna Be Sorry* (062764-1, 20 March 1941)

A COMPLEX MAN

Fats Waller clearly had a most complex personality. One might say there were two Fats Wallers; the outrageously outgoing extrovert of public knowledge and the deeply sensitive, shy inner man, known only to his family and closest associates. Even many who were quite close to him failed to see the second, and I well remember talking with Eva Taylor, who had been a close neighbour as well as being involved with him musically through her husband Clarence Williams who said, "Fats Waller, he was my boy. He always carried his own private party with him wherever he went." That he was 'Happy-go-lucky' and also extravagent and totally unreliable is common knowledge, and his antics are the subjects of hundreds of anecdotes, some of which are found in these pages. But there are other aspects of the Waller character.

Like many who knew hardship in their youth, he was an over-indulgent parent, and both Maurice Waller and Spencer Williams (son of Eva and Clarence) confirmed that the Waller boys, who grew up with the Williams children, had more money than was good for them and had only to mention that they wanted something, and it was there. Maurice recounted how his father was going to be away on tour at his graduation, but that before leaving had asked what he would like if successful, and he replied, "A horse". On graduation day a horse duly arrived, even though there was no pasture or stable space available anywhere near where they lived. "When dad was home, we always had a ball." Maurice said. Spencer recalled that his own more sensible parents insisted that they performed some small task before getting pocket money, but "Maurice and Ronnie always had enough for all of us."

Waller's generosity, one might even say profligacy, exteded to others too, both in money and gifts and in other acts of generosity and several are noted in these pages. Finding work for Mary Lou Williams and Harry 'The Hipster' Gibson are but two examples, whilst his teaching of Count Basie as related in *Good Morning Blues* (pages 69-71) and his kindness to Hazel Mundell in Brighton provide further testimony. But perhaps the most telling facts are that he paid tax on an income comparable to that paid to the U.S. President, but left such a small sum at the end of his life

One of the tragedies of his life was being born black in a society that only allowed members of his race to play out fixed stereotypes in the entertainment world. He was well schooled in the classics and had a deep love and reverence for them. His sometimes light hearted treatment of Bach, Beethoven and Brahms was merely a guise to cover what he really felt. He instilled this love in his sons, particularly Maurice, who told us that his father had got him a job as a music demonstrator at Macy's when he was quite young. His father always insisted on daily practice and if ever he tried to swing or improvise on one of the classics, his father would bawl out to him, "Stop that, Maurice!" His organ session in Paris remained one of the most moving musical experiences of his whole life. Not, I suspect, only because of what was played, but because he was treated as an equal, probably for the first time in his life. There are many accounts of after hours sessions from those who were his musical associates, and the sort of phrase I've heard so often is, "You don't know Fats Waller", or, "You've never heard the real Fats Waller", and I would then be told of hours spent through the night in hotel rooms listening to Fats play the most beautiful music — sometimes the classics, but at other times, similar things which he tossed off on the spot. One such account which dwells heavily on aspects of the Waller character is given by Franz Jackson in *An Autobiography Of Black Jazz* and is worth quoting in full:

> *I worked with Fats Waller in a little pick-up band around New York City, and was also in the last big band that he took on a Southern road trip. We played in huge tobacco warehouses to accommodate the large crowds that wanted to hear Fats play his latest recordings. His records were extremely popular during the period of 1941 and 1942. There was another tenor man in Fats Waller's band named Eugene "Baby Bear" Cedric. Fats would constantly push us into jam sessions. Fats liked the excitement. Although Fats would always do his numbers on the piano, he would leave a lot of room for his soloists. He would say, "What are you guys going to do?" He would back you up with some solid accompaniment. He would never try to outplay you. Whatever he was doing it was helping the band.*
>
> *Fats was a very emotional person. He could turn his personality on and off like a light. When he was at the piano, he was a different fellow than when he was seated on the bus, where he generally remained very quiet. He was very pensive. He had to have someone with him all the time. He had a fellow who traveled with him as a companion. This fellow would go out and get whiskey, food or girls for Fats when he did not feel like leaving his room. When Fats couldn't sleep, he would send for me to come up to his room: My presence was all that he needed to start playing the organ. This private musical concert would sometimes last until daybreak. He had to have somebody to sit down and listen to what he was doing. He needed a person to play to.*
>
> *Fats Waller was a lonely man and frequently needed a pacifier. His companion and road manager attempted to fill that need when Fats would get homesick and lonesome in the middle of a successful tour and threaten to go*

> *home. His companion usually managed to talk him out of that notion. However, there were times when Fats would ignore the tour schedules. He would stop the bus and throw his suitcases into his chauffeur-driven Lincoln and scream "Holland Tunnel" to his chauffeur, Buster Shepherd. Off they would go to Harlem, leaving his manager Ed Kirkeby behind to deal with the irate promoters and theater owners. Offstage, Fats was shy and alone in the midst of a crowd.*
>
> *New melodies bubbled out of Fats Waller's creative brain like water spouting out of the head of a whale. He wrote songs with such ease that he never fully realized the value of his musical contributions. He wrote "I Can't Give You Anything But Love, Baby" and "On the Sunny Side of the Street" without ever getting any royalties or credits. In the summer of 1929 he sold the rights to 21 of his songs, including the ones from the musical hit, 'Hot Chocolates', to Irving Mills for $500. Fats Waller was so creative that he could have set the phone book to music. Unfortunately, he did not have a head for the bulk of business that he created.*

Although he was devoted to classical music, Waller was also serious about his role as entertainer and instilled this in his sidemen, saying they should always remember that people had paid to be entertained, not to be made aware of personal problems. He clearly lived by this credo himself and even when he might start playing something serious for himself a shout of "Come on Fats, swing it!" would bring the broad grin and an immediate response.

Franz Jackson, among others, mentions that he was essentially a very shy person and phrases like 'alone in a crowd' and he often seemed a 'million miles away' when travelling with the band on long bus journeys are often used by his sidemen. And yet, when the mood was on him, he would join in the gambling and other fun and games that were part of life on the road.

I have been struck by the number of references I've had to all night sessions and Waller's ability to keep going for days on end without sleep, often paying people to keep him company through the night while he played. He seems to have forced himself to keep going until he dropped, a point which took him far past that at which ordinary mortals would have collapsed, and I wonder if perhaps he had a fear of sleep. Had he possibly had a disturbing experience in his youth — or perhaps a premonition of his own passing?

Fats was a deeply religious man, not perhaps in the formal sense, although he would often claim in interviews that he did go to church. This may have been for public consumption and may indeed have been so, but no-one I've spoken with, family, friends or travelling companions, ever mentioned Fats going into a church. However, he did read religious works, but despite this undoubted sincerity, was quite able to equate these feelings with his behaviour which, even by the standards accepted in the musical profession of the time, was quite outrageous. It seems that sex was regarded as an essential of life, like food and drink and no-one expected a man to be abstemious whilst on the road. Back home, however, it was a different matter. But not for Fats. Ernie Anderson notes a fling with a lusty chorus girl in the Apollo dressing room and that after his Carnegie Hall concert he sent his wife and family home while he was going out to have some fun. And I've had even more graphic accounts of amorous encounters in New York which need not be repeated.

Yes, Fats Waller had a most complex personality, one that would have tested the most thorough analysis. So many contradictory aspects, often on display in rapid succession. He was no doubt frustrated, but equally he enjoyed and loved life, and if we remember him for the happiness he spread and rejoice in it, that is perhaps what he would have wanted. But perhaps we should also ponder the unrecorded and undocumented Fats that appears 'between the lines'.

FATS WALLER'S MUSIC

The following pages attempt to list all compositions in which Fats Waller can be shown to have had an interest The list is divided into two sections; an alphabetical listing of compositions, and a chronological listing of copyrights and renewal registrations. The compilation of the first of these has been very much a combined effort and thanks are due to a number of people: firstly to Peter L. T. Stroud and Howard Rye, who researched the files of the American Society of Composers, Authors & Publishers (ASCAP), The Performing Rights Society (PRS) and the Library of Congress Copyright entries; secondly to Catherine Harvey and Roy Rhodes who scoured published literature and checked record labels for clues to unsuspected Waller tunes. Items noted in this way have almost all been cross-checked against the three main file sources, but a small body remains and these are listed as a supplement. Thirdly, Roy Cooke and Max Abrams also sent listings which have been checked against the main file.

This first listing is presented in column format, with the first and second columns giving the tune title and and co-authors, if any. The third column gives the publisher, identified according to the key which follows. Then will be found the first copyright date and the date that Waller himself recorded the tune. If not recorded by Fats, it has sometimes been possible to indicate a version by another artist, but this list is by no means exhaustive and should be regarded purely as additional flavouring.

Items showing George Marion or George Marion, Jr. as co-composer (they are assumably the same person) are almost certainly tunes intended for the show *Early To Bed*. Waller is reputed to have written the music to thirteen numbers for this, but only those so indicated are definitely from the show.

Where a posthumous copyright or other date is shown, it may be assumed in the absence of any note to the contrary that the actual date of composition is unknown. It is quite likely that previously unknown Waller tunes will continue to be published. Irving Mills told me that he had "a drawer full of Waller manuscripts" and when Bruce Bastin researched Joe Davis's papers he found a number of unpublished Waller tunes. These are hardly likely to be isolated cases.

The copyright file is the work of Howard Rye alone and he contributes the following note in explanation:

Under the 1909 Copyright Act, the Copyright Office of the Library of Congress maintained a Register of Copyrights, to which an index was published entitled *The Library of Congress Catalog of Copyright Entries*. The *Catalog* entry reproduces the essential facts concerning the registration, which are transcribed in the 'Chronological List of Fats Waller Copyrights' which follows, in the order: title; authorship details; whether registered as published or unpublished; date of copyright; copyright registration number; copyright claimant, with place of domicile or publication. For unknown reasons, the last-mentioned information was not recorded by the Copyright Office between March 1932 and June 1934 inclusive and is therefore omitted from registrations recorded during this period. It should be noted that in a few cases where a composition was the subject of (presumably) contractual arrangements between publishers, the name of a publisher not the copyright claimant may appear after the author details, registering the other concern's interest in the composition. In the one case in which it has been possible to check published sheet music in the British Library collection, the publisher whose interest was registered proved to be the publisher of the sheet music rather than the publisher claiming copyright.

The claimant of copyright in an unpublished work was required to deposit one copy with the Copyright Office; this frequently took the form of a lead-sheet. The date of copyright in an unpublished work is the date on which this copy was received. The date of copyright of a published work is the date of publication. The claimant of copyright in a published work was required to deposit two copies; the date of receipt, though recorded by the Copyright Office, is omitted here.

The Copyright Office assigned a registration number to deposited items as received. Up to September 1928, music registrations were prefixed E-. From October 1928, published and unpublished music were distinguished by the prefixes EUSP- and EUSU- respectively. The 'US' was dropped the following month and thereafter the two series were prefixed Epub- and Eunpub-, abbreviated in renewal records to EP- and EU-, which form is used here. Foreign claims were allocated their own EFor- (EF-) series, without any indication of whether published or unpublished. Where given here, publication information is derived from other sources. Other types of copyright material were allocated different prefixes but these do not concern us here.

Published music was not protected by a previous registration of the same composition un- published, and this accounts for some of the multiple registrations of the same title. In other cases, it will be clear from the information given that some modification had been made for which it was desired to secure protection, or that it was desired to record the rights of a further author or claimant. It was possible to claim copyright in an arrangement or other modification or variation in its own right. In later years this was frequently specified explicitly with the abbreviation 'NM' (for 'new material'), which is used here. Posthumous copyrights of new material added by others have been listed where they have been located, but are not cross-referenced except where the claimant included a cross-reference in the copyright registration.

Copyright once secured ran for twenty-eight years, after which it could be renewed for a further twenty-eight years. If no renewal application was made, the composition passed into the public domain after twenty-eight years. The Copyright Office maintained a register of renewals, allocating registration numbers prefixed R-. It is clear that recording of renewal applications was entirely uncritical, disputes between claimants being a matter for the courts rather than the librarians. There was evidently no barrier to the registration of copyright renewals by persons long deceased, and there was presumably equally little barrier to the impersonation of the living. Despite this the renewal records can often be of great value and all located renewals are included. Readers may form their own conclusions as to which renewal applications were made by the individuals named on them, and which by proprietors seeking to safeguard their own claims, with or without the authorization of authors or their descendants, but in some instances internal evidence points clearly to renewals being made by ill-informed sources!

The status claimed by renewal applicants is indicated in the Catalog by a series of abbreviations, of which the following appear here: A: Author; C: Child or Children of the Author; NK: Next of Kin; PPW: Proprietor of a Posthumous Work; PWH: Proprietor of a

Copyright Work made for hire; W: Widow .

This system for the recording of copyrights and renewals was changed by the Copyright Act 1976, which came into effect on 1 January 1978. The records have been systematically searched only up to June 1977, though one later registration has been located and is included.

In addition to information derived from the Library of Conress Copyright Records, the copyright file also includes additional information derived in the main from published sheet music held by the British Library. Where the B.L. holds the American edition, as is most often the case, this information appears in square brackets after the main copyright data. Details of British editions and other notes appear following renewals and preceded by "BL"

It is unlikely that full information on British editions in Waller's lifetime has been obtained by this means. The British copyright deposit system was much laxer than the United States system and in the case of popular music difficulties are further compounded by the decision of the British Museum Library, as it then was, not to catalogue what the librarians then regarded as 'non-permanent music', which was merely stored in bundles in alphabetical order of first-named composer, after being first loosely (and often incorrectly divided into 'vocal' and 'instrumental'. No cross-reference to joint authorship exists, but the bundles have been searched under Waller and Spencer Williams. No attempt has been made to locate editions published after Waller's death.

Key to publishers

A	Alfred Music Co. Inc.
AA	American Academy of Music Inc.
Ad	Advanced Music Corporation
B	Bourne Inc. (now Bourne Co.)
BA	Bud Allen Music Co.
Be	Best Music Inc.
BVC	Bregman, Vocco & Conn Inc.
C	Chappell & Co. Inc.
CC	Con Conrad Music Publisher Inc. (now Ltd.)
CR	C.R. Publishing Co.
CW	Clarence Williams Music Publishing Co. Inc.
DB	Dorsey Brothers Music Inc.
DCE	Davis, Coots & Engel Inc.
DDG	Donaldson, Douglas & Gumble Inc. E Equitable Music Corp.
EBM	E.B. Marks Music Corp.
Ex	Exclusive Publications Inc.
FBH	F.B. Haviland Publishing Co.
FC	Frank Clark Music
G	Georgia Music Corp.
GMS	Gotham Music Service Inc.
H	Harms Inc.
IB	Irving Berlin Inc.
IC	Irving Caesar Inc.
J	Joy Music Inc.
JD	Joe Davis (Music Co.) Inc.
JG	Jack Glogau
JM	Jack Mills Inc.
KE	Keit-Engel Inc.
KP	Keith Prowse Music Publishing Co. Ltd.
L	Lawrence Music Publishers Inc.
LF	Leo Feist Inc.
M	Majestic Music Co.
Ma	Marlo Music Corp.
M-A	Melo-Art Music Publishers
Mf	Mayfair Music Corp.
Mi	Miller Music Inc.
MM	Mills Music Inc.
NS	Natrass Schenk Inc.
P	George & Arthur Piantodosi Inc.
PaP	Paull-Pioneer Music Corp.
Pi	Pickwick Music Corp.
PK	Phil Kornheiser Inc.
PM	The Peter Maurice Music Co. Ltd.
PP	Philip L. Ponce Inc.
R	Robbins Music Corp.
Re	Remick Music Corp.
R-E	Robbins-Engel Inc.
Ro	Royal Music Co.
RS	Red Star Songs Inc.
RSP	Ralph S. Peer
S	Southern Music Publishing Co. Inc.
Sa	Editions Salabert, Paris
SB	Santly Bros Inc.
SF	Sam Fox Publishing Co. Inc.
ShB	Shapiro, Bernstein & Co. Inc.
SJS	Santly-Joy-Select Inc.
SM	Schuster & Miller Inc.
SP	Stept & Powers Inc.
Su	Superior Music Inc.
TH	Tune-House Inc.
Tr	Triangle Music Publishing Co. Ltd.
W	M. Witmark & Sons
WWM	World Wide Music Co. Ltd.
WW	Williams & Waller
*	Non vocal item
—	Never assigned to a publisher

An Alphabetical Listing of known Waller Compositions

Title	Co-Writer(s)	Original Publisher	Copyright date or as indicated	Date recorded by Fats Waller or as indicated
Abakadabra		see Moppin' And Boppin'		
Ace In The Hole [arranger only]	Bartley Costello, Frank Crumit	FBH	24 Jan 34	—
African Ripples (In *Fats Waller's Inimitable Piano Styles*)*		JD	20 Apr 31	16 Nov 34
Ah I Have Sighed To Rest Me (Miserere) (From Trovatore)*	Verdi [arr. Waller]	see *Fats Waller Swingin' The Operas*		
Ah So Pure (From Marta)*	Flotow [arr. Waller]	see *Fats Waller Swingin' The Operas*		
Ain't-cha' Glad	Andy Razaf	KE	8 Aug 33	(Horace Henderson, 3 Oct 33)
Ain't Misbehavin'	Andy Razaf, Harry Brooks	MM	8 Jul 29	2 Aug 29
All Alone (No One Cares)	—	CW	14 Aug 23	—
All God's Chillun Got Wings*	Trad [arr. Waller]	PM	ASCAP 1961	21 Aug 38
Alligator Crawl*	—	Tr	18 Apr 27	16 Nov 34
Previously known as *House Party Stomp* and *Charleston Stomp*		see also *Fats Waller's Inimitable Piano Styles*		
All That Meat And No Potatoes	Ed Kirkeby	LF	19 Jun 41	20 Mar 41
And That Is Life	Andy Razaf	IB	8 Sep 33	—
Shown in U.S.A. Copyright Renewals as *And This Is Life*.				
And This Is Life		see *And That Is Life*		
Angeline	George Brown (= Billy Hill)	L	5 Aug 32	(Cab Calloway, 7 Jun 32)
Anita	—	MM	28 Oct 39	28 Jun 39
Annie Laurie*	Trad [arr. Waller]	see *Fats Waller's Swingtime In Scotland*		
Anybody Here Want To Try My Cabbage	Andy Razaf	T	15 Sep 24	(Maggie Jones, 10 Dec 24)
Any Day The Sun Don't Shine	Andy Razaf	CW	4 Dec 24	—
Published in *Fats Waller's Own Original Tunes.*				
The Apple Of My Eye	Joe Young	IB	1 Jul 32	—
An Armful Of You*	—	S	11 May 54	
Asbestos (In *Fats Waller's Inimitable Piano Styles*)*		Mf	ASCAP 1945	—
At Twilight	Anita Waller	CR	16 Nov 44	12 Jan 40
Auld Lang Syne*	Trad [arr. Waller]	see *Fats Waller's Swingtime In Scotland*		
An Awful Lot My Gal Ain't Got (But What She's Got, She's Got An Awful Lot)	Spencer Williams	IB	4 Oct 24	—
Bach Up To Me (also in *Fats Waller Swingcopations*)		PP	2 Sep 36	8 Jun 36
Ball And Chain Blues	Andy Razaf	TH	28 Mar 25	—
Beethoven's Sangwattni*	—	CW	26 May 26	—
Be Modern, There's Happiness In Store For You	Alexander Hill	JD	3 Dec 30	—
Benny Sent Me	Spencer Williams	R	1 Jun 36	—
Bessie, Bessie, Bessie	Ed Kirkeby	CR	16 Nov 44	1 Oct 41
Bird Doggin' The Chicks		see *Mandy I'm Just Wild About You*		
Black And Blue		see *What Did I Do To Be So Black And Blue*		
Black Cat Rag	—	CR	ASCAP 1947	
Black Maria [revison/arrangement only]	Andy Razaf, J.C. Johnson, Fred Rose	PaP	1 Feb 40	12 Jan 40
Black Raspberry Jam (also in *Fats Waller Swingcopations*)*		PP	2 Sep 36	8 Jun 36
Bloody Razor Blues	Spencer Williams	JD	27 Oct 24	(Helen Gross, Oct .'24)
Blowin' Of The Breeze (Blew You Into My Arms), The	Spencer Williams	Re	12 Aug 32	—
Blue Bells Of Scotland*	Trad [arr. Waller]	see *Fats Waller's Swingtime In Scotland*		

Blue Black Bottom*	Mike Jackson	S	23 Jun 65	16 Feb 27
Bluer Than The Ocean Blues	Spencer Williams, Tommie Connor	WW	UK © 1933	—
This composition was published and registered with ASCAP in 1938.				
Blues Idiom*	—	MM	ASCAP 1945	—
Blues Never Die*	—	CW	2 Oct 23	—
Blue, Turning Grey Over You	Andy Razaf	JD	3 Dec 29	11 Mar 35
Blue Velvet	Spencer Williams	—	13 Mar 41	—
Bond Street* [from *London Suite*]	—	PM	10 Apr 40	12 Jun 39
Bonny Mary Of Argyle*	Trad [arr. Waller]	see *Fats Waller's Swingtime In Scotland*		
Boogie Woogie Blues*		see *Fats Waller's Boogie Woogie*		
Boogie Woogie Jump*		see *Fats Waller's Boogie Woogie*		
Boogie Woogie Rag * (also known as Boogie Woogie Drag)		see *Fats Waller's Boogie Woogie*		
Boogie Woogie Stomp*		see *Fats Waller's Boogie Woogie*		
Boogie Woogie Suite*		see *Fats Waller's Boogie Woogie*		
Boogie Woogie With Fats Waller [Piano Album]		MM	29 Jan 41	
Contents not known.				
Breakin' My Heart	Spencer Williams	JG	14 Jul 32	—
Breezin'*	—	S	11 May 54	—
Date of composition not known				
Brother Ben	Spencer Williams	CW	4 Jun 25	(Sara Martin, 25 Mar 26)
Published in *Fats Waller's Own Original Tunes.*				
Buddie	Andy Razaf	W	15 Feb 32	—
Bullet Wound Blues	Spencer Williams	JD	27 Oct 24	—
By Heck [transcribed & arranged only]	S.R. Henry, L. Wolfe Gilbert	EBM	7 Sep 38	—
Call The Plumber In	Andy Razaf	CW	1 Nov 24	—
Published in *Fats Waller's Own Original Tunes.*				
The Campbells Are Comin'*	Trad [arr. Waller]	see *Fats Waller's Swingtime In Scotland*		
Camp Meetin' Stomp*	—	CW	16 Oct 25	—
Candied Sweets	Jack Pettis	R	2 Mar 28	(Jack Pettis, 22 Dec 27)
Can't We Get Together	Andy Razaf, Harry Brooks	MM	7 Aug 29	—
Cash For Your Trash		see *Get Some Cash For Your Trash*		
Caught (In *Fats Waller's Inimitable Piano Styles*)*		Mf	date unknown	—
Charleston Hound	Eddie Rector, Clarence Williams, Spencer Williams	CW	1 Jun 26	(Blue Grass Foot Warmers, 16 Jun 26)
This would appear to be the same composition as *Swingin' Hound* .				
Charleston Stomp		see *Alligator Crawl*		
Charlie Is My Darling*	Trad [arr. Waller]	see *Fats Waller's Swingtime In Scotland*		
Chelsea*		see *London Suite*		
China Jumps (in *Fats Waller's Piano Antics*)*		G	3 Jan 41	—
Chinese Blues	Irving Mills	JM	17 Apr 26	(Original Memphis Five, 23 Jan 26)
© Sam Coslow, Irving Mills, Jimmy McHugh, but credited to;'Waller-Mills' on record.				
Chocolate Bar [from *Keep Shufflin'*]		CR	ASCAP 1947	—
Choo Choo	Andy Razaf, Eugene Sedric	Ex	15 Mar 39	—
ASCAP, U.S.A. Copyright Entries and PRS all show 'Eugene Seebic', but ASCAP confirm this is Eugene Sedric.				
Clothes Line Ballet *	—	JD	9 Mar 34	16 Nov 34
Also published in *Fats Waller's Inimitable Piano Styles.*				
Come And Get It	Ed Kirkeby	CR	16 Nov 44	1 Jul 41
Come On And Stomp, Stomp, Stomp	Chris Smith, Irving Mills	JM	27 Dec 27	(Johnny Dodds, 8 Oct 27)
Comin' Thro' The Rye*	Trad [arr. Waller]	see *Fats Waller's Swingtime In Scotland*		
Concentratin' On You	Andy Razaf	SB	2 Sep 31	(Blanche Calloway, 18 Nov 31)

Title	Co-writer(s)	Publisher	Date	
Connie's Hot Chocolates (musical production) .				
Compositions:	Ain't Misbehavin'			
	Can't We Get Together			
	Dixie Cinderella			
	Off-Time			
	That Rhythm Man			
	Say It With Your Feet			
	Sweet Savannah Sue			
	What Did I Do To Be So Black And Blue?			
Congo Lou*	—	CW	26 May 26	—
Cottage In The Rain	Spencer Williams	WoW	22 Nov 38	12 Jun 39
Crazy 'Bout That Man I Love	Clarence Williams, Spencer Williams	CW	18 Jun 26	—
Published in *Fats Waller's Own Original Tunes.*				
Crumbs Of Your Love, The	Andy Razaf, Minto Cato	SB	2 Sep 31	—
Darkie's Lament, A*	—	GMS	12 Jul 27	—
Dear Little Mountain Sweetheart	Ed Kirkeby	C	16 Nov 44	—
Shown in Library of Congress Copyright Entries as written by Kirkeby and Lew Cobey (not Waller); ASCAP indicates as above.				
Deep River*	Trad [arr. Waller]	PM	published 1938	21 Aug 38
Did-Ja?	Ed Kirkeby	CR	12 Nov 46	—
The Digah's Stomp*	—	RSP	8 May 28	1 Dec 27
Supposedly based on *The Dream* by Jess Pickett (or *The Digah's Dream*)				
Dixie Cinderella	Andy Razaf, Harry Brooks	MM	2 Jul 29	—
Doin' What I Please	Andy Razaf	L	20 Feb 33	(6 Oct 32, Don Redman)
Do Me A Favor, Lend Me A Kiss	Andy Razaf, Spencer Williams	IB	27 Jun 32	—
This is not the same work as *Do Me A Favo(u)r*, recorded by Fats Waller.				
Done Gone Mad*	—	CW	2 Oct 23	—
Don't Give Me That Jive, Come On With The Come On	Ed Kirkeby	CR	16 Nov 44	26 Dec 41
Don't Want You No More*	—	CW	2 Oct 23	—
Down On The Delta	Spencer Williams, Sam Stept	SP	24 Sep 32	—
Do You Have To Go	Anita Waller	CR	16 Nov 44	20 Mar 41
Early To Bed (Musical Production)				
Compositions:	Hi De Hi Ho In Harlem			
	The Ladies Who Sing With A Band			
	Slightly Less Than Wonderful			
	There's A Man In My Life (There's A Gal In My Life)			
	This Is So Nice It Must Be Illegal			
	When The Nylons Bloom Again			
	? There's "Yes" In The Air (not confirmed)			
Easy Living		see *The Short Trail Became The Long Trail*		
Effervescent*	—	JD	10 Dec 34	—
Also published in *Fats Waller's Inimitable Piano Styles.*				
E Flat Blues		see *Fats Waller's Original E Flat Blues*		
Every Sweetie That I Get, Somebody Takes Her From Me	Spencer Williams	CW	19 Sep 24	—
Falling Castle (in *Fats Waller's Piano Antics*)*		G	3 Jan 41	—
Farewell Blues [arranger only]	Elmer Schoebel et al	MM	1 Sep 36	—
Fat Man Blues*	—	GMS	12 Aug 27	—
Fats Waller Et Le Swing*	—	Sa	ASCAP 1942	—
Fats Waller Piano Pranks		See *Fats Waller's Inimitable Piano Styles*		

Fats Waller's Boogie Woogie (Suite for Piano)* — MM 9 Apr 45 —
Contents:
Boogie Woogie Blues
Boogie Woogie Stomp
Boogie Woogie (D)rag
Boogie Woogie Jump
Copyrighted as Boogie Woogie Suite.

Fats Waller's Boogie Woogie Conceptions Of Popular Favorites (Piano Album) MM 21 Jun 43
Contents not known.

Fats Waller Compositions, Piano Solos arranged by Eddie James* SM 1955
Contents:
Handful Of Keys
Gladyse
Numb Fumblin'
Valentine Stomp
Smashing Thirds
Harlem Fuss

Fats Waller's Inimitable Piano Styles (Piano Album)* Mf 21 Apr 55 (Rev. Ed.)
Contents:
African Ripples
Clothes Line Ballet
Alligator Crawl
Effervescent
Asbestos
Keepin' Out Of Mischief Now
Caught
Viper's Drag
Rev. ed. copyrighted as *Fats Waller Piano Pranks*. No © traced of original edition.

Fats Waller's Musical Rhythms (Piano Album) compiled & arr. Waller R 8 Jan 43
Contents:
All That Meat And No Potatoes (Waller, Kirkeby)
Pennsylvania 6-5000 (Gray, Sigman)
I'm Nobody's Baby (Davis, Ager, Santly)
At Sundown (Donaldson)
Swinging Down The Lane (Isham Jones, Gus Kahn)
Changes (Donaldson)
I'm More Than Satisfied (Waller, Klages)
Lost (Oman, Mercer, Teetor)

Fats Waller's Original E Flat Blues (E Flat Blues) Ed Kirkeby CR 16 Nov 44 11 Mar 35

Fats Waller's Original Piano Conceptions (Piano Album) [arr. Waller] MM 14 Dec 35
Contents:
Dinah (Akst, Lewis, Young)
Margie (Davis, Robinson, Conrad)
Who's Sorry Now (Kalmar, Snyder)
For Me And My Girl (Meyer, Leslie, Goetz)
Mary Lou (Lyman, Waggner, Robinson)
Tonight You Belong To Me (Lee, Rose)
Just A Baby's Prayer At Twilight (Jerome, Lewis, Young)
My Honey's Lovin' Arms (Meyer, Ruby)
When You're Smiling (Fisher, Goodwin, Shay)
Just Try To Picture Me Down Home In Tennessee (Donaldson, Jerome)

Fats Waller's Original Piano Conceptions No.2 MM 1/16 Sep 36
Contents not known.

Fats Waller's Own Original Tunes (Piano Album) CW 10 Nov 37
Contents:
Squeeze Me
I'm Not Worrying
Wallerlng Around
Midnight Stomp
Call The Plumber In
The Short Trail Became A Long Trail
The Heart That Once Belonged To Me

Swingin' Hound
Wild Cat Blues
Any Day The Sun Don't Shine
Senorita Mine
Brother Ben
Crazy 'Bout That Man Of Mine (I Love)
Lonesome One
Old Folks Shuffle

Fats Waller's Piano Antics* G 3 Jan 41
Contents:
China Jumps
Sneakin' Home
Palm Garden
Wand'rin' Aroun'
Falling Castle

Fats Waller's Swing Sessions For The Piano (Piano Album)* [arr. Waller] MM 7 Sep 37
Contents:
Stardust (Carmichael, Parish)
Singing The Blues (Conrad, Robinson)
Happy As The Day Is Long (Arlen, Koehler)
The Sheik Of Araby (Smith, Snyder, Wheeler)
Shoe Shine Boy (Cahn, Chaplin)
Jealous (Little, Finch, Malie)
Truckin' (Bloom, Koehler)
How Come You Do Me Like You Do (Austin, Bergere)
I Surrender Dear (Barris, Clifford)
When It's Sleepy Time Down South (Muse, Leon Rene, Otis Rene)

Fats Waller's Swingtime In Scotland (Piano Album)* Trad [arr. Waller] MM 4 May 38
Contents:
Loch Lomond 20 Nov 39
Annie Laurie 20 Nov 39
The Campbells Are Comin'
Auld Lang Syne
Blue Bells Of Scotland
Robin Adair
My Love Is Like A Red Red Rose
Charlie Is My Darling
Bonny Mary Of Argyle
Comin' Thro' The Rye

Fats Waller's Victor Record Song Hits (Piano Album) arr. Waller JD 12 Nov 36
Contents:
Armful O' Sweetness (Hill)
Baby Brown (Hill)
Big Chief De Sota (Arbelo, Razaf)
Breakin' The Ice (McCarthy, Cavanaugh, Weldon)
Brother, Seek And Ye Shall Find (Crum, Stewart)
Christopher Columbus (Berry, Razaf)
Cinders (Kogen, Holzer)
Garbo Green (Fisher)
Georgia May (Denniker, Razaf)
Georgia Rockin' Chair (Fisher)
How Can You Face Me? (Waller, Razaf)
I Ain' Got Nobody (S. Williams, Razaf)
I Just Made Up With That Old Girl Of Mine (Little, Pease, McConnell)
I'm Crazy 'bout My Baby (Waller, Hill)
Moon Rose (Rose, Fisher)
Porter's Love Song To A Chambermaid (Johnson, Razaf)
Rosetta (Hines, Woode)
S'posin' (Denniker, Razaf)
Woe! Is Me (Emmerich, Cavanaugh, Sanford)
You've Been Taking Lessons In Love (Tharp, Watts)

Fats Waller Stomp*	Thomas Morris, Charlie Irvis	RSP	21 Oct 27	20 May 27
'Cirein' on record labels is an obvious corruption of C. IRVIS.				
Fats Waller Swingopations (Piano Album)*		SF	16 Feb 38 (© under individual titles)	
Contents:	Bach Up To Me			
	Black Raspberry Jam			
	Fractious Fingering			
	Latch On			
	Lounging At The Waldorf			
	Paswonky			
Fats Waller Swingin' The Operas (Piano Album)* [arr. Waller]		MM	17 Jan 39	
Contents:	Ah I Have Sighed To Rest Me (Miserere) (from Il Trovatore) (Verdi)			
	Ah So Pure (from Marta) (Flotow)			20 Nov 39
	Intermezzo (from Cavalleria Rusticana) (Mascagni)			20 Nov 39
	My Heart At Thy Sweet Voice (from Samson And Delilah) (Saint-Saens)			20 Nov 39
	Over The Summer Sea (from ?) (Verdi)			
	Serenade (from Les Millions D'arlequin) (Drigo)			
	Sextet (from Lucia Di Lammermoor) (Donizetti)			20 Nov 39
	Swaltzing (from Faust) (Gounod) (recorded and in MM ed. at BL as *Waltz from Faust*)			20 Nov 39
	Then You'll Remember Me (from Bohemian Girl) (Balfe)			20 Nov 39
	Vesti La Giubba (from Pagliacci) (Leoncavallo)			
Find Out What They Like, And How They Like It	Andy Razaf	JD	18 Nov 29	—
Flat Tire Papa, Mama's Gonna Give You Air	Spencer Williams	M	8 Nov 24	—
Compare *Ice Cold Papa Mama's Gonna Melt You Down.*				
Florida Low Down	J. Fred Coots, Jo Trent	FC	6 Apr 26	(Original Indiana Five, 9 Apr 26)
Also known as *That Florida Low Down* .				
Foolin' Myself	Andy Razaf	MM	22 Jun 55	—
Date of composition is not known.				
Fractious Fingering*	—	PP	2 Sep 36	8 Jun 36
Also published in *Fats Waller Swingcopations.*				
Freeze Out*	—	CW	13 Jan 28	(Clarence Williams, 19 Dec 28)
Friendless Blues*	—	CW	21 Feb 24	—
There are also compositions with this title by W. C. Handy and others.				
Functionizin'	Irving Mills	Ex	22 Jan 35	1 Dec 35
(from 'Harlem Living Room Suite')				(previously by Alex Hill, 10 Sep 34)
Fussin' Around*	—	MM	ASCAP 1945	—
Georgia Bo-bo	Jo Trent	ShB	23 Apr 26	(Lill's Hot Shots, 28 May 26)
Get Away Young Man	George Marion	Mf	ASCAP 1941	—
Get Some Cash For Your Trash	Ed Kirkeby	LF	13 Feb 42	26 Dec 41
Also known as *Cash For Your Trash..*				
Girl Should Never Ripple When She Bends, A	George Marion	Mf	ASCAP 1943	—
Also known as *A Girl Who Doesn't Ripple When She Bends.*				
Gladyse*	—	S	26 Dec 29	2 Aug 29
First published in 1955.				
Goddess Of Rain	Harry Brooks, Andy Razaf	MM	ASCAP 1929	—
Go Down Moses*	Trad [arr. Waller]	PM	ASCAP 1961	21 Aug 38
Goin' About	—	S	23 Jun 65	4 Nov 29
Gone	Harry Link, Andy Razaf	SB	23 Nov 29	—
Got Myself Another Jockey Now	Andy Razaf	H	29 Feb 28	—
Gotta Be, Gonna Be Mine	Andy Razaf	L	29 Jul 32	(Washboard Rhythm Kings, 14 Dec 32)

Great Scott	Henry Troy	TH	2 Feb 26	(Troy Harmonists, Mar 26)
Handful Of Keys*	—	S	29 Dec 30	1 Mar 29
First published in 1955.				
Happy Feeling*	—	G	26 Jan 40	—
Harlem Fuss*	—	S	17 Dec 30	1 Mar 29
First published in 1955.				
Harlem Living Room Suite				
Contents:	Functionizin' Corn Whiskey Cocktail/ Scrimmage			
For details of Functionizin' see individual title; the other two titles do not appear to have been registered, either at the Library of Congress or with ASCAP.				
Heart Of Stone	Alex Hill	DDG	24 Jan 31	—
Heart That Once Belonged To Me, Belongs To Someone Else, The	Clarence Williams	CW	7 Jul 25	—
Also published in *Fats Waller's Own Original Tunes*.				
Heavy Sugar	Andy Razaf	JD	18 Nov 29	—
Hello Atlanta Town	Jo Trent, Clarence Williams	CW	4 Apr 24	—
Hi De Hi Ho In Harlem	George Marion Jr.	Ad	ASCAP, 1943	—
Hog Maw Stomp*	—	CW	12 Mar 24	16 Feb 27
Also known as *Hog Man Stomp*.		RSP	5 Nov 28	
Hold My Hand	J. C. Johnson	SM	20 May 38	12 Apr 38
Home Alone Blues	John Holmes	TH	18 Oct 24	—
Honey Hush	Ed Kirkeby	IB	18 Jul 39	28 Jun 39
Honeysuckle Rose	Andy Razaf	SB	11 Sep 29	7 Nov 34
Hopeless Love Affair	Andy Razaf	PP	6 Jan 38	7 Oct 37
House Party Stomp*	—	Tr	14 Nov 25	—
Said to be identical to *Alligator Crawl*.				
How Can I, With You In My Heart	J. C. Johnson	PP	6 Jan 38	7 Oct 38
How Can You Face Me	Andy Razaf	JD	8 Feb 32	11 Mar 35
Additional lyrics by Reg Howard, © 1934.				
How Jazz Was Born	Andy Razaf	H	29 Feb 28	—
How Ya Baby	J. C. Johnson	PP	6 Jan 38	7 Oct 37
Hungry	Joe Young, Andy Razaf	IB	16 Jun 32	—
I Can See You All Over The Place	Clarence Williams	CW	6 Jan 36	(Clarence Williams, 9 Feb 35)
I Can't Forgive You	J. C. Johnson	MM	24 Oct 38	—
I'd Rather Be Blue Than Green	Clarence Williams, Spencer Williams, Andy Razaf	CW	4 Aug 24	(Sara Martin, c.26 Sep 24)
I Didn't Dream It Was Love	Elliott Grennard, Con Conrad	CC	11 Jul 32	—
I Got Love	Spencer Williams	KP	21 Oct 38	—
I Had To Do It	Andy Razaf	BVC	1 Nov 38	(Benny Godman, 13 Oct 38)
I Hate To Leave You Now	Dorothy Dick	J	18 Jul 57 (ASCAP 1949)	(Louis Armstrong, 28 Dec 32)
I Hope You're Satisfied	Clarence Williams	CW	13 Jan 28	—
Compare *I'm More Than Satisfied*.				
I'm Crazy 'Bout My Baby And My Baby's Crazy 'Bout Me	Alex Hill	JD	14 Feb 31	5 Mar 31 (with Ted Lewis)
I'm Goin' Huntin'	J. C. Johnson	GMS	24 Sep 27	(Jimmy Bertrand, 21 Apr 27)
I'm Goin' Right Along	Jo Trent	CW	28 Apr 24	—

Title	Lyricist	Publisher	Date	Recorded
I'm Gonna Fall In Love (And Marry You)	Spencer Williams	WW	UK© 1933	—
This composition was published and registered with ASCAP in 1938.				
I'm Just Wild About You	Andy Razaf	P.	1 Aug 29	—
I'm Looking For A Rainbow*	—	MM	ASCAP 1945	—
I'm More Than Satisfied	Ray Klages	R	14 Sep 27	(Chicago Loopers, Oct 27)
Compare *I Hope You're Satisfied.* Sources are not unanimous re Klages's contribution, but see © entry.				
I'm Not Worrying	Clarence Williams	CW	1 Jul 29	(Clarence Williams, 16 Apr 29)
Also published in *Fats Waller's Own Original Tunes*.				
I'm Now Prepared To Tell The World It's You	Andy Razaf	MM	8 Jul 32	—
I'm Savin' Up My Pennies*	—	R	22 Dec 38	—
I May Be A Little Green, But I Ain't No Fool	Spencer Williams	CW	1 Nov 24	—
I Need Someone Like You	—	S	7 Dec 29	30 Sep 29
I Repent	—	G	5 Feb 41	2 Jan 41
I've Got A Feeling I'm Falling	Billy Rose, Harry Link	SB	14 Mar 29	27 Jun 29 [with Gene Austin]
I've Got You Where I Want You	Spencer Williams	WW	ASCAP/UK© 1933	—
Ice Cold Papa Mama's Gonna Melt You Down	Andy Razaf	TH	15 Sep 24	—
Compare *Flat Tire Papa, Mama's Gonna Give You Air.*				
Ice Man Lives In An Ice House, The (In A Village By The Sea)	Ricardo Duromo (Hardman), Elmer S. Hughes (Eliott Shapiro)	PM	30 Jun 31	—
If I Had Waited For You	Andy Razaf	IB	8 Dec 33	—
If I Meant Something To You	J. C. Johnson	ShB	14 Jul 38	—
If It Ain't Love	Andy Razaf, Don Redman	DCE	19 Feb 32	(Chick Webb, 6 Jul 34)
The compositiom with a similar title recorded by Waller is *If It Isn't Love* (Burton, Jason)				
If You Can't Be Good Be Careful	Andy Razaf	MM	27 Mar 53	—
If You Like Me, Like I Like You	Clarence Williams, Spencer Williams	CW	9 Apr 29	21 Dec 28
In Harlem	Jo Trent	CW	28 Apr 24	—
In Harlem's Araby	Jo Trent	E	24 Jul 24	early 1924 [with Porter Grainger]
In My Baby's Eyes (You're My Baby Doll)	Jo Trent	CW	10 Jun 24	—
In The Evening By The Moonlight	Spencer Williams	Re	ASCAP 1946	—
In The Springtime	Jo Trent	CW	28 Apr 24	—
Inside		see *Inside This Heart Of Mine*		
Inside This Heart Of Mine (Inside)	J. C. Johnson	MM	8 Jul 38	12 Apr 38
Intermezzo (from "Cavalleria Rusticana")*	Mascagni [arr. Waller]	see *Fats Waller Swingin' The Operas*		
It Pays To Advertise*	—	AA	ASCAP 1942	—
It Seems To Me*	—	CW	14 Jul 23	—
Jealous Of Me	Andy Razaf	PP	6 Jan 38	7 Oct 37
Jitterbug Tree	Andy Razaf, J. C. Johnson, Fred Rose	PaP	2 Dec 38	—
Waller revised Fred Rose's music; he was not an original writer of this work.				
Jitterbug Waltz*		R	16 Oct 42	16 Mar 42
Jitterbug Waltz	Maxine Manners, Charles Grean	?	unknown date	—
John Henry, That Superman	Andy Razaf	IB	5 Aug 33	—
Also known as *John Henry*.				
Joint Is Jumpin'	Andy Razaf, J. C. Johnson	PP	6 Jan 38	7 Oct 37
This compositiom was not published until 1940.				
Jo-Jo-Josephine	Billy Moll	ShB	21 Oct 30	—
Juarez (Musical Production) Compositions	My Mamasita (see *Mamacita*]			
Jungle Jamboree		see *That Jungle Jamboree* .		
Keep A Song In Your Soul	Alex Hill	JD	8 Dec 30	(Fletcher Henderson, 2 Dec 30)

Keep Shufflin' (Musical Production)				
Compositions:	Chocolate Bar			
	Got Myself Another Jockey Now			
	How Jazz Was Born			
	Labor Day Parade (may not be by Waller)			
	Willow Tree			
Keepin' Out Of Mischief Now	Andy Razaf	CC	10 Feb 32	11 Jun 37 (previously by Louis Armstrong, 11 Mar 32)
Also published in *Fats Waller's Inimitable Piano Styles.*				
Kiss Ma Again	Clarence Williams	CW	28 Apr 25	—
Shown on the British publisher's list as *Kiss Me Again.*				
Ladies Who Sing With The Band, [The]	George Marion Jr.	Ad	1 Jun 43	23 Sep 43
Latch On (also in *Fats Waller Swingcopations*)*		RR	2 Sep 36	8 Jun 36
Laughing Water	Harry Brooks, Andy Razaf	MM	ASCAP 1929	—
Lay Your Head Upon My Shoulder	—	—	21 Jun 33	—
Leaving Me	Andy Razaf	MM	22 Jun 55	(Jimmie Lunceford, 20 Mar 34)
Lenox Avenue Blues*	—	RSP	8 Aug 27	17 Nov 26
Levee Land (Opening Chorus)	—	*CW	3 May 26	—
Limehouse		see *London Suite*		
Lion's Roar, The	—	*CW	13 Jan 28	—
Little Brown Betty	Alex Hill	RS	21 Jan 31	—
Load Of Coal (musical production)				
Compositions:	Honeysuckle Rose			
	Zonky			
Loch Lomond*	Trad [arr. Waller]	see *Fats Waller's Swingtime In Scotland*		
London Suite*	—	PM	7 Feb 47	12 Jun 39
Contents:	Whitechapel			
	Limehouse			
	Soho			
	Piccadilly			
	Chelsea			
	Bond Street (previous © 10 May 40)			
Copyrighted in U.S.A. as *Fats Waller's Famous London Suite.*				
Lonesome Me	Andy Razaf, Con Conrad	CC	31 May 32	2 Aug 39
Lonesome One	Clarence Williams, Andy Razaf	CW	3 May 26	—
Williams and Razaf are only indicated as co-writers by ASCAP, but were not named in the © entry. Published in *Fats Waller's Own Original Tunes.*				
Long, Deep And Wide*	—	CW	10 Feb 27	(Clarence Williams, Aug 28)
Long Time No Song	George Marion Jr.	Mf	ASCAP 1943	? (on Ristic LP)
Look-A-Here*	—	MM	ASCAP 1945	—
Lookin' Good But Feelin' Bad	Lester A. Santly	SB	30 Sep 29	18 Dec 29
Lost Love	Andy Razaf	MM	6 Aug 37	9 Jun 37
Loungin' At The Waldorf (first published in *Fats Waller Swingcopations*)*		PP	2 Sep 36	8 Jun 36
Lovie Lee	Andy Razaf	GMS	31 Mar 28	—
Mamacita	Buddy Kaye	DB	5 Feb 41	2 Jan 41
Also known as *My Mamacita*				
Mandy I'm Just Wild About You	Jo Trent, Clarence Williams	CW	28 Apr 24	—
Also known as *Bird Doggin' The Chicks*. The composition *Mandy* which Waller recorded was written by Irving Berlin.				
March Of The Spades*	—	MM	ASCAP 1945	—
Martinique (from *Early To Bed* (?))	George Marion Jr.	Ad	?	23 Sep 43
Me And My Old World Charm	George Marion Jr.	Mf	ASCAP 1943	—
Also known as *My Old World Charm.*				

Meditation*	—	Tr	28 Nov 27	—
Messin' Around With The Blues*	Phil Worde	RSP	21 Jul 27	14 Jan 27
Midnight Stomp*	Clarence Williams	CW	16 Oct 25	(Clarence Williams, c. Nov 28)
First copyrighted as *Mid Night Stomp* by Waller only. Published in *Fats Waller's Own Original Tunes*.				
Mighty Fine	Andy Razaf	G	9 Jan 40	12 Jan 40
Minor Drag, The*	—	S	17 Dec 30	1 Mar 29
Monkey Talk*	—	CW	13 Jan 28	—
Moonlight Mood	J. C. Johnson	MM	16 Sep 38	—
Moppin' And Boppin'	Benny Carter, Ed Kirkeby	MM	11 Dec 46	23 Jan 43
Also known as *Abakadabra*. Shown in U.S. Copyright Entries as included in film *'Stormy Weather'*.				
My Baby's Coming Back Home	Jo Trent	CW	28 Apr 24	—
My Fate Is In Your Hands	Andy Razaf	SB	11 Sep 29	25 Nov 29
My Feelin's Are Hurt*	—	S	23 Mar 31	4 Sep 29
My Gift Of Dreams	Andy Razaf, Edgar Dowell	SB	25 Jun 32	—
My Heart At Thy Sweet Voice (from "Samson And Delilah")*	Saint-Saens/arr. Waller	see *Fats Waller Swinging The Operas*		
My Heart's At Ease	Joe Young	IB	5 May 32	—
My Jamaica Love	Andy Razaf	CW	25 Jul 24	—
My Love Gets Hungry Too	Ed Kirkeby	CR	12 Nov 46 (ASCAP 1945)	—
My Love Is Like A Red Red Rose*	Trad/arr. Waller	see *Fats Waller's Swingtime In Scotland*		
Shown by ASCAP as *O My Love Is Like A Red Red Rose.*				
My Mamacita		see *Mamacita*		
My Man Cures The Blues	Jo Trent	CW	28 Apr 24	—
My Man Is Good For Nothin' But Love	Andy Razaf, Harry Brooks	MM	31 Dec 29	—
My Old World Charm		see *Me And My Old World Charm*		
My Song Of Hate	Andy Razaf	AA	ASCAP 1942	—
My Sweet Baby Irene	Andy Razaf, Spencer Williams	CW	4 Aug 24	—
Also known as *My Sweet Babe Irene.*				
Never Heard Of Such Stuff*	—	MM	1 Apr 53	—
Date of composition not known.				
Nobody Knows (How Much I Love You)	Bud Allen, Bennett Carter	BA	26 Dec 27	17 Jan 28 [with J. Thompson]
Not There, Right There	Spencer Williams	WoW	22 Nov 38	12 Jun 39
No Wonder	Morey Davidson	SB	23 Oct 29	—
Numb Fumblin'*	—	S	29 Dec 30	1 Mar 29
First published 14 Aug 35.				
Off-Time	Andy Razaf, Harry Brooks	MM	2 Jul 29	—
Oh Baby, Sweet Baby	Ed Kirkeby	CR	16 Nov 44	1 Oct 41
Oh! You Sweet Thing	Andy Razaf	L	29 Jul 32	(Billy Banks, 18 Aug 32)
Also known as *You Sweet Thing*. This is not the same composition as *Sweet Thing* recorded by Waller .				
Old Fashioned Susie's Blues	Andy Razaf, Clarence Williams	CW	12 Jun 24	(Sara Martin, 26 Sep 24)
Recorded by Sara Martin as *Old Fashioned Sara's Blues*.				
Old Folks Shuffle	Clarence Williams	CW	18 Jun 26	(Blue Grass Foot Warmers, 21 Jun 26)
Also published in *Fats Waller's Own Original Tunes*.				
Old Grand Dad	—	DB	12 Apr 40	11 Apr 40
Also known as *Old Grandad* .				
Old Yazoo	—	L	8 Aug 32	(Baron Lee, 17 Aug 32)
O My Love Is Like A Red Red Rose		see *My Love Is Like A Red Red Rose*		
One O'clock Blues*	Bud Allen, Walter Bishop	BA	3 Aug 28	—
Onion Time*	—	MM	ASCAP 1945	—
Only Sometimes	Joe Young	IB	9 Jul 32	—

Title	Co-writer(s)	Publisher	Date	Recorded
On Rainy Days	Andy Razaf	MM	8 Jul 38	—
On Sunday When We Gathered 'Round The Organ	Andy Razaf, Alex Hill	IB	8 Dec 33	—
On Your Mark	George Marion Jr.	Mf	ASCAP 1943	—
Oriental Tones*	—	CW	21 Feb 24	—
Doubtful evidence has it that Clarence Williams wrote this work, though it was copyrighted in Waller's name.				
Our Love Was Meant To Be	Alex Hill	PK	23 Dec 30	7 Sep 37
Some sources indicate Joe Davis as co-writer with Waller and Hill.				
Over The Summer Sea (from ?)*	Verdi/arr. Waller	see *Fats Waller Swingin' The Operas*		
Palm Garden (in *Fats Waller's Piano Antics*)*		G	3 Jan 41	—
The Panic Is On	Geo. Clarke, Bert Clarke, Winston Tharp	B	ASCAP 1935	1 Feb 36
Paraphernalia*	—	MM	ASCAP 1945	—
Paswonky (first published in *Fats Waller Swingcopations*)*		PP	2 Sep 36	8 Jun 36
Patty Cake Patty Cake (Baker Man)	Andy Razaf, J.C. Johnson	SF	28 Dec 38	7 Dec 38
Peekin' In Seek*	—	MM	ASCAP 1945	—
Piccadilly*		see *London Suite*		
Please Take Me Back	Jo Trent	CW	7 Jul 24	—
Please Take Me Out Of Jail*	Thomas Morris	RSP	19 May 28	1 Dec 27
Please Tell Me Why	Ed. Adams	GMS	26 Nov 24	—
Prisoner Of Love	Andy Razaf	JD	18 Nov 29	—
Radio Papa, Broadcastin' Mama	Andy Razaf	JD	18 Nov 29	—
Railroad Rhythm	—	CW	2 Mar 29	(ClarenceWilliams, 26 Sep 29)
Also known as *Touchdown*, and copyrighted under that title (confirmed by CW catalog).				
Ramblin' Papa Blues	Spencer Williams	TH	15 Sep 24	—
Rhythm Man		see *That Rhythm Man*		
Ridin' But Walkin'*	—	S	9 Apr 30	18 Dec 29
Robin Adair*	Trad/arr. Waller	see *Fats Waller's Swingtime In Scotland*		
Rock Me Just Like A Sweet Daddy Should	Andy Razaf	CW	25 Jul 24	—
Shown by ASCAP as *Rock Me Just As A Sweet Daddy Should.*				
Rollin' Down The River	R. Stanley Adams	SB	2 Apr 30	(Ben Pollack, 23 Jun 30)
Rump, Steak Serenade	Ed Kirkeby	CR	16 Nov 44	1 Jul 41
Russian Fantasy	—	?S	ASCAP 1935	11 Mar 35
Rusty Pail Blues*	—	RSP	2 May 27	14 Jan 27
Recorded under the title *The Rusty Pail.*				
Sad Sapsucker [Am I]	Ed Kirkeby	CR	16 Nov 44	13 May 41
St. Louis Blues [transcription only]	Handy [arr. Waller]	A	20 Nov 28	—
St. Louis Shuffle	Jack Pettis	RE	8 Mar 27	(Fletcher Henderson, 23 Mar 27)
Previously recorded by Jack Pettis, Dec 26.				
Savannah Blues*	Thomas Morris	RSP	18 Aug 27	20 May 27
Say It With Your Feet	Andy Razaf, Harry Brooks	MM	27 Jul 29	—
Say Yes	J. C. Johnson, Andy Razaf	C	27 Feb 939	—
Scram Scoundrel, Scram	Ned Washington	AA	ASCAP 1943	?6 Nov 40 (as *Scram!*)
Senorita Mine	Eddie Rector, Spencer Williams, Clarence Williams	CW	31 May 26	(Blue Grass Foot Warmers, 16 Jun 26)
Also publshed in *Fats Waller's Own Original Tunes.*				
Serenade (from "Les Millions D'arlequin")*	Drigo/arr. Waller	see *Fats Waller Swingin' The Operas*		
Shake Your Feet	Irving Mills	GMS	27 Dec 27	—
Shakin' It All Night Long	Spencer Williams	R	1 Jun 36	—
Sheltered By The Stars, Cradled By The Moon	Joe Young	IB	19 May 32	—
Some sources give the title as *Sheltered By The Stars, Cradled By The Moon, Covered By The Night .*				
Shet Yo' Mouf	Andy Razaf	CW	19 Sep 24	?Jan 1927 (as *Shut Your Mouth)*

Title	Lyricist	Publisher	Copyright	Recorded
The Short Trail Became The Long Trail (published in *Fats Waller's Own Original Tunes*)	Andy Razaf	CW	1924 (© not traced)	—
Also known as *The Short Trail Became A Long Trail and Easy Living.*				
Since Won Long Hop Took One Long Hop To China	Jack Meskill	MARLO	20 Feb 32	—
Sing Out	Manny Kurtz	AA	ASCAP 1942	—
Sittin' Up Waitin' For You	Andy Razaf	Su	27 Jun 33	—
Six Or Seven Times	Irving Mills	GMS	22 Nov 29	12 Sep 29
Slaving	Clarence Williams	CW	21 Feb 24	—
Slightly Less Than Wonderful	George Marion Jr.	Ad	1 Jun 43	23 Sep 43
Sloppy Water Blues*	—	RSP	21 Jan 27	14 Jan 27
Slower Than Molasses	Andy Razaf	IB	4 Aug 33	—
Smashing Thirds*	—	S	23 Mar 31	24 Sep 29
First published in 1955.				
Smother Me With Your Love*	—	R	ASCAP 1939	—
Snake Hip Dance (from "Hot Chocolates")	Andy Razaf, Harry Brooks	MM	27 Sep 29	(Wilton Crawley, 3 Oct 29)
Sneakin' Home (from *Fats Waller's Piano Antics*)*		G	3 Jan 41	—
Soho*		see *LondonS uite*		
Solid Eclipse	J. C. Johnson	SM	14 Jun 38	—
Soothin' Syrup Stomp*	—	RSP	21 Jan 27	14 Jan 27
Spades Are Trump's (musical production)				
Compositions:	Rollin' Down The River			
Spider And The Fly (Poor Fly, Bye Bye)	Andy Razaf, J. C. Johnson	SJS	29 Oct 38	7 Dec 38
Squeeze Me	Clarence Williams	CW	31 Jul 25	10 Aug 39
Also published in *Fats Waller's Own Original Tunes*)				
Stayin' At Home, Happy To Be By Myself	Andy Razaf	Be	19 Jul 40	16 Jul 40
Stealin' Apples	Andy Razaf	Ex	10 Jul 36	(Fletcher Henderson, 27 Mar 36)
Strange As It Seems	Andy Razaf	L	5 Jul 32	Adelaide Hall, 5 Aug 32)
Strivers Row	Jack Ryan	TH	18 Oct 24	—
Strollin' Roun' The Town	Jo Trent	CW	4 Apr 24	—
Sugar Rose	Phil Ponce	C	11 Mar 36	1 Feb 36
Sunshine	Al Koppell, Jean Herbert	IC	5 Dec 33	—
Supple Couple	George Marion Jr.	Mf	ASCAP 1943	—
Swaltzing (from "Faust")*	Gounod [arr. Waller]	see *Fats Waller Swingin' The Operas*		
Sweet Baby	Clarence Williams	CW	14 Jan 24	—
Sweetie Don't Grow Sour On Me	Charles O'Flynn	CW	10 Jun 24	—
Sweet Savannah Sue	Andy Razaf, Harry Brooks	MM	22 Jul 29	2 Aug 29
Swingin' Hound (in *Fats Waller's Own Original Tunes*)	Eddie Rector, Clarence Williams, Spencer Williams	Pi	ASCAP 1937	—
Swing On Mississippi	Ned Washington	MA	10 May 34	—
Swing Out To Victory	Ed Kirkeby	CR	16 Nov 44	13 Jul 42
Take It From Me I've Taken To You	R. Stanley Adams	SB	2 Apr 30	—
Also known as *(Take It From Me (I'm Takin' To You).*				
Tall Timber	Andy Razaf	Mi	7 Aug 33	—
Tan Town Topics (musical production)				
Compositions	Charleston Hound Senorita Mine			
That Blue Strain	Spencer Williams	CW	19 Sep 24	—
That Florida Low Down		see *Florida Low Down*		
That Gets It, Mister Joe	J.C. Johnson	—	29 Oct 69	1 Oct 41
That Jungle Jamboree	Andy Razaf, Harry Brooks	MM	17 Sep 29	(Jungle Band, 29 Jul 29)
Also known as *Jungle Jamboree.*				

That Rhythm Man	Andy Razaf, Harry Brooks	MM	26 Jun 29	(Louis Armstrong, 22 Jul 29)
Also known as *(That) Rhythm Man.*				
That's All*	—	S	21 Feb 31	24 Aug 29
That's My Man	Jo Trent	CW	11 Apr 24	—
That Struttin' Eddie Of Mine	Eddie Rector, Clarence Williams, Spencer Williams	CW	18 Jun 26	—
That's Where The South Begins	Billy Hill (as George Brown)	L	29 Jul 32	—
That Was My Own Idea	Billy Moll	ShB	21 Sep 29	—
Then You'll Remember Me (from "The Bohemian Girl")*	Balfe [arr. Waller]	see *Fats Waller Swingin' The Operas*		
There'll Come A Time When You'll Need Me	Joe Davis	JD	24 Sep 27	—
Re-copyrighted 27 Mar 53 with Irving Mills as co-writer; compare *There'll Come A Time When You'll Want Me*.				
There'll Come A Time When You'll Want Me	Clarence Williams	CW	18 Jun 26	—
Compare *There'll Come A Time When You'll Need Me.*				
There's A Gal In My Life		see *There's A Man In My Life*		
There's A Man In My Life	George Marion Jr.	Ad	1 Jun 43	23 Sep 43 (as *There's A Gal In My Life*)
There's "Yes" In The Air	George Marion Jr.	Mf	ASCAP 1943	—
This Is So Nice [It Must Be Illegal]	George Marion Jr.	Ad	1 Jun 43	23 Sep 43
Touch-Down*	—	CW	2 Mar 29	(Clarence Williams, 16 Apr 29)
Also known as *Railroad Rhythm.*				
Trouble*	—	JD	18 Nov 29	(Clarence Williams, 28 Jun 34)
Undercurrent*	—	Ex	28 Oct 38	—
Up Jumped You With Love	Ed Kirkeby	CR	16 Nov 44	13 Jul 42
Valentine Stomp*	—	S	26 Dec 29	2 Aug 2
First published 1955.				
Vesti La Giubba (from "Pagliacci")	Leoncavallo [arr. Waller]	see *Fats Waller Swingin' The Operas*		
Viper's Drag*	—	JD	19 Nov 30	16 Nov 34
Also published in *Fats Waller's Inimitable Piano Styles.*				
Wait And See	Andy Razaf	JD	16 Mar 36	28 Jun 39
Waiting For You To Begin	Joe Young	IB	16 Sep 32	—
Walkin' The Floor	Andy Razaf	IB	16 Jun 32	—
Wallering Around (published in *Fats Waller's Own Original Tunes*)*	—	CW/Pi	1924 (© not traced)	—
Waltz Divine	Andy Razaf, Harry Brooks	MM	ASCAP 1929	—
Wand'rin' Aroun' (from *Fats Walleris Piano Antics*)*		G	3 Jan 41	—
We Need A Little Love That's All	Ed Kirkeby	CR	16 Nov 44	16 Mar 42
What A Pretty Miss	Spencer Williams	WoW	22 Nov 38	8 Jun 39
What Can Be Wrong With Me	Jo Trent	CW	4 Apr 24	—
What Did I Do To Be So Black And Blue	Andy Razaf, Harry Brooks	MM	20 Aug 29	(Louis Armstrong, 22 Jul 29)
What's Your Name	J. C. Johnson	SM	14 Jun 38	—
What Will I Do In The Morning	J. C. Johnson	PP	6 Jan 38	7 Oct 37
When Gabriel Blows His Horn	Andy Razaf	NS	10 Feb 32	—
When The Nylons Bloom Again	George Marion Jr.	Ad	26 Jul 43	—
When You're Tired Of Me Just Let Me Know	Andy Razaf	CW	12 Jun 24	(Eva Taylor, c.16 May 24)
Where The Dew Drops Kiss The Morning Glories Good Mornin'	Spencer Williams	Re	24 Aug 32	—
Also known as *When The Dew Drops Kiss The Morning Glories Good Mornin'*.				
Where The Honeysuckle Grows	George Thorne II	S	ASCAP 1953	—
Whitechapel		see *London Suite*		
Whiteman Stomp	Jo Trent	R	14 Sep 27	11 May 27 with Fletcher Henderson
Clarence Williams (not Trent) shown by ASCAP as co-writer. Columbia record shows Trent, Waller & Whiteman.				

Title	Lyricist / Co-composer	Publisher	Date	Recorded
Why Am I Alone With No One To Love	Spencer Williams, Andy Razaf	Tr	18 Feb 29	—
Why Do We Hurt The Ones We Love	Andy Razaf, Al Jolson	IB	8 Sep 33	—
Wild Cat Blues	Clarence Williams	CW	24 Sep 23	(Clarence Williams, 30 Jul 23)
This is believed to be Waller's first published composition and was also published in *Fats Waller's Own Original Tunes.*				
Willow Tree	Andy Razaf	H	29 Feb 28	27 Mar 28 with La Sugar Babes
Described as "A Musical Misery"				
Won't You Get Off It, Please*	—	S	9 Apr 30	18 Dec 29
Workin' Woman's Blues	Spencer Williams	Tr	24 Jan 25	—
Wringin' And Twistin'	Jo Trent, Frank Trumbauer	R	20 Oct 27	(Bix-Tram-Lang, 17 Sep 27)
Yacht Club Swing	Herman Autry, J. C. Johnson	BVC	22 Oct 38	13 Oct 38
Yes Suh		see *Yow Sah*		
You Can't Have Your Cake And Eat It	Spencer Williams	PM	15 Jun 45	12 Jun 39
Notified to PRS by Peter Maurice Music Co. Ltd., London, 15 Jul 39.				
You Gotta Swing It*	—	AA	ASCAP 1942	—
You Must Be Losin' Your Mind	Ed Kirkeby	CR	16 Nov 44	16 Mar 42
You're Breakin' My Heart	Spencer Williams	Ro	8 May 33	—
You're My Baby Doll		see *In My Baby's Eyes*		
You're My Ideal	Spencer Williams	ShB	23 Jul 32	(Lionel Hampton, 18 Jan 38)
You Sweet Thing		see *Oh You Sweet Thing*		
Yow Sah	Joe Young	IB	10 Aug 33	(Wbd. Rh. Kings, 14 Dec 32)
Recorded as *Yes Suh!* by The Rhythmakers, 26 Jul 32.				
Zonky	Andy Razaf	SB	11 Sep 29	11 Mar 35

Titles Listed In Various Sources As Fats Waller Compositions

When a major artist is believed, as Fats Waller is believed, to have sold compositions outright for others to claim authorship, it is inevitable that attempts will be made by well-wishers and others to identify the lost works. The following titles are known to have been claimed for Fats at some time or other, but without corroboration by ASCAP, the Library of Congress, or PRS. Documented credits, where known, are indicated in parentheses. Additional details, including copyright registrations, are given where they have been located, though in the nature of the case these cannot prove that Fats had no hand in authorship of the compositions. This list is entirely uncritical and may include genuine Waller compositions which for some reason were never formally claimed, as well as some (e.g. *Tea For Two*) whose attribution to Waller by persons claiming special knowledge seems wholly fanciful. One composition, *Chinese Blues*, which was attributed to Waller on a record label before being copyrighted by others, has been included in the main list, though without prejudice as to any alterations which may have been introduced in the meantime.

It is startling that this list includes so many compositions which were apparently featured in shows but were not copyrighted (by anyone). It would be a good guess that these already appear in the list of compositions under other titles and were reused in the shows with only minor modifications, or possibly just a change of title.

All That's Not Of Jesus Will Go Down
Anywhere Sweetie Goes (I'll Be There) (Clarence Williams), © 7 Nov 27, CW, New York (E678499)
B Flat Blues
Black Bottom Is The Latest Fad
The Boy In The Boat (Boston Blues)

Chinese Blues — included in main list
Confessin' (Lookin' For Another Sweetie). See *Lookin' For Another Sweetie.*
Corn Whisky Cocktail
The Crack
18th Street Strut (Bennie Moten) , © 25 Feb 26, Tr, New York (E636040)
Everybody's Happy In Jimtown (from *Keep Shufflin'*)
Harlem Living Room Suite
Hop Off (Clarence Williams), © 23 Jan 28, CW, New York (E686068)
I Can't Give You Anything But Love (Jimmy McHugh, Dorothy Fields), © 6 Mar 28, "from *Harry Delmar's Revels*", JM, New York (E687442)
I'm A Stationary Woman, Lookin' For A Permanent Man (Andy Razaf, Spencer Williams) , © 10 Feb 30, G, New York (Eunp 16983)
I'm Livin' In A Great Big Way (Jimmy McHugh, Dorothy Fields), © 6 Feb 35, as Got A Snap In My Finger, I'm Livin' In A Great Big Way & 11 Apr 35, IB, New York, as "from *Hooray For Love*". (Eunp 99341; Epub 47562)
Keep Shufflin'
Labour Day Parade
Lookin' For Another Sweetie (Confessin') (Louis Smith, Sterling Grant), © 10 Feb 30, S, New York (Eunp 16937) (Alternative title not mentioned in © entry)
Mean To Me (Roy Turk, Fred Ahlert), © 5 Jan 29 & 1 Feb 29, DeSylva, Brown & Henderson, Inc (Eunp 2556 & Epub 3212)
Muscle Shoals Blues (George W. Thomas), © 8 Feb 19 (Muscleshoals Blues), Geo. W. Thomas, New Orleans (E442895)
My Gal Is Good For Nothing But Love [probably the same as My Man Is Good For Nothing But Love in main list.]
My Handy Man Ain't Handy No More (Andy Razaf, Eubie Blake), © 26 Aug 30 & 6 Oct 30, ShB, New York (Eunp 27043 & Epub 18211)
Piccaninny Land (from *Hot Chocolates*)
Poolroom Papa
Redskinland (from *Hot Chocolates*)
Reefer Song (If You're A Viper) (Rozetta Howard, Horace Malcolm & Herbert Moren) *[all sic]*, © 8 Jan 38 (as *If You're A Viper*), State Street music publishing co, Chicago (Eunp 158514)
Scrimmage (Jack Beaver)
Song Of The Cotton Fields (from *Hot Chocolates*)
Sposin' (Andy Razaf, Paul Denniker), © 23 Sep 29, Tr, New York (Epub 9430)
Stompin' The Bug (Mercedes Gilbert, Phil Worde) , © 21 Jul 27, Ralph Peer, New York (E672294)
Sweet Devilish Thing
Sweetie Pie (John Jacob Loeb) , © 16 Jun 34, 26 Jul 34, 31 Jul 34, LF, New York [Eunp88902; Epub42984; Epub43158]
Tea For Two (Vincent Youmans, Irving Caesar), © 10 Jun 24 [from *No No Nannette*], H, New York [E589297]
That's What The Bird Said To Me
There's Gonna Be The Devil To Pay
Thundermug Stomp [allegedly retitled Hot Mustard (Fletcher Henderson), © 21 Feb 27, GMS, New York (E660469)]
Top And Bottom Stomp (retitled The Henderson Stomp (Fletcher Henderson), © 18 Dec 26 & 11 Apr 27 (as *Henderson Stomp*, in arrangement by Frank Skinner), R-E, New York (E652950; E661652)]
Traffic In Harlem
Turn On The Heat (B.G. De Sylva (pseud of George Gard De Sylva), Lew Brown & Ray Henderson), © 18 Jun 29 & 29 Jul 29 (from *Sunnyside Up*), DeSylva, Brown & Henderson, New York (Eunp8126; Epub8018)
Variety Stomp (Abel Green, Jo Trent, Fletcher Henderson), © 29 Mar 27 & 1 Oct 27 (as by Jo Trent & Fletcher Henderson, in orchestration by Leonard Hayton), R-E, New York (E659470; E671833)
Waiting At The End Of The Road (Irving Berlin), © 30 Apr 29 & 10 Jun 29, IB, New York (Eunp 6223; Epub6663)
Waller Jive
Wedding Of The Rabbi And The Bear
West Wind (Milton Ager, Murray Mencher & Charles Newman) , © 22 Jan 36, Ager, Yellen & Bernstein, inc., New York (Epub 52999)
You Slay Me (Maceo Pinkard, William Tracey), © 21 Mar 31 & 22 Apr 31, Pinkard inc, New York [Eunp36784; Epub22787]

A Chronological listing of Fats Waller Copyrights Compiled by Howard Rye

1921-1922: No entries have been found in the copyright records for these years.

1923

IT SEEMS TO ME, melody by Thos. Waller.
unpublished 14 Jul 23 E563823 CW, New York
no renewal traced.

ALL ALONE, words & melody by Theo. (Fats) Waller.
unpublished 14 Aug 23 E568618 CW, New York
no renewal traced.

WILD CAT BLUES, words & melody by Thomas Waller & Clarence Williams
unpublished 24 Sep 23 E569581 CW, New York
renewed: 25 Sep 50 by Clarence Williams (A): R67755.
see also 11 Oct 23.

BLUES NEVER DIE, melody by Thomas Waller.
unpublished 2 Oct 23 E571487 CW, New York
no renewal traced.

DONE GONE MAD, melody by Thomas Waller.
unpublished 2 Oct 23 E571488 CW, New York
no renewal traced.

DON'T WANT YOU NO MORE, melody by Thomas Waller.
unpublished 2 Oct 23 E571489 CW, New York
no renewal traced.

WILD CAT BLUES, by Thomas Waller & Clarence Williams; arranged by H. Qualli Clark, pianoforte, Quarto.
published 11 Oct 23 E576352 CW, New York
renewed: 11 Oct 50 by Clarence Williams (A): R68177.
see also 24 Sep 23.

1924

SWEET BABY, words by C. Williams, melody by Thomas Waller.
unpublished 14 Jan 24 E580660 *[sic]* CW, New York
renewed: 11 Jan 52 by Edith Hatcher Waller (W): R88609.

FRIENDLESS BLUES, melody by Thomas Waller.
unpublished 21 Feb 24 E579693 CW, New York
renewed: 23 Jan 52 by Edith Hatcher Waller (W): R89330.

ORIENTAL TONES, melody by Thomas Waller.
unpublished 21 Feb 24 E579701 CW, New York
renewed: 23 Jan 52 by Edith Hatcher Waller (W): R89331.

SLAVING, words & melody by Thomas Waller & Clarence Williams.
unpublished 21 Feb 24 E579706 CW, New York
renewed: 21 Feb 51 by Clarence Williams (A): R75074.

HOG MAW STOMP, melody by Thomas Waller.
unpublished 12 Mar 24 E584357 CW, New York
renewed: 23 Jan 52 by Edith Hatcher Waller (W): R89332.

WHAT CAN BE WRONG WITH ME, words by Joseph Trent, melody by Thomas Waller.
unpublished 4 Apr 24 E585071 CW, New York
renewed: 4 Apr 51 by Joseph Trent (A of words): R76370.

HELLO ATLANTA TOWN, words by Joseph Trent & Clarence Williams, melody by Thomas Waller.
unpublished 4 Apr 24 E585074 CW, New York
renewed: 4 Apr 51 by Joseph Trent & Clarence Williams (A's of words): R76373.

STROLLIN' ROUN' THE TOWN, words by Joseph Trent, melody by Thomas Waller.
unpublished 4 Apr 24 E585076 CW, New York
renewed: 4 Apr 51 by Joseph Trent (A of words): R76375.

THAT'S MY MAN, words by Joseph Trent, melody by Thomas Waller
unpublished 11 Apr 24 E585321 CW, New York
renewed: 11 Apr 51 by Joseph Trent (A of words): R76947.

IN HARLEM, words by Joseph Trent, melody by Thomas Waller.
unpublished 28 Apr 24 E585866 CW, New York
renewed: 30 Apr 51 by Joseph Trent (A of words): R77976.
MY MAN CURES THE BLUES, words by Joseph Trent, melody by Thomas Waller.
unpublished 28 Apr 24 E585867 CW, New York
renewed: 30 Apr 51 by Joseph Trent (A of words): R77977.
IN THE SPRINGTIME, words by Joseph Trent, melody by Thomas Waller
unpublished 28 Apr 24 E585868 CW, New York
renewed: 30 Apr 51 by Joseph Trent (A of words): R77978.
MY BABY'S COMING BACK HOME, words by Joseph Trent, melody by Thomas Waller.
unpublished 28 Apr 24 E585869 CW, New York
renewed: 28 May 51 by Joseph Trent (A of words): R79118.
I'M GOIN' RIGHT ALONG, words by Joseph Trent, melody by Thomas Waller.
unpublished 28 Apr 24 E585870 CW, New York
renewed: 30 Apr 51 by Joseph Trent (A of words): R77979.
MANDY, I'M JUST WILD ABOUT YOU, words by Joseph Trent & Clarence Williams, melody by Thomas Waller.
unpublished 28 Apr 24 E585876 CW, New York
renewed: 30 Apr 51 by Joseph Trent & Clarence Williams (A's of words): R77985.
SWEETIE DON'T GROW SOUR ON ME, words by Charles O'Flynn, melody by Thomas Waller.
unpublished 10 Jun 24 E589098 CW, New York
renewed: 11 Jun 51 by Charles O'Flynn (A of words): R79515.
IN MY BABY'S EYES, words by Joseph H. Trent, melody by Thomas Waller.
unpublished 10 Jun 24 E589101 CW, New York
renewed: 11 Junr 51 by Joseph Trent (A of words): R79518.
WHEN YOU'RE TIRED OF ME JUST LET ME KNOW, words by Andrea Razaf, melody by Thomas Waller.
unpublished 12 Jun 24 E589148 CW, New York
renewed: 12 Jun 51 by Andy Razaf (A): R79450.
renewed: 12 Jun 51 by Andrea Razaf (A of words): R79566.
OLD FASHIONED SUSIE'S BLUES, words & melody by Andrea Razaf, Tom Waller & Clarence Williams.
unpublished 12 Jun 24 E589150 CW, New York
renewed: 12 Jun 51 by Andy Razaf (A): R79439.
renewed: 12 Jun 51 by Clarence Williams & Andrea Razaf (A's of words): R79588.
PLEASE TAKE ME BACK, words by Joseph H. Trent, melody by Thomas Waller.
unpublished 7 Jul 24 E589744 CW, New York
renewed: 9 Jul 51 by Joseph H. Trent (A of words): R80748.
IN HARLEM'S ARABY, words & music by Jo Trent & Tom (Fats) Waller.
published 24 Jul 24 E594173 E, New York
renewed: 23 Jan 52 by Edith Hatcher Waller (W): R89333.
ROCK ME JUST LIKE A SWEET DADDY SHOULD, words by Andrea Razaf, melody by Thomas Waller.
unpublished 25 Jul 24 E594224 CW, New York
renewed: 23 Jul 51by Andy Razaf (A): R81444.
MY JAMAICA LOVE, words by Andrea Razaf, melody by Thomas Waller.
unpublished 25 Jul 24 E594225 CW, New York
renewed: 23 Jul 51by Andy Razaf (A): R81445.
MY SWEET BABY IRENE, words by Andrea Razaf & Spencer Williams, melody by Thomas Waller.
unpublished 4 Aug 24 E594552 CW, New York
renewed: 6 Aug 51 by Andy Razaf (A): R81845.
renewed: 6 Aug 51 by Spencer Williams (A): R81846.
I'D RATHER BE BLUE THAN GREEN, words & melody by C. Williams, Spencer Williams, Andrea Razaf & Thomas Waller
unpublished 4 Aug 24 E594554 CW, New York
renewed: 6 Aug 51 by Spencer Williams (A): R81847.
renewed: 6 Aug 51 by Andy Razaf (A): R81848.
renewed: 31 Aug 51 by Clarence Williams & Spencer Williams (A's): R82839.
RAMBLIN' PAPA BLUES, words by Spencer Williams, melody by Thos. Waller.
unpublished 15 Sep 24 E597414 TH, New York
renewed: 17 sep 51 by Spencer Williams (A of words): R83286.
ANYBODY HERE WANT TO TRY MY CABBAGE, words by Andrea Razaf, melody by Thos. Waller.
unpublished 15 Sep 24 E597415 TH, New York
renewed: 27 Nov 51 by Andy Razaf (A): R86433.
see also 6 Sep 25.

ICE COLD PAPA MAMA'S GONNA MELT YOU DOWN, words by Andrea Razaf, melody by Thomas Waller.
unpublished 15 Sep 24 E597416 TH, New York
renewed: 27 Nov 51 by Andy Razaf (A): R86434.

SHET YO' MOUF, words & melody by Andrea Razaf & Tom Waller.
unpublished 19 Sep 24 E597572 CW, New York
renewed: 27 Nov 51 by Andy Razaf (A): R86436.

EVERY SWEETIE THAT I GET, SOMEBODY TAKES HER FROM ME, words & melody by Thomas Waller & Spencer Williams.
unpublished 19 Sep 24 E597573 CW, New York
renewed: 19 Sep 51 by Spencer Williams (A): R83332.

THAT BLUE STRAIN, words & melody by Thomas Waller & Spencer Williams.
unpublished 19 Sep 24 E597574 CW, New York
renewed: 19 Sep 51 by Spencer Williams (A): R83333.

AWFUL (AN) LOT MY GAL AIN'T GOT, BUT WHAT SHE'S GOT, SHE'S GOT AN AWFUL LOT, words & melody by Thomas Waller & Spencer Williams.
unpublished 4 Oct 24 E602134 IB, New York
renewed: 6 Oct 51 by Spencer Williams (A): R84020.
see also 19 May 25.

STRIVERS ROW, words by Jack Moore [pseud. of Jack Ryan], music by Tom Brown [pseud. of Tom Waller].
published 18 Oct 24 E602448 TH, New York
renewed: 23 Jan 52 by Edith Hatcher Waller (W): R89883.

HOME ALONE BLUES, words by John Holmes, music by Thomas Waller.
published 18 Oct 24 E602449 TH, New York
renewed: 23 Jan 52 by Edith Hatcher Waller (W): R89884.

BLOODY RAZOR BLUES, words & melody by Spencer Williams & Thomas Waller; arranged by Arthur Ray.
unpublished 27 Oct 24 E600909 JD, New York
renewed: 29 Oct 51 by Spencer Williams (A): R85083.
renewed: 16 Nov 51 by Spencer Williams (A) & Edith Waller (W): R86364.

BULLET WOUND BLUES, words & melody by Spencer Williams & Thomas Waller; arranged by Arthur Ray.
unpublished 27 Oct 24 E600910 JD, New York
renewed: 29 Oct 51 by Spencer Williams (A): R85084.
renewed: 16 Nov 51 by Spencer Williams (A) & Edith Waller (W): R86365.

CALL THE PLUMBER IN, words & melody by Andrea Razaf & Thomas Waller.
unpublished 1 Nov 24 E602775 CW, New York
renewed: 2 Nov 51 by Andrea Razaf (A): R85568.
renewed: 27 Nov 51 by Andy Razaf (A): R86439.

I MAY BE A LITTLE GREEN BUT I AIN'T NO FOOL, words & melody by Thomas Waller & Spencer Williams.
unpublished 1 Nov 24 E602778 CW, New York
renewed: 1 Nov 51 by Spencer Williams (A): R85414.

FLAT TIRE PAPA, MAMA'S GONNA GIVE YOU AIR, words & music by Spencer Williams & Thomas Waller.
published 8 Nov 24 E601763 M, New York
renewed: 8 Nov 51 by Spencer Williams (A): R85827.

PLEASE TELL ME WHY, words & music by Ed Adams & Thomas Waller.
published 26 Nov 24 E603829 GMS, New York
renewed: 23 Jan 52 by Edith Hatcher Waller (W): R89885.

ANY DAY THE SUN DON'T SHINE, words & melody by Andrea Razaf & Thomas Waller.
unpublished 4 Dec 24 E601952 CW, New York
renewed: 4 Dec 51 by Andy Razaf (A): R86454.
renewed: 5 Dec 51 by A. Razaf [sic] (A): R87074.

1925

WORKIN' WOMAN'S BLUES, words & melody by Spencer Williams & Thomas Waller, arranged by Merle T. Kendrick.
unpublished 24 Jan 25 E605273 Tr, New York
renewed: 24 Jan 52 by Spencer Williams (A): R89239.
renewed: 24 Jan 52 by Edith L. Waller (W): R89240.

BALL AND CHAIN BLUES, words by Andrea Razaf, melody by Thomas Waller
unpublished 28 Mar 25 E610786 TH, New York
renewed: 30 Apr 52 by Edith L. Waller (W): R94108.
renewed: 3 Jun 52 by Andy Razaf (A): R95742.

ANYBODY HERE WANT TO TRY MY CABBAGE, words by Andrea Razaf, melody by Thomas Waller
published 6 Apr 25 E610996 TH, New York
renewed: 8 Apr 52 by Edith L. Waller (W): R93270.
renewed: 3 Jun 52 by Andy Razaf (A): R95743.
see also 15 Sep 24.

KISS MA AGAIN, words & music by Clarence Williams & Thomas Waller
published 28 Apr 25 E611540 CW., New York
renewed: 28 Apr 52 by Edith L. Waller (W): R94092.
renewed: 28 Apr 52 by Clarence Williams (A): R94236.

AWFUL (AN) LOT MY GAL AIN'T GOT, BUT WHAT SHE'S GOT SHE'S GOT AN AWFUL LOT, words & music by Thomas Waller & Spencer Williams.
published 19 May 25 E616194 IB, New York
renewed: 19 May 52 by Edith L. Waller (W): R94857.
renewed: 19 May 52 by Spencer Williams (A): R94858.
see also 4 Oct 24.

BROTHER BEN, words & melody by Thomas Waller & Spencer Williams
unpublished 4 Jun 25 E616384 CW, New York
renewed: 4 Jun 52 by Spencer Williams (A): R95809.
renewed: 4 Jun 52 by Edith L. Waller (W): R95810.

HEART (THE) THAT ONCE BELONGED TO ME, BELONGS TO SOMEONE ELSE words & music by Clarence Williams & Thomas Waller; pianoforte acc. with ukulele arranged by Dick Konter
published 7 Jul 25 E619927 CW, New York
renewed: 7 Jul 52 by Clarence Williams (A): R97437.
renewed: 16 Jul 52 by Edith L. Waller (W): R97608.

SQUEEZE ME, words & m Clarence Williams & Thomas Waller; pianoforte acc. with u. arranged by Dick Konter
published 31 Jul 25 E627848 CW, New York
renewed: 31 Jul 52 by Clarence Williams (A): R98496.
renewed: 22 Oct 52 by Edith L. Waller (W): R101184.

CAMPMEETIN' STOMP, melody by Thomas Waller
unpublished 16 Oct 25 E621709 CW, New York
renewed: 22 Oct 52 by Edith L. Waller (W): R101173.

MID NIGHT STOMP, melody by Thomas Waller
unpublished 16 Oct 25 E621708 CW, New York
renewed: 22 Oct 52 by Edith L. Waller (W): R101172.
see also 26 Nov 26.

HOUSE PARTY STOMP, by Thos. (Fats) Waller, pianoforte.
unpublished 14 Nov 25 E626757 Tr., New York
renewed: 2 Dec 52 by Edith L. Waller (W): R103382.

1926

GREAT SCOTT, words & melody by by Henry Troy & Thomas Waller.
unpublished 2 Feb 26 E634308 TH, New York.
renewed: 16 Feb 53 by Edith Hatcher Waller (W): R107583.
renewed: 18 Aug 53 by Henry Troy (A): R116177.

FLORIDA LOW DOWN, words & music by J. Fred Coots, Jo Trent & Fats Waller; pianoforte acc. with ukelele arrangement by May Singhi Breen. (Cover Title: THAT FLORIDA LOW DOWN)
published 6 Apr 26 E636738 F C, New York
renewed: 7 Apr 53 by Edith Hatcher Waller (W): R110011.

CHINESE BLUES, words by Sam Coslow, music by Irving Mills & Jimmy Hugh [as James Francis McHugh in renewals], pianoforte acc. with ukulele arrangeement by M. Kalua.
published 17 Apr 26 E640304 JM, New York
renewed: 15 Apr 54 by Sam Coslow, Irving Mills & Jimmy McHugh (A's): R128849
This entry is included because it is credited to 'Waller-Mills' on the Original Memphis Five recording of 23 Jan 26.

GEORGIA BO-BO, words & music by Jo Trent & Fats Waller [pseud. of Thomas Waller]
published 23 Apr 26 E637273 ShB, New York
renewed: 23 Apr 53 by Edith Hatcher Waller (W): R110578.
renewed: 23 Apr 53 by Jo Trent (A): R110587.

LONESOME ONE, melody by Thomas (Fats) Waller.
unpublished 3 May 26 E640606 CW, New York
renewed: 6 May 53 by Edith Hatcher Waller (W): R111686.

LEVEE LAND, opening chorus, melody by Thomas (Fats) Waller
unpublished 3 May 26 E640609 CW, New York
renewed: 6 May 53 by Edith Hatcher Waller (W): R111687.
BEETHOVEN'S SANGWATTNI, melody by Thomas (Fats) Waller
unpublished 26 May 26 E641182 CW, New York
renewed: 27 May 53 by Edith Hatcher Waller (W): R112649.
CONGO LOU, melody by Thomas (Fats) Waller.
unpublished 26 May 26 E641184 CW, New York
renewed: 27 May 53 by Edith Hatcher Waller (W): R112650.
SENORITA MINE, Spanish fox-trot, from *Tan Town Topics* revue, words by Spencer Williams & Eddie Rector, music by Clarence Williams & Thomas (Fats) Waller; pianoforte acc. with ukelele arrangement by Gus Horsley.
published 31 May 26 E642487 CW, New York
renewed: 1 Jun 53 by Edith Hatcher Waller (W): R112909.
renewed: 1 Jun 53 by Spencer Williams (A): R112931.
renewed: 2 Jun 53 by Spencer Williams, Eddie Rector & Clarence Williiams (A's): R112837.
CHARLESTON HOUND, from *Tan Town Topics* revue, words by Eddie Rector & Spencer Williams, music by Clarence Williams & Thomas (Fats) Waller; pianoforte acc. with ukelele acrangement by Hannibal McGuire.
published 1 Jun 26 E642488 CW, New York
renewed: 11 Jun 53 by Spencer Williams (A): R113244.
renewed: 12 Jun 53 by Edith Hatcher Waller (W): R113428.
THAT STRUTTIN' EDDIE OF MINE, words by Eddie Rector & Spencer Williams, melody by Clarence Williams & Thomas Waller.
unpublished 18 Jun 26 E642477 CW, New York
renewed: 18 Jun 53 by Spencer Williams (A): R113517.
renewed: 18 Jun 53 by Eddie Rector, Spencer Williams & Clarence Williiams (A's): R113635.
renewed: 19 Jun 53 by Edith Hatcher Waller (W): R113646.
CRAZY 'BOUT THAT MAN I LOVE, words & melody by Spencer Williams, Thomas Waller & Clarence Williams.
unpublished 18 Jun 26 E642479 CW, New York
renewed: 18 Jun 53 by Spencer Williams (A): R113518.
renewed: 18 Jun 53 by Spencer Williams & Clarence Williiams (A's): R113635.
renewed: 19 Jun 53 by Edith Hatcher Waller (W): R113647.
see also 2 Feb 27.
THERE'LL COME A TIME WHEN YOU WANT ME, words & melody by Clarence Williams & Thomas Waller.
unpublished 18 Jun 26 E642483 CW, New York
renewed: 18 Jun 53 by Spencer Williams (A): R113640.
renewed: 19 Jun 53 by Edith Hatcher Waller (W): R113648.
renewals as THERE'LL COME A TIME WHEN YOU WANT ME, BUT I WON'T BE WAITING FOR YOU.
OLD FOLKS SHUFFLE, melody by Thomas Waller & Clarence Williams.
unpublished 18 Jun 26 E642484 CW, New York
renewed: 18 Jun 53 by Clarence Williams (A): R113641.
renewed: 19 Jun 53 by Edith Hatcher Waller (W): R113649.
OLD FOLKS SHUFFLE, black bottom fox-trot by Clarence Williams & Thomas (Fats) Waller; pianoforte.
published 26 Nov 26 E651969 CW, New York
renewed: 27 Nov 53 by Clarence Williams (A): R121396.
MIDNIGHT STOMP, by C. Williams & Fats Waller [pseud. of Thomas Waller]; pianoforte.
published 26 Nov 26 E654832 CW, New York
renewed: 17 Nov 53 by Clarence Williams (A): R121397.
renewed: 30 Nov 53 by Edith Hatcher Waller (W): R121537.
see also 16 Oct 25.

1927

SOOTHIN' SYRUP STOMP, melody by Thomas Waller.
unpublished 21 Jan 27 E655656 RSP, New York
renewed: 23 Jan 54 by Edith Hatcher Waller (W): R125052.
SLOPPY WATER BLUES, melody by Thomas Waller.
unpublished 21 Jan 27 E655658 RSP, New York
renewed: 25 Jan 54 by Edith Hatcher Waller (W): R125053.

CRAZY 'BOUT THAT MAN I LOVE, words & melody by Spencer Williams, Thomas Waller & Clarence Williams.
unpublished 10 Feb 27 E658140 CW, New York
renewed: 10 Feb 54 by Spencer Williams & Clarence Williams (A's): R125560
renewed: 11 Feb 54 by Spencer Williams (A): R125636.
renewed: 12 Feb 54 by Edith Hatcher Waller (W): R125541.
see also 18 Jun 26.

LONG, DEEP AND WIDE, melody by Thomas Waller.
unpublished 10 Feb 27 E658146 CW, New York
renewed: 12 Feb 54 by Edith Hatcher Waller (W): R125522.

ST. LOUIS SHUFFLE, by Jack Pettis & Thomas Waller; scored by Al Goering, orch. quarto.
published 8 Mar 27 E661069 R-E., New York
renewed: 19 Mar 54 by Jack Pettis (A), Edith Waller (W) & Robbins music corp (PWH of A. Goering): R127272.

ALLIGATOR CRAWL, blues fox-trot by Fats Waller [pseud. of Thomas Waller]; arranged by Frank L. Ventre, orch quarto.
published 18 Apr 27 E661814 Tr., New York
renewed: 20 Apr 54 by Edith Waller (W): R129192.
see also 17 Dec 34 & 30 Aug 37 & 27 Sep 37.

RUSTY PAIL BLUES, melody by Fats Waller [i.e. Thomas Waller].
unpublished 2 May 27 E664284 RSP, New York
renewed: 4 May 54 by Edith Hatcher Waller (W): R129933.

DARKIE'S (A) LAMENT, by Thomas Waller, pianoforte.
published 12 Jul 27 E672242 GMS, New York
renewed: 14 Jul 54 by Edith Hatcher Waller (W): R133338.
renewed: 12 Aug 54 by Edith L. Waller (W): R134408.

MESSIN' AROUND WITH THE BLUES, by Phil Worde & Thomas Waller; arranged by Phil Worde, pianoforte.
unpublished 21 Jul 27 E672293 RSP, New York
renewed: 22 Jul 54 by Edith Hatcher Waller (W): R133666.
renewed: 12 Aug 54 by Edith L. Waller (W): R134409.

LENOX AVENUE BLUES, melody by Thos. Waller.
unpublished 8 Aug 27 E672785 RSP, New York
renewed: 12 Aug 54 by Edith Hatcher Waller (W): R134341.
renewed: 12 Aug 54 by Edith L. Waller (W): R134410.

FAT MAN BLUES, by Thomas Waller; pianoforte.
published 12 Aug 27 E670898 GMS, New York
renewed: 12 Aug 54 by Edith L. Waller (W): R134406.

SAVANNAH BLUES, melody by Thomas Waller & Thomas Morris.
unpublished 18 Aug 27 E670844 RSP, New York
renewed: 19 Aug 54 by Edith Hatcher Waller (W): R134770.
renewed: 7 Sep 54 by Edith L. Waller (W): R135577.

I'M MORE THAN SATISFIED, words by Raymond Klages, melody by Thomas Waller.
unpublished 14 Sep 27 E674143 R, New York
renewed: 14 Sep 54 by Edith L. Waller (W): R135649.
renewed: 15 Sep 54 by May E. Klages (W): R135665 & R135797 (identical registrations).
see also 14 Nov 27.

WHITEMAN STOMP, melody by Jo Trent & Thomas Waller.
unpublished 14 Sep 27 E674144 R, New York
renewed: 14 Sep 54 by Edith L. Waller (W): R135650.
renewed: 14 Sep 54 by Jo Trent (A): R135865.
see also 14 Feb 28.

THERE'LL COME A TIME WHEN YOU'LL NEED ME, words & melody by Joe Davis & Fats Waller [pseud. of Thomas Waller]
unpublished 24 Sep 27 E671588 JD, New York
renewed: 27 Sep 54 by Edith L. Waller (W): R136360.
renewed: 27 Sep 54 by Edith Waller (W) & Joseph M. Davis (A): R136445.
renewals as THERE'LL COME A TIME WHEN YOU'LL NEED ME, THEN I WON'T HAVE TIME FOR YOU.

I'M GOIN' HUNTIN', by Thos. Waller & J.C. Johnson; pianoforte.
published 24 Sep 27 E671847 GMS, New York
renewed: 24 Sep 54 by Edith L. Waller (W): R136226.
renewed: 24 Sep 54 by J.C. Johnson (A): R136227.

WRINGIN' AND TWISTIN', words by Jo Trent, melody by Thomas W. Waller & Frank Trumbauer.
unpublished 20 Oct 27 E674925 R, New York
renewed: 20 Oct 54 by Edith Waller (W): R137515.
renewed: 20 Oct 54 by Jo Trent & Frank Trumbauer (A's): R137679.

FATS WALLER STOMP, melody by T.Waller, T. Mooris & C. Irvis.
unpublished 21 Oct 27 E674913 RSP, New York
renewed: 21 Oct 54 by Edith L. Waller (W): R137523.

I'M MORE THAN SATISFIED, words by Ray Klages, mus Thomas Waller; pianoforte acc. with ukelele arrangement by Hank Linet
published 14 Nov 27 E675399 R, New York
renewed: 15 Nov 54 by Edith L. Waller (W): R139057.
renewed: 17 Nov 54 by May E. Klages (W): R139084.
see also 14 Sep 27.

MEDITATION, by Fats Waller [pseud. of Thomas Waller], pianoforte.
published 28 Nov 27 E675774 Tr., New York
renewed: 29 Nov 54 by Edith L. Waller (W): R139928.

NOBODY KNOWS, words by B. Allen, music by Thomas Waller & Bennett Carter; pianoforte & ukelele acc.
published 26 Dec 27 E682754 BA., New York
renewed: 30 Dec 54 by Edith Hatcher Waller (W): R141785.
renewed: 17 Jan 55 by Thomas W. Waller, Jr. (C): R143278.
renewals as NOBODY KNOWS HOW MUCH I LOVE YOU.

COME ON AND STOMP, STOMP, STOMP, words & music by Chris Smith, Thomas Waller & Irving Mills; pianoforte acc. with ukelele acc. by M. Kalua.
published 27 Dec 27 E681048 JM, New York
renewed: 28 Dec 54 by Dora Smith (W): R141783.
renewed: 30 Dec 54 by Edith Hatcher Waller (W): R141783.
renewed: 17 Jan 55 by Thomas W. Waller, Jr. (C): R143276.

SHAKE YOUR FEET, by Irving Mills & Thomas Waller; pianoforte.
published 27 Dec 27 E682385 GMS, New York
renewed: 30 Dec 54 by Edith Hatcher Waller (W): R141784.
renewed: 17 Jan 55 by Thomas W. Waller, Jr. (C): R143277.

1928

I HOPE YOU'RE SATISFIED, words by Clarence Williams, melody by Thos. Waller.
unpublished 13 Jan 28 E681159 CW, New York
renewed: 13 Jan 55 by Clarence Williams (A): R143339.
renewed: 17 Feb 55 by Thomas W. Waller, Jr. (C): R144855.
renewed: 2 Mar 55 by Clarence Williams (A): R145408.

MONKEY TALK, melody by Thomas Waller.
unpublished 13 Jan 28 E681160 CW, New York
renewed: 17 Feb 55 by Thomas W. Waller, Jr. (C): R144857.

FREEZE OUT, melody by Thos. Waller,
unpublished 13 Jan 28 E681161 CW, New York
renewed: 17 Feb 55 by Thomas W. Waller, Jr. (C): R144858.

LION'S (THE) ROAR, melody by Thomas Waller
unpublished 13 Jan 28 E681162 CW, New York
renewed: 17 Feb 55 by Thomas W. Waller, Jr. (C): R144859.

WHITEMAN STOMP, by Jo Trent & Thomas Waller; arranged by Leonard Hayton, orch quarto.
published 14 Feb 28 E683179 R, New York
renewed: 14 Feb 55 by Thomas W. Waller, Jr. (C): R144401.
renewed: 17 Feb 55 by Robbins music corp, (PWH of L. Hayton): R144548.
renewed: 17 Feb 55 by Thomas W. Waller, Jr. (C): R144856.
see also 14 Sep 27.

WILLOW TREE, from *Keep Shufflin'*, words & music by Andy Razaf & Thomas Waller; pianoforte & ukelele acc.
published 29 Feb 28 E683823 H, New York
renewed: 1 Mar 55 by Thomas W. Waller, Jr. (C): R145383.
renewed: 1 Mar 55 by Anita Rutherford Waller (W) & Andy Razaf (A): R145834.

GOT MYSELF ANOTHER JOCKEY NOW, from *Keep Shufflin'*, words by Andy Razaf, music by Thomas Waller; pianoforte & ukelele acc.
published 29 Feb 28 E683825 H, New York
renewed: 1 Mar 55 by Thomas W. Waller, Jr. (C): R145385.
renewed: 1 Mar 55 by Andy Razaf (A): R145386.
renewed: 1 Mar 55 by Andy Razaf (A) & Anita Rutherford Waller (W) : R145835.

HOW JAZZ WAS BORN, from *Keep Shufflin'*, words by Andy Razaf, music by Thomas Waller; pianoforte & ukelele acc.
published 29 Feb 28 E683826 H, New York
renewed: 1 Mar 55 by Andy Razaf (A): R145387.
renewed: 1 Mar 55 by Thomas W. Waller, Jr. (C): R145388.
renewed: 1 Mar 55 by Andy Razaf (A) & Anita Rutherford Waller (W) : R145836.

CANDIED SWEETS, stomp, by Jack Pettis & Thomas Waller; arranged by Al Goering, orch quarto.
published 2 Mar 28 E686539 R., New York
renewed: 2 Mar 55 by Jack Pettis (A): R145862.
renewed: 4 Mar 55 by Thomas W. Waller, Jr. (C): R146402.

LOVIE LEE, words & music by Andy Razaf [Andy Paul Pazaf in renewals] & Thomas Waller.
published 31 Mar 28 E688820 GMS, New York
renewed: 31 Mar 55 by Andy Razaf (A): R147147
renewed: 1 Apr 55 by Thomas W. Waller, Jr. (C): R147455

DIGAH'S (THE) STOMP, by Thomas (Fats) Waller; pianoforte.
unpublished 8 May 28 E691907 RSP, New York
renewed: 10 May 55 by Thomas W. Waller, Jr. (C): R149616.

PLEASE TAKE ME OUT OF JAIL, melody by T. Morris & T. Waller.
unpublished 19 May 28 E690735 RSP, New York
renewed: 20 May 55 by Thomas W. Waller, Jr. (C): R150194.

ONE O'CLOCK BLUES, by Bud Allen, Walter Bishop & Thomas Waller [melody only]
unpublished 3 Aug 28 E696731 BA, New York
renewed: 3 Aug 55 by Walter Bishop (A): R153859.
renewed: 5 Aug 55 by Thomas W. Waller, Jr. (C): R154307.

HOG MAN STOMP, by Thomas Waller [melody only]
unpublished 5 Nov 28 EU857 RSP, New York
renewed: 10 Nov 55 by Thomas W. Waller, Jr. (C): R159599.

ST. LOUIS BLUES, by W.C. Handy, transcribed by Thomas Waller, organ.
published 20 Nov 28 EPI460 Alfred & co., New York
renewed: 23 Nov 55 by William C. Handy (PWH): R160064.

1929

WHY AM I ALONE WITH NO ONE TO LOVE, words & music by Spencer Williams, Andy Razaf & Thomas Waller.
published 18 Feb 29 EP3591 Tr, New York
renewed: 20 Feb 56 by Andy Razaf (A): R165141.
renewed: 20 Feb 56 by Spencer Williams (A): R165142.
renewed: 20 Feb 56 by Thomas W. Waller, Jr. (C): R165305.

TOUCH-DOWN, by Thomas (Fats) Waller [melody only].
unpublished 2 Mar 29 EU4230 CW, New York
renewed: 2 Mar 56 by Maurice Rutherford Waller, Ronald Rutherford Waller & Thomas W. Waller, Jr. (C): R165776.
renewed: 5 Mar 56 by Anita Rutherford Waller (W): R166218.

I'VE GOT A FEELING I'M FALLING, words & music by Billy Rose, Harry Link & Fred Waller *[sic]* [words & melody only]. [Renewals correct composer name to Thomas Waller.]
unpublished 14 Mar 29 EU4730 SB, New York
renewed: 27 Mar 56 by Billy Rose, Harry Link (A's), by Thomas W. Waller, Jr., Maurice Waller & Ronald Rutherford Waller(C): R167649
renewed: 14 Mar 56 by Harry Link (A): R167461.
renewed :14 Mar 56 by Billy Rose (A): R166462.

I'VE GOT A FEELING I'M FALLING, words by Billy Rose, music by Harry Link & Thomas Waller.
published 1 Apr 29 EP4715 SB, New York
renewed: 2 Apr 56 by Billy Rose (A): R167518.
renewed: 2 Apr 56 by Harry Link (A): R167519.
renewed: 2 Apr 56 by Billy Rose, Harry Link (A's), by Thomas W. Waller, Jr., Maurice Waller & Ronald Rutherford Waller(C): R167649

IF YOU LIKE ME, LIKE I LIKE YOU, words & music by Clarence Williams, Thomas Fats Waller & Spencer Williams; pianoforte acc. with ukelele arrangement by Ben Garrison.
published 9 Apr 29 EP5584 CW, N.Y
renewed: 9 Apr 56 by Spencer Williams (A): R168102.
renewed: 11 Apr 56 by Maurice Rutherford Waller, Ronald Rutherford Waller & Thomas W. Waller, Jr. (C): R168536.
renewed: 27 Apr 56 by Clarence Williams (A) & Anita Rutherford Waller (W): R169740.

THAT RHYTHM MAN, from *Connie's Hot Chocolates*, lyrics by Andy Razaf, music by Thomas Waller & Harry Brooks, pianoforte acc. with ukelele arrangement by M. Kalua
published 26 Jun 29 EP7300 MM, New York
renewed: 26 Jun 56 by Andy Razaf (A): R172904.
renewed: 27 Jun 56 by Andy Razaf, Harry Brooks (A's), Thomas Waller, Jr., Maurice Rutherford Waller & Ronald Rutherford Waller (C): R173056.

I'M NOT WORRYING, words & mus Clarence Williams & Thomas Waller; pianoforte & ukelele acc.
published 1 Jul 29 EP7708 CW, New York
renewed: 3 Jul 56 by Clarence Williams (A), Thomas W. Waller, Jr., Maurice Rutherford Waller & Ronald Rutherford Waller (C): R173269.
renewed: 5 Jul 56 by Clarence Williams (A) & Anita Rutherford Waller (W): R173346.
renewed: 18 Oct 56 by Clarence Williams (A): R178588.

DIXIE CINDERELLA, from *Connie's Hot Chocolates*, lyr Andy Razaf, music by Thomas Waller & Harry Brooks; pianoforte acc. with ukelele arrangement by M. Kalua.
published 2 Jul 29 EP7893 MM, New York
renewed: 2 Jul 56 by Andy Razaf (A): R173155.
renewed: 3 Jul 56 by Andy Razaf, Harry Brooks (A's), Thomas W. Waller, Jr., Maurice Rutherford Waller & Ronald Rutherford Waller (C): R173270.

OFF-TIME, from *Connie's Hot Chocolates*, lyr Andy Razaf, music by Thomas Waller & Harry Brooks; pianoforte acc.with ukelele arrangement by M. Kalua.
published 2 Jul 29 EP7894 MM, New York
renewed: 2 Jul 56 by Andy Razaf (A): R173156.
renewed: 3 Jul 56 by Andy Razaf, Harry Brooks (A's), Thomas W. Waller, Jr., Maurice Rutherford Waller & Ronald Rutherford Waller (C): R173271.

AIN'T MISBEHAVIN', from *Connie's Hot Chocolatess*, lyr Andy Razaf, music by Thomas Waller & Harry Brooks; pianoforte & ukelele acc.
published 8 Jul 29 EP8110 MM, New York
renewed: 9 Jul 56 by Thomas W. Waller, Jr. (C): R173567.
renewed: 9 Jul 56 by Andy Razaf (A): R173568.
renewed: 11 Jul 56 by Thomas W. Waller, Jr., Maurice Rutherford Waller & Ronald Rutherford Waller (C): R173947.

SWEET SAVANNAH SUE, from *Connie's Hot Chocolates*, lyr Andy Razaf, music by Thomas Waller & Harry Brooks; pianoforte acc. with ukelele arrangement by M. Kalua.
published 22 Jul 29 EP8679 MM, New York
renewed: 23 Jul 56 by Andy Razaf (A): R174272.
renewed: 11 Jul 56 by Maurice Rutherford Waller, Ronald Rutherford Waller & Thomas W. Waller, Jr. (C): R175206.

SAY IT WITH YOUR FEET, from *Connie's Hot Chocolates*, lyr Andy Razaf, music by Thomas Waller & Harry Brooks, pianoforte acc. with ukelele arrangement by M. Kalua.
published 27 Jul 29 EP8678 MM, New York
renewed: 27 Jul 56 by Andy Razaf (A): R174560.
renewed: 11 Jul 56 by Thomas W. Waller, Jr., Ronald Rutherford Waller & Maurice Rutherford Waller (C): R175208.

I'M JUST WILD ABOUT YOU, lyr Andy Razaf, music by Thomas Waller [words & melody only]
unpublished 1 Aug 29 EU9413 George & Arthur Piantadosi, inc., New York
renewed: 1 Aug 56 by Andy Razaf (A): R174874.
renewed: 2 Aug 56 by Andy Razaf (A) & Anita Rutherford Waller (W): R174778.
renewed: 2 Aug 56 by Thomas W. Waller, Jr., Maurice Rutherford Waller & Ronald Rutherford Waller (C): R175593.

CAN'T WE GET TOGETHER, from *Connie's Hot Chocolates*, lyr Andy Razaf, music by Thomas Waller & Harry Brooks; pianoforte acc. by M. Kalua.
published 7 Aug 29 EP8680 MM, New York
renewed: 7 Aug 56 by Andy Razaf (A)): R175124.
renewed: 8 Aug 56 by Thomas W. Waller, Jr., Maurice Rutherford Waller & Ronald Rutherford Waller (C): R175207.

WHAT DID I DO TO BE SO BLACK & BLUE, from *Connie's Hot Chocolates*, lyrics by Andy Razaf, music by Thomas Waller & Harry Brooks pianoforte & ukelele acc.
published 20 Aug 29 EP8913 MM, New York
renewed: 20 Aug 56 by Andy Razaf (A)): R175584.
renewed: 21 Aug 56 by Thomas W. Waller, Jr., Maurice Rutherford Waller & Ronald Rutherford Waller (C): R175903.
see also 30 Oct 40.

ZONKY, words by Andy Razaf, music by Thomas Waller [words & melody only]
unpublished 11 Sep 29 EU10783 SB, New York
renewed: 11 Sep 56 by Thomas W. Waller, Jr. (C): R176626.
renewed: 11 Sep 56 by Andy Razaf (A): R176627.
renewed: 12 Sep 56 by Andy Razaf (A), by Maurice Rutherford Waller, Thomas W. Waller, Jr., & Ronald Rutherford Waller (C): R176737.
see also 11 Oct 29.

HONEYSUCKLE ROSE, words by Andy Razaf, music by Thomas Waller [words & melody only].
unpublished 11 Sep 29 EU10784 SB, New York
renewed: 11 Sep 56 by Thomas W. Waller, Jr. (C): R176628.
renewed: 11 Sep 56 by Andy Razaf (A): R176629.
renewed: 12 Sep 56 by Andy Razaf (A), by Maurice Rutherford Waller, Thomas Waller, Jr., & Ronald Rutherford Waller (C): R176738.
see also 20 Nov 29 & 9 Jan 62.

MY FATE IS IN YOUR HANDS, words by Andy Razaf, music by Thomas Waller [words & melody only].
unpublished 11 Sep 29 EU10785 SB, New York
renewed: 11 Sep 56 by Andy Razaf (A): R176630.
renewed: 11 Sep 56 by Thomas W. Waller, Jr. (C): R176631.
renewed: 12 Sep 56 by Andy Razaf (A), by Maurice Rutherford Waller, Thomas W. Waller, Jr., & Ronald Rutherford Waller (C): R176739.
see also 11 Oct 29.

THAT JUNGLE JAMBOREE, lyrics by Andy Razaf; music by Thomas Waller & Harry Brooks.
unpublished 17 Sep 29 EU11050 MM, New York
renewed: 17 Sep 56 by Andy Razaf (A)): R176946.
renewed: 19 Sep 56 by Thomas W. Waller, Jr., Ronald Rutherford Waller, Maurice Rutherford Waller (C): R177124.

THAT WAS MY OWN IDEA, words by Billy Moll, music by Thomas Waller [words & melody only].
unpublished 21 Sep 29 EU11214 ShB, New York
renewed: 24 Sep 56 by Thomas W. Waller, Jr., Maurice Rutherford Waller & Ronald Rutherford Waller (C): R177250.
renewed: 25 Sep 56 by Shapiro Bernstein & co, Inc (PWN of B. Moll) & Thomas Waller, Jr. (C): R177739.

SNAKE HIP DANCE, lyr Andy Razaf, music by Thomas Waller & Harry Brooks; pianoforte score by Harold Potter; pianoforte. acc. w. ukelele arrangement by M. Kalua.
published 27 Sep 29 EP9831 MM, New York
renewed: 27 Sep 56 by Andy Razaf (A)): R177447.
renewed: 10 Oct 56 by Thomas W. Waller, Jr., Maurice Rutherford Waller & Ronald Rutherford Waller (C): R179248.

LOOKIN' GOOD BUT FEELIN' BAD, lyr Lester A. Santly, music by Thomas Waller [words & melody only].
unpublished 30 Sep 29 EU11511 SB, New York
renewed: 10 Oct 56 by Lester A. Santley (A), Thomas W. Waller, Jr., Maurice Rutherford Waller & Ronald Rutherford Waller (C): R179246.

MY FATE IS IN YOUR HANDS, lyr Andy Razaf, music by Thomas Waller; pianoforte & ukelele acc.
published 11 Oct 29 EP10041 SB, New York
renewed: 15 Oct 56 by Andy Razaf (A), Thomas W. Waller, Jr., Maurice Rutherford Waller & Ronald Rutherford Waller (C): R179242.
renewed: 8 Nov 56 by Andy Razaf (A): R179891.
BL: also published by Campbell Connelly, London, n.d.
see also 11 Sep 29.

ZONKY, from *Load Of Coal*, lyr Andy Razaf, music by Thomas Waller; pianoforte & ukelele acc.
published 11 Oct 29 EP10042 SB. New York
renewed: 8 Oct 56 by Andy Razaf (A): R179892.
renewed: 15 Oct 56 by Andy Razaf (A),Thomas W. Waller, Jr., Maurice Rutherford Waller & Ronald Rutherford Waller (C): R179243.
BL: also published by Editions Campbell Connelly, Paris, 1931.
see also 11 Sep 29.

NO WONDER, words by Morey Davidson, music by Thomas Waller [words & melody only].
unpublished 23 Oct 29 EU12397 SB, New York
renewed: 23 Oct 56 by Morey Davidson (A), Thomas W. Waller, Jr., Maurice Rutherford Waller & Ronald Rutherford Waller (C): R179447.

TROUBLE, melody by Thomas Waller.
unpublished 18 Nov 29 EU13346 JD, New York
renewed: 23 Oct 56 by Thomas W. Waller, Jr. (C): R180884.
renewed: 23 Oct 56 by Thomas W. Waller, Jr., Maurice Rutherford Waller & Ronald Rutherford Waller (C): R181829.

FIND OUT WHAT THEY LIKE, AND HOW THEY LIKE IT, words by Andy Razaf, music by Thomas Waller [words & melody only]
unpublished 18 Nov 29 EU13368 JD, New York
renewed: 19 Nov 56 by Andy Razaf (A): R180580.
renewed: 21 Nov 56 by Thomas W. Waller, Jr., Maurice Rutherford Waller & Ronald Rutherford Waller (C): R181830.

HEAVY SUGAR, words by Andy Razaf, music by Thomas Waller [words & melody only].
unpublished 18 Nov 29 EU13369 JD, New York
renewed: 19 Nov 56 by Andy Razaf (A): R180581.
renewed: 21 Nov 56 by Andy Razaf (A) & Thomas W. Waller, Jr. (C): R180887.
renewed: 21 Nov 56 by Thomas W. Waller, Jr., Maurice Rutherford Waller & Ronald Rutherford Waller (C): R181831.

PRISONER OF LOVE, words by Andy Razaf, music by Thomas Waller [words & melody only].
unpuplished 18 Nov 29 EU13370 JD, New York
renewed: 19 Nov 56 by Andy Razaf (A): R180582.
renewed: 21 Nov 56 by Andy Razaf (A) & Thomas W. Waller, Jr. (C): R180888.
renewed: 21 Nov 56 by Thomas W. Waller, Jr., Maurice Rutherford Waller & Ronald Rutherford Waller (C): R181832.
see also 20 Jan 30.

RADIO PAPA, BROADCASTIN' MAMA, words by Andy Razaf, music by Thomas Waller [words & melody only].
unpublished 18 Nov 29 EU13371 JD, New York
renewed: 19 Nov 56 by Andy Razaf (A): R180583.
renewed: 21 Nov 56 by Thomas W. Waller, Jr., Maurice Rutherford Waller & Ronald Rutherford Waller (C): R181833.
see also 14 Mar 32.

HONEYSUCKLE ROSE, from *Load of Coal*, lyrics by Andy Razaf, music by Thomas Waller; pianoforte & ukelele acc.
published 20 Nov 29 EP10915 SB, New York
renewed: 20 Nov 56 by Thomas Waller, Jr. (C): R180749.
renewed: 20 Nov 56 by Andy Razaf (A): R180750.
renewed: 21 Nov 56 by Andy Razaf (A), by Maurice Rutherford Waller, Thomas W. Waller, Jr., & Ronald Rutherford Waller (C): R181835.
see also 1 Sep 29.

SIX OR SEVEN TIMES, words & music by Irving Mils & Thomas Waller.
published 22 Nov 29 EP11370 GMS, N.Y
no renewal traced.

GONE, lyrics by Andy Razaf, music by Harry Link & Thomas Waller [words & melody only].
unpublished 23 Nov 29 EU13641 SB, New York
renewed: 23 Nov 56 by Andy Razaf (A): R180795.
renewed: 23 Nov 56 by Dorothy Link (W): R180796.
renewed: 26 Nov 56 by Andy Razaf (A), Dorothy Dick Link (W), Thomas W. Waller, Jr., Maurice Rutherford Waller & Ronald Rutherford Waller (C): R181834.
see also 24 Jan 30.

BLUE, TURNING GREY OVER YOU, words by Andy Razaf, music by Thomas Waller [words & melody only].
unpublished 3 Dec 29 EU13958 JD, New York
renewed: 3 Dec 56 by Andy Razaf (A): R181661.
renewed: 4 Dec 56 by Thomas W. Waller, Jr., Maurice Rutherford Waller & Ronald Rutherford Waller (C): R182360.
renewed: 17 Dec 56 by Thomas W. Waller, Jr. (C): R182557.
renewed: 18 Dec 56 by Andy Razaf (A) & Thomas W. Waller, Jr. (C): R183190.
see also 20 Jan 30.

I NEED SOMEONE LIKE YOU, words & music by Thomas Waller [words & melody only]
unpublished 7 Dec 29 EU14145 S, New York
renewed: 7 Dec 56 by Thomas W. Waller, Jr., Maurice Rutherford Waller & Ronald Rutherford Waller (C): R182359.
renewed: 17 Dec 56 by Thomas W. Waller, Jr. (C): R182558.

GLADYSE, melody by Thomas Waller.
unpublished 26 Dec 29 EU14961 S, New York
renewed: 26 Dec 56 by Thomas W. Waller, Jr. (C): R183109.
renewed: 27 Dec 56 by Thomas W. Waller, Jr., Maurice Rutherford Waller & Ronald Rutherford Waller (C): R184121.

VALENTINE STOMP, melody by Thomas Waller.
unpublished 26 Dec 29 EU14975 S, New York
renewed: 26 Dec 56 by Thomas W. Waller, Jr. (C): R183110.
renewed: 27 Dec 56 by Thomas W. Waller, Jr., Maurice Rutherford Waller & Ronald Rutherford Waller (C): R184122.

MY MAN IS GOOD FOR NOTHIN' BUT LOVE, lyrics by Andy Razaf, music by Thomas Waller & Harry Brooks; pianoforte acc. with ukelele arrangement by M. Kalua.
published 31 Dec 29 EP12480 MM, New York
renewed: 31 Dec 56 by Thomas W. Waller, Jr. (C): R183437.
renewed: 31 Dec 56 by Andy Razaf (A): R183438.
renewed: 2 Jan 57 by Thomas W. Waller, Jr., Maurice Rutherford Waller & Ronald Rutherford Waller (C): R184500.

1930

BLUE TURNING GREY OVER YOU, words by Andy Razaf, music by Thomas Waller; New York, Triangle music publishing co., inc.
published 20 Jan 30 EP12676 JD, New York
renewed: 22 Jan 57 by Thomas W. Waller, Jr. (C): R184878.
renewed: 22 Jan 57 by Andy Razaf (A) & Thomas W. Waller, Jr. (C): R185385.
renewed: 23 Jan 57 by Thomas W. Waller, Jr., Maurice Rutherford Waller & Ronald Rutherford Waller (C): R185641.
renewed: 28 Jan 57 by Andy Razaf (A): R185457.
BL holds two different editions published by Tr, New York, 1930, also Lawrence Wright, London, 1930, 'featured by Bert Ambrose at the Mayfair Hotel [London]'.
see also 3 Dec 29.

PRISONER OF LOVE, lyrics by Andy Razaf, music by Thomas Waller; New York, Triangle music publishing co., inc.
published 20 Jan 30 EP12677 JD, New York
see also 18 Nov 29.
renewed: 22 Jan 57 by Thomas W. Waller, Jr. (C): R184879.
renewed: 22 Jan 57 by Andy Razaf (A) & Thomas W. Waller, Jr. (C): R185386.
renewed: 23 Jan 57 by Thomas W. Waller, Jr., Maurice Rutherford Waller & Ronald Rutherford Waller (C): R185642.
renewed: 28 Jan 57 by Andy Razaf (A): R185456.

GONE, words & music by Harry Link, Andy Razaf & Thomas Waller; pianoforte & ukelele acc.
published 24 Jan 30 EP12794 SB, New York
renewed: 25 Jan 57 by Dorothy Link (W): R185146.
renewed: 22 Jan 57 by Thomas W. Waller, Jr. (C): R185147.
renewed: 28 Jan 57 by Andy Razaf (A): R185455.
renewed: 29 Jan 57 by Dorothy Dick Link (W), Andy Razaf (A), Thomas W. Waller, Jr., Maurice Rutherford Waller & Ronald Rutherford Waller (C): R185639.
see also 23 Nov 29.

TAKE IT FROM ME I'VE TAKEN TO YOU, lyrics by R. Stanley Adams, melody by Thomas Waller.
unpublished 2 Apr 30 EU19560 SB, New York
renewed: 2 Apr 57 by Stanley R. Adams (A): R188961,
renewed: 3 Apr 57 by R. Stanley Adams (A), Thomas W. Waller, Jr., Maurice Rutherford Waller & Ronald Rutherford Waller (C): R190257,
renewed: 24 Mar 58 by Thomas W. Waller, Jr. (C): R211038.
see also 11 Jun 31 (Take It From Me, I'm Takin' To You).

ROLLIN' DOWN THE RIVER, lyrics by R. Stanley Adams, melody by Thomas Waller.
unpublished 2 Apr 30 EU19561 SB, New York
renewed: 2 Apr 57 by Stanley R. Adams (A): R188962,
renewed: 3 Apr 57 by R. Stanley Adams (A), Thomas W. Waller, Jr., Maurice Rutherford Waller & Ronald Rutherford Waller (C): R190258,
renewed: 24 Mar 58 by Thomas W. Waller, Jr. (C): R211039.
see also 25 Apr 30.

RIDIN' BUT WALKIN', melody by Thos. Waller.
unpublished 9 Apr 30 EU19978 S, New York
renewed: 10 Apr 57 by Thomas W. Waller, Jr., Maurice Rutherford Waller & Ronald Rutherford Waller (C): R190509.
renewed: 24 Mar 58 by Thomas W. Waller, Jr. (C): R211040.
see also 22 Dec 30.

WON'T YOU GET OFF IT, PLEASE, melody by Thos. Waller.
unpublished 9 Apr 30 EU19979 S, New York
renewed: 10 Apr 57 by Thomas W. Waller, Jr., Maurice Rutherford Waller & Ronald Rutherford Waller (C): R190510.
renewed: 24 Mar 58 by Thomas W. Waller, Jr. (C): R211041.

ROLLIN' DOWN THE RIVER, from *Spades are trump [sic]*, lyrics by R. Stanley Adams, music by Thomas Waller; pianoforte & ukelele accompaniment. [Featured in Connie's Revue *Spades Are Trumps*.]
published 25 Apr 30 EP15016 SB, New York
renewed: 25 Apr 57 by Stanley R. Adams (A): R190749,
renewed: 25 Apr 57 by R. Stanley Adams (A), Thomas W. Waller, Jr., Maurice Rutherford Waller & Ronald Rutherford Waller (C): R191558,
renewed: 24 Mar 58 by Thomas W. Waller, Jr. (C): R211042.
BL: also published by Campbell Connolly, London, n.d.
see also 2 Apr 30.

JO-JO-JOSEPHINE, words & melody by Billy Moll & Thomas Waller.
unpublished 21 Oct 30 EU29466 ShB, New York
renewed: 23 Oct 57 by Thomas W. Waller, Jr., Maurice Rutherford Waller & Ronald Rutherford Waller (C): R201557.
renewed: 29 Oct 57 by Shapiro, Bernstein & co. (PWH of B. Moll): R203059.
renewed: 19 Mar 58 by Thomas W. Waller, Jr. (C): R210952.

VIPER'S DRAG, by Thomas Waller, pianoforte.
unpublished 19 Nov 30 EU30874 JD, New York
renewed: 20 Nov 57 by Thomas W. Waller, Jr. (C): R203226.
renewed: 22 Nov 57 by Thomas W. Waller, Jr., Maurice Rutherford Waller& Ronald Rutherford Waller (C): R203697, as VIPER'S DRAG (from *Piano Pranks*).
renewed: 19 Mar 58 by Thomas W. Waller, Jr. (C): R210953.
see also 17 Dec 34.

BE MODERN, THERE'S HAPPINESS IN STORE FOR YOU, words & melody by Thomas Waller & Alexander Hill.
unpublished 3 Dec 30 EU31525 JD, New York
renewed: 4 Dec 57 by Maurice Rutherford Waller, Ronald Rutherford Waller & Thomas W. Waller, Jr. (C): R203898.
renewed: 18 Dec 57 by Thomas W. Waller, Jr. (C): R205126.
renewed: 30 Dec 57 by Viola Hill (W), Yvonne Hill (C) & Thomas Waller (C): R208510.

KEEP A SONG IN YOUR SOUL, words & music by Thomas Waller & Alexander Hiill.
published 8 Dec 30 EP19528 JD, New York
renewed: 9 Dec 57 by Thomas W. Waller, Jr., Maurice Rutherford Waller & Ronald Rutherford Waller (C): R204330.
renewed: 18 Dec 57 by Thomas W. Waller, Jr. (C): R205125.
renewed: 31 Dec 57 by Viola Hill (W), Yvonne Hill (C) & Thomas Waller (C): R208495.
BL holds two different editions published by JD, New York City, 1930; also published by Lawrence Wright, London, sung by Roy Barbour in *On With The Show 1931* at the North Pier Pavilion, Blackpool.

HARLEM FUSS, melody by Thomas Waller.
unpublished 17 Dec 30 EU32294 S, New York
renewed: 18 Dec 57 by Thomas W. Waller, Jr. (C): R204405.

MINOR (THE) DRAG, melody by Thomas Waller.
unpublished 17 Dec 30 EU32295 S, New York
renewed: 18 Dec 57 by Thomas W. Waller, Jr. (C): R204402.

RIDIN' BUT WALKIN', by Fats Waller [pseud. of Thomas Waller]; arranged by Brewster-Raph, orch pts.quarto. [Southern Music Hot Tune of The Month Club No.8 (Victor record V38119).]
published 22 Dec 30 EP20355 S, New York
renewed: 23 Dec 57 by Thomas W. Waller, Jr. (C): R205007.
renewed: 23 Dec 57 by Thomas W. Waller, Jr., Maurice Rutherford Waller & Ronald Rutherford Waller (C): R205655.
see also 9 Apr 30.

OUR LOVE WAS MEANT TO BE, words by Alexander Hill, melody by Thomas Waller.
unpublished 23 Dec 30 EU32414 PK, New York
renewed: 23 Dec 57 by Thomas W. Waller, Jr. (C): R205012.
renewed: 23 Dec 57 by Thomas W. Waller, Jr., Maurice Rutherford Waller & Ronald Rutherford Waller (C): R205654.
renewed: 17 Feb 58 by Viola Hill (W), Yvonne Hill (C) & Thomas W. Waller (C): R208689.
see also 12 Jul 37.

HANDFUL OF KEYS, melody by Thomas Waller.
unpublished 29 Dec 30 EU32615 S, New York
renewed: 30 Dec 57 by Thomas W. Waller, Jr. (C): R205248.
renewed: 30 Dec 57 by Thomas W. Waller, Jr., Maurice Rutherford Waller & Ronald Rutherford Waller (C): R208093.
see also 14 Jul 33.

NUMB FUMBLIN', melody by Thomas Waller.
unpublished 29 Dec 30 EU32616 S, New York
renewed: 30 Dec 57 by Thomas W. Waller, Jr. (C): R205249.
renewed: 30 Dec 57 by Maurice Rutherford Waller, Ronald Rutherford Waller & Thomas W. Waller, Jr. (C): R208092.
see also 14 Aug 35

1931

LITTLE BROWN BETTY, words & music by Alex Hill & Fats Waller [pseud. of Thos. Waller]; arranged by Helmy Kresa; with ukelele arrangement.
published 21 Jan 31 EP20686 Red Star music co., inc., New York
renewed: 21 Jan 58 by Thomas W. Waller, Jr. (C): R206966.
renewed: 29 Jan 58 by Viola Hill (W) & Yvonne Hill (C): R208111.
renewed: 26 Feb 58 by Thomas W. Waller, Jr., Maurice Rutherford Waller & Ronald Rutherford Waller (C): R209946.

HEART OF STONE, lyrics by Alexander Hill, music by Thomas Waller; w. ukelele arrangement.
published 24 Jan 31 EP20741 DDG., New York
renewed: 24 Jan 58 by Thomas W. Waller, Jr. (C): R207467.
renewed: 28 Jan 58 by Alexander Hill (A): R208007.

I'M CRAZY 'BOUT MY BABY AND MY BABY'S CRAZY 'BOUT ME, words & melody by Thomas Waller & Alexander Hill.
unpublished 14 Feb 31 EU34757 JD, New York
renewed: 20 Feb 58 by Viola Hill (W), Thomas W. Waller & Yvonne Hill (C): R209375.
renewed: 26 Feb 58 by Thomas W. Waller, Jr., Maurice Rutherford Waller & Ronald Rutherford Waller (C): R209944.
renewed: 19 Mar 58 by Thomas W. Waller, Jr. (C): R210594.
see also 2 Mar 31.

THAT'S ALL, melody by Thomas Waller.
unpublished 21 Feb 31 EU35576 S, New York
renewed: 26 Feb 58 by Thomas W. Waller, Jr., Maurice Rutherford Waller & Ronald Rutherford Waller (C): R209943.
renewed: 19 Mar 58 by Thomas W. Waller, Jr. (C): R210595.

I'M CRAZY 'BOUT MY BABY AND MY BABY'S CRAZY 'BOUT ME, words by Alexander Hill, music by Thomas Waller.
published 2 Mar 31 EP21419 JD, New York
renewed: 3 Mar 58 by Thomas W. Waller, Jr., Maurice Rutherford Waller & Ronald Rutherford Waller (C): R210099.
renewed: 12 Mar 58 by Thomas W. Waller (C), Viola Hill (W) & Yvonne Hill (C): R211079.
renewed: 19 Mar 58 by Thomas W. Waller, Jr. (C): R210591.
BL: also published by Laurance Wright *[sic]*, London, 1931, featured by Roy Fox and His Decca Recording Orchestra at the Monseigneur Restaurant [London].
see also 14 Feb 31.

SMASHING THIRDS, melody by Thomas Waller.
unpublished 23 Mar 31 EU37807 S, New York
see also 1 Jan 36.
renewed: 24 Mar 58 by Thomas W. Waller, Jr. (C): R211060.
renewed: 24 Mar 58 by Thomas W. Waller, Jr., Maurice Rutherford Waller & Ronald Rutherford Waller (C): R211215.

MY FEELIN'S ARE HURT, melody by Thomas Waller.
unpublished 23 Mar 31 EU37808 S, New York
renewed: 24 Mar 58 by Thomas W. Waller, Jr. (C): R211061.
renewed: 24 Mar 58 by Thomas W. Waller, Jr., Maurice Rutherford Waller & Ronald Rutherford Waller (C): R211216.

AFRICAN RIPPLES, by Fats Waller [pseud. of Thomas Waller], pianoforte.
published 20 Apr 31 EP22487 JD, New York
renewed: 21 Apr 58 by Thomas W. Waller, Jr. (C): R213165.
renewed: 21 Apr 58 by Thomas W. Waller, Jr., Maurice Rutherford Waller & Ronald Rutherford Waller (C): R214156, as AFRICAN RIPPLES (novelty piano solo).
BL: Also published by KP, London, in *Rhythmic Piano Solos* series.

TAKE IT FROM ME, I'M TAKIN' TO YOU, lyrics by R. Stanley Adams, music by Thomas Waller; with ukelele arrangement by May Singhi Breen. [Featured by Leo Reisman and His Victor Recording Orchestra.]
published 11 Jun 31 EP23388 SB, New York
renewed: 11 Jun 58 by Thomas Waller, Jr. (C): R216213.
renewed: 12 Jun 58 by R. Stanley Adams, Thomas Waller., Maurice Rutherford Waller & Ronald Rutherford Waller (C): R216131.
see also 2 Apr 30 (Take It From Me, I've Taken To You).

ICE (THE) MAN LIVES IN AN ICE HOUSE, words by Ricardo Duromo [pseud. of R. Hardman] & Elmer S. Hughes [pseud. of Elliott Shapirol, music by Thomas Waller.
published 30 Jun 31 EF19167 Richard Hardman, Tolworth, Surrey, England
renewed: 30 Jun 58 by Thomas W. Waller, Jr. (C): R217093.
renewed: 2 Jul 58 by Maurice Rutherford Waller, Ronald Rutherford Waller & Thomas W. Waller, Jr. (C): R217205.
BL: also published as THE ICE MAN LIVES IN AN ICE HOUSE (IN A VILLAGE BY THE SEA), PM, London, n.d., featured by Henry Hearty.

CRUMBS (THE) OF YOUR LOVE, lyrics by Andy Razaf, melody by Thomas Waller & Minto Cato.
unpublished 2 Sep 31 EU44361 SB, New York
renewed: 2 Sep 58 by Andy Razaf (A): R220569.
renewed: 3 Sep 58 by Andy Razaf, Minto Cato (A's), Thomas Waller., Maurice Rutherford Waller & Ronald Rutherford Waller (C): R220793.
renewed: 4 Sep 58 by Thomas W. Waller, Jr. (C): R220838.

CONCENTRATIN' ON YOU, lyrics by Andy Razaf, melody by Thomas Waller.
unpublished 2 Sep 31 EU44362 SB, New York
renewed: 2 Sep 58 by Andy Razaf (A): R220570.
renewed: 3 Sep 58 by Andy Razaf (A), Thomas Waller., Maurice Rutherford Waller & Ronald Rutherford Waller (C): R220794.
renewed: 4 Sep 58 by Thomas W. Waller, Jr. (C): R220839.

CONCENTRATIN' ON YOU, words by Andy Razaf, music by Thomas Waller; ukelele arrangement by May Singhi Breen.
published 13 Oct 31 EP25800 SB, New York
renewed: 13 Oct 58 by Thomas W. Waller, Jr. (C): R222784.
renewed: 15 Oct 58 by Andy Razaf (A), Thomas Waller., Maurice Rutherford Waller & Ronald Rutherford Waller (C): R223019.
renewed: 31 Oct 58 by Andy Razaf (A): R223808.

1932

HOW CAN YOU FACE ME, fox-trot, words by Andy Razaf, music by Thomas Waller.
published 8 Feb 32 EP28324 JD, New York
renewed: 9 Feb 59 by Maurice Rutherford Waller & Ronald Rutherford Waller (C): R230546.
renewed: 9 Feb 59 by Thomas W. Waller, Jr. (C): R231792.
renewed: 9 Feb 59 by Andy Razaf (A): R231793.
renewed: 19 Feb 59 by Andy Razaf (A) & Thomas Waller, Jr. (C): R231616.
BL: HOW CAN YOU FACE ME? (Fox-Trot Ballad), additional lyric by Reg Howard, Irvin Dash, London, n.d (claiming © JD, New York City, 1934] (no corresponding U.S. © has been traced).

KEEPIN' OUT OF MISCHIEF NOW, words by Andy Razaf, music by Thomas Waller; w. ukelele acc.
published 10 Feb 32 EP28394 CC, New York
renewed: 10 Feb 59 by Andy Razaf (A): R230456.
renewed: 10 Feb 59 by Thomas W. Waller, Jr. (C): R230457.
renewed: 12 Feb 59 by Maurice Rutherford Waller & Ronald Rutherford Waller (C): R231133.

WHEN GABRIEL BLOWS HIS HORN, lyrics by Andy Razaf, music by Thomas Waller; pianoforte treble.
unpublished 10 Feb 32 EU51445 NS, New York
renewed: 10 Feb 59 by Thomas W. Waller, Jr. (C): R230450.
renewed: 10 Feb 59 by Andy Razaf (A): R230451.
renewed: 12 Feb 59 by Maurice Rutherford Waller & Ronald Rutherford Waller (C): R231132.
see also 26 Mar 32.

BUDDIE, lyrics by Andy Razaf, music by Thomas Waller; with ukelele arrangement by Geo. J. Trinkaus.
published 15 Feb 32 EP28473 W, New York
renewed: 16 Feb 59 by Andy Razaf (A): R231052.
renewed: 16 Feb 59 by Thomas W. Waller, Jr., Maurice Rutherford Waller & Ronald Rutherford Waller (C): R232429.

IF IT AIN'T LOVE, words & melody by Andy Razaf, Donald Redman & Thomas Waller.
unpublished 19 Feb 32 EU 51940 DCE, New York
renewed: 19 Feb 59 by Andy Razaf (A): R231423.
renewed: 19 Feb 59 by Thomas W. Waller, Jr. (C): R231424.
renewed: 19 Feb 59 by Donald Matthew Redman (A): R231611.
renewed: 24 Feb 59 by Thomas W. Waller, Jr., Maurice Rutherford Waller & Ronald Rutherford Waller (C): R232839.
see also 2 Mar 32 & 8 Mar 32.

SINCE WON LONG HOP TOOK ONE LONG HOP TO CHINA, words by Jack Meskill, music by Thomas Waller.
unpublished 20 Feb 32 EU52467 Ma
renewed: 20 Feb 59 by Thomas W. Waller, Jr. (C): R231447.

IF IT AIN'T LOVE, words & music by Andy Razaf, Donald Redman & Thomas Waller; with ukelele arrangement by May Singhi Breen.
published 2 Mar 32 EP28824 DCE, New York
renewed: 2 Mar 59 by Andy Razaf (A): R232128.
renewed: 4 Mar 59 by Thomas W. Waller, Jr., Maurice Rutherford Waller & Ronald Rutherford Waller (C): R232430.
renewed: 12 Mar 59 by Donald Matthew Redman (A): R233174.
see also 19 Feb 32 & 8 Mar 32.

IF IT AIN'T LOVE, words & music by Andy Razaf, Donald Redman & Thomas Waller; arranged by Paul Weirich, with male trio arranged by R.H. Noeltner.
published 8 Mar 32 EP28940 DCE, New York
renewed: 23 Jul 59 by Paul Weinrich (A): R240223.
see also 19 Feb 32 & 2 Mar 32.

RADIO PAPA, BROADCASTIN' MAMA, words by Andy Razaf, m Thomas Waller; pianoforte with words.
published 14 Mar 32 EP28971 JD
renewed: 16 Mar 59 by Andy Razaf (A): R232892.
renewed: 16 Mar 59 by Thomas W. Waller, Jr., Maurice Rutherford Waller & Ronald Rutherford Waller (C): R233155.
renewed: 11 Mar 60 by Thomas W. Waller, Jr. (C of Thomas Waller): R253364.
see also 18 Nov 29.

WHEN GABRIEL BLOWS HIS HORN, words by Andy Razaf, music by Thomas Waller; with ukelele arrangement by May Singhi Breen.
published 26 Mar 32 EP29364 NS, New York
renewed: 26 Mar 59 by Andy Razaf (A): R233645.
renewed: 27 Mar 59 by Thomas W. Waller, Jr., Maurice Rutherford Waller & Ronald Rutherford Waller (C): R234679.
renewed: 11 Mar 60 by Thomas W. Waller, Jr. (C of Thomas Waller): R253363.
see also 10 Feb 32.

MY HEART'S AT EASE, words by Joe Young, melody by Fats Waller.
unpublished 5 May 32 EU55792 IB
renewed: 6 May 59 by Thomas W. Waller, Jr., Maurice Rutherford Waller & Ronald Rutherford Waller (C): R236271.
renewed: 7 May 59 by Ruth Young Grundberg (W of Joe Young): R236624.
renewed: 15 May 59 by Anita Waller (W): R237262.
renewed: 11 Mar 60 by Thomas W. Waller, Jr. (C of Thomas Waller): R253359.
see also 31 May 32.

SHELTERED BY THE STARS, CRADLED BY THE MOON, words by Joe Young, melody by Thomas Waller.
unpublished 19 May 32 EU56532 IB
renewed: 20 May 59 by Thomas W. Waller, Jr., Maurice Rutherford Waller & Ronald Rutherford Waller (C): R237123.
renewed: 26 May 59 by Anita Waller (W): R237400.
renewed: 27 May 59 by Ruth Young Grundberg (W of Joe Young): R237522.
renewed: 11 Mar 60 by Thomas W. Waller, Jr. (C of Thomas Waller): R253358.
see also 29 Jun 32.

MY HEART'S AT EASE, words by Joe Young, music by Thomas Waller; pianoforte & ukelele arr, Helmy Kresa.
published 31 May 32 EP30394 IB
renewed: 2 Jun 59 by Thomas W. Waller, Jr., Maurice Rutherford Waller & Ronald Rutherford Waller (C): R237380.
renewed: 12 Jun 59 by Anita Waller (W): R238499.
renewed: 11 Mar 60 by Thomas W. Waller, Jr. (C of Thomas Waller): R253362.
see also 5 May 32.

LONESOME ME, words by Andy Razaf, music by Thomas Waller & Con Conrad; with ukelele arrangement.
published 31 May 32 EP30445 CC
renewed: 16 Jun 59 by Andy Razaf (A): R238027.
renewed: 22 Sep 59 by Reserve Music Inc. (PWH of Con Conrad): R242518.
renewed: 11 Mar 60 by Thomas W. Waller, Jr. (C of Thomas Waller): R253361.

WALKIN' THE FLOOR, words by Andy Razaf, melody by Thomas Waller.
unpublished 16 Jun 32 EU57659 IB
renewed: 16 Jun 59 by Andy Razaf (A): R238021.
renewed: 17 Jun 59 by Thomas W. Waller, Jr., Maurice Rutherford Waller & Ronald Rutherford Waller (C): R238417.
see also 23 Aug 33.

HUNGRY, words by Joe Young & Andy Razaf, melody by Thomas Waller.
unpublished 16 Jun 32 EU57663 IB
renewed: 16 Jun 59 by Andy Razaf (A): R238022.
renewed: 16 Jun 59 by Ruth Young Grunberg (W): R238127.
renewed: 17 Jun 59 by Thomas W. Waller, Jr., Maurice Rutherford Waller & Ronald Rutherford Waller (C): R238418.
renewed: 8 Jul 59 by Andy Razaf (A) & Anita Waller (W): R239640.

MY GIFT OF DREAMS, words by Andy Razaf, melody by Thomas Waller & Edgar Dowell.
unpublished 25 Jun 32 EU58111 SB
renewed: 25 Jun 59 by Andy Razaf (A): R238489.
renewed: 26 Jun 59 by Andy Razaf (A), Thomas W. Waller, Jr., Maurice Rutherford Waller & Ronald Rutherford Waller (C): R238665.

DO ME A FAVOR, LEND ME A KISS, words by Andy Razaf & Spencer Williams, melody by Thomas Waller.
unpublished 27 Jun 32 EU58152 IB
renewed: 29 Jun 59 by Spencer Williams (A): R238575 & R238576 [identical renewals].
renewed: 30 Jun 59 by Thomas W. Waller, Jr., Maurice Rutherford Waller & Ronald Rutherford Waller (C). R238802.
renewed: 8 Jul 59 by Andy Razaf, Spencer Williams (A's) & Anita Waller (W): R239367.

SHELTERED BY THE STARS, CRADLED BY THE MOON, words by Joe Young, music by Thomas Waller; pianoforte & ukelele arrangements by Helmy Kresa.
published 29 Jun 32 EP30922 IB
renewed: 30 Jun 59 by Thomas W. Waller, Jr., Maurice Rutherford Waller & Ronald Rutherford Waller (C): R238804.
see also 19 May 32.

APPLE (THE) OF MY EYE, words by Joe Young, melody by Fats Waller.
unpublished 1 Jul 32 EU58303 IB
renewed: 2 Jul 59 by Thomas W. Waller, Jr., Maurice Rutherford Waller & Ronald Rutherford Waller (C): R238803.
renewed: 5 Aug 59 by Ruth Young Grunberg (W of Joe Young): R240709.
see also 24 Aug 32.

STRANGE AS IT SEEMS, words by Andy Razaf, music by Thomas Waller; with ukelele arrangement. [Introduced by Art Jarrett.]
published 5 Jul 32 EP31275 L
renewed: 6 Jul 59 by Andy Razaf (A): R239449.
renewed: 7 Jul 59 by Thomas W. Waller, Jr., Maurice Rutherford Waller & Ronald Rutherford Waller (C): R239415.

I'M NOW PREPARED TO TELL THE WORLD IT'S YOU, words by Andy Razaf, music by Thos. Waller.
published 8 Jul 32 EP31232 MM
renewed: 8 Jul 59 by Andy Razaf (A): R239596.

ONLY SOMETIMES, words by Joe Young, melody by Thomas Waller,
unpublished 9 Jul 32 EU58698 IB
renewed: 10 Jul 59 by Thomas W. Waller, Jr., Maurice Rutherford Waller & Ronald Rutherford Waller (C): R239998.
renewed: 5 Aug 59 by Ruth Young Grunberg (W of Joe Young): R241151.

I DIDN'T DREAM IT WAS LOVE, words & music by Elliott Grennard, Thomas Waller & Con Conrad; with ukelele arrangement.
published 11 Jul 32 EP31147 CC
renewed: 13 Jul 59 by Thomas W. Waller, Jr., Maurice Rutherford Waller & Ronald Rutherford Waller (C): R239999.
renewed: 25 Aug 59 by Reserve Music, Inc. (PWH of Con Conrad & Elliott Grennard): R241392.

BREAKIN' MY HEART, words by Spencer Williams, melody by Thomas Waller.
unpublished 14 Jul 32 EU58875 JG
renewed: 14 Jul 59 by Spencer Williams (A): R239920.
renewed: 16 Jul 59 by Thomas W. Waller, Jr., Maurice Rutherford Waller & Ronald Rutherford Waller (C): R240000.

YOU'RE MY IDEAL, words by Spencer Williams, melody by Thomas Waller.
unpublished 23 Jul 32 EU59242 ShB
renewed: 23 Jul 59 by Spencer Williams (A): R240344.
renewed: 27 Jul 59 by Thomas W. Waller, Jr., Maurice Rutherford Waller & Ronald Rutherford Waller (C): R240467.
renewed: 31 Jul 59 by Spencer Williams (A), Maurice Rutherford Waller, Ronald Rutherford Waller & Thomas Waller, Jr. (C):: R240674.
see also 28 Jan 38.

GOTTA BE, GONNA BE MINE, words by Andy Razaf, music by Thomas Waller; with ukelele arrangement.
published 29 Jul 32 EP31631 L
renewed: 29 Jul 59 by Andy Razaf (A): R240316.
renewed: 30 Jul 59 by Thomas W. Waller, Jr., Maurice Rutherford Waller & Ronald Rutherford Waller (C): R240606.

OH! YOU SWEET THING, words by Andy Razaf, music by Thomas Waller; with ukelele arrangement.
published 29 Jul 32 EP31632 L
renewed: 29 Jul 59 by Andy Razaf (A): R240317.
renewed: 30 Jul 59 by Thomas W. Waller, Jr., Maurice Rutherford Waller & Ronald Rutherford Waller (C): R240607.
BL: also published by J.R. Lafleur & Co., London, 1934, featured & broadcast by Harry Roy and His Band; and arranged by T. Conway Brown for Boosey & Hawkes Military Dance Club, published by J.R. Lafleur & Son, London, 1934.

THAT'S WHERE THE SOUTH BEGINS, words by George Brown, m Thomas Waller; with ukelele arrangement. [Renewals indicate that George Brown is a pseudonym of Billy Hill.]
published 29 Jul 32 EP31633 L
renewed: 29 Jul 59 by Lee DeDette Taylor (C of Billy Hill): R240318.
renewed: 30 Jul 59 by Thomas W. Waller, Jr., Maurice Rutherford Waller & Ronald Rutherford Waller (C): R240608.

NGELINE, words by George Brown, music by Thomas Waller; with ukelele arrangement. [Renewals indicate that George Brown is a pseudonym of Billy Hill.]
published 5 Aug 32 EP31845 L
renewed: 6 Aug 59 by Thomas W. Waller, Jr., Maurice Rutherford Waller & Ronald Rutherford Waller (C): R240971.
renewed: 7 Aug 59 by Lee DeDette Taylor (C of Billy Hill): R240693.

LD YAZOO, words & music by Thomas Waller; with ukelele arrangement.
published 8 Aug 32 EP31951 L
renewed: 13 Aug 59 by Thomas W. Waller, Jr., Maurice Rutherford Waller & Ronald Rutherford Waller (C): R241191.

LOWIN' (THE) OF THE BREEZE BLEW YOU INTO MY ARMS, words by Spencer Williams, music by Thomas Waller; with ukelele arrangement by Geo. F. Trinkaus.
published 12 Aug 32 EP31646 Re
renewed: 12 Aug 59 by Spencer Williams (A): R240826.
renewed: 17 Aug 59 by Thomas W. Waller, Jr., Maurice Rutherford Waller & Ronald Rutherford Waller (C): R241192.

PPLE (THE) OF MY EYE, words by Joe Young, music by Thomas Waller; with ukelele arrangement by Helmy Kresa.
published 24 Aug 32 EP31833 IB
renewed: 25 Aug 59 by Thomas W. Waller, Jr., Maurice Rutherford Waller & Ronald Rutherford Waller (C): R241636.
see also 1 Jul 32.

HERE THE DEW DROPS KISS THE MORNING GLORIES GOOD MORNIN', words by Spencer Williams, music by Thomas Waller; with ukelele arrangement by Geo. F. Trinkaus.
published 24 Aug 32 EP31924 Re
renewed: 24 Aug 59 by Spencer Williams (A): R241345, as WHEN THE DEW DROPS KISS THE MORNING GLORIES GOOD MORNIN'
renewed: 25 Aug 59 by Thomas W. Waller, Jr., Maurice Rutherford Waller & Ronald Rutherford Waller (C): R241635.

AITING FOR YOU TO BEGIN, words by Joe Young, melody by Fats Waller.
unpublished 16 Sep 32 EU61433 IB
renewed: 17 Sep 59 by Thomas W. Waller, Jr., Maurice Rutherford Waller & Ronald Rutherford Waller (C): R242562.
renewed: 21 Sep 59 by Ruth Young Grunberg (W of Joe Young): R242780.

OWN ON THE DELTA, words by Spencer Williams, melody by Thomas Waller & Sam H. Stept; pianoforte treble.
unpublished 24 Sep 32 EU61827 SP
renewed: 23 Sep 59 by Thomas W. Waller, Jr., Maurice Rutherford Waller & Ronald Rutherford Waller (C): R243001.
renewed: 24 Sep 59 by Spencer Williams (A): R242702.
see also 17 Feb 33.

933

OWN ON THE DELTA, fox-trot, words by Spencer Williams, m Thomas Waller; with ukelele arrangement.
published 17 Feb 33 EF28394 Irvin Dash music co., ltd.
renewed: 17 Feb 60 by Spencer Williams (A): R252315.
renewed: 21 Apr 60 by Thomas W. Waller, Jr., Maurice Rutherford Waller & Ronald Rutherford Waller (C): R255814.
renewed: 13 Feb 61 by Thomas W. Waller, Jr. (C): R270981.
BL: vocal fox-trot featured by Carroll Gibbons & The Savoy Hotel Orpheans, Irvin Dash, London, 1933.
see aslo 24 Sep 32.

OIN' WHAT I PLEASE, words by Andy Razaf, music by Thomas Waller.
published 20 Feb 33 EP35021 L
renewed: 21 Apr 60 by Thomas W. Waller, Jr., Maurice Rutherford Waller & Ronald Rutherford Waller (C): R255813.
renewed: 19 Jul 60 by Andy Razaf (A): R260289.
renewed: 13 Feb 61 by Thomas W. Waller, Jr. (C): R270973.

'OU'RE BREAKIN' MY HEART, words by Spencer Williams, music by Thomas Waller, with ukelele arrangement.
published 8 May 33 EP36145 Ro
renewed: 9 May 60 by Spencer Williams (A): R256861.
renewed: 9 May 60 by Thomas W. Waller, Jr., Maurice Rutherford Waller & Ronald Rutherford Waller (C): R257500.
renewed: 13 Feb 61 by Thomas W. Waller, Jr. (C): R270974.

LAY YOUR HEAD UPON MY SHOULDER, valse song. [no other details] [renewals specify: words & music by Thomas Waller].
unpublished 21 Jun 33 EU73058 Thomas Walle
renewed: 23 Jun 60 by Thomas W. Waller, Jr., Maurice Rutherford Waller & Ronald Rutherford Waller (C): R259014.
renewed: 13 Feb 61 by Thomas W. Waller, Jr. (C): R270959.

SITTIN' UP WAITIN' FOR YOU, words by Andy Razaf, melody by Thomas Waller.
unpublished 27 Jun 33 EU74211 S
renewed: 19 Jul 60 by Andy Razaf (A): R260286.
renewed: 28 Jul 60 by Thomas W. Waller, Jr., Maurice Rutherford Waller & Ronald Rutherford Waller (C): R260890.
renewed: 16 Aug 60 by Anita Rutherford Waller (W), Thomas Waller, Jr., Maurice Waller (C) & Andy Razaf (A): R261693.
renewed: 13 Feb 61 by Thomas W. Waller, Jr. (C): R270960.
see also 21 Aug 33.

HANDFUL OF KEYS, by Thomas Waller; modern pianoforte arrangement by Frank Weldon.
published 14 Jul 33 EP37324 S
renewed: 20 Jul 60 by Thomas W. Waller, Jr., Maurice Rutherford Waller & Ronald Rutherford Waller (C): R260435.
renewed: 13 Feb 61 by Thomas W. Waller, Jr. (C): R270975.
see also 29 Dec 30.

SLOWER THAN MOLASSES, words by Andy Razaf, music by Thomas Waller.
unpublished 4 Aug 33 EU74562 IB
renewed: 4 Aug 60 by Andy Razaf (A): R261043.
renewed: 5 Aug 60 by Thomas W. Waller, Jr., Maurice Rutherford Waller & Ronald Rutherford Waller (C): R261106.
renewed: 13 Feb 61 by Thomas W. Waller, Jr. (C): R270961.

JOHN HENRY, THAT SUPERMAN, words by Andy Razaf, melody by Thomas Waller.
unpublished 5 Aug 33 EU74618 IB
renewed: 5 Aug 60 by Andy Razaf (A): R261333.
renewed: 8 Aug 60 by Thomas W. Waller, Jr., Maurice Rutherford Waller & Ronald Rutherford Waller (C): R261107.
renewed: 13 Feb 61 by Thomas W. Waller, Jr. (C): R270962.

TALL TIMBER, words by Andy Razaf, music by Thomas Waller; with ukelele arrangement.
published 7 Aug 33 EP37369 Mi
renewed: 8 Aug 60 by Andy Razaf (A): R261363, as TALL TIMBER, with recitation.
renewed: 8 Aug 60 by Andy Razaf (A) & Edith L. Waller (W): R261391.
renewed: 12 Aug 60 by Thomas W. Waller, Jr., Maurice Rutherford Waller & Ronald Rutherford Waller (C): R261486.
renewed: 13 Feb 61 by Thomas W. Waller, Jr. (C): R270976.

AIN'T-CHA' GLAD, words by Andy Razaf, music by Thomas Waller; pianoforte arranged by R.N. Noeltner.
published 8 Aug 33 EP37406 KE
renewed: 8 Aug 60 by Andy Razaf (A): R261359.
renewed: 12 Aug 60 by Thomas W. Waller, Jr., Maurice Rutherford Waller & Ronald Rutherford Waller (C): R261487.
renewed: 13 Feb 61 by Thomas W. Waller, Jr. (C): R270977.

YOW SAH, words by Joe Young, melody by Thomas Waller.
unpublished 10 Aug 33 EU74859 IB
renewed: 12 Aug 60 by Thomas W. Waller, Jr., Maurice Rutherford Waller & Ronald Rutherford Waller (C): R261488.
renewed: 15 Aug 60 by Ruth Young Grunberg (W of Joe Young): R261333.
renewed: 13 Feb 61 by Thomas W. Waller, Jr. (C): R270963.

SITTIN' UP WAITIN' FOR YOU, words by Andy Razaf, music by Thomas Waller.
published 21 Aug 33 EP37471 Su
renewed: 22 Aug 60 by Andy Razaf (A): R261927.
renewed: 22 Aug 60 by Andy Razaf (A), Anita Rutherford (W of Thomas Waller), Thomas Waller, Jr. & Maurice Waller (C): R261963.
renewed: 22 Aug 60 by Thomas W. Waller, Jr., Maurice Rutherford Waller & Ronald Rutherford Waller (C): R262001.
renewed: 13 Feb 61 by Thomas Waller, Jr. (C): R270978.
see also 27 Jun 33.

WALKIN' THE FLOOR, words by Andy Razaf, music by Thomas Waller; with ukelele arrangement.
published 23 Aug 33 EP37553 IB
renewed: 26 Aug 59 by Andy Razaf (A): R241670 (quoting © date as 23 Aug 32).
renewed: 23 Aug 60 by Andy Razaf (A): R261975.
renewed: 24 Aug 60 by Thomas W. Waller, Jr., Maurice Rutherford Waller & Ronald Rutherford Waller (C): R262025.
renewed: 13 Feb 61 by Thomas W. Waller, Jr. (C): R270979.
see also 16 Jun 32.

AND THAT IS LIFE, words by Andy Razaf, melody by Thomas Waller.
unpublished 8 Sep 33 EU76055 IB
renewed: 12 Sep 60 by Thomas W. Waller, Jr., Maurice Rutherford Waller & Ronald Rutherford Waller (C): R262983.
renewed: 13 Feb 61 by Thomas W. Waller, Jr. (C): R270964.

WHY DO WE HURT THE ONES WE LOVE, words by Al Jolson & Andy Razaf, melody by Thomas Waller.
unpublished 8 Sep 33 EU76056 IB
renewed: 9 Sep 60 by Erle Johnson Krasna (W of Al Jolson): R262615.
renewed: 12 Sep 60 by Thomas W. Waller, Jr., Maurice Rutherford Waller & Ronald Rutherford Waller (C): R262984.
renewed: 18 Oct 60 by Andy Razaf (A): R264345.
renewed: 13 Feb 61 by Thomas W. Waller, Jr. (C): R270965.

SUNSHINE, words by Al Koppell & Jean Herbert, melody by Thomas Waller.
unpublished 5 Dec 33 EU79718 IC
renewed: 7 Dec 60 by Thomas W. Waller, Jr., Maurice Rutherford Waller & Ronald Rutherford Waller (C): R267620.
renewed: 13 Feb 61 by Thomas W. Waller, Jr. (C): R270966.
renewed: 22 Aug 61 by Alfred B. Koppell (A): R280642.

ON SUNDAY WHEN WE GATHERED 'ROUND THE ORGAN, words by Alexander Hill & Andy Razaf, melody by Thomas Waller.
unpublished 8 Dec 33 EU79789 IB
renewed: 9 Dec 60 by Thomas W. Waller, Jr., Maurice Rutherford Waller & Ronald Rutherford Waller (C): R267559.
renewed: 6 Jan 61 by Andy Razaf (A): R268929.
renewed: 13 Feb 61 by Thomas W. Waller, Jr. (C): R270967.

IF I HAD WAITED FOR YOU, words by Andy Razaf, melody by Thomas Waller.
unpublished 8 Dec 33 EU79790 IB
renewed: 9 Dec 60 by Thomas W. Waller, Jr., Maurice Rutherford Waller & Ronald Rutherford Waller (C): R267560.
renewed: 6 Jan 61 by Andy Razaf (A): R268930.
renewed: 13 Feb 61 by Thomas W. Waller, Jr. (C): R270968.
renewed: 17 Apr 61 by Andy Razaf (A): R274537.

The three following compositions were copyrighted in the United Kingdom in 1933, according to sheet music published by Spencer Williams & Thomas Waller, New York & London, received by the British Library in July 1938, which may be a better guide to the actual date of publication than the inconsistently presented dates printed on them. No United States copyrights of these compositions have been traced. United Kingdom law does not require deposit of unpublished material as a condition of copyright.

BLUER THAN THE OCEAN BLUES, written & composed by Spencer Williams, Tommie Connor & Thomas "Fats" Waller.
[Featured, Broadcast and Recorded by "Fats Waller" *[sic]* The King of Swing Pianists.]
published © 1933 (cover)/1938 (music) see head note above

I'M GONNA FALL IN LOVE (AND MARRY YOU), written & composed by Spencer Williams & Thomas "Fats" Waller.
published © 1933 (cover)/1938 (music) see head note above

I'VE GOT YOU WHERE I WANT YOU, Song, written & composed by Spencer Williams & Thomas "Fats" Waller.
[Featured, Broadcast and Recorded by "Fats Waller" *[sic]* The King of Swing Pianists.]
published © 1933 (cover & music) see head note above

1934

ACE IN THE HOLE, words by Bartley Costello & Frank Crumit, music arranged by Thomas Waller; with arrangement for ukulele, etc. [Editon states 'modern arrangement by Thomas Waller'].
published 24 Jan 34 EP40171 FBH
renewed: 24 Jan 61 by Jane B. Costello (NK): R270455.
renewed: 13 Feb 61 by Thomas W. Waller, Jr. (C): R270980.
renewed: 20 Feb 61 by Thomas W. Waller, Jr., Maurice Rutherford Waller & Ronald Rutherford Waller (C): R271930.

CLOTHES LINE BALLET, by Thomas Fats Waller; pianoforte.
unpublished 9 Mar 34 EU83953 JD
renewed: 9 Mar 61 by Thomas W. Waller, Jr. (C): R272062.
renewed: 9 Mar 61 by Thomas W. Waller, Jr., Maurice Rutherford Waller & Ronald Rutherford Waller (C): R272319.
renewed: 14 Mar 61 by Thomas Waller, Jr. (C): R272950.
see also 10 Dec 34.

SWING ON MISSISSIPPI, words by Ned Washington, music by Thomas Waller; with guitar arrangement.
published 10 May 34 EP42094 M-A
renewed: 10 May 61 by Ned Washington (A): R275682.
renewed: 10 May 61 by Thomas W. Waller, Jr., Maurice Rutherford Waller & Ronald Rutherford Waller (C): R275785.
renewed: 14 Dec 61 by Thomas W. Waller, Jr. (C): R286902.

CLOTHES LINE BALLET, by Thomas Fats Waller; pianoforte.
published 10 Dec 34 EP45236 JD, New York
renewed: 13 Dec 61 by Thomas Waller, Jr. (C): R286758.
renewed: 14 Dec 61 by Thomas W. Waller, Jr. (C): R286904.
see also 9 Mar 34.

EFFERVESCENT, by Thomas Fats Waller; pianoforte.
published 10 Dec 34 EP45237 JD, New York
renewed: 13 Dec 61 by Thomas Waller, Jr. (C): R286757.
renewed: 14 Dec 61 by Thomas W. Waller, Jr. (C): R286905.

ALLIGATOR CRAWL, by Fats Waller; pianoforte.
published 17 Dec 34 EP45374 JD, New York
renewed: 18 Dec 61 by Thomas W. Waller, Jr. (C): R286931.
see also 18 Apr 27 & 30 Aug 37 & 27 Sep 37.

VIPER'S DRAG, by Fats Waller, pianoforte.
published 17 Dec 34 EP45375 JD, New York
renewed: 18 Dec 61 by Thomas W. Waller, Jr. (C): R286932.
see also 19 Dec 30.

1935

FUNCTIONIZIN', by Fats Waller & Irving Mills; pianoforte.
published 22 Jan 35 EP46220 Ex, New York
renewed: 18 Jan 63 by Irving Mills (A): R309159.
renewed: 22 Jan 62 by Thomas W. Waller, Jr. (C): R289343.

NUMB FUMBLIN', by Thomas (Fat's) Waller *[sic]*; pianoforte.
published 14 Aug 35 EF42031 S, London
renewed: 14 Aug 62 by Thomas W. Waller, Jr. (C): R299939.
renewed: 23 Jan 63 by Thomas Waller, Jr. (C): R309035.
see also 29 Dec 30.

WALLER'S (FATS) ORIGINAL PIANO CONCEPTIONS; special pianofore arrangements by Fats Waller.
published 14 Dec 35 EP52924 MM, New York
renewed: 17 Dec 62 by Thomas W. Waller, Jr. (C): R309017.
renewed: 23 Jan 63 by Thomas Waller, Jr. (C): R309029.
renewed: 11 Dec 63 by Mills Music, Inc. (PWH): R334224.
BL: FATS WALLER'S ORIGINAL PIANO CONCEPTIONS No.1, Feldman, London, n.d.

1936

SMASHING THIRDS, by Thomas (Fats) Waller; pianoforte.
published 1 Jan 36 EF43142 *[sic]* S, New York
renewed: 4 Jan 63 by Thomas W. Waller, Jr. (C): R308179.
renewed: 23 Jan 63 by Thomas Waller, Jr. (C): R309036.
see also 23 Mar 31.

CAN SEE YOU ALL OVER THE PLACE, words by Clarence Williams, music by C. Williams & Thomas (Fats) Waller; with guitar arrangement.
published 6 Jan 36 EP54822 CW, New York
renewed: 7 Jan 63 by Clarence Williams (A): R307973.
renewed: 23 Jan 63 by Thomas Waller, Jr. (C): R309743.

UGAR ROSE, words by Phil Ponce, music by Fats Waller; with arrangement for guitar, etc., and special transcription for pianoforte. [Cover has photo of Fats and cites Victor 25266.]
published 11 Mar 36 EP53945 C, New York
renewed: 11 Mar 63 by Dorothy Verkamp & Ethel Ponce Fenley (C of Phil Ponce): R312199.
renewed: 12 Mar 63 by Thomas W. Waller, Jr. (C): R312657.
renewed: 10 Jan 64 by Thomas W. Waller, Jr. (C): R329214.
BL: also published by Chappell, London, 1936, with photo of Fats and citing HMV BD5062.

VAIT AND SEE, fox trot, words by Andy Razaf, music by Thomas (Fats) Waller.
published 16 Mar 36 EP54038 JD, New York
renewed: 18 Mar 63 by Andy Razaf (A): R312405.
renewed: 3 Apr 63 by Maurice Rutherford Waller(C): R313391.
renewed: 22 Apr 53 by Andy Razaf (A) & Thomas Waller, Jr. (C): R315313.
renewed: 10 Jan 64 by Thomas W. Waller, Jr. (C): R329215.

ENNY SENT ME, words & music by Spencer Williams & Thomas Waller.
unpublished 1 Jun 36 EU125508 R, New York
renewed: 3 Jun 63 by Spencer Williams (A): R316647.
renewed: 3 Jun 63 by Spencer Williams (A) & Thomas W. Waller, Jr. (C): R316770.
renewed: 10 Jan 64 by Thomas W. Waller, Jr. (C): R329206.

HAKIN' IT ALL NIGHT LONG, words by Spencer Williams, music byThomas Waller.
unpublished 1 Jun 36 EU125509 R, New York
renewed: 3 Jun 63 by Spencer Williams (A): R316648.
renewed: 3 Jun 63 by Spencer Williams (A) & Thomas W. Waller, Jr. (C): R316769.
renewed: 10 Jan 64 by Thomas W. Waller, Jr. (C): R329207.

TEALIN' APPLES, words by Andy Razaf, music by Thomas (Fats) Waller.
published 10 Jul 36 EP56288 Ex, New York
renewed: 10 Jul 63 by Andy Razaf (A): R318208.
renewed: 10 Jul 63 by Thomas W. Waller, Jr. (C): R318815.
renewed: 10 Jan 64 by Thomas W. Waller, Jr. (C): R329217.

VALLER'S (FATS) ORIGINAL PIANO CONCEPTIONS, No.2; new arrangements by Fats Waller.
published 1 Sep 36 EP57287 MM, New York
renewed: 10 Jan 64 by Thomas W. Waller, Jr. (C): R329218.
renewed: 31 Aug 64 by Mills Music, Inc. (PWH): R345131.
see also 16 Sep 36.

AREWELL BLUES, by Elmer Schoebel, Paul Mares & Leon Rappolo *[sic]*; arranged by Fats Waller; pianoforte.
published 1 Sep 36 EP57288 MM, New York
renewed: 11 Dec 63 by Thomas Waller, Jr. (C): R327542.
renewed: 10 Jan 64 by Thomas W. Waller, Jr. (C): R329218.
see also 16 Sep 36.

ATCH ON, by Thomas Waller; pianoforte.
unpublished 2 Sep 36 EU131265 PP, New York
renewed: 9 Sep 63 by Thomas Waller, Jr. (C): R321974.
renewed: 15 Nov 63 by Anita Rutherford Waller (W) & Maurice Waller (C): R326141.
renewed: 10 Jan 64 by Thomas W. Waller, Jr. (C): R329208.
see also 16 Feb 38.

ASWONKY, by Thomas Waller, pianoforte.
unpublished 2 Sep 36 EU131366 PP, New York
renewed: 9 Sep 63 by Thomas Waller, Jr. (C): R321975.
renewed: 15 Nov 63 by Anita Rutherford Waller (W) & Maurice Waller (C): R326142.
renewed: 10 Jan 64 by Thomas W. Waller, Jr. (C): R329209.
see also 16 Feb 38.

BLACK RASPBERRY JAM, by Thomas Waller, pianoforte.
unpublished 2 Sep 36 EU131267 PP, New York
renewed: 9 Sep 63 by Thomas Waller, Jr. (C): R321976.
renewed: 15 Nov 63 by Anita Rutherford Waller (W) & Maurice Waller (C): R326143.
renewed: 10 Jan 64 by Thomas W. Waller, Jr. (C): R329210.
see also 16 Feb 38.

BACH UP TO ME, by Thomas Waller, pianoforte.
unpublished 2 Sep 36 EU131268 PP, New York
renewed: 9 Sep 63 by Thomas Waller, Jr. (C): R321977.
renewed: 15 Nov 63 by Anita Rutherford Waller (W) & Maurice Waller (C): R326144.
renewed: 10 Jan 64 by Thomas W. Waller, Jr. (C): R329211.
see also 16 Feb 38.

FRACTIOUS FINGERING, by Thomas Waller, pianoforte.
unpublished 2 Sep 36 EU131269 PP, New York
renewed: 9 Sep 63 by Thomas Waller, Jr. (C): R321978.
renewed: 15 Nov 63 by Anita Rutherford Waller (W) & Maurice Waller (C): R326145.
renewed: 10 Jan 64 by Thomas W. Waller, Jr. (C): R329212.
see also 16 Feb 38.

LOUNGING AT THE WALDORF, by Thomas Waller, pianoforte.
unpublished 2 Sep 36 EU131270 PP, New York
renewed: 9 Sep 63 by Thomas Waller, Jr. (C): R321979.
renewed: 15 Nov 63 by Anita Rutherford Waller (W) & Maurice Waller (C): R326146.
renewed: 10 Jan 64 by Thomas W. Waller, Jr. (C): R329213.
see also 16 Feb 38.

WALLER'S (FATS) ORIGINAL PIANO CONCEPTIONS, No.2; new arrangements by Fats Waller.
published 16 Sep 36 EP57546 MM, New York
renewed: 10 Jan 64 by Thomas W. Waller, Jr. (C): R329219.
renewed: 14 Sep 64 by Mills Music, Inc. (PWH): R348179.
see also 1 Sep 36.

WALLER'S (FATS) VICTOR RECORD SONG HITS; 20 songs; new arrangements, compiled & edited by Joe Davis.
published 12 Nov 36 EP60328 JD, New York
no renewal traced.

1937

OUR LOVE WAS MEANT TO BE, words by Alex Hill & Joe Davis, music by Thomas (Fats) Waller. [Featured by Jack & Loretta Clemens.]
published 12 Jul 37 EP63101 JD, New York
renewed: 13 Jul 64 by Thomas W. Waller, Jr. (C): R341380.
renewed: 23 Jul 64 by Viola Hill (W), Yvonne Hill & Thomas W. Waller, Jr. (C): R342055.
renewed: 18 Jan 65 by Thomas Waller, Jr. (C): R343943.
see also 23 Dec 30.

LOST LOVE, words by Andy Razaf, m Thomas (Fats) Waller; with guit.ar arrangement. [Featured by June Robbins with Gus Arnheim's Orcehstra.]
published 6 Aug 37 EP64031 MM, New York
renewed: 6 Aug 64 by Andy Razaf (A): R342596.
renewed: 6 Aug 64 by Thomas W. Waller, Jr. (C): R343045.
renewed: 18 Jan 65 by Thomas Waller, Jr. (C): R343944.

ALLIGATOR CRAWL, fox-trot, Thomas (Fats) Waller; arranged by Ralph Gordon; orch. pts.
published 30 Aug 37 EP63921 JD, New York
renewed: 18 Jan 65 by Joy Music, Inc. (PWH of Ralph Gordon): R353116.
BL: also published by KP, London, 1937.
see also 18 Apr 27 & 17 Dec 34 & 27 Sep 37.

WALLER'S (FATS) SWING SESSIONS FOR THE PIANO, arranged by Fats [i.e. Thomas] Waller; pianoforte.
published 7 Sep 37 EP64227 MM, New York
renewed: 18 Jan 65 by Thomas Waller, Jr. (C): R343945.
renewed: 7 Sep 65 by Mills Music, Inc. (PWH): R371852, as FATS WALLER'S SWING SESSIONS FOR THE PIANO; the popular classics in original piano versions plus Fats Waller's sensational swing interpretations, arrangements: Thomas Waller (Fats Waller). NM: arrangements.

ALLIGATOR CRAWL, fox-trot, Thomas (Fats) Waller, pianoforte.
published 27 Sep 37 EP64347 JD, New York
renewed: 25 Nov 64 by Maurice Rutherford Waller(C): R349977.
renewed: 18 Jan 65 by Thomas Waller, Jr. (C): R343946.

ALLIGATOR CRAWL, words by Andy Razaf & Joe Davis, music by Thomas (Fats) Waller.
published 27 Sep 37 EP64348 JD, New York
renewed: 28 Sep 64 by Andy Razaf (A): R345451.
renewed: 25 Nov 64 by Maurice Rutherford Waller(C): R349978.
renewed: 18 Jan 65 by Thomas Waller, Jr. (C): R343947.
see also 18 Apr 27 & 17 Dec 34 & 30 Aug 37.

FATS WALLER'S OWN ORIGINAL TUNES; SWING SONG FOLIO, words by Andy Razaf, Spencer Williams & others, music by Clarence Williams & Thomas (Fats) Waller.
published 10 Nov 37 EP66333 CW, New York
renewed: 10 Nov 64 by Clarence Williams (A): R348092.
renewed: 10 Nov 64 by Andy Razaf (A): R348093.
renewed: 10 Nov 64 by Spencer Williams (A): R348094.
renewed: 18 Jan 65 by Thomas Waller, Jr. (C): R343948.

1938

HOW CAN I, WITH YOU IN MY HEART, words by J.C. Johnson, melody by Thomas Waller.
unpublished 6 Jan 38 EU157729 PP, New York
renewed: 6 Jan 65 by J.C. Johnson (A): R352740.
renewed: 6 Jan 65 by Thomas W. Waller, Jr. (C): R353275.
renewed: 18 Jan 65 by Thomas Waller, Jr. (C): R355306.

JEALOUS OF ME, words by Andy Razaf, melody by Thomas Waller.
unpublished 6 Jan 38 EU157730 PP, New York
renewed: 6 Jan 65 by Andy Razaf (A): R352720.
renewed: 6 Jan 65 by Thomas W. Waller, Jr. (C): R353274.
renewed: 18 Jan 65 by Thomas Waller, Jr. (C): R353953.

WHAT WILL I DO IN THE MORNING, words by J.C. Johnson, melody by Thomas Waller.
unpublished 6 Jan 38 EU157731 PP, New York
renewed: 6 Jan 65 by J.C. Johnson (A): R352741.
renewed: 18 Jan 65 by Thomas W. Waller, Jr. (C): R355307.

HOW YA BABY, words by J.C. Johnson, melody by Thomas Waller.
unpublished 6 Jan 38 EU157732 PP, New York
renewed: 6 Jan 65 by J.C. Johnson (A): R352742.
renewed: 6 Jan 65 by Thomas W. Waller, Jr. (C): R353276.
renewed: 18 Jan 65 by Thomas Waller, Jr. (C): R355308.

JOINT IS JUMPIN', words by Andy Razaf & J.C. Johnson, melody by Thomas Waller.
unpublished 6 Jan 38 EU157733 PP, New York
renewed: 6 Jan 65 by Andy Razaf (A): R352722.
renewed: 6 Jan 65 by J.C. Johnson (A): R352739.
renewed: 6 Jan 65 by Thomas W. Waller, Jr. (C): R353277.
renewed: 18 Jan 65 by Thomas Waller, Jr. (C): R353954.

HOPELESS LOVE AFFAIR, words by Andy Razaf, melody by Thomas Waller.
unpublished 6 Jan 38 EU157734 PP, New York
renewed: 6 Jan 65 by Andy Razaf (A): R352721.
renewed: 6 Jan 65 by Thomas W. Waller, Jr. (C): R353278.
renewed: 18 Jan 65 by Thomas Waller, Jr. (C): R353955.

YOU'RE MY IDEAL, words by Spencer Williams, music by Thomas Waller.
published 28 Jan 38 EP67322 ShB, New York
renewed: 28 Jan 65 by Spencer Williams (A): R355046.
renewed: 28 Jan 65 by Thomas W. Waller, Jr. (C): R355126.
renewed: 29 Jan 65 by Spencer Williams (A): R354724.
renewed: 29 Jan 65 by Thomas W. Waller, Jr. (C): R354725.
see also 23 Jul 32.

BACH UP TO ME, swingopation, Thomas Fats Waller; transcribed Ken Macomber; pianoforte.
published 16 Feb 38 EP67357 SF, Cleveland.
renewed: 16 Feb 65 by Thomas Waller, Jr. (C): R355657.
see also 2 Sep 36.

BLACK RASPBERRY JAM, swingopation, Thomas Fats Waller; transcribed Ken Macomber; pianoforte.
published 16 Feb 38 EP67358 SF, Cleveland.
renewed: 16 Feb 65 by Thomas Waller, Jr. (C): R355658.
see also 2 Sep 36.

FRACTIOUS FINGERING, swingopation, Thomas Fats Waller; transcribed Ken Macomber; pianoforte.
published 16 Feb 38 EP67359 SF, Cleveland.
renewed: 16 Feb 65 by Thomas Waller, Jr. (C): R355659.
see also 2 Sep 36.
LATCH ON, swingopation, Thomas Fats Waller; transcribed Ken Macomber; pianoforte.
published 16 Feb 38 EP67360 SF, Cleveland.
renewed: 16 Feb 65 by Thomas W. Waller, Jr. (C): R355660.
see also 2 Sep 36.
LOUNGING AT THE WALDORF, swingopation, Thomas Fats Waller; transcribed Ken Macomber; pianoforte.
published 16 Feb 38 EP67361 SF, Cleveland.
renewed: 16 Feb 65 by Thomas W. Waller, Jr. (C): R355661.
see also 2 Sep 36.
PASWONKY, swingopation, Thomas Fats Waller; transcrined Ken Macomber; pianoforte.
published 16 Feb 38 EP67362 SF, Cleveland.
renewed: 16 Feb 65 by Thomas W. Waller, Jr. (C): R355662.
see also 2 Sep 36.
WALLER'S (FATS) SWINGTIME IN SCOTLAND; special arrangements by Fats [i.e. Thomas] Waller; pianoforte.
published 4 May 38 EP69235 MM, New York
renewed: 5 May 65 by Thomas W. Waller, Jr. (C): R360561.
renewed: 24 Nov 65 by Thomas Waller, Jr. (C): R376350.
renewed: 2 May 66 by Mills Music, Inc. (PWH): R391308.
BL: also published by Feldman, London, n.d.
HOLD MY HAND, words by J.C. Johnson, music by Thomas (Fats) Waller.
published 20 May 38 EP69515 SM, New York
renewed: 20 May 65 by Thomas W. Waller, Jr. (C): R361963.
renewed: 24 Nov 65 by Thomas W. Waller, Jr. (C): R376351.
WHAT'S YOUR NAME, words by J.C. Johnson, melody by Thomas (Fats) Waller.
unpublished 14 Jun 38 EU169294 SM, New York
renewed: 14 Jun 65 by Thomas W. Waller, Jr. (C): R363155.
renewed: 14 Jun 65 by J.C. Johnson (A): R363225.
renewed: 24 Nov 65 by Thomas W. Waller, Jr. (C): R376345.
SOLID ECLIPSE, words by J.C. Johnson, melody by Thomas (Fats) Waller.
unpublished 14 Jun 38 EU169295 SM, New York
renewed: 14 Jun 65 by Thomas W. Waller, Jr. (C): R363156.
renewed: 14 Jun 65 by J.C. Johnson (A): R363226.
renewed: 24 Nov 65 by Thomas W. Waller, Jr. (C): R376346.
INSIDE THIS HEART OF MINE, words by J.C. Johnson, music by Thomas (Fats) Waller. [Featured by Sammy Kaye and His Orchestra] [Renewals state: 'Piano Score by Buzz Adlam'.]
published 8 Jul 38 EP70327 MM, New York
renewed: 8 Jul 65 by Thomas W. Waller, Jr. (C): R364381.
renewed: 9 Jul 65 by J.C. Johnson (A): R366030.
renewed: 24 Nov 65 by Thomas W. Waller, Jr. (C): R376352.
ON RAINY DAYS, words & music by Andy Razaf & Thomas (Fats) Waller. [Renewals state: 'Piano Score by Buzz Adlam'.]
published 8 Jul 38 EP70331 MM, New York
renewed: 8 Jul 65 by Andy Razaf (A): R364308.
renewed: 8 Jul 65 by Thomas W. Waller, Jr. (C): R364380.
renewed: 24 Nov 65 by Thomas W. Waller, Jr. (C): R376353.
IF I MEANT SOMETHING TO YOU, words by J.C. Johnson, melody by Thomas (Fats) Waller.
unpublished 14 Jul 38 EU171576 ShB., New York
renewed: 14 Jul 65 by Thomas W. Waller, Jr. (C): R365002.
renewed: 14 Jul 65 by J.C. Johnson (A): R366042.
renewed: 24 Nov 65 by Thomas W. Waller, Jr. (C): R376347.
BY HECK, eccentric fox-trot, transcribed & arranged by Thomas (Fats) Waller.
published 7 Sep 38 EP71354 Edward B. Marks music corp., New York
renewed: 7 Sep 65 by Edward B. Marks Music Corp. (PWH of Thomas Waller): R367874, as BY HECK, tempo josh de swing, eccentric fox-trot, music by S.R. Henry, transcribed & arranged by Thomas (Fats) Waller. NM: swing jazz arrangement for piano.
renewed: 24 Nov 65 by Thomas W. Waller, Jr. (C): R440718 (also specifies 'music by S.R. Henry').

MOONLIGHT MOOD, words by J.C. Johnson, music by Thomas (Fats) Waller. [Featured by Russ Morgan.]
published 16 Sep 38 EP71647 MM, New York
renewed: 16 Sep 65 by J.C. Johnson (A): R368082.
renewed: 17 Sep 65 by Thomas W. Waller, Jr. (C): R370328.
renewed: 24 Nov 65 by Thomas W. Waller, Jr. (C): R376354.

I GOT LOVE, words & music by Spencer Williams & Thomas (Fats) Waller. [Featured, broadcast and recorded by Fats Waller.]
published 21 Oct 38 EF56520 Keith, Prowse & co., ltd., London *[sic]*
renewed: 22 Oct 65 by Thomas W. Waller, Jr. (C): R371068.
renewed: 24 Nov 65 by Thomas W. Waller, Jr. (C): R376356.
see also 9 Dec 38.

YACHT CLUB SWING, words & melody by Herman Autre [sic], J.C. Johnson & Thomas Fats Waller.
unpublished 22 Oct 38 EU180150 BVC, New York
renewed: 26 Oct 65 by Herman Autre, a.k.a. Herman Autrey & Herman Autry, J.C. Johnson (A's), Edith Hatcher Waller (W), Thomas W. Waller, Jr. & Maurice Waller(C): R370942.
renewed: 19 Nov 65 by J.C. Johnson (A): R3373292.
renewed: 24 Nov 65 by Thomas W. Waller, Jr. (C): R376348.
see also 15 May 45.

I CAN'T FORGIVE YOU, lyrics by J.C. Johnson, music by Thomas (Fats) Waller. [Featured by Vincent Lopez and His Orchestra.]
published 24 Oct 38 EP72491 MM, New York
renewed: 25 Oct 65 by J.C. Johnson (A): R370902.
renewed: 25 Oct 65 by Thomas W. Waller, Jr. (C): R371067.
renewed: 24 Nov 65 by Thomas W. Waller, Jr. (C): R376355.

UNDERCURRENT, fox-trot, Thomas (Fats) Waller; small swing band parts. [Jitterbug Series arrangements for small swing bands.]
published 28 Oct 38 EP72596 Ex, New York
renewed: 29 Oct 65 by Thomas W. Waller, Jr. (C): R372729.
renewed: 24 Nov 65 by Thomas W. Waller, Jr. (C): R376361.

SPIDER AND THE FLY, words & melody by Thomas (Fats) Waller, Andy Razaf & J.C. Johnson.
unpublished 29 Oct 38 EU180500 SJS, New York
renewed: 29 Oct 65 by Andy Razaf (A): R371890.
renewed: 29 Oct 65 by J.C. Johnson (A): R371900.
renewed: 3 Nov 65 by Thomas W. Waller, Jr. (C) & Andy Razaf (A): : R373378.
renewed: 24 Nov 65 by Thomas W. Waller, Jr. (C): R376349.
see also 2 Dec 38.

I HAD TO DO IT, words by Andy Razaf, music by Thomas (Fats) Waller.
published 1 Nov 38 EP72577 BVC, New York
renewed: 1 Nov 65 by Andy Razaf (A): R371963.
renewed: 19 Nov 65 by Andy Razaf (A), Edith Hatcher Waller (W), Thomas W. Waller, Jr. & Maurice Waller (C): R373632
renewed: 24 Nov 65 by Thomas W. Waller, Jr. (C): R376360.

NOT THERE, RIGHT THERE, words & music by Thomas (Fats) Waller & Spencer Williams. [A World Wide Hit.]
published 22 Nov 38 EF57063 WWM, London
renewed: 22 Nov 65 by Thomas W. Waller, Jr. (C): R374472.
renewed: 24 Nov 65 by Thomas W. Waller, Jr. (C): R376358.

COTTAGE IN THE RAIN, words & music by Thomas (Fats) Waller & Spencer Williams. [A World Wide Hit.]
published 22 Nov 38 EF57064 WWM, London
renewed: 22 Nov 65 by Thomas W. Waller, Jr. (C): R374473.
renewed: 24 Nov 65 by Thomas W. Waller, Jr. (C): R376359.

WHAT A PRETTY MISS, words & music by Thomas (Fats) Waller & Spencer Williams. [A World Wide Hit.]
published 22 Nov 38 EF57065 WWM, London
renewed: 29 Nov 65 by Thomas W. Waller, Jr. (C): R375776.
renewed: 24 Nov 65 by Thomas W. Waller, Jr. (C): R376357.

SPIDER AND THE FLY, POOR FLY, BYE-BYE, words & music by Thomas (Fats) Waller, Andy Razaf & J.C. Johnson.
published 2 Dec 38 EP73215 SJS, New York
renewed: 2 Dec 65 by J.C. Johnson (A): R374805.
renewed: 2 Dec 65 by Andy Razaf (A): R374811.
renewed: 2 Dec 65 by Thomas W. Waller, Jr. (C) & Andy Razaf (A): : R375777.
renewed: 3 Dec 65 by Thomas W. Waller, Jr. (C): R376344.
BL holds two different editions published by SJS, New York City, 1938; also published by Campbell Connelly, London, n.d.
see also 29 Oct 38.

JITTERBUG TREE, words by Andy Razaf & J.C. Johnson, melody by Fred Rose, revised by Thomas (Fats) Waller). [Renewals specifiy 'melody from Fred Rose's *Black Maria*, words by Andy Razaf & J.C. Johnson, music by Fred Rose & Fats Waller (Thomas Waller), rev. by Thomas 'Fats' Waller'. NM: revision of music.]
unpublished 2 Dec 38 EU181642 PaP, New York
renewed: 6 Dec 65 by Thomas W. Waller, Jr. (C): R375775.
renewed: 6 May 66 by Andy Razaf (A): R411455.
renewed: 18 Feb 66 by Thomas Waller, Jr. (C): R381199.
renewed: 23 Nov 66 by Andy Razaf & J.C. Johnson (A's): R397818.
see also 19 Jan 39.

I GOT LOVE, by Spencer Williams & Thomas (Fats) Waller; arranged by Phil Cardew; orch. pts.
published 9 Dec 38 EF56952 Keith, Prowse & co., ltd., London *[sic]*
renewed: 25 Apr 66 by Keith Prowse Music Publishing Co. Ltd. (PWH of Phil Cardew): R384914.
see also 21 Oct 38.

I'M SAVIN' UP MY PENNIES, by Fats Waller; pianoforte. treble.
unpublished 22 Dec 38 EU183263 R, New York
renewed: 23 Dec 65 by Thomas W. Waller, (C): R376510.

PATTY CAKE, PATTY CAKE, BAKER MAN, words & music by Andy Razaf, J.C. Johnson & Thomas "Fats" Waller.
published 28 Dec 38 EP73753 SF, Cleveland
renewed: 28 Dec 65 by Thomas W. Waller, Jr. (C): R376362.
renewed: 28 Dec 65 by Andy Razaf (A): R376413.
renewed: 28 Dec 65 by J.C. Johnson (A): R376466.

Note: The Library of Congress did not publish a composer-index to the Catalog of Copyright Records for the years 1939 to 1943 inclusive. As a consequence, only those copyright registrations which were the subject of renewals, or are adjacent to registrations which were the subject of renewals, have been located.

1939

WALLER (FATS) SWINGIN' THE OPERAS, arranged by Thomas (Fats) Waller; pianoforte.
published 17 Jan 39 EP74403 MM, New York
renewed: 17 Jan 66 by Thomas W. Waller, Jr. (C): R378183.
renewed: 22 Apr 66 by Thomas W. Waller, Jr. (C): R384655.

JITTERBUG TREE, words by Andy Razaf & J.C. Johnson, melody from Fred Rose's *Black Maria*, revised by Thomas (Fats) Waller; pianoforte score by Ted Eastwood. [Renewals as JITTERBUG TREE (THAT "BLACK MARIA" STRAIN) NM: new words, revised music & arrangement.]
published 19 Jan 39 EP74333 PaP, New York
see also 2 Dec 38.
renewed: 19 Jan 66 by Andy Razaf (A): R380700.
renewed: 20 Jan 66 by Thomas W. Waller, Jr. (C): R379085.
renewed: 22 Apr 66 by Thomas W. Waller, Jr. (C): R385908.
renewed: 23 Nov 66 by Andy Razaf, J.C. Johnson (A's) & Shawnee Press, Inc. (PWH of Ted Eastwood): R397819.

SAY YES, words & music by Andy Razaf, J.C. Johnson & Thomas (Fats) Waller.
published 27 Feb 39 EP75369 C, New York
renewed: 28 Feb 66 by J.C. Johnson (A): R381122.
renewed: 28 Feb 66 by Andy Razaf (A): R381133.
renewed: 28 Feb 66 by Andy Razaf & J.C. Johnson (A's): R381226.
renewed: 28 Feb 66 by Thomas W. Waller, Jr. (C): R382043.
renewed: 22 Apr 66 by Thomas W. Waller, Jr. (C): R384656.

CHOO CHOO, words by Andy Razaf, music by Eugene Seebic *(sic)* & Thomas Waller.
published 15 Mar 39 EP75751 Ex., New York
renewed: 15 Mar 66 by Thomas W. Waller, Jr. (C): R382268.
renewed: 12 Apr 66 by Andy Razaf (A): R384178.
renewed: 22 Apr 66 by Thomas Waller, Jr. (C): R384657.

HONEY HUSH, words by Ed Kirkeby, melody by Thomas (Fats) Waller.
unpublished 18 Jul 39 EU200442 IB, New York
renewed: 7 Oct 66 by Thomas W. Waller, Jr. (C): R395276.
ANITA, words & music by Fats Waller. [Featured by Gray Gordon's Tic-Toc Rhythm Orchestra.]
published 28 Oct 39 EP80708 MM, New York
renewed: 28 Oct 66 by Thomas Waller, Jr. (C): R397090.

1940

MIGHTY FINE, words by Andy Razaf, music by Thomas (Fats) Waller.
published 9 Jan 40 EP82085 G, New York
renewed:9 Jan 67 by Andy Razaf (A): R401865.
renewed: 10 Jan 67 by Andy Razaf (A): R401960.
renewed: 21 Feb 67 by Thomas W. Waller, Jr. (C): R404857.
HAPPY FEELING, by Thomas (Fats) Waller; pianoforte.
published 26 Jan 40 EP82450 G, New York
renewed: 21 Feb 67 by Thomas W. Waller, Jr. (C): R404856.
BLACK MARIA, new words by Andy Razaf & J.C. Johnson, music by Fred Rose, arranged by Fats Waller. [NM: new lyrics & revised piano arrangement.]
published 1 Feb 40 EP82848 PaP, New York
renewed : 1 Feb 67 by Andy Razaf (A): R404197.
renewed: 21 Feb 67 by Andy Razaf (A): R404855.
BLACK MARIA, jam fox-trot, new lyrics by Andy Razaf & J.C. Johnson, music by Fred Rose, revised by Thomas (Fats) Waller; orch. parts.
published 27 Feb 40 EP83434 PaP, New York
no renewal traced.
BOND STREET, from London Suite, by Thomas Waller; pianoforte.
published 10 Apr 40 EP84708 PM, London.
renewed: 18 Dec 67 by Thomas W. Waller, Jr. (C): R424933.
OLD GRAND DAD, words & melody by Fats [i.e. Thomas] Waller.
unpublished 12 Apr 40 EU220223 G, New York
renewed: 18 Dec 67 by Thomas Waller, Jr. (C): R424929.
OLD GRAND DAD, words & melody by Fats [i.e. Thomas] Waller.
unpublished 9 May 40 EU222242 G, New York
no renewal traced.
STAYIN' AT HOME, words by Andy Razaf, melody by Fats [i.e. Thomas] Waller.
unpublished 19 Jul 40 EU226996 Be, New York
renewed: 19 Jul 67 by Andy Razaf (A): R414254.
renewed: 18 Dec 67 by Thomas W. Waller, Jr. (C): R424931.
STAYIN' AT HOME, HAPPY TO BE BY MYSELF, words by Andy Razaf, m usic byFats [i.e. Thomas] Waller.
published 18 Oct 40 EP88492 Be, New York
renewed: 18 Oct 67 by Andy Razaf (A): R420028.
renewed: 18 Dec 67 by Thomas W. Waller, Jr. (C): R424935.
WHAT DID I DO TO BE SO BLACK AND BLUE, by Andy Razaf, Thomas Waller & Harry Brooks, arranged by Jimmy Dale; orch. parts.
published 30 Oct 40 EP89590 MM, New York
renewed: 24 Apr 68 by Mills Music, Inc. (PWH of Jimmy Dale):R434394.
see also 20 Aug 29.

1941

WALLER'S (FATS) PIANO ANTICS; 5 compositions; Fats [i.e. Thomas] Waller; pianoforte.
published 3 Jan 41 EP91291 G, New York
renewed: 4 Jan 68 by Thomas Waller, Jr. (C): R426390, as FATS WALLER'S PIANO ANTICS; 5 new original novelty piano solos.
BOOGIE WOOGIE WITH FATS WALLER; folio; arranged by Fats [i.e. Thomas] Waller; pianoforte.
published 29 Jan 41 EP103910 MM, New York
renewed: 29 Jan 68 by Mills Music, Inc. (PWH): R428693.
I REPENT, words & music by Fats [i.e. Thomas] Waller; pianoforte.
unpublished 5 Feb 41 EU245732 G, New York
renewed: 7 Feb 68 by Thomas W. Waller, Jr. (C): R429225.
renewed: 5 Aug 68 by Thomas W. Waller, Jr. (C): R441150.

MY MAMASITA, from *Juarez*, by Fats [i.e. Thomas] Waller; pianoforte. treble.
unpublished 5 Feb 41 EU245733 G, New York
renewed: 20 Jun 68 by Thomas W. Waller, Jr. (C): R437588.
renewed: 5 Aug 68 by Thomas W. Waller, Jr. (C): R441151.
see also 20 Aug 41.

BLUE VELVET, words & music by Thomas Waller & Spencer Williams. [Renewals as BLUE VELVET; Chanson cerulean].
13 Mar 41 EF65025 Spencer Williams, London
renewed: 14 Mar 68 by Agnes Bage Williams (W), Della M. Smith & Lindy I. Goodwin (C of Spencer Williams): R431532.
renewed: 20 Jun 68 by Thomas W. Waller, Jr. (C): R437589.
renewed: 5 Aug 68 by Thomas W. Waller, Jr. (C): R441162.

ALL THAT MEAT AND NO POTATOES, words & music by Fats [i.e. Thomas] Waller & Ed Kirkeby.
published 19 Jun 41 EP95470 LF, New York
renewed: 20 Jun 68 by Thomas W. Waller, Jr. (C): R437587.
renewed: 5 Aug 68 by Thomas W. Waller, Jr. (C): R441155.

MAMACITA, words by Buddy Kaye, music by Fats [i.e. Thomas] Waller.
published 20 Aug 41 EP96949 G, New York
renewed: 20 Aug 68 by Thomas W. Waller, Jr. (C): R442106.
renewed: 21 Aug 68 by Buddy Kaye (A): R442049.
renewed: 18 Aug 69 by Buddy Kaye (A): R467050, as MAMACITA, novelty song.
see also 5 Feb 41.

1942

GET SOME CASH FOR YOUR TRASH, words by Ed Kirkeby, music by Thomas (Fats) Waller.
published 13 Feb 42 EP109558 LF, New York
renewed: 13 Feb 69 by Thomas W. Waller, Jr. (C): R455686.
renewed: 14 Feb 69 by Ed Kirkeby (A) & Thomas W. Waller, Jr. (W)*[sic]*: R456568.

JITTERBUG WALTZ, by Thomas Fats Waller; pianoforte.
published 16 Oct 42 EP108665 R, New York
renewed: 17 Oct 69 by Thomas W. Waller, Jr. (C): R470790, as THE JITTERBUG WALTZ., piano solo.
renewed: 6 Nov 69 by Thomas Waller, Jr. (C): R472448.

1943

WALLER (THOMAS(FATS)) MUSICAL RHYTHMS, compiled & arranged by Fats [i.e. Thomas] Waller; pianoforte.
published 8 Jan 43 EP111206 R, New York
renewed: 12 Jan 70 by Robbins Music Corp. (PWH): R477095.
renewed: 5 Feb 70 by Thomas W. Waller, Jr. (C): R496455.

SLIGHTLY LESS THAN WONDERFUL; from *Early To Bed*, words by George Marion, jr., music by Fats [i.e. Thomas] Waller
published 1 Jun 43 EP114155 Ad, New York
renewed: 1 Jun 70 by Thomas W. Waller, Jr. (C): R485475.
renewed: 3 Jun 70 by Dorothy Marion (W) & Georgette Marion Collier (C): R485836.

THERE'S A MAN IN MY LIFE; from *Early To Bed*, words by George Marion, jr., music by Fats [i.e. Thomas] Waller.
published 1 Jun 43 EP114156 Ad, New York
renewed: 1 Jun 70 by Thomas W. Waller, Jr. (C): R485476.
renewed: 3 Jun 70 by Dorothy Marion (W) & Georgette Marion Collier (C): R485837.

LADIES WHO SING WITH THE BAND; from *Early To Bed*, words by George Marion, jr., music by Fats [i.e. Thomas] Waller.
published 1 Jun 43 EP114157 Ad, New York
renewed: 1 Jun 70 by Thomas W. Waller, Jr. (C): R485477.
renewed: 3 Jun 70 by Dorothy Marion (W) & Georgette Marion Collier (C): R485838.

THIS IS SO NICE; from *Early To Bed*, words by George Marion, jr., music by Fats [i.e. Thomas] Waller.
published 1 Jun 43 EP114158 Ad, New York
renewed: 1 Jun 70 by Thomas W. Waller, Jr. (C): R485478.
renewed: 3 Jun 70 by Dorothy Marion (W) & Georgette Marion Collier (C): R485839.

WHEN THE NYLONS BLOOM AGAIN; from *Early To Bed*, words by George Marion, jr., music by Fats [i.e. Thomas] Waller.
published 26 Jul 43 EP115316 Ad, New York
renewed: 27 Jul 70 by Thomas W. Waller, Jr. (C): R488828.
renewed: 30 Jul 70 by Dorothy Marion (W) & Georgette Marion Collier (C): R488799.

WALLER'S (FATS) BOOGIE WOOGIE CONCEPTIONS OF POPULAR FAVORITES; arranged by Thomas (Fats) Waller.
published 21 Jun 43 EP116523 MM, New York
renewed: 23 Jun 70 by Thomas W. Waller, Jr. (C): R486683.
renewed: 19 May 71 by Mills Music, Inc. (PWH): R538129.

1944

AIN'T MISBEHAVIN', by Andy Razaf, Fats [i.e. Thomas] Waller & Harry Brooks, arranged by Ted Mossman; pianoforte.
published 10 Jul 44 EP124007 MM, New York
renewed: 5 Apr 72 by Ted Mossman (A): R626510, AIN'T MISBEHAVIN' (piano solo); NM: simplified arrangement.
see also 8 Jul 29 & 9 Mar 45.

DEAR LITTLE MOUNTAIN SWEETHEART, words by Ed Kirkeby, melody by Lew Cobey.
unpublished 16 Nov 44 EU398026 CR, New York
Included because listed by ASCAP as by Ed Kirkeby & Fats Waller.

SAD SAPSUCKER, words by Ed Kirkeby, melody by Fats [i.e. Thomas] Waller.
unpublished 16 Nov 44 EU400422 CR, New York
renewed: 18 Nov 71 by Thomas W. Waller, Jr. (C): R516985.

YOU MUST BE LOSIN' YOUR MIND, words by Ed Kirkeby, melody by Fats [i.e. Thomas] Waller.
unpublished 16 Nov 44 EU400423 CR, New York
renewed: 18 Nov 71 by Thomas W. Waller, Jr. (C): R516986.

WALLER'S (FATS) ORIGINAL E FLAT BLUES, words by Ed Kirkeby, melody by Fats [i.e. Thomas] Waller.
unpublished 16 Nov 44 EU400424 CR, New York
renewed: 18 Nov 71 by Thomas W. Waller, Jr. (C): R516987.

DO YOU HAVE TO GO?, words by Anita Waller, melody by Fats [i.e. Thomas] Waller.
unpublished 16 Nov 44 EU400425 CR, New York
renewed: 18 Nov 71 by Thomas W. Waller, Jr. (C): R516998.

AT TWILIGHT, words by Anita Waller, melody by Fats [i.e. Thomas] Waller.
unpublished 16 Nov 44 EU400426 CR, New York
renewed: 18 Nov 71 by Thomas W. Waller, Jr. (C): R516989.

UP JUMPED YOU WITH LOVE, words by Ed Kirkeby, melody by Fats [i.e. Thomas] Waller.
unpublished 16 Nov 44 EU400427 CR, New York
renewed: 18 Nov 71 by Thomas W. Waller, Jr. (C): R516990.

DON'T GIVE ME THAT JIVE, COME ON WITH THE COME ON, words by Ed Kirkeby, melody by Fats [i.e. Thomas] Waller.
unpublished 16 Nov 44 EU400428 CR, New York
renewed: 18 Nov 71 by Thomas W. Waller, Jr. (C): R516991.

BESSIE, BESSIE, BESSIE, words by Ed Kirkeby, melody by Fats [i.e. Thomas] Waller.
unpublished 16 Nov 44 EU400429 CR, New York
renewed: 18 Nov 71 by Thomas W. Waller, Jr. (C): R516992.

COME AND GET IT, words by Ed Kirkeby, melody by Fats [i.e. Thomas] Waller.
unpublished 16 Nov 44 EU400430 CR, New York
renewed: 18 Nov 71 by Thomas W. Waller, Jr. (C): R516993.

OH BABY – SWEET BABY, words by Ed Kirkeby, melody by Fats [i.e. Thomas] Waller.
unpublished 16 Nov 44 EU400431 CR, New York
renewed: 18 Nov 71 by Thomas W. Waller, Jr. (C): R516994.

SWING OUT TO VICTORY, words by Ed Kirkeby, melody by Fats [i.e. Thomas] Waller.
unpublished 16 Nov 44 EU400432 CR, New York
renewed: 18 Nov 71 by Thomas W. Waller, Jr. (C): R516995.

RUMP STEAK SERENADE, words by Ed Kirkeby, melody by Fats [i.e. Thomas] Waller.
unpublished 16 Nov 44 EU400433 CR, New York
renewed: 18 Nov 71 by Thomas W. Waller, Jr. (C): R516996.

WE NEED A LITTLE LOVE THAT'S ALL, words by Ed Kirkeby, melody by Fats [i.e. Thomas] Waller.
unpublished 16 Nov 44 EU400434 CR, New York
renewed: 18 Nov 71 by Thomas W. Waller, Jr. (C): R516997.

1945

AIN'T MISBEHAVIN', by Andy Razaf, Thomas Waller & Harry Brooks; arranged by Jimmy Dale. 60¢ © arrangement. Piano-conductor acore (orchestra) and parts.
published 9 Mar 45 EP1595 MM, New York
renewed: 14 Jul 72 by Jimmy Dale (A): R533156; NM: arrangement for dance orchestra.
see also 8 Jul 29 & 10 Jul 44.

BOOGIE WOOGIE SUITE, by Fats [i.e. Thomas] Waller; pianoforte.
published 9 Apr 45 EP130539 MM, New York
renewed: 10 Apr 72 by Thomas W. Waller, Jr. (C): R526862.
YACHT CLUB SWING, words & music by Fats [i.e. Thomas] Waller, J.C. Johnson & Herman Autry (sic).
published 15 May 45 EP131430 BVC, New York
renewed: 15 May 72 by Thomas W. Waller, Jr. (C): R528938.
renewed: 19 May 72 by J.C. Johnson (A): R529327.
renewed: 26 May 72 by J.C. Johnson, Herman Autry (A), Edith Hatcher Waller (W), Thomas W. Waller, Jr. & Maurice Waller (C): R530088.
renewed: 8 Jun 72 by Herman Autrey (A): R529865.
see also 22 Oct 38.
YOU CAN'T HAVE YOUR CAKE AND EAT IT, words & music by Fats [i.e. Thomas] Waller & Spencer Williams.
published 15 Jun 45 EP133743 Peter Maurice, inc., New York
renewed: 16 Jun 72 by Agnes Bage Williams (W), Della M. Smith & Lindy I. Goodwin (C of Spencer Williams): R530955.
renewed: 10 Jul 72 by Thomas Waller, Jr. (PWH): R531630.
renewed: 12 Jul 72 by Thomas W. Waller, Jr. (PPW of Thomas Waller): R531479.

1946

DID-JA?, words by Ed Kirkeby, music by Thomas Waller.
unpublished 12 Nov 46 EU45170 CR, New York
renewed: 12 Dec 73 by Thomas W. Waller, Jr. (C): R565601.
MY LOVE GETS HUNGRY TOO!, words by Ed Kirkeby, music by Thomas Waller.
unpublished 12 Nov 46 EU45176 CR, New York
renewed: 12 Dec 73 by Thomas W. Waller, Jr. (C): R565602.
STORMY WEATHER: MOPPIN' AND BOPPIN' [excerpt][words & music] by T "Fats" Waller, Benny Carter land] Ed Kirkeby. For voice and piano, with chord symbols.
published 11 Dec 46 EP6285 MM, New York, publisher *[sic]*
renewed: 12 Dec 73 by Thomas W. Waller, Jr. (C): R565605.
renewed: 2 May 74 by Benny Carter (A): R577134.
renewals as MOPPIN' AND BOPPIN' From the picture *Stormy Weather*.

1947 [The Catalog of Unpublished Music for 1947 has not been available, but no renewals have been located.]
"FATS" WALLER'S FAMOUS LONDON SUITE; for the piano.
published 7 Feb 47 EF5170 The Peter Maurice Music Co. Ltd., New York
renewed: 30 Jan 75 by Thomas Waller & Maurice Waller (C): R596878.
AIN'T MISBEHAVIN', by Andy Razaf, Thomas Waller & Harry Brooks; arranged by 'Zep' Meissner. Piano-conductor score (orchestra) & parts. © on arrangement.
published 21 Apr 47 EP6846 MM, New York
renewed: 31 Jan 75 by Zep Meissner (A): R596990.
AIN'T MISBEHAVIN', minuet by Thomas Waller & Harry Brooks; transcribed by Eddy Rogers. Score (violin & piano) & part.
published 12 Dec 47 EP23306 MM, New York; on arrangement
renewed: 2 Jun 75 by Dorothy W. Rogers (W): R605309.
THE MINOR DRAG, by Thomas "Fats" Waller, arranged by Jimmy Dale. New York Sole selling agent, Southern Music Pub. Co. Piano-conductor score (orchestra) & parts.
published 9 Dec 47 EP24073 Peer International Corp.
no renewal traced.

1948-1952 No entries have been located in the Catalog of Published Music for these years. The Catalog of Unpublished Music for these years has not been available, but no renewals have been located. Renewals have not been checked beyond June 1977.

1953

IF YOU CAN'T BE GOOD, BE CAREFUL, words & music by Andy Razaf & Thomas (Fats) Waller.
published 27 Mar 53 EP71556 MM, New York
THERE'LL COME A TIME WHEN YOU'LL NEED ME, words & music by Thomas "Fats" Waller & Irving Mills.
published 27 Mar 53 EP71566 MM, New York

PATTY CAKE, PATTY CAKE, BAKER MAN, words & music by Andy Razaf, J.C. Johnson & Thomas "Fats" Waller; arranged by F. Henri Klickmann (in Klickmann, F.H., *Tunes For Tots*, p.10-11 [For piano]
Appication cites previous registration on 28 Dec 38: EP73753.
published 30 Mar 53 EP71155 SF; on arrrangement

NEVER HEARD OF SUCH STUFF, piano solo by Thomas (Fats) Waller. 60¢
published 1 Apr 53 EP71505 MM, New York

PATTY CAKE, PATTY CAKE, BAKER MAN, words & music by Andy Razaf, J.C. Johnson & Thomas "Fats" Waller; arranged by F. Henri Klickmann (in Klickmann, F.H., *Tunes For Tots*, p.10-11 [For accordion, ukelele words].
Application cites previous registration on 28 Dec 38: EP73753.
published 23 Dec 53 EP77703 SF. NM: arrangement

1954

OH BABY, SWEET BABY, words & music by Thomas "Fats" Waller & Ed Kirkeby. 40¢
published 1 May 54 EP80806 CR, N.Y

BREEZIN', by Thomas "Fats" Waller [melody & chord symbols]
unpublished 11 May 54 EU358257 S

AN ARMFUL OF YOU, by Thomas "Fats" Waller [melody, chords in treble clef & chord symbols].
unpublished 11 May 54 EU358258 S

1955 [The Catalog of Unpublished Music for 1955 has not been available]

FATS WALLER PIANO PRANKS; Fats Waller inimitable piano styles, arranger: Stanley Applebaum, 31p. $1. Appl. author: Mayfair Music Corp., employed for hire of Stanley Applebaum. NM: rev. ed. inc. 3 new mumbers.
published 21 Apr 55 EP89237 Mf, New York

FOOLIN' MYSELF, words by Andy Razaf, music by Thomas Waller.
published 22 Jun 55 EP90844 MM, New York

LEAVING ME, words by Andy Razaf, music by Thomas Waller.
published 22 Jun 55 EP90843 MM, New York

1956 No entries have been located in the Catalogs of Published or Unpublished Music for 1956 .

1957

I HATE TO LEAVE YOU NOW, words by Dorothy Dick, music by Harry Link & Fats Waller.
unpublished 18 Jul 57 EU486939 J

SQUEEZE ME; original words & music by Thomas 'Fats' Waller & Clarence Williams, revised words by Clarence Williams. NM: revised words.
published 18 Dec 57 EP114989 Pi

1958-1961: No entries have been located in the Catalogs of Published or Unpublished Music for these years.

1962

HONEYSUCKLE ROSE, from *Load of Coal*, music by Thomas Waller, arranged by Joy Music, Inc. NM: arrangement.
unpublished 9 Jan 62 EU701514 J

1963-1964: No entries have been located in the Catalogs of Published or Unpublished Music for these years.

1965

GOIN' ABOUT, worda & music by Mike Jackson & Thomas 'Fats' Waller.
published 23 Jun 65 EP204704 S

BLUE BLACK BOTTOM, worda & music by Mike Jackson & Thomas 'Fats' Waller [without words] *[sic]*
published 23 Jun 65 EP206196 S

1966-1968: No entries have been located in the Catalogs of Published or Unpublished Music for these years.

1969

THAT GETS IT, MISTER JOE, words by J.C. Johnson, music by Thomas (Fats) Waller; 2p.
unpublished 29 Oct 69 EU143359 © J.C. Johnson & Estate of Thomas (Fats) Waller by Thomas W. Waller, Jr.

1970-1971: No entries have been located in the Catalogs of Published or Unpublished Music for these years.

1972 (© registered in 1974)
HANDFUL OF KEYS, Paroles françaises de Jean Eigel, musique de Fats Waller. France, 4p. Additional title: OU EST PASSÉE MA CLÉ? Application cites previous publication, 14 Jul 33: EP37324; NM: French words.
published 5 Nov 72 EF38582 Societe des Editions Musicales Internationales

1973-1976: No entries have been located in the Catalogs of Published or Unpublished Music for these years.

1977
THE JOINT IS JUMPIN', by Thomas Waller, Andy Razaf & J.C. Johnson. In *From Rags To Jazz*, p.32-33. Appl au arranged by Dorsey Brothers Music div. Music Sales Corporation, employer for hire.
Application cites previous registration on 6 Jan 38: EU178833. NM: arrangement
published 15 Dec 76 EP364371 DB, a div. of Music Sales Corporation
MIGHTY FINE, by Thomas Waller & Andy Razaf. In From Rags To Jazz, p.32-33. Appl au: arranged by Dorsey Brothers Music div. Music Sales Corporation, employer for hire.
Application cites previous registration on 9 Jan 40: EP82085. NM: arrangement
published 15 Dec 76 EP364372 DB, a div. of Music Sales Corporation

1978
AIN'T MISBEHAVIN', for S.S.A.T.B. & accompaniment for piano & rhythm section of guitar, bass & drums; music by Thomas Waller & Harry Brooks, lyrics by Andy Razaf; arranged by Chuck Cassey; Melville, N. Y., Belwin Mills Publishing Corporation, c.1978. 12p. Jazz ensembles for advancing choirs.
Application cites previous registration in 1929, renewed in 1957.
published in Oct-Dec 78 cat. PA17-221 MM, piano/vocal ed.

A FATS WALLER SCRAPBOOK

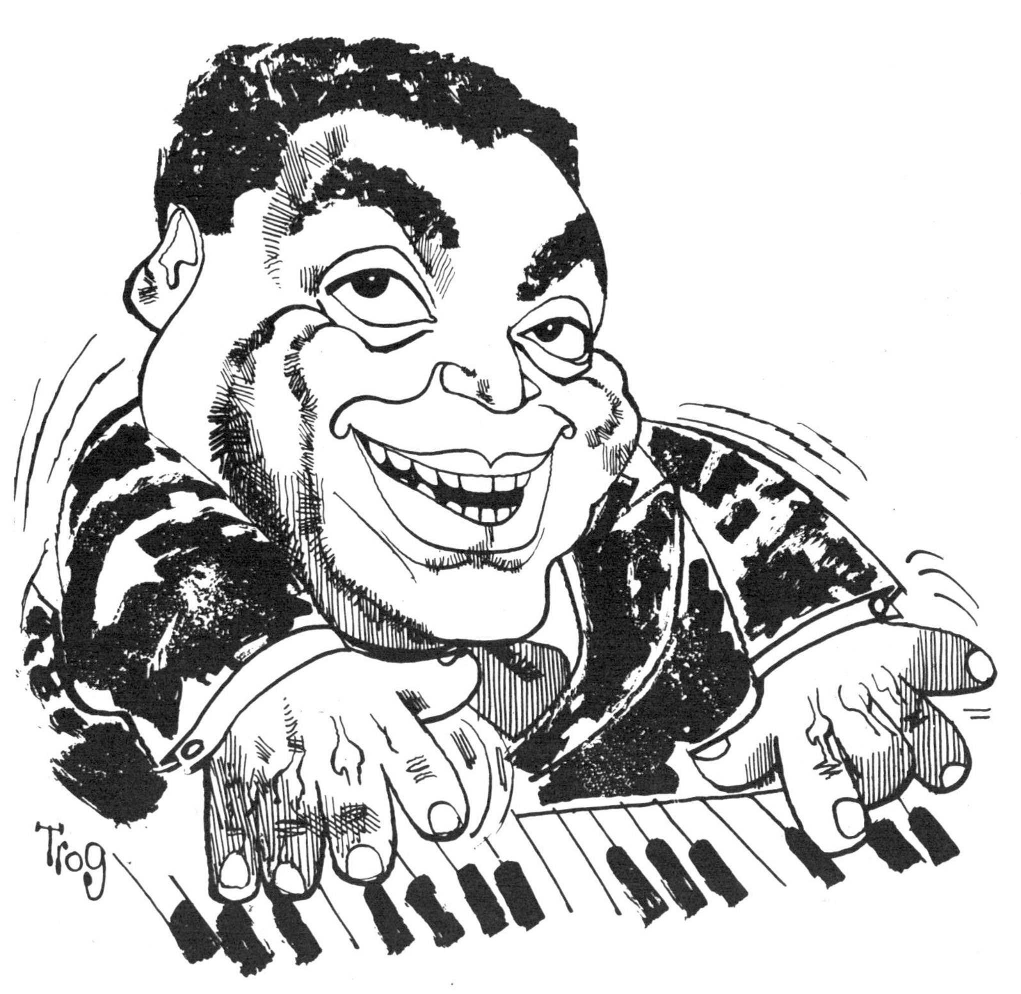

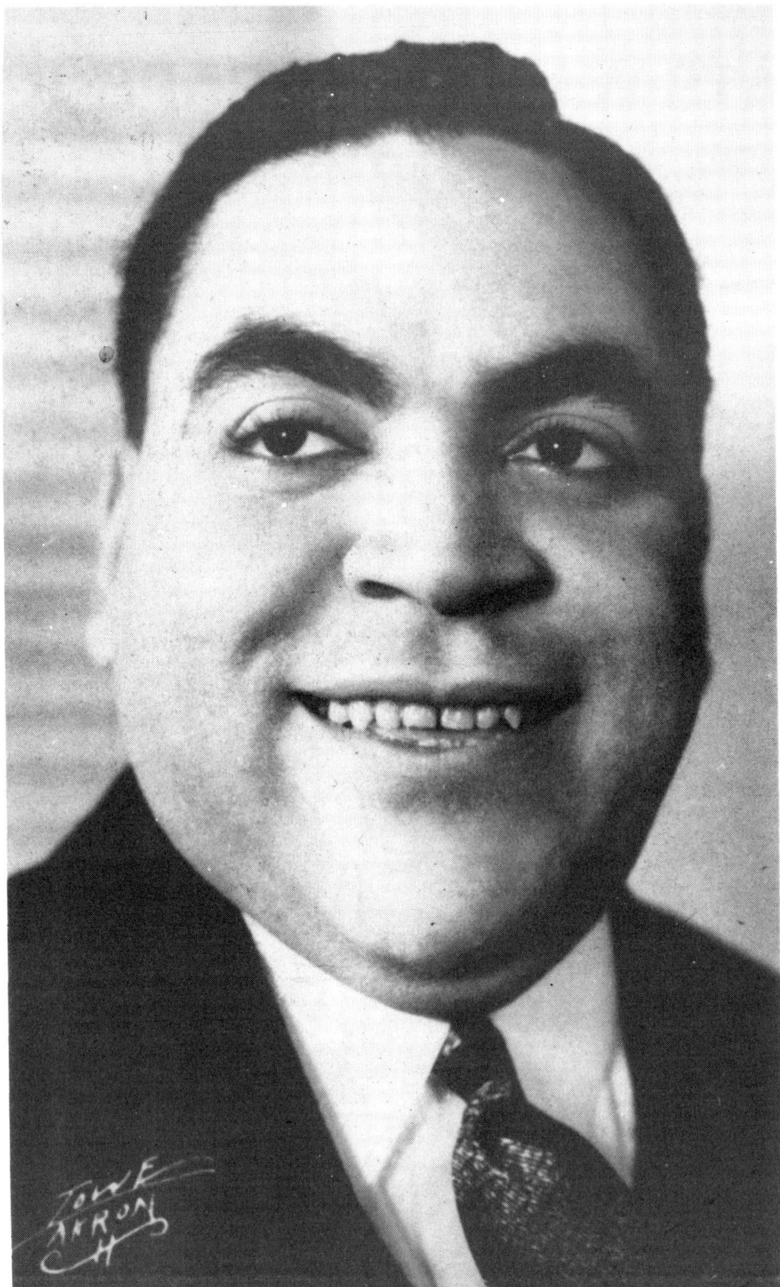
TOWE
AKRON

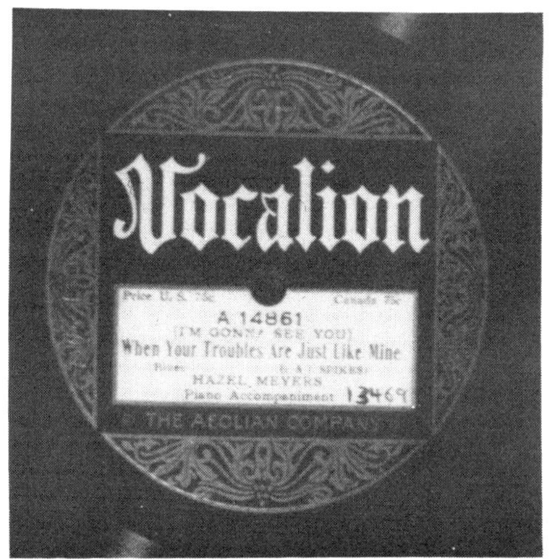

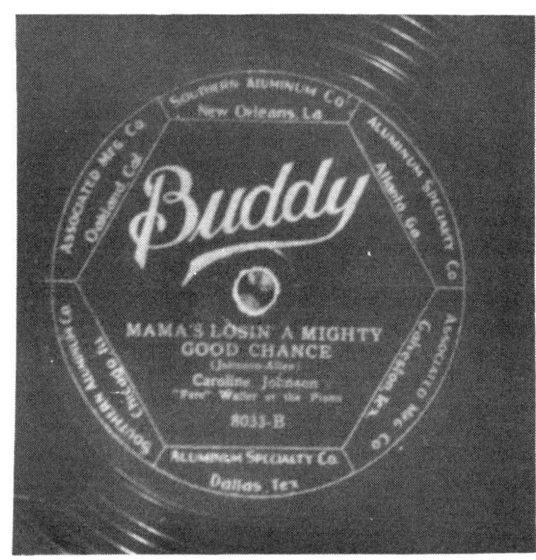

Above: Two labels from the early recording days.
Left: Fats around 1933/4.
Below: Two samples of sheet music covers of Waller compositions.

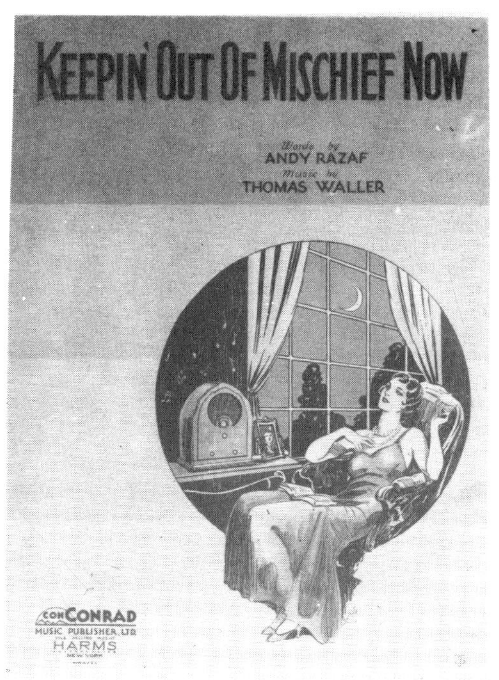

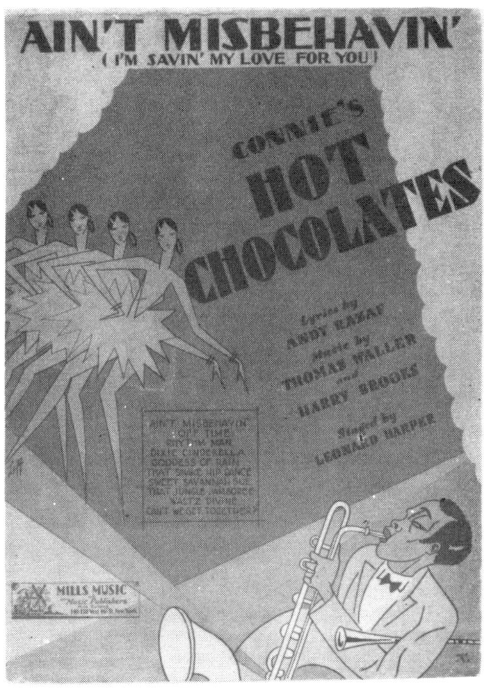

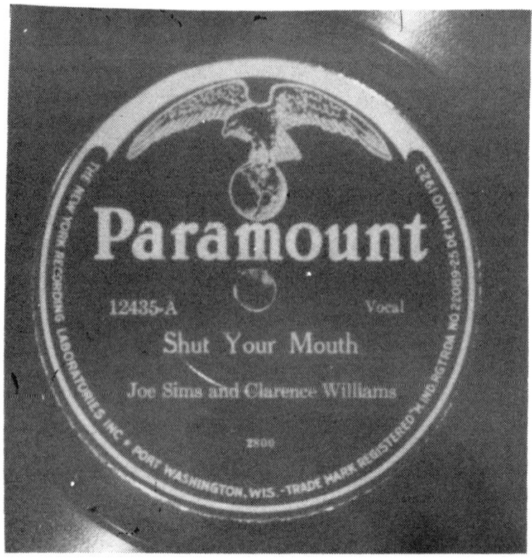

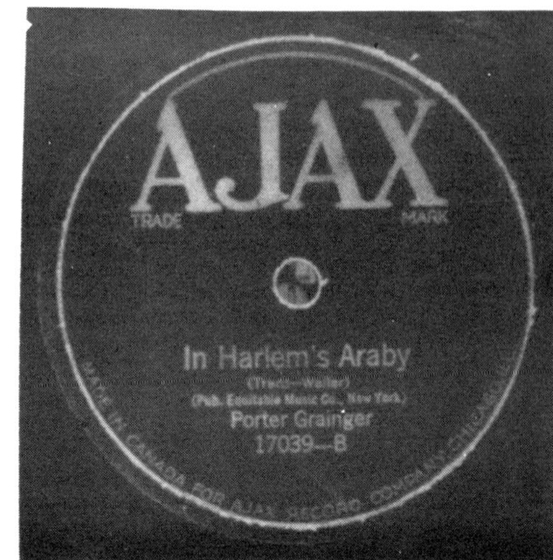

Above: Two more early Waller record labels.
Below: Two more sheet music covers.

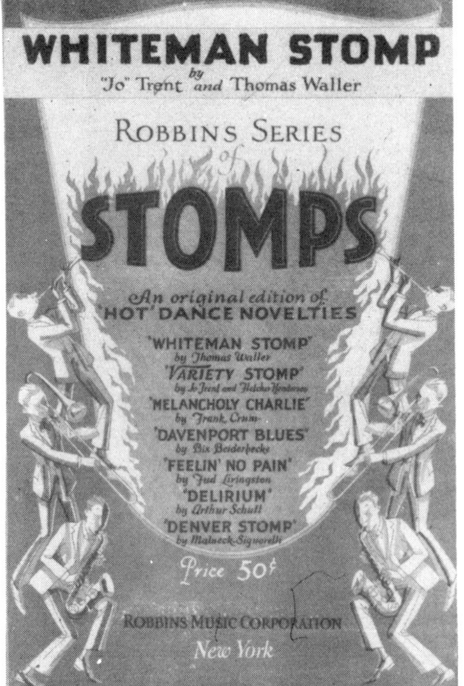

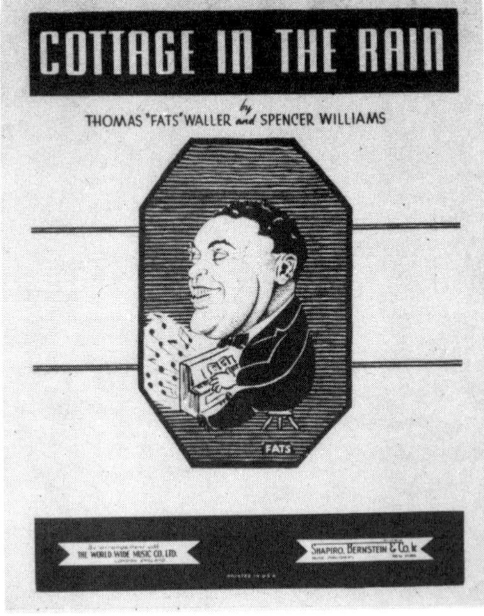

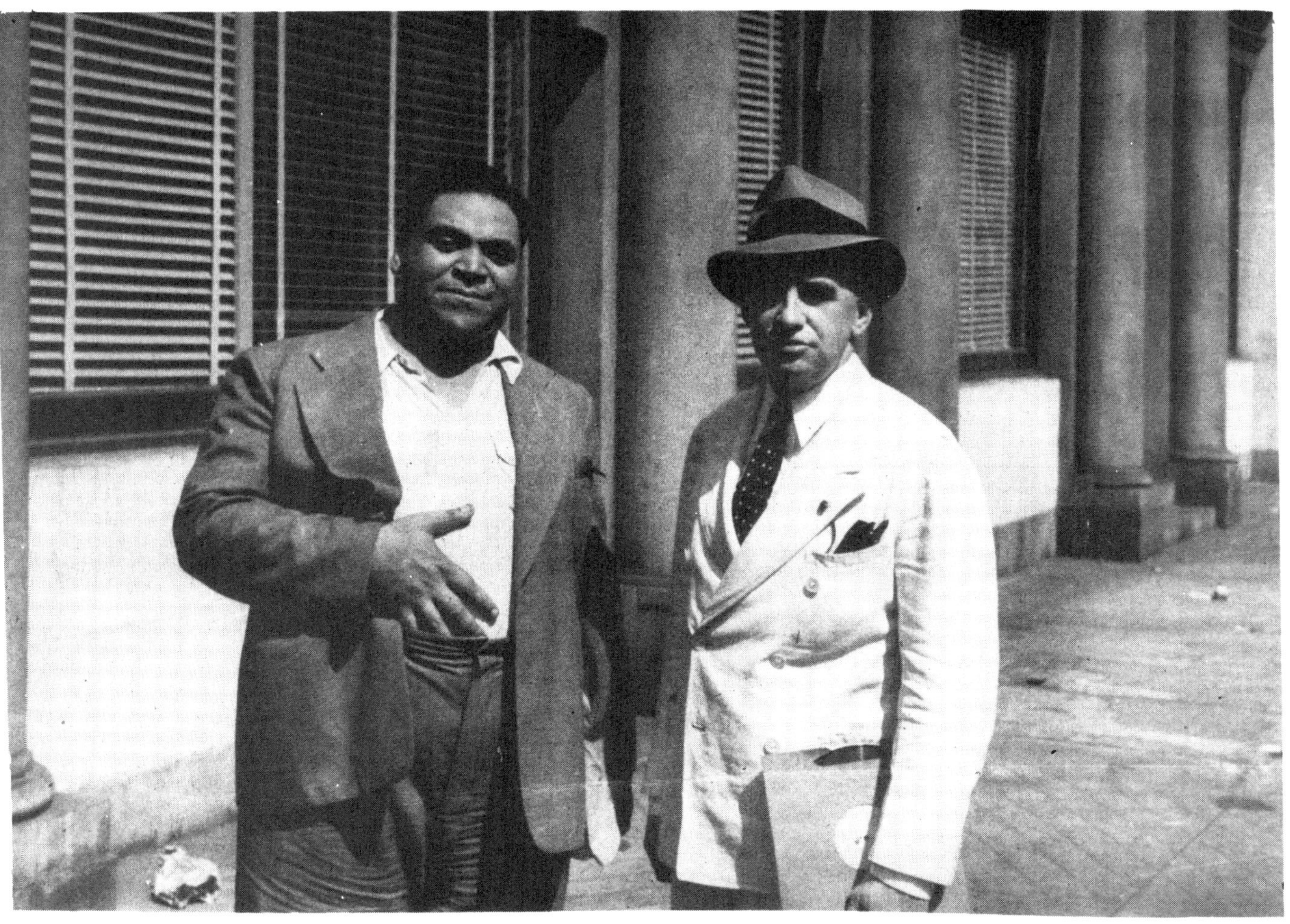

Waller with manager Phil Ponce in 1936. Ponce appears to be carrying a test pressing.

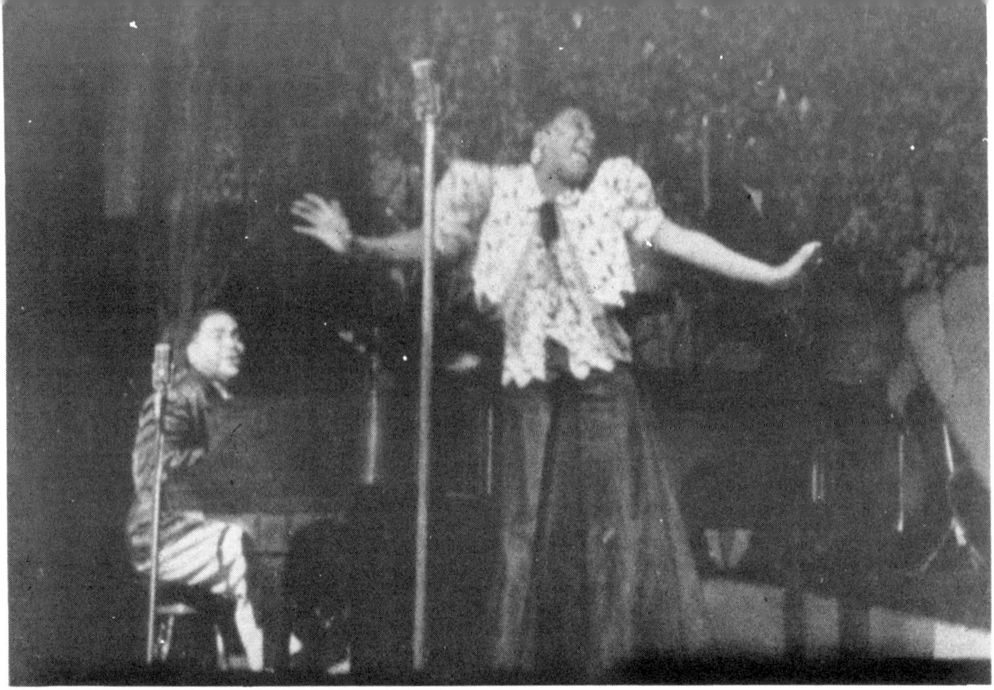

Four action snapshots of the Orchestra.

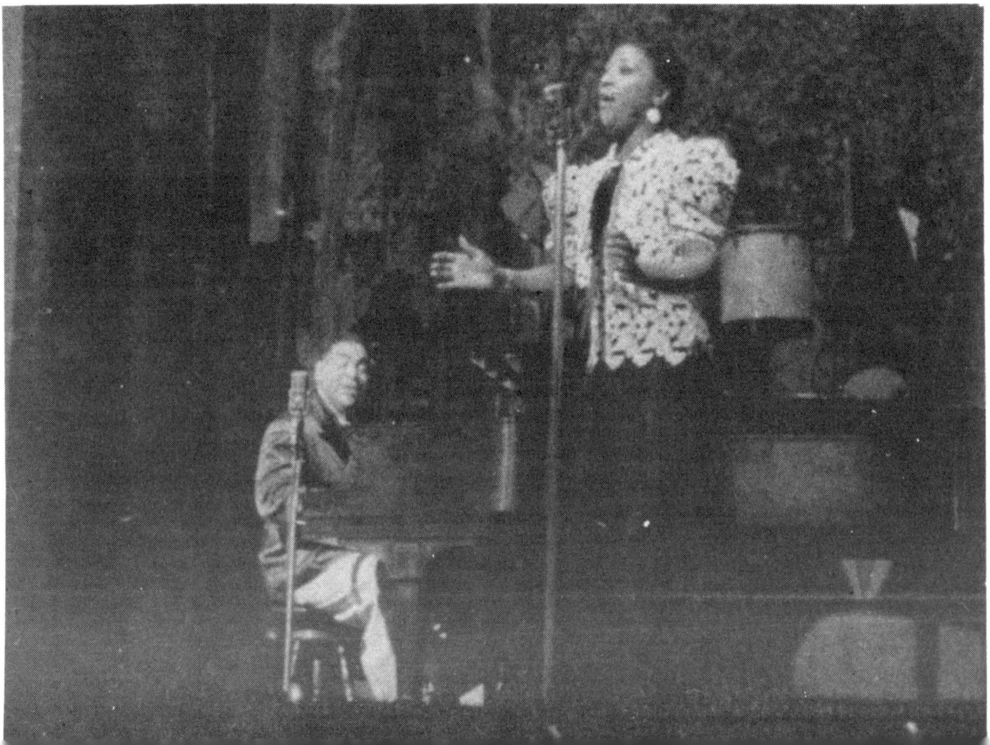

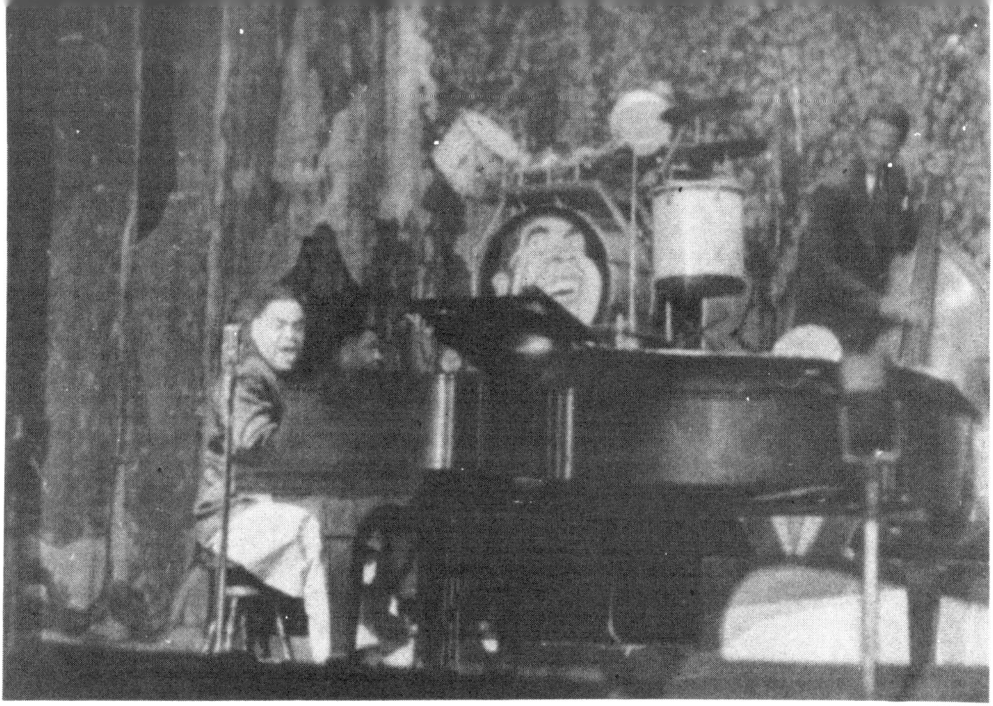

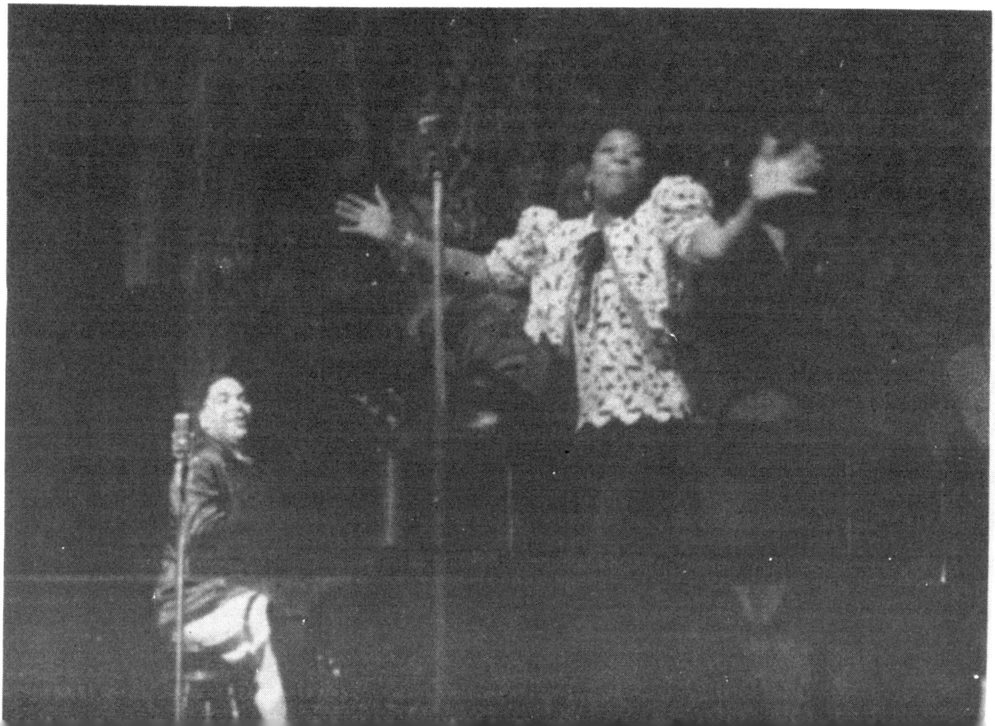

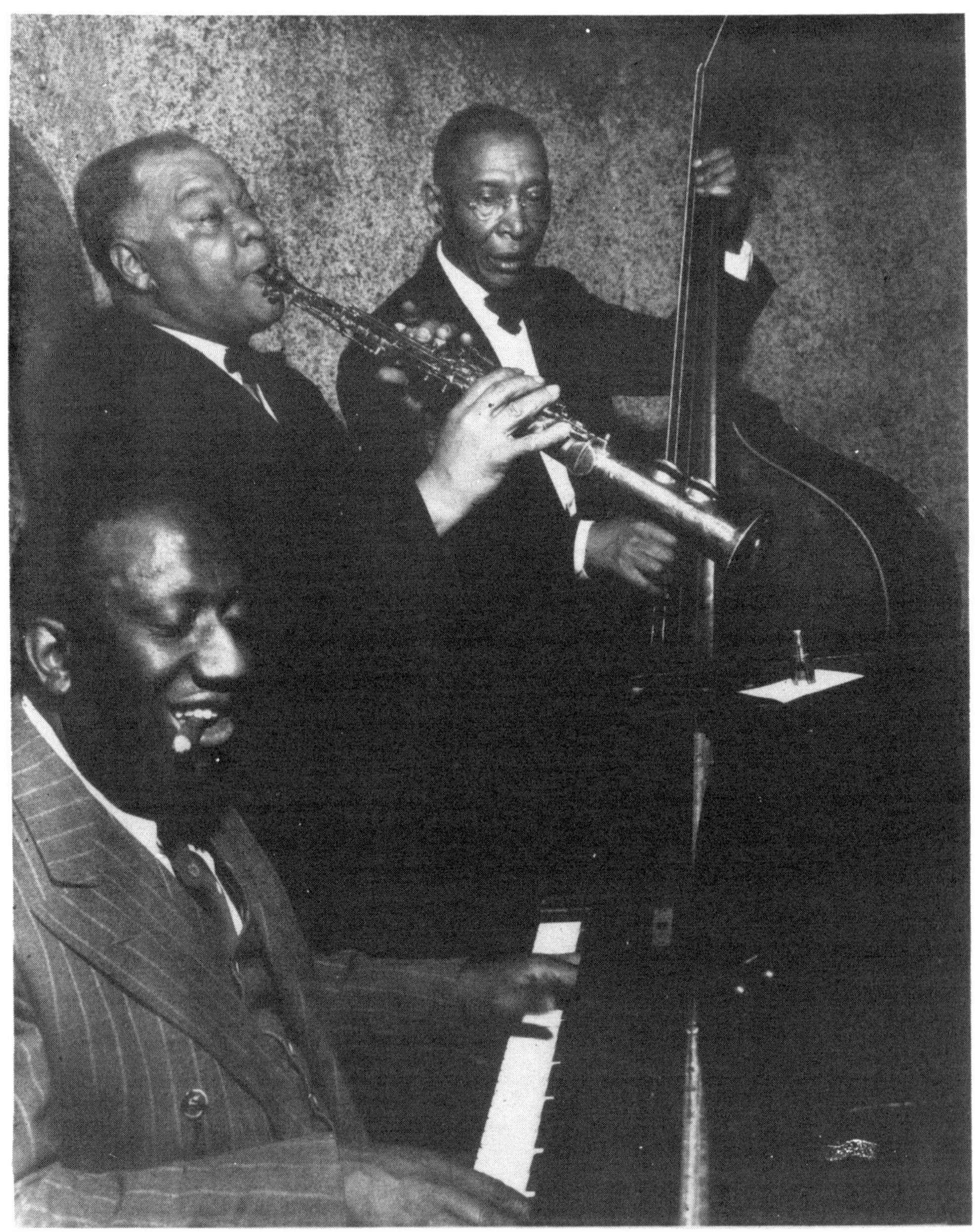

A fine action shot of James P. Johnson with Sidney Bechet and Pops Foster.

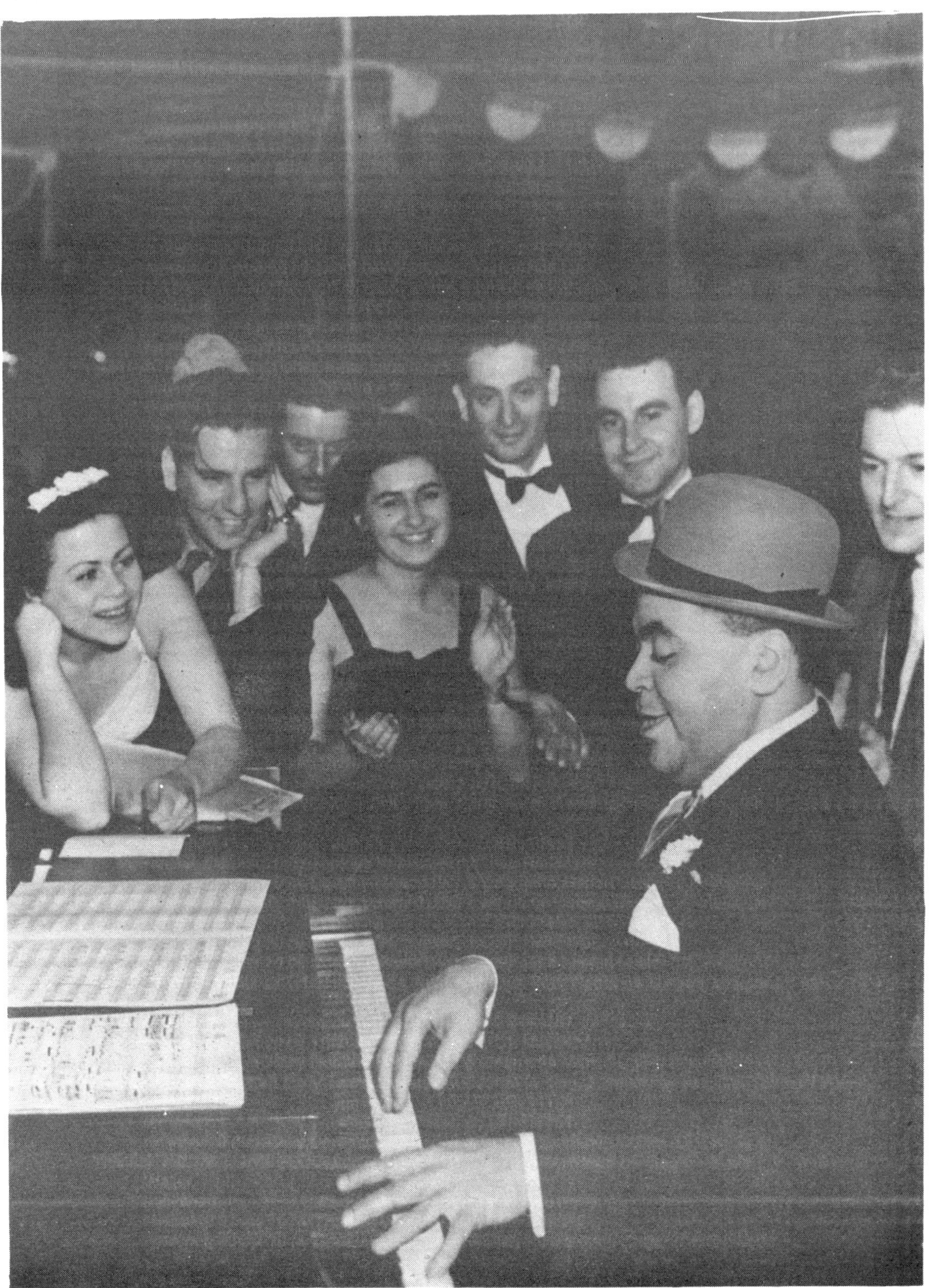

Fats in action with a group of admirers looking on.

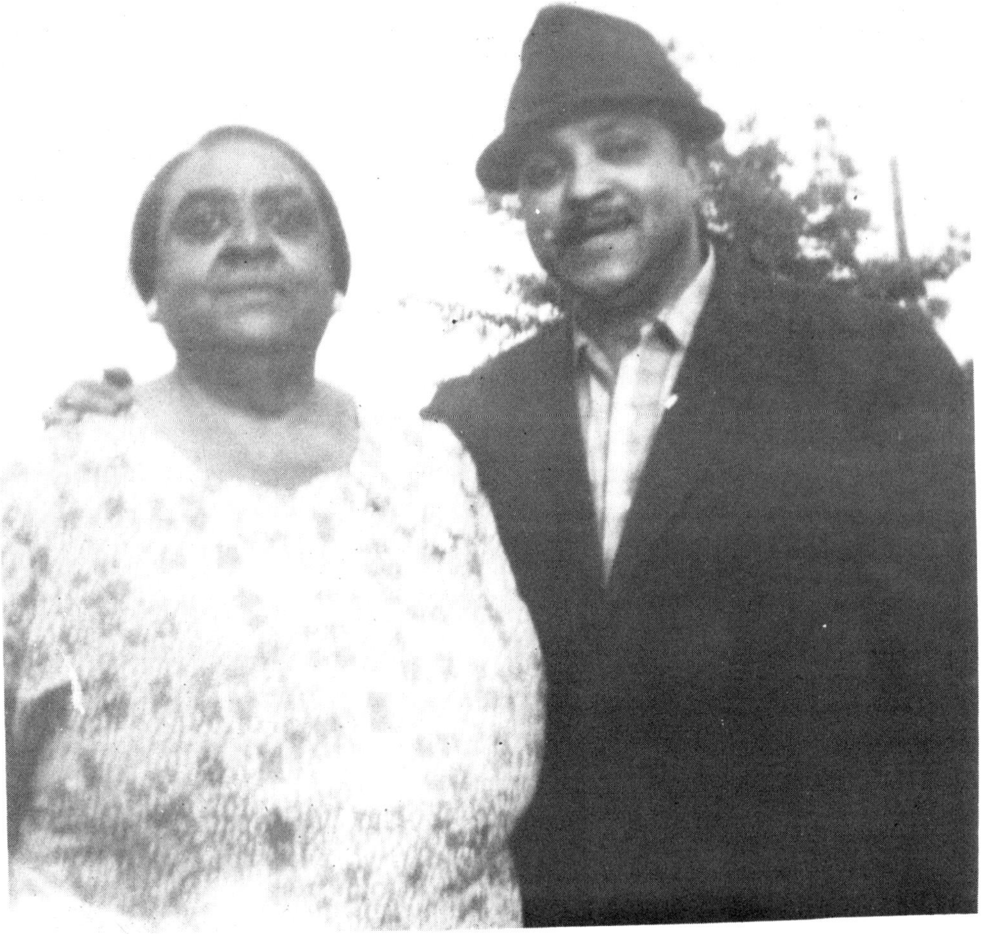

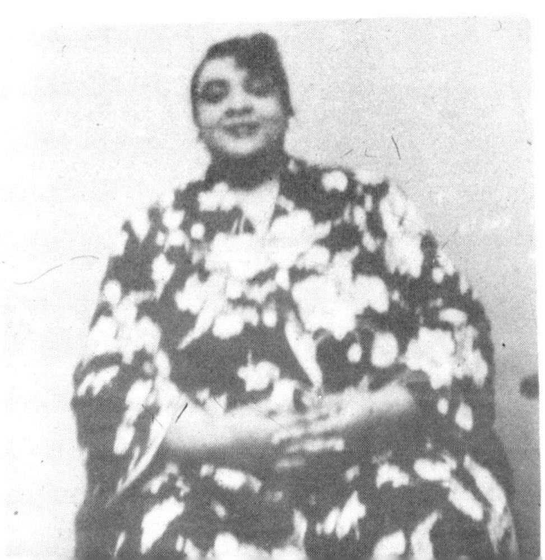

Some family members.
Above: Naomi Waller Washington (Fats's sister) with Henry Parker on 6 May 1968.
Left: An earlier snapshot of Naomi from 1948.
Right: Henry Parker with Thomas Waller, Jr., on 8 June 1968.

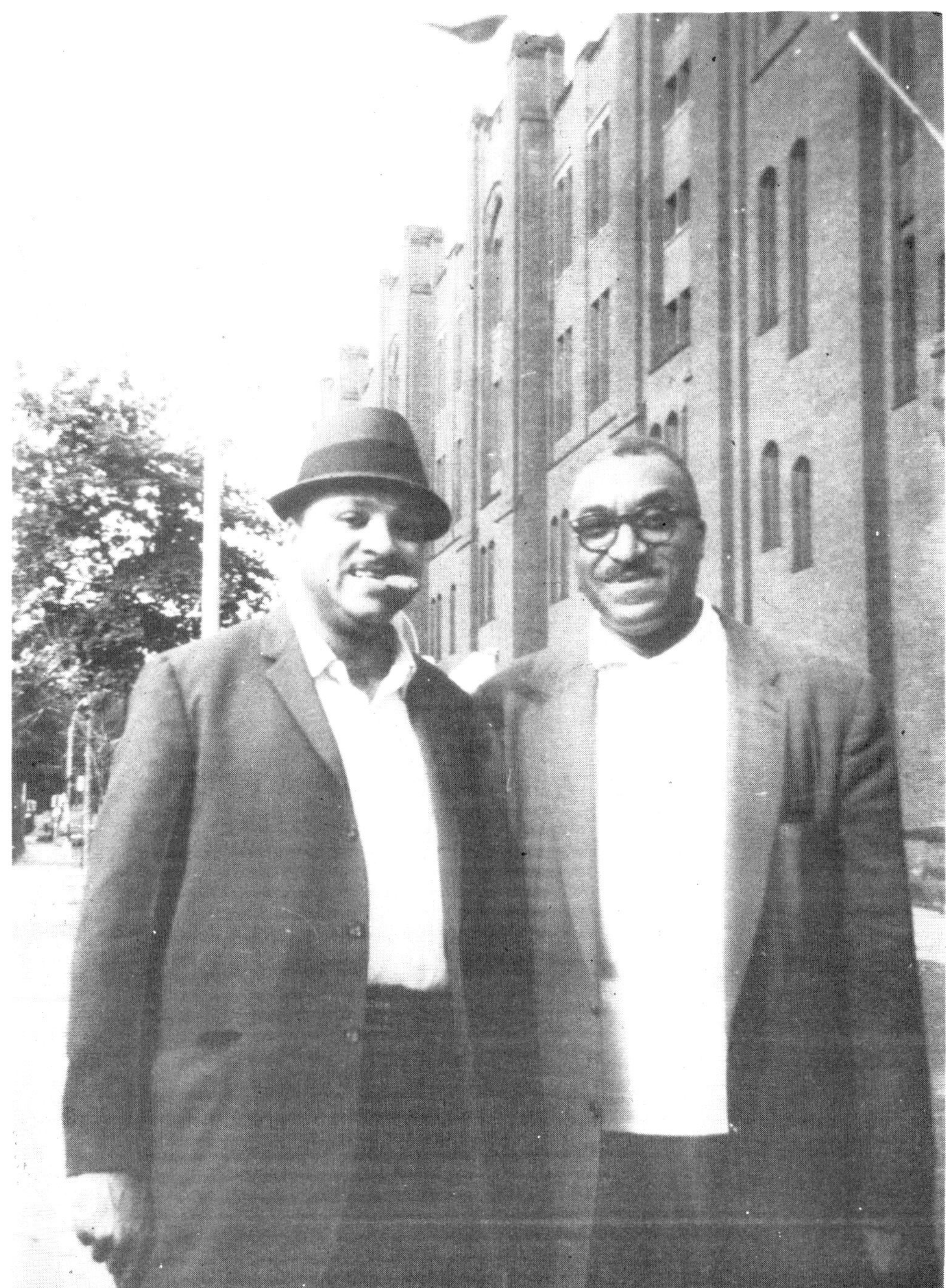

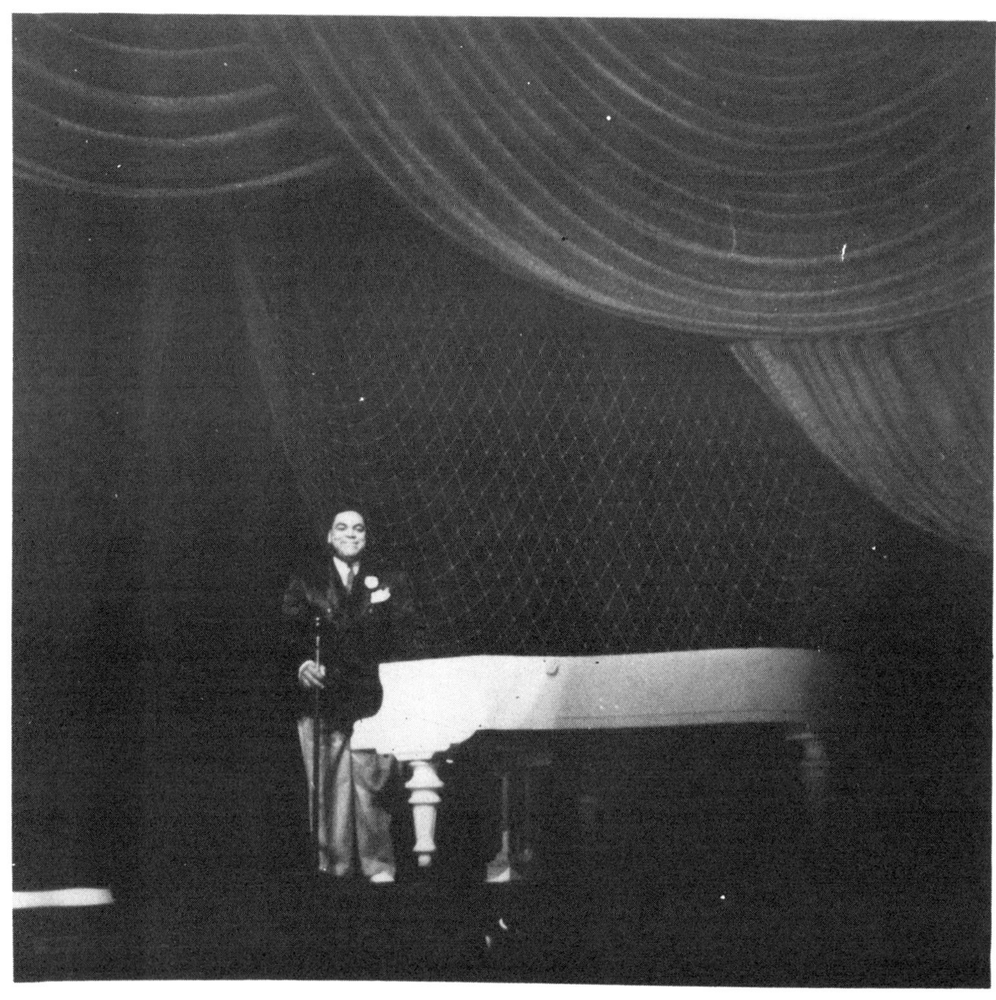

Two shots of Fats on stage at the London Palladium during his first week.

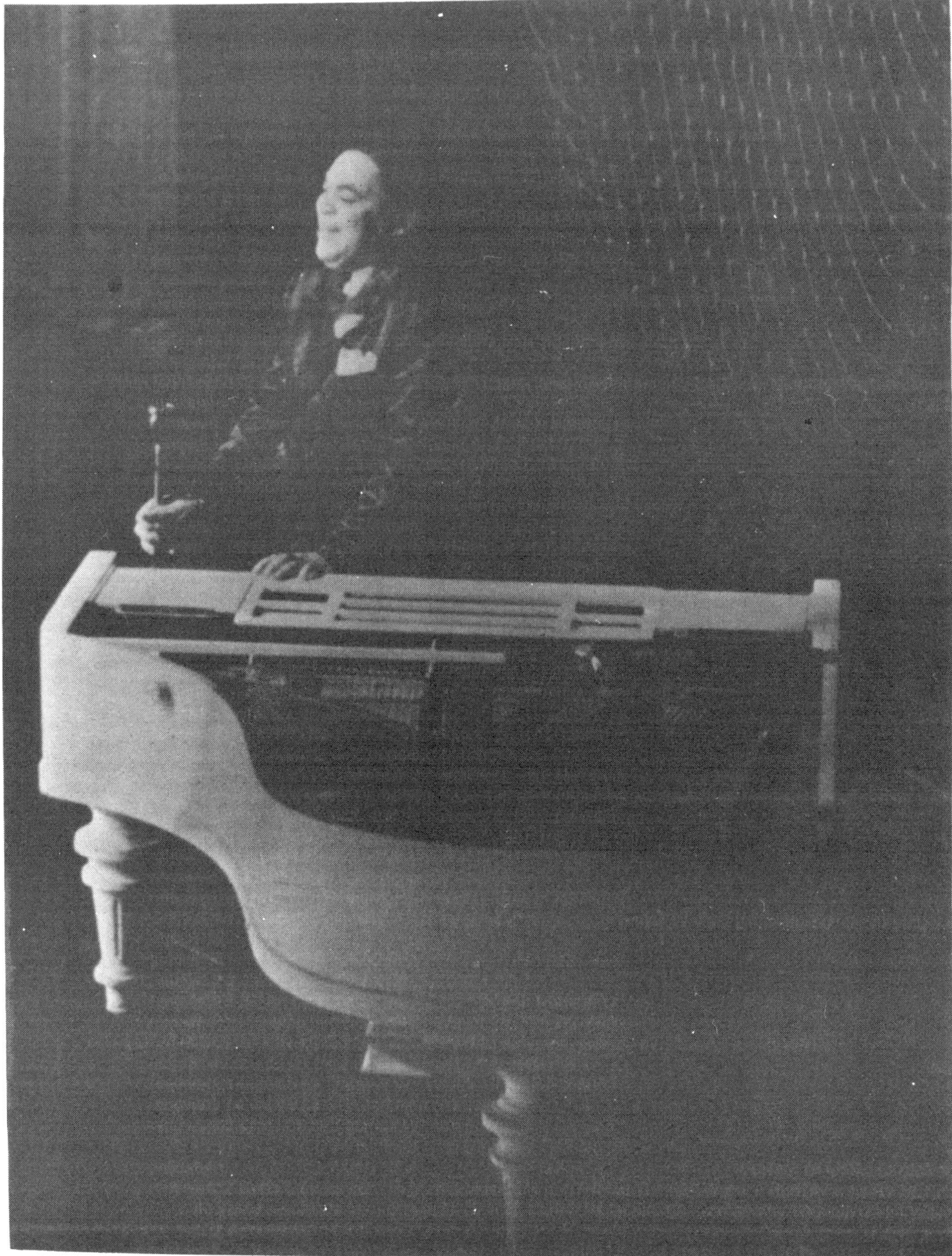

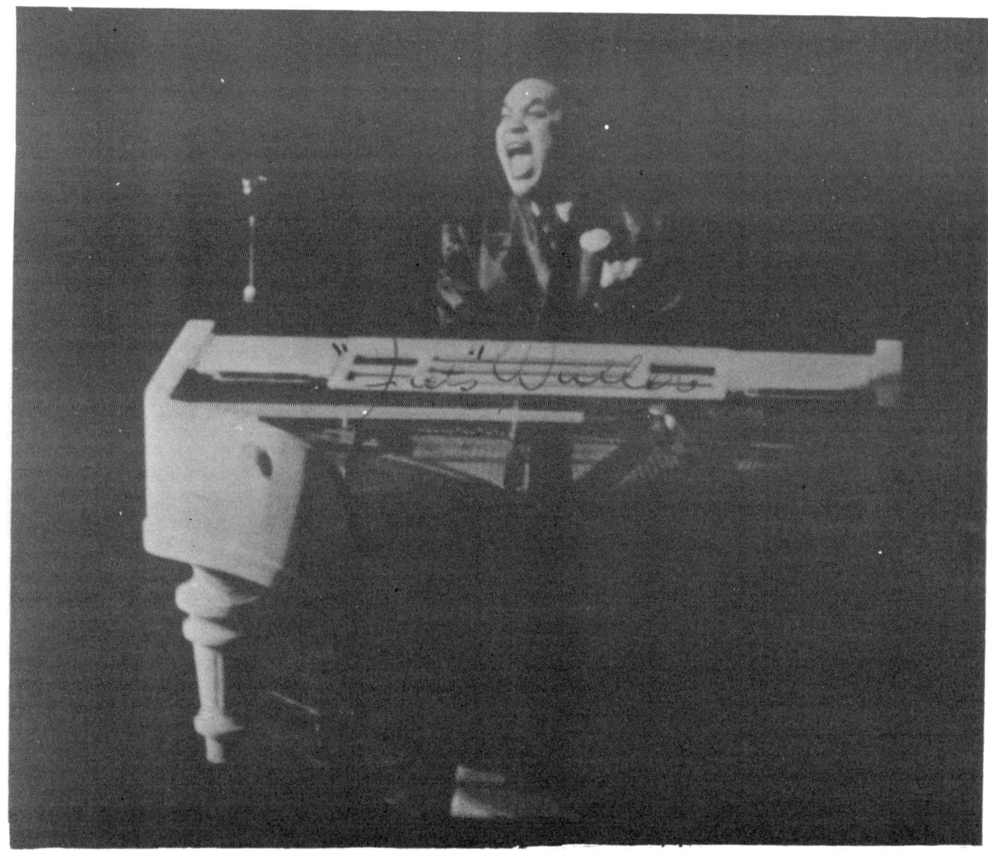

7. First Time in England

LOWE, HITE and STANLEY

"Extremes of Fun"

8. First Time in England

"FATS" WALLER

The World's Greatest Rhythm Pianist

Walter Winchell, in the New York "Daily Mirror"—says:—

"The present controversy between Benny Goodman and Louis Armstrong over the title 'King of Swing' is belittled by musicians . . . they contend that neither of them plays an instrument of rhythm . . . "FATS" WALLER however, 'toys' with a piano, and if we were the committee of one to decide matters—"FATS" would certainly get the title."

Matinées—WEDNESDAY and THURSDAY at 2.30 p.m.

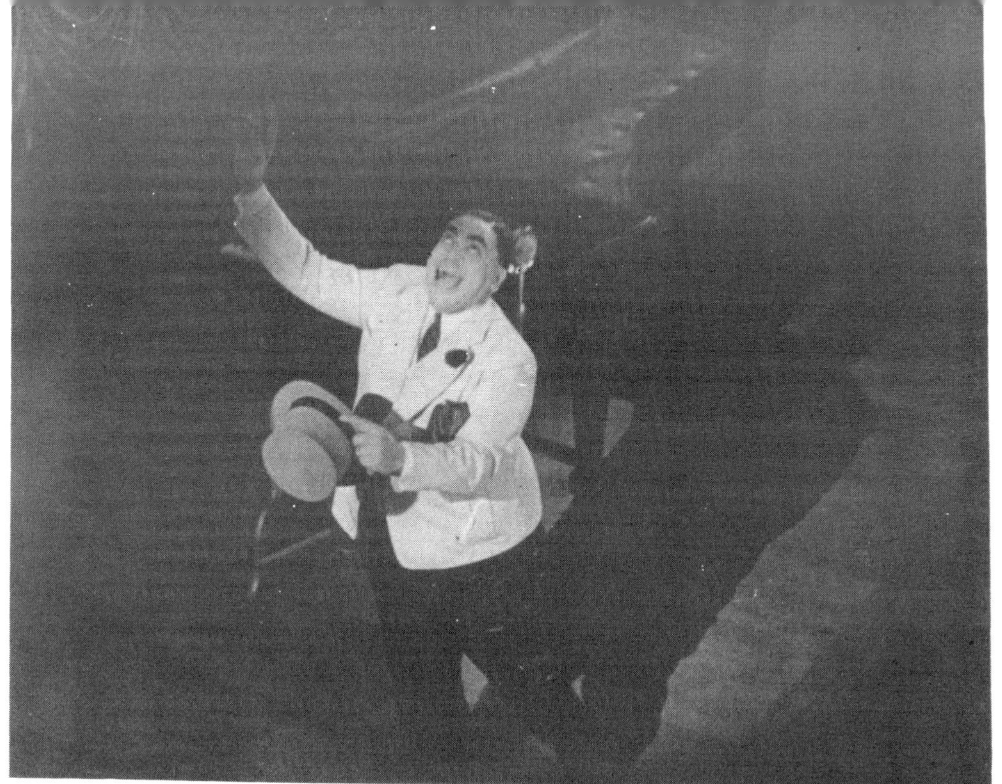

Left: Another shot from the first week, this one autographed by Fats, and above, one from the second, complete with grey topper.

At the time of Waller's visit, Palladium programmes were small books, largely given over to advertising and with a standard cover design. For both weeks, Fats closed the first half and the two respective panels are shown left and below.

7. EDDIE RIO and BROTHERS

Comedy Features from R.K.O. "New Faces of 1938"

8. "FATS" WALLER

The World's Greatest Rhythm Pianist

Walter Winchell, in the New York "Daily Mirror"—says:—

"The present controversy between Benny Goodman and Louis Armstrong over the title 'King of Swing' is belittled by musicians . . . they contend that neither of them plays an instrument of rhythm . . . "FATS" WALLER however, 'toys' with a piano, and if we were the committee of one to decide matters—"FATS" would certainly get the title."

This Theatre is fully licensed. Bars open till 11 p.m.

Matinées—WEDNESDAY and THURSDAY at 2.30 p.m.

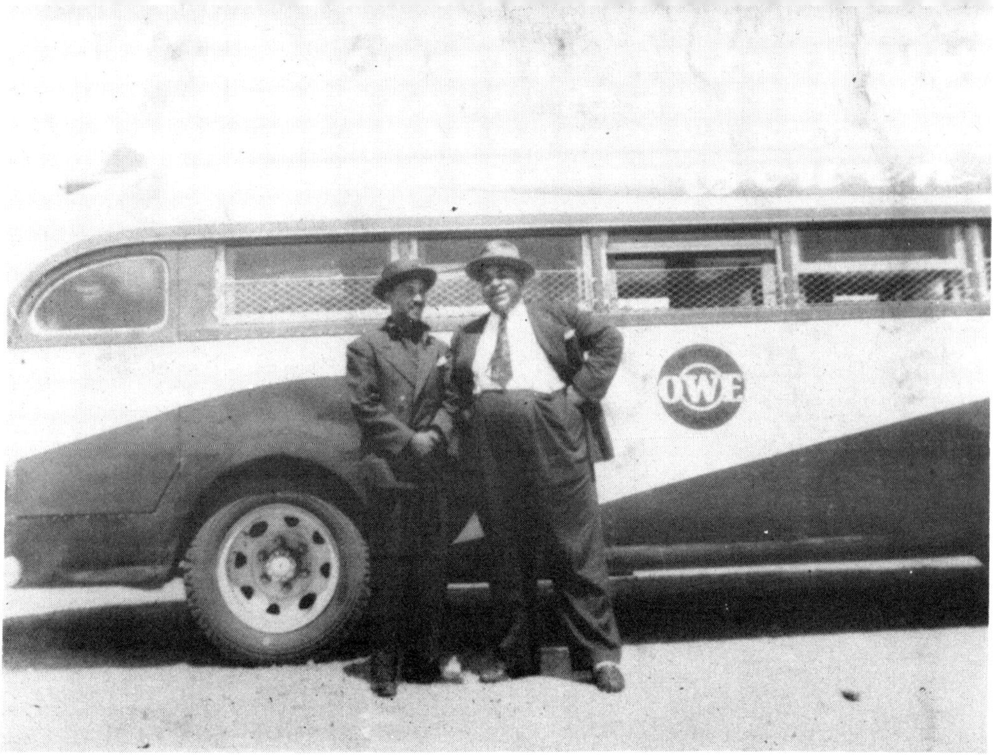

OWE

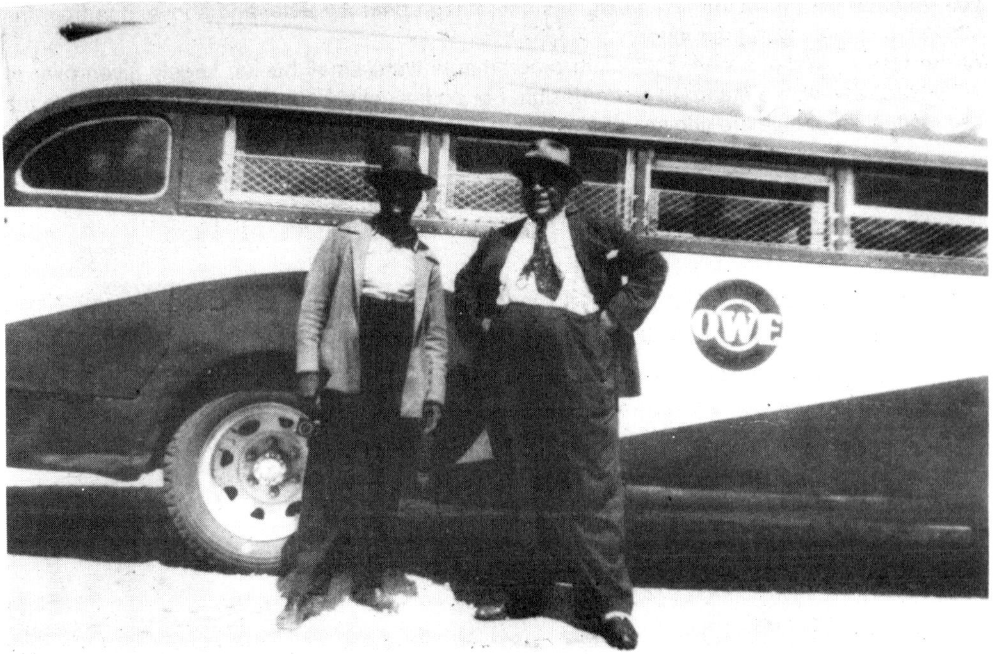

OWE

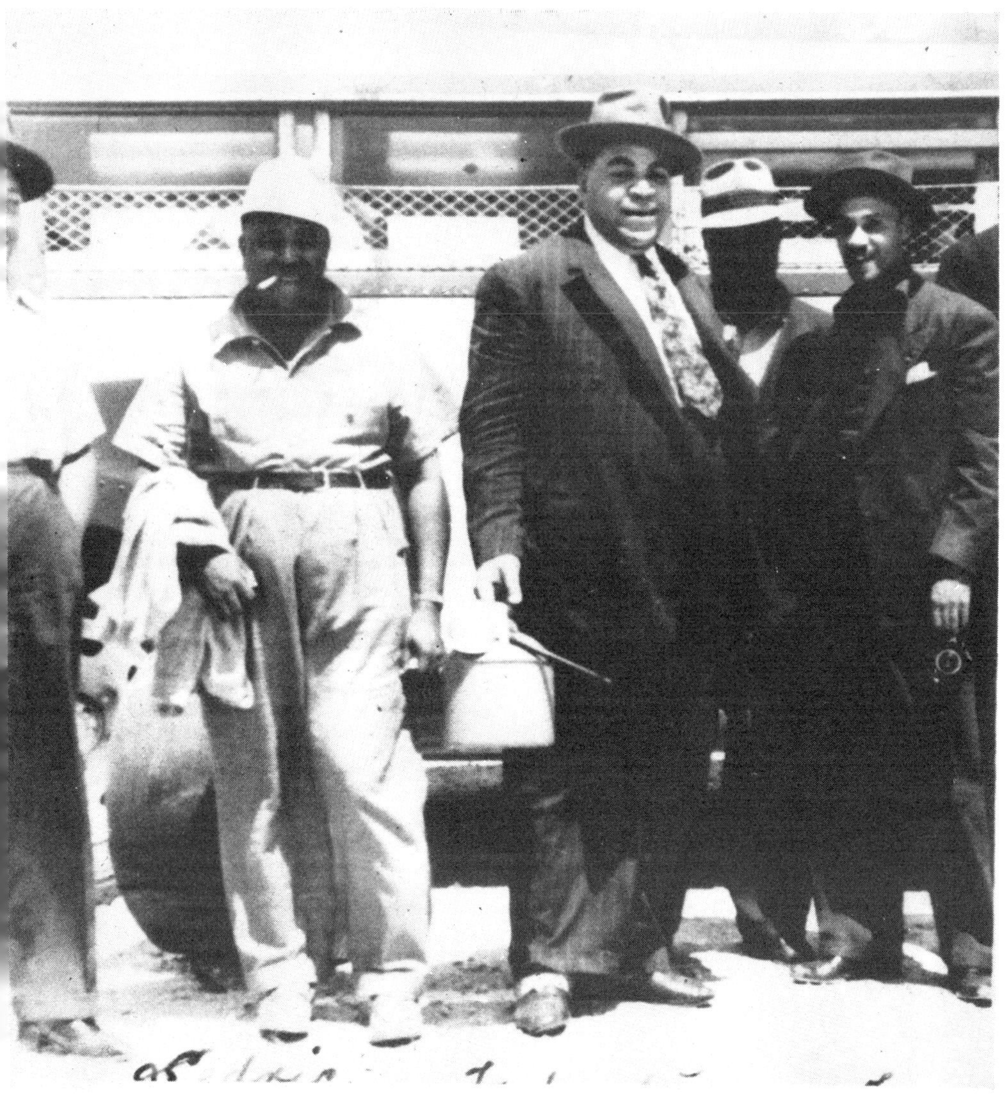

Above: Gene Sedric, Fats, George Wilson and Freddie Skerritt in front of the band bus in El Paso, Texas, on 25 May 1940.
Left: Two shots probably on the same day, but marked only "Texas 1940". Skerritt is with Fats in the top shot, but the musician in the bottom shot is unidentified.

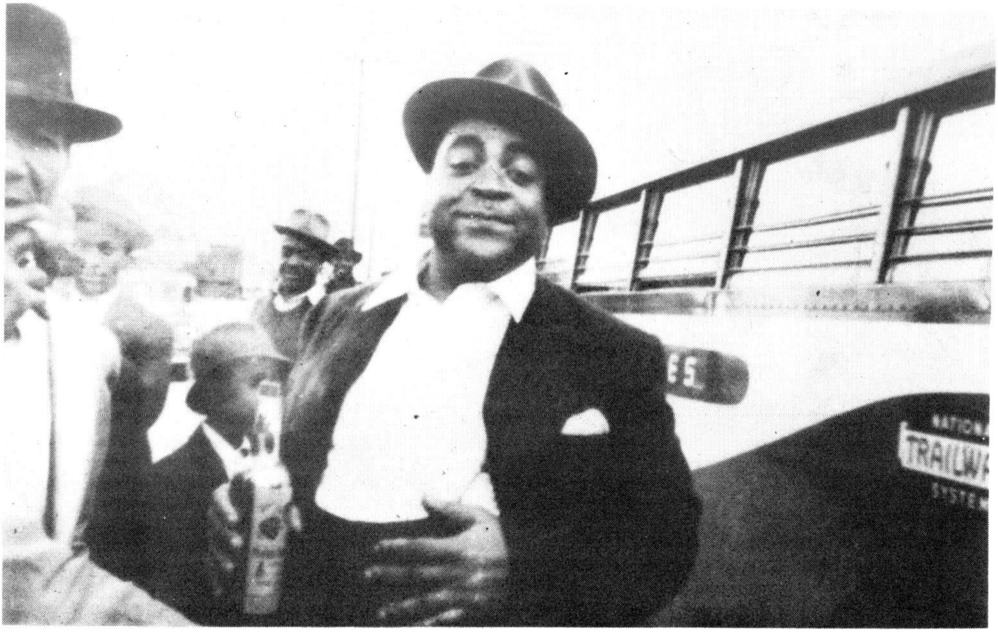

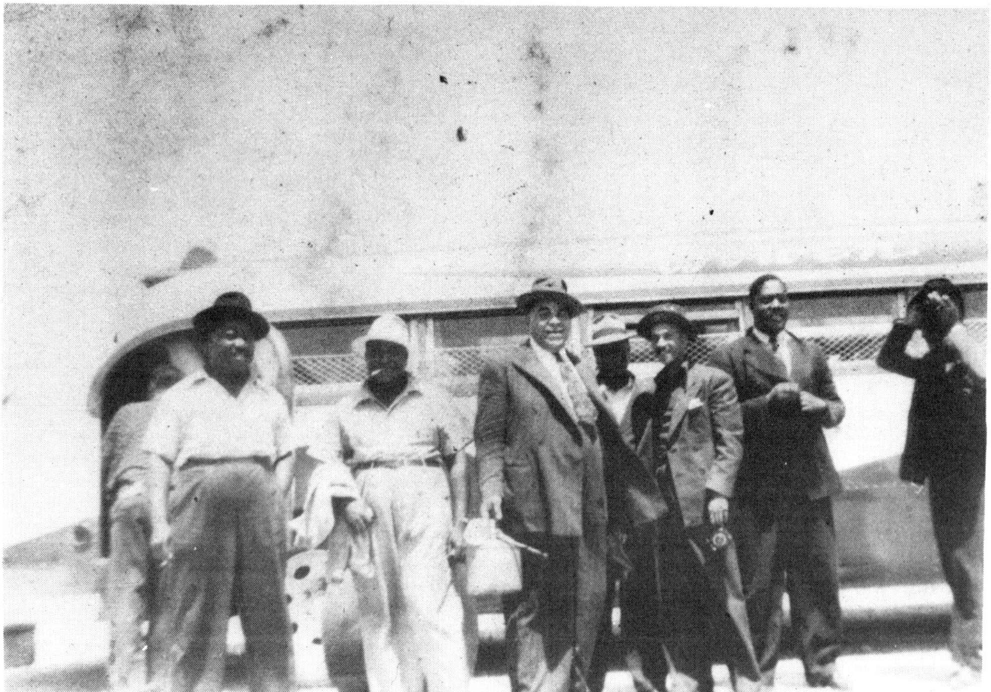

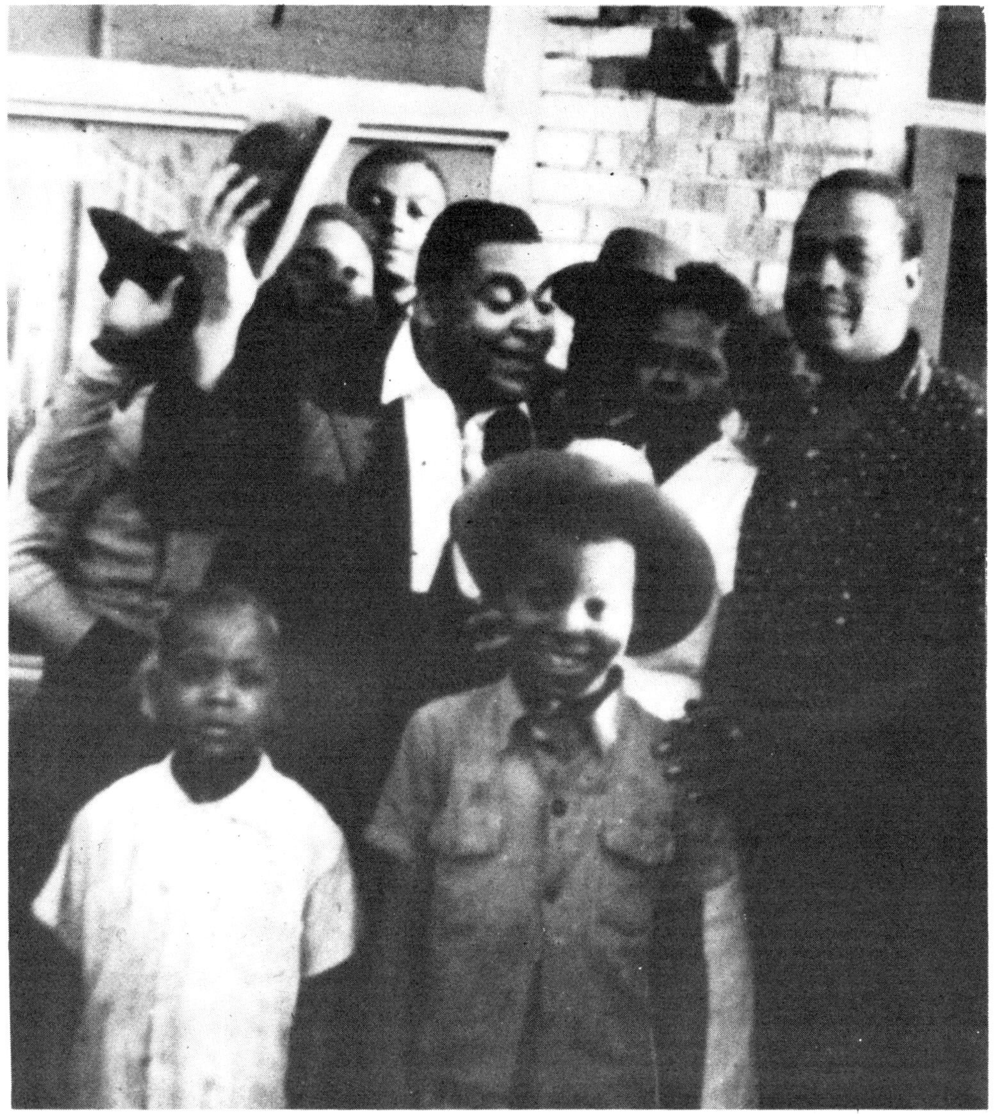

Above: Fats and John Hamilton with fans, "Texas, 1940."
Left top: Fats 'Feeling no pain' in Wichita Falls, Texas, on 23 May 1940.
Bottom: Don Donaldson, Gene Sedric, Fats, George Wilson Freddie Skerritt and 'Slim' Moore in front of the bus in El Paso, Texas, 25 May 1940.

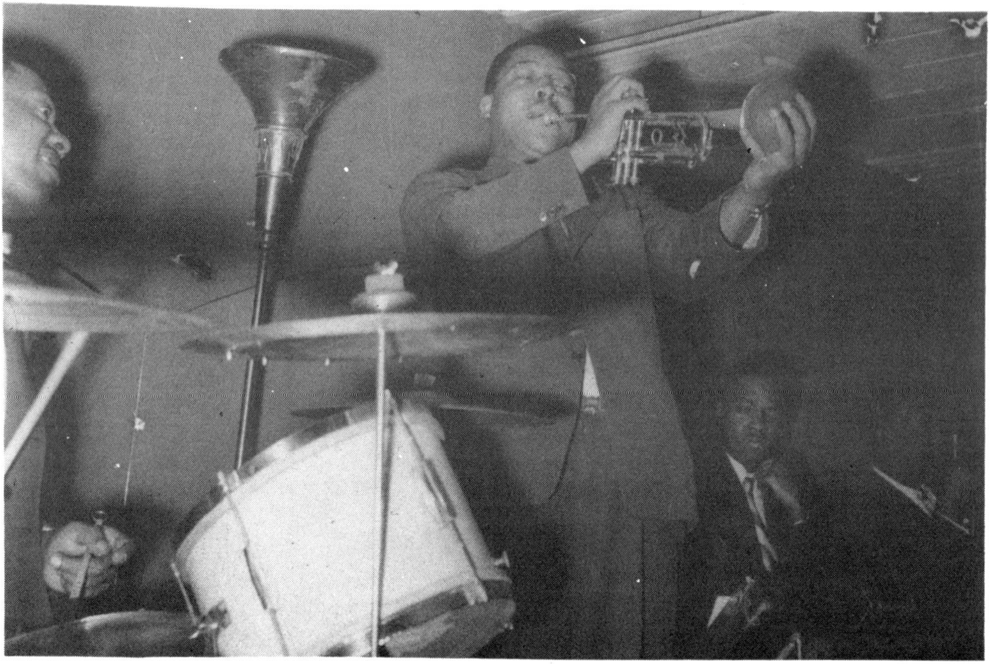

Some former Waller sidemen. Above: John Hamilton. Below: Franc Williams and George James. Right top: Bobby Williams. Right bottom: Al Casey.

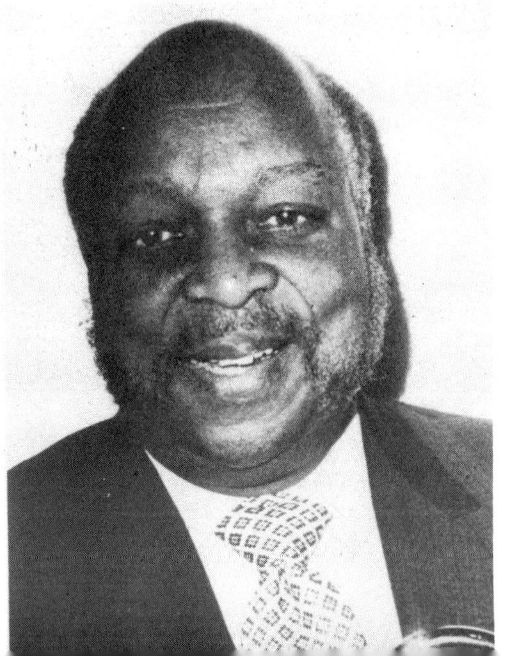

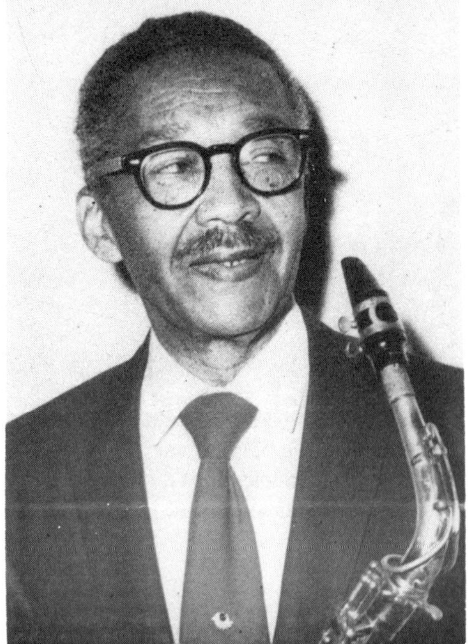

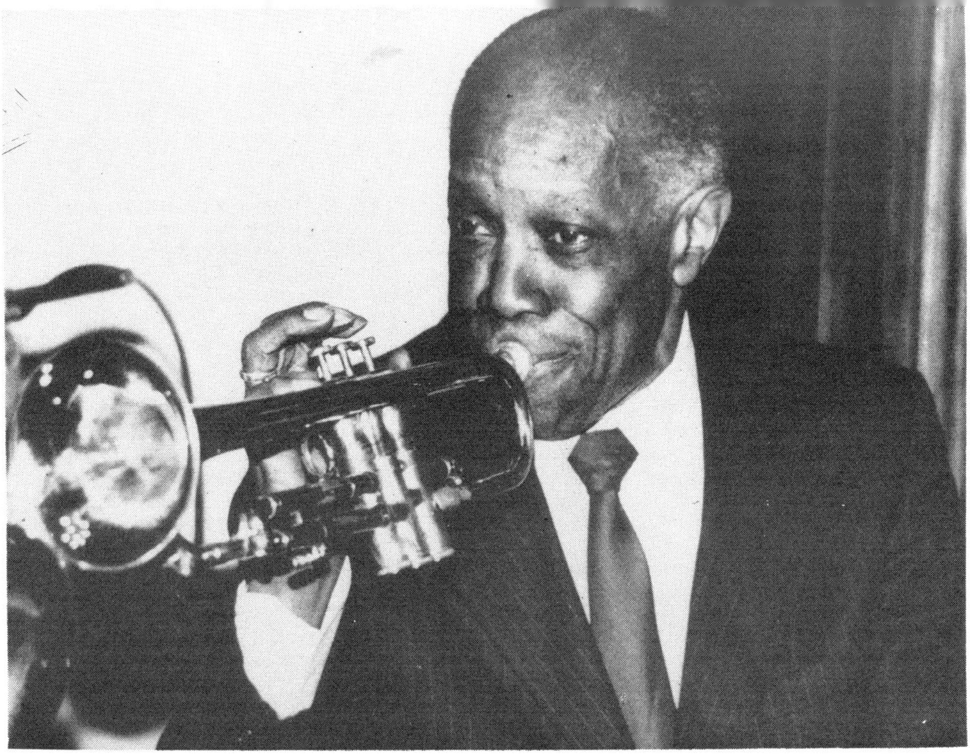

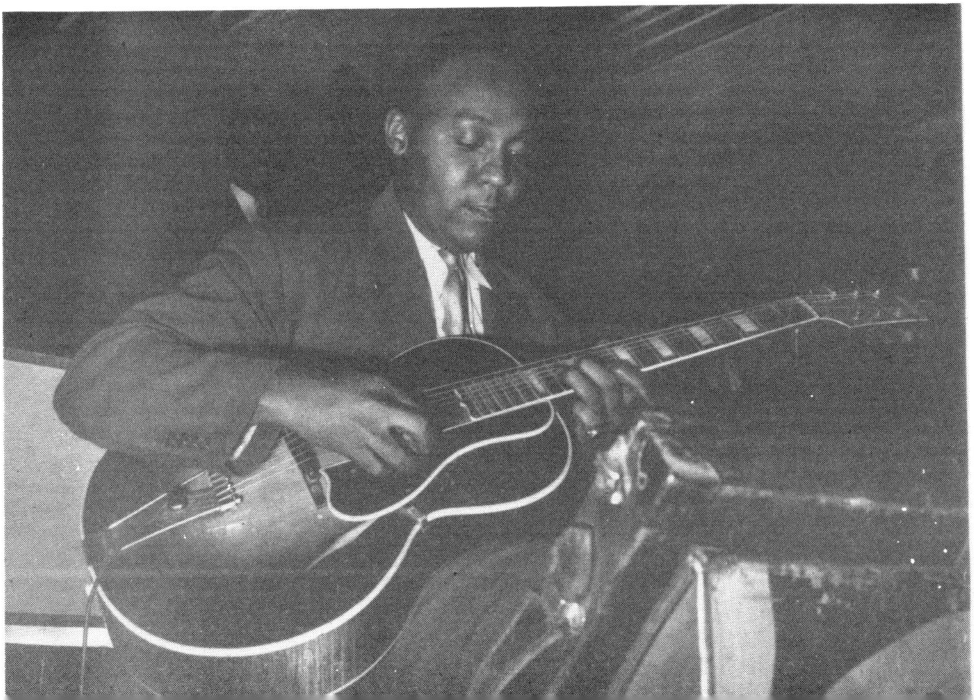

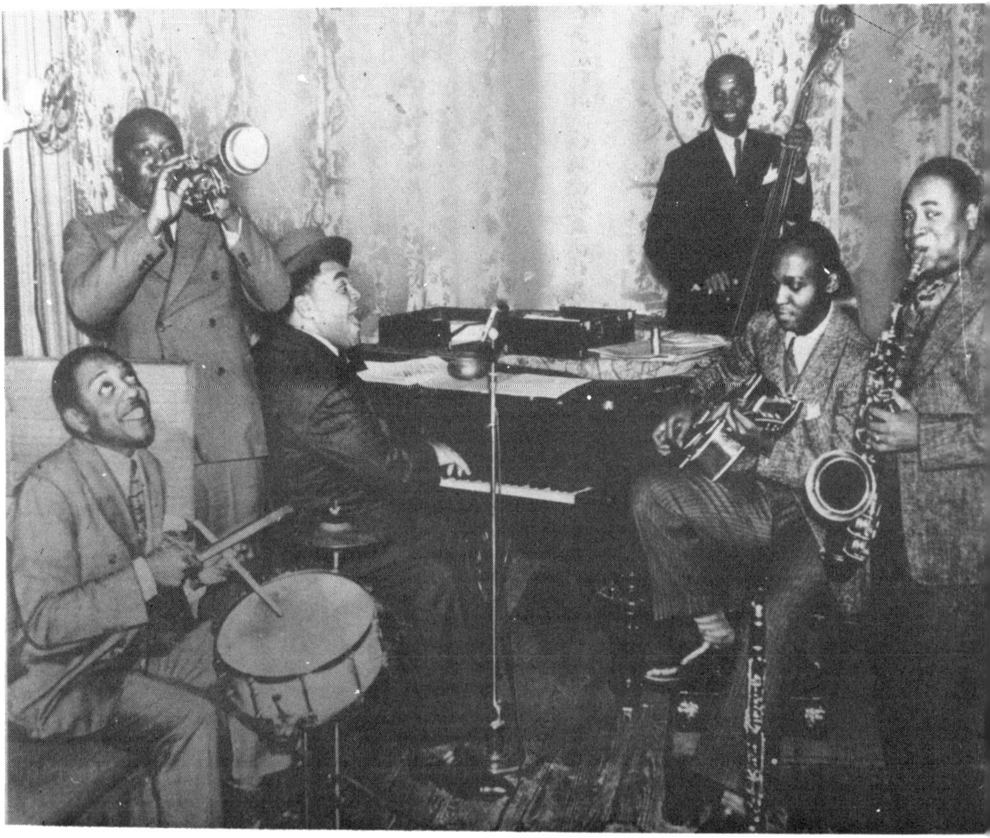

The 1938 "Rhythm" of Slick Jones, Herman Autrey, Fats, Cedric Wallace, Al Casey and Gene Sedric in action. Below: Victors from Argentina and China.

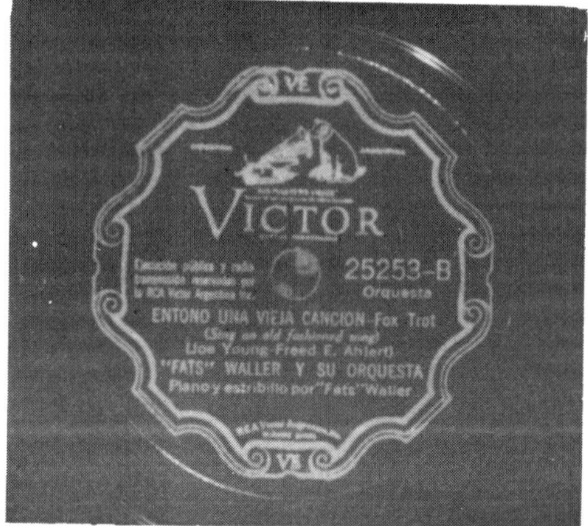

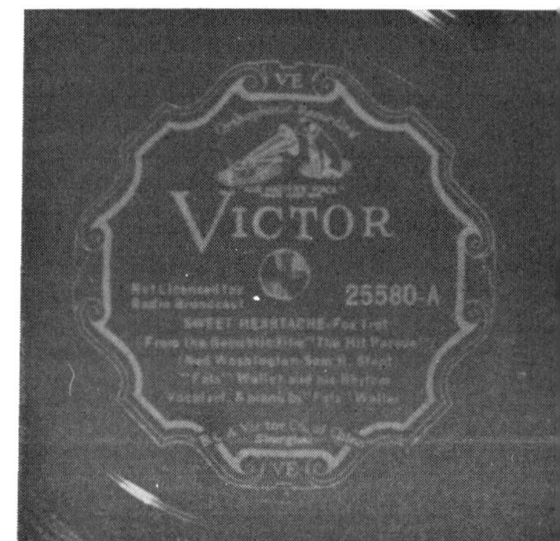

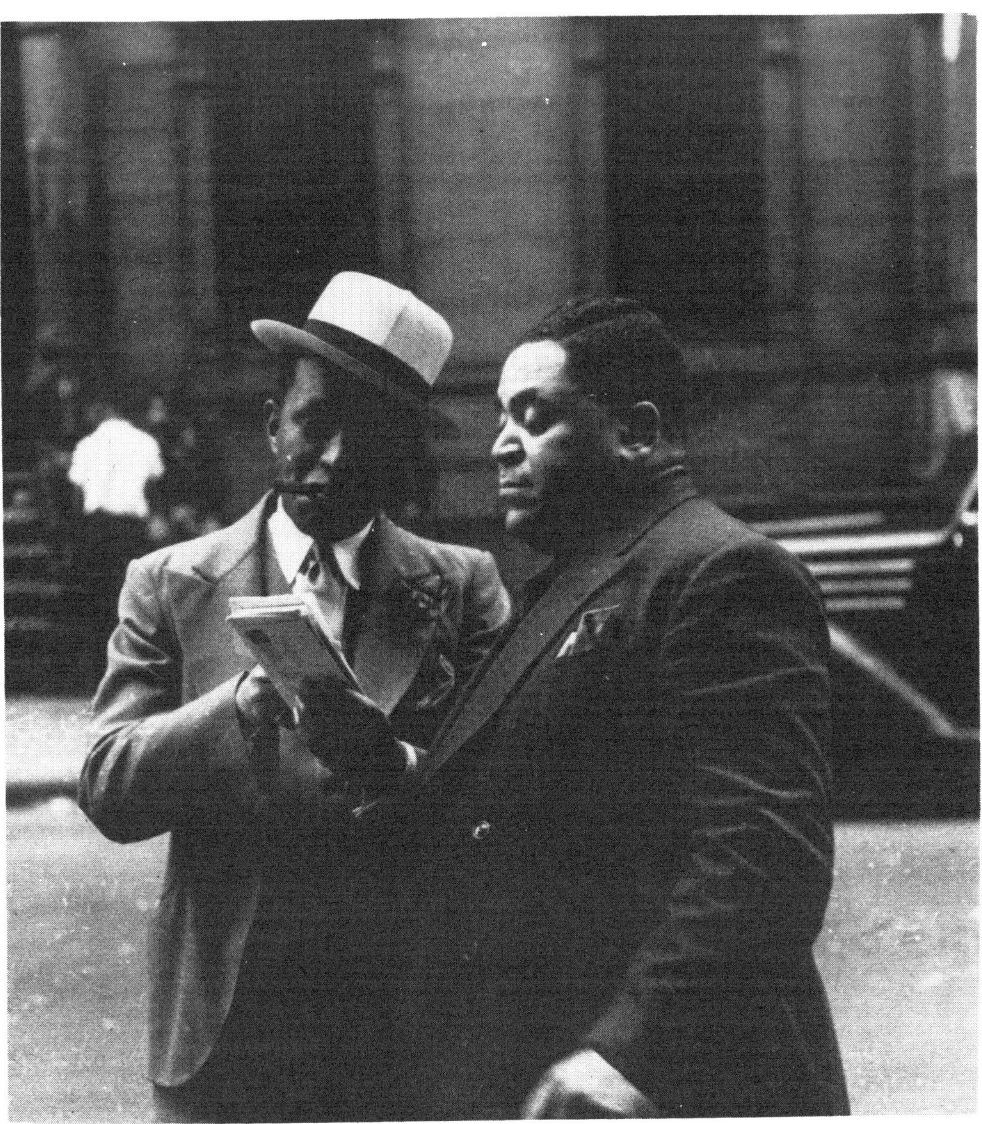

This shot of Fats and Willie 'The Lion' Smith in serious discussion, plus the six on the next three pages were taken by Charles Peterson on the street behind the Apollo theatre in May 1937 when Fats was celebrating his birthday. and headlining at the theatre. He is seen patronising the food stalls on the street, with his fellow artists, inspecting some suiting material, and with his arm round his neice.

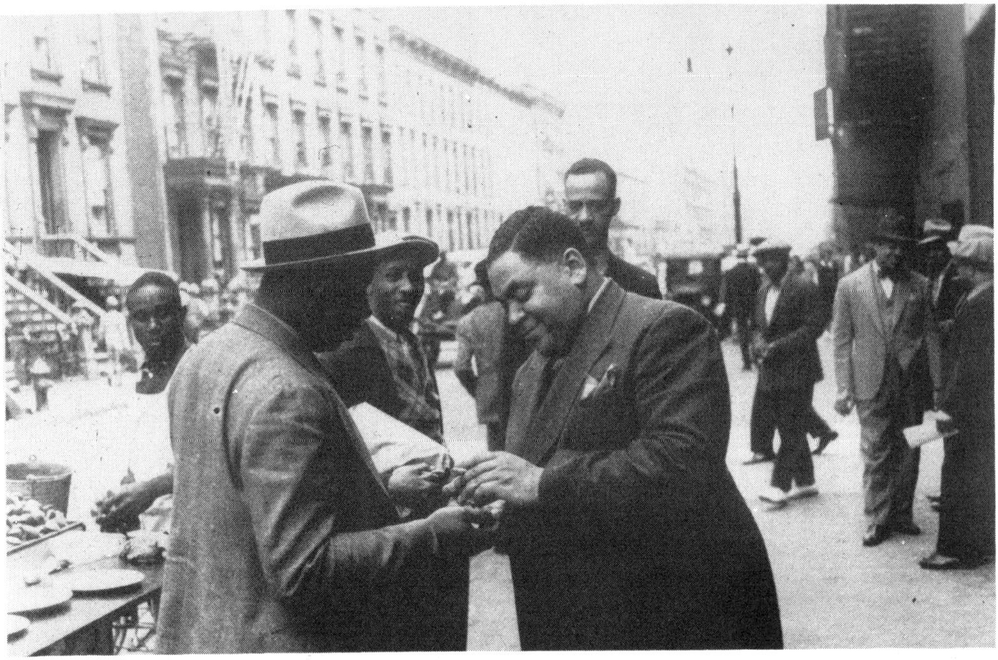

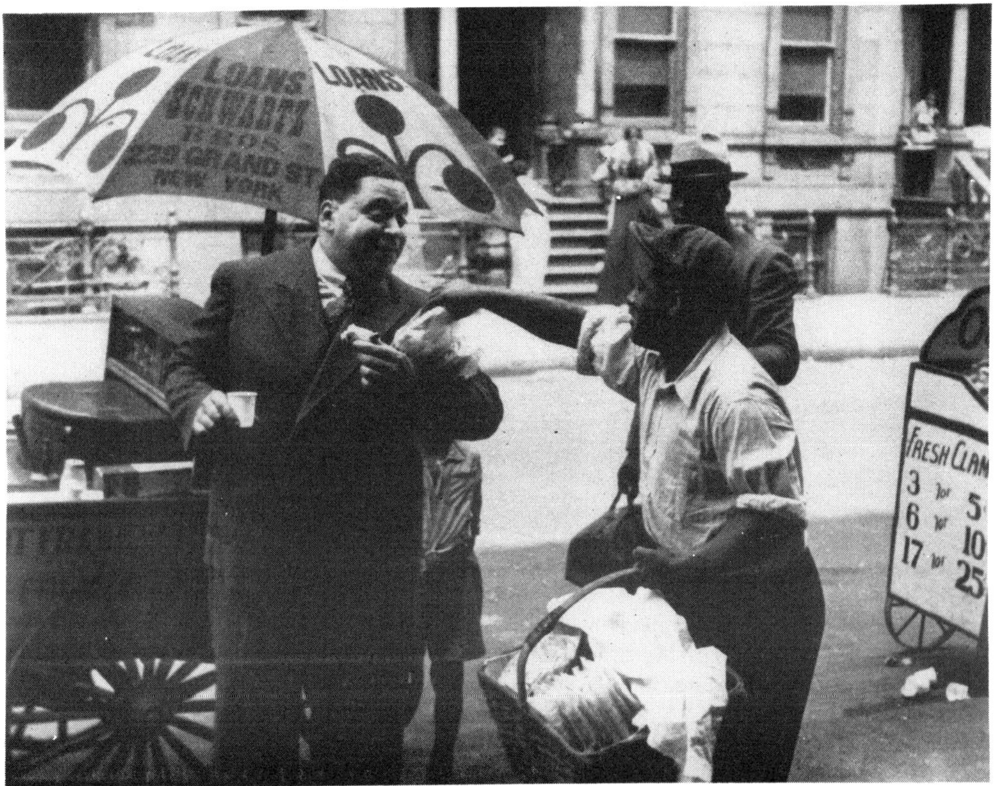

LOANS LOANS
SCHWARTZ
229 GRAND ST
NEW YORK
FRESH CLAM
3 for 5
6 for 10
17 for 25

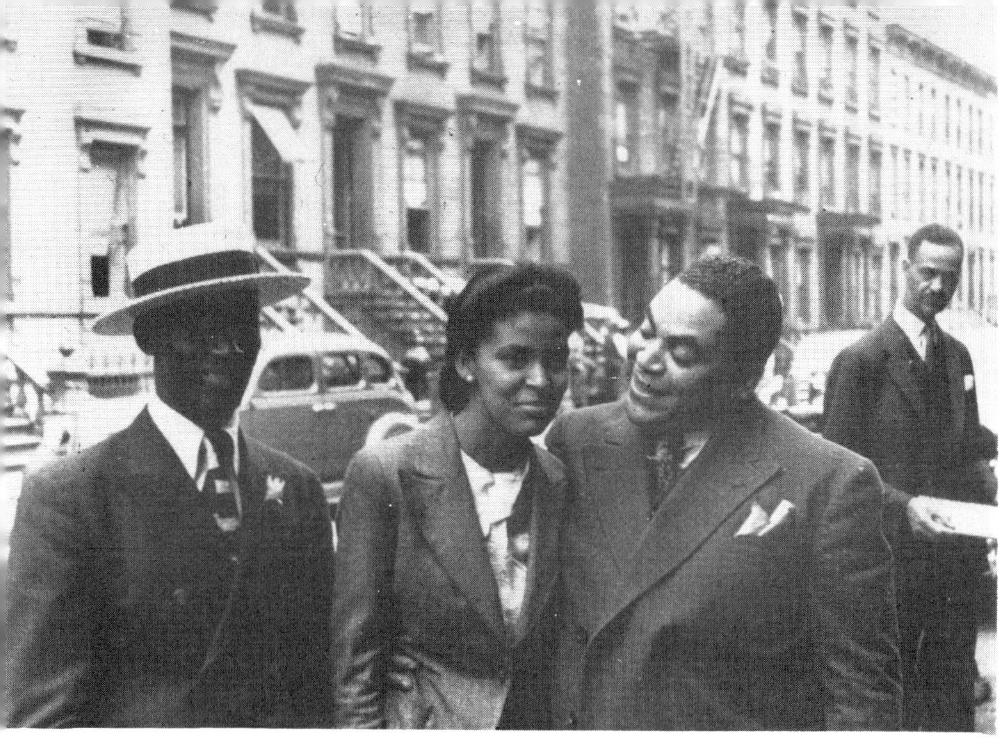

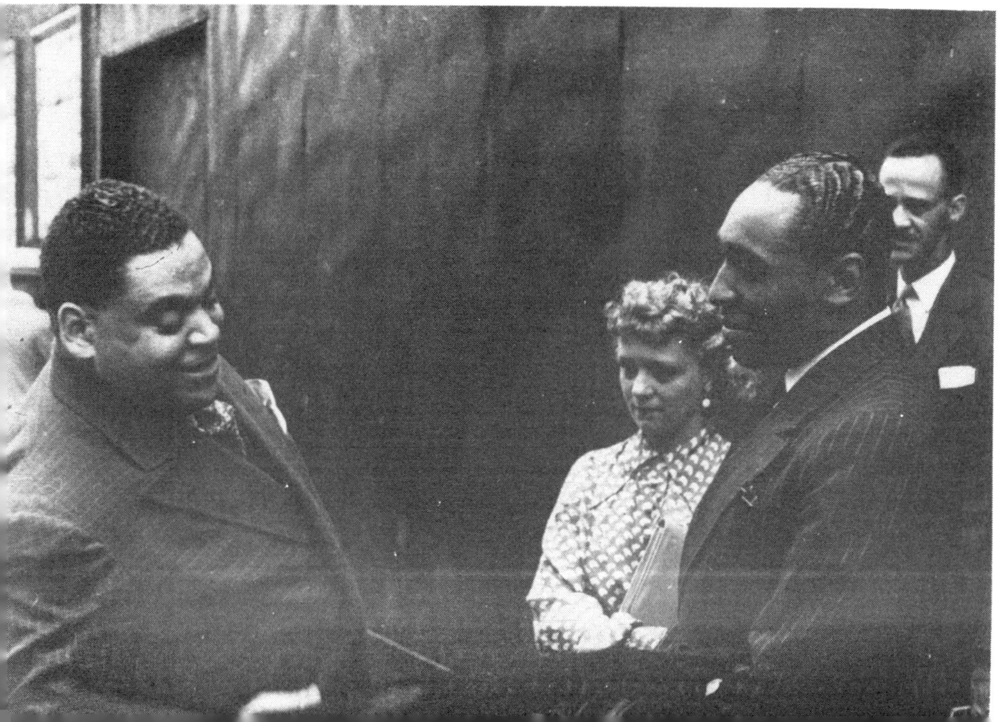

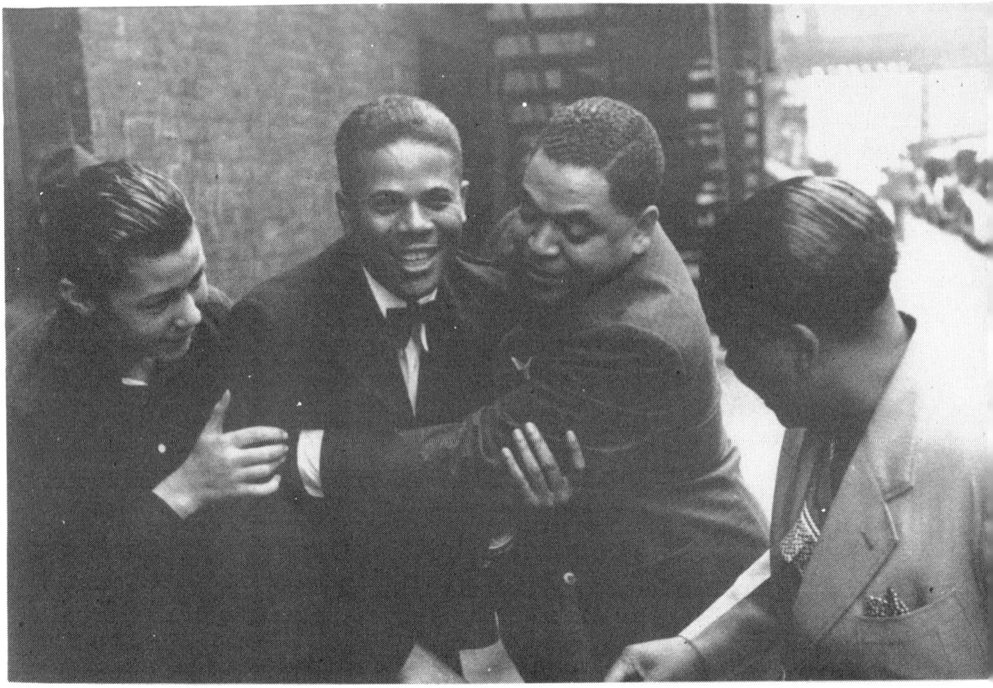

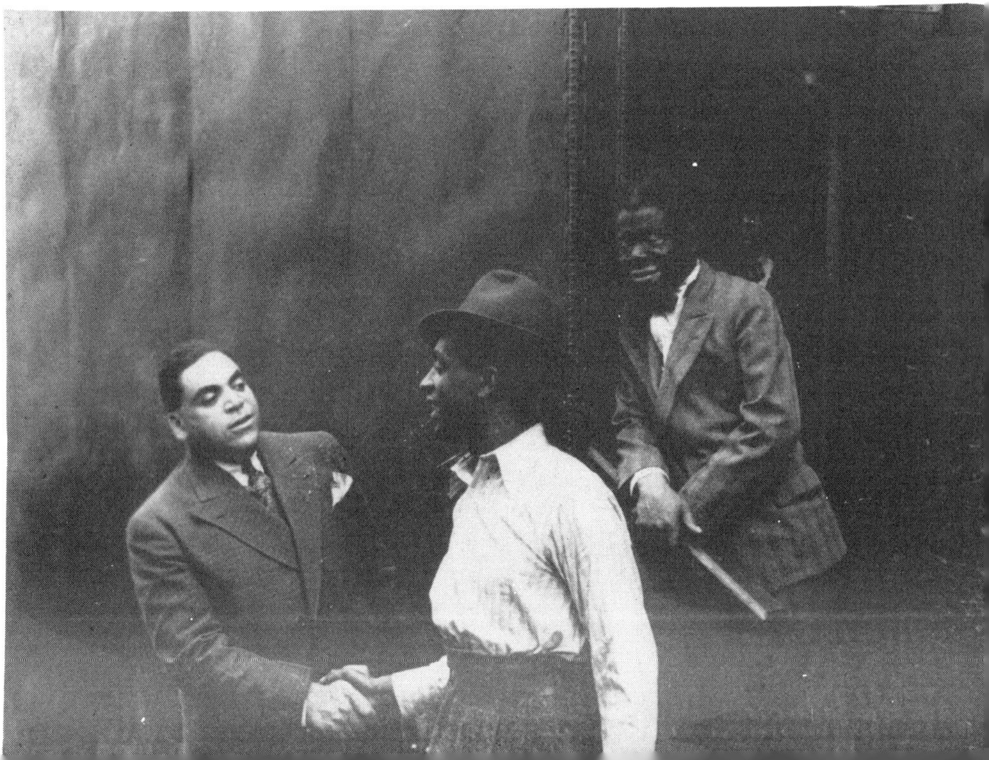

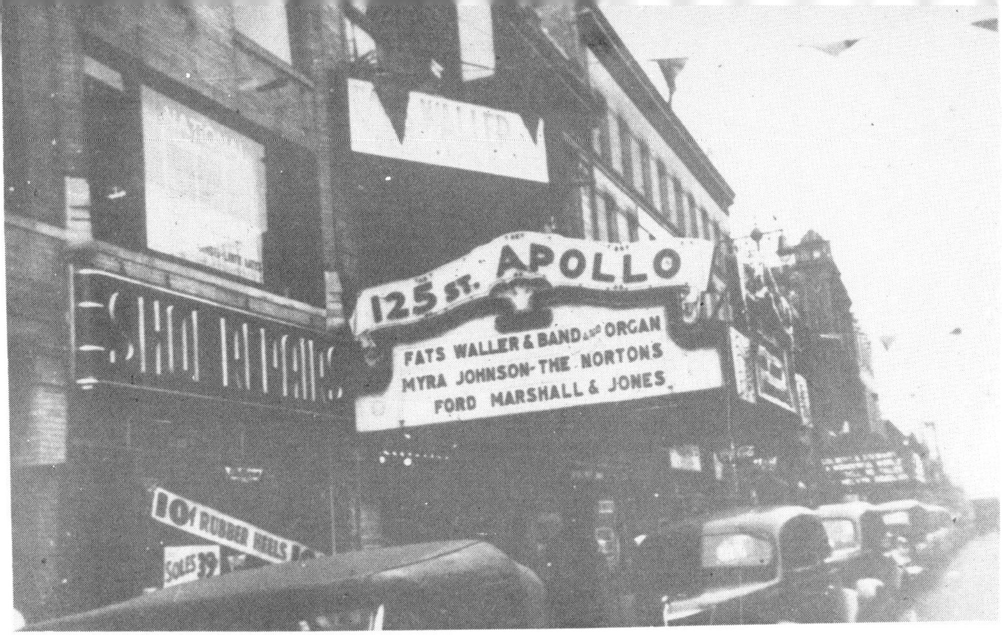

Above: The front of the Apollo at a later date. Below: Fats flies United.

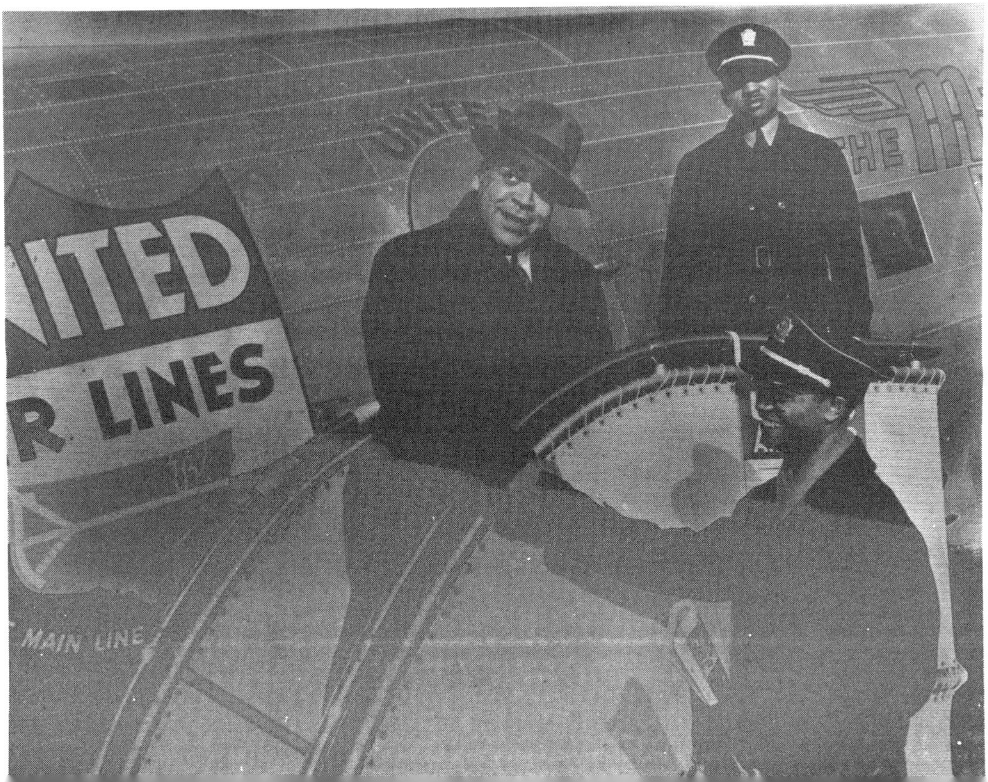

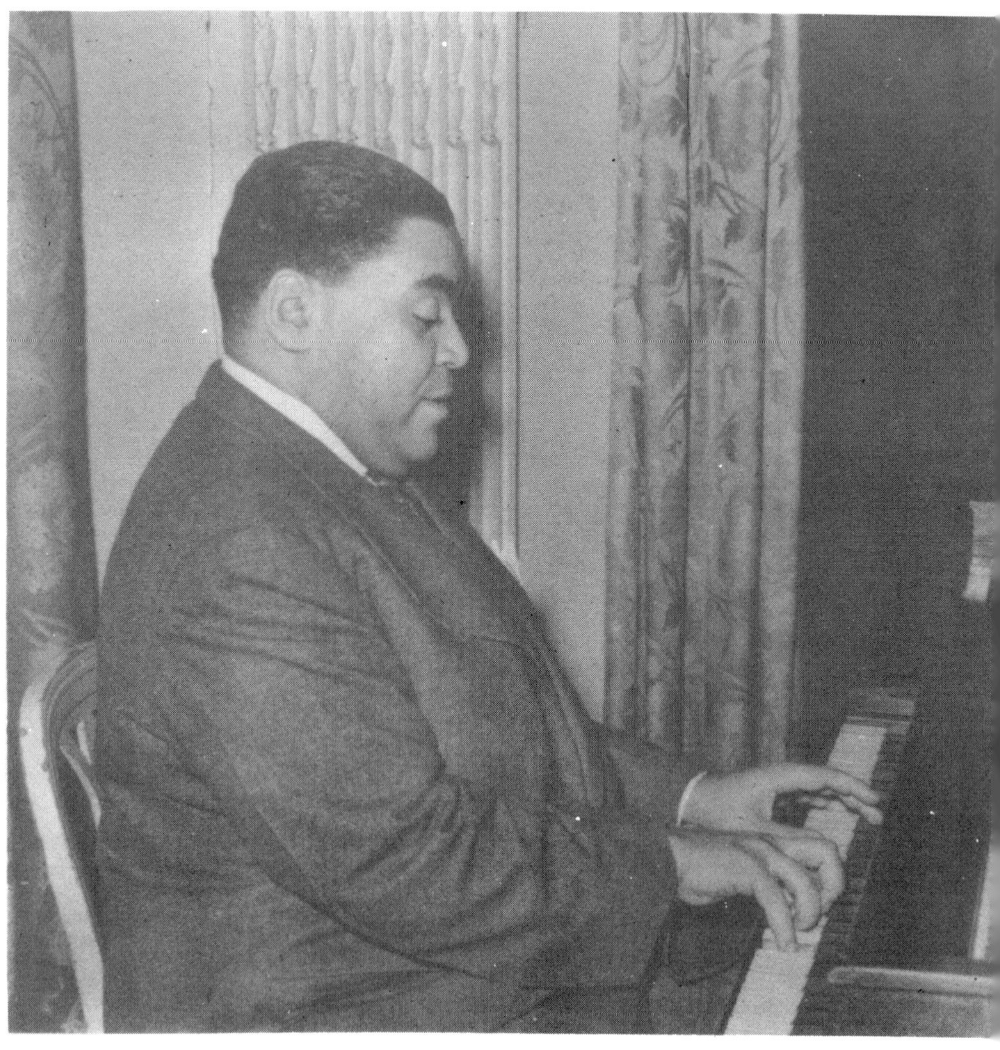

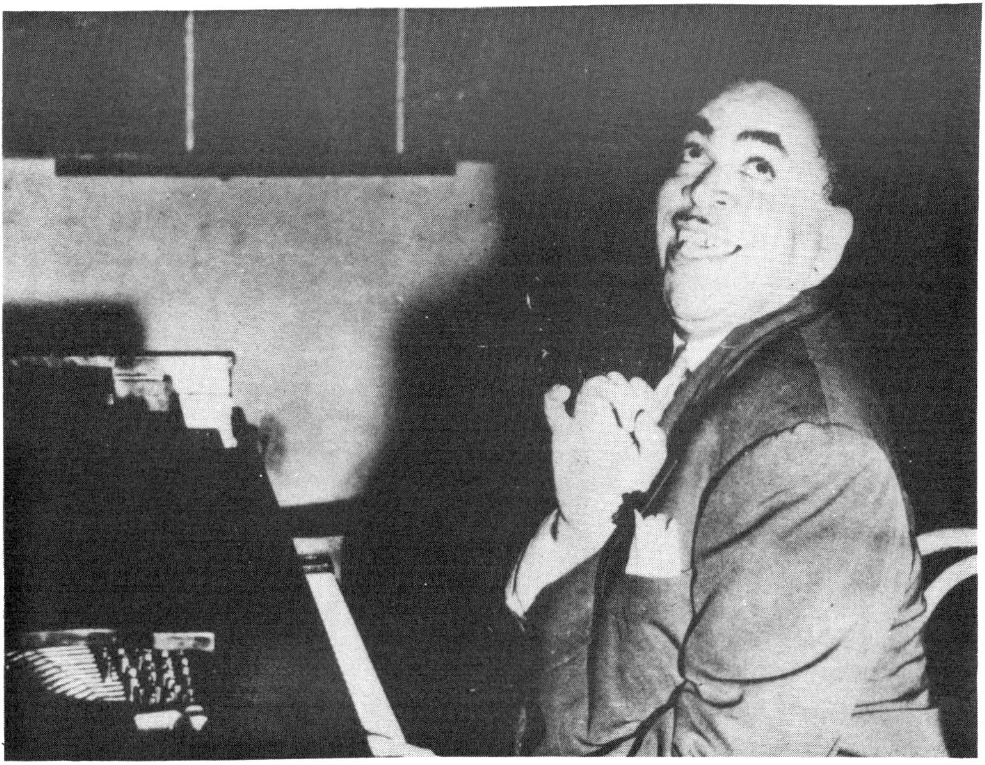

Above: The public image of Waller and on the left the more serious private person.
Below: Two Victor 'Special' labels.

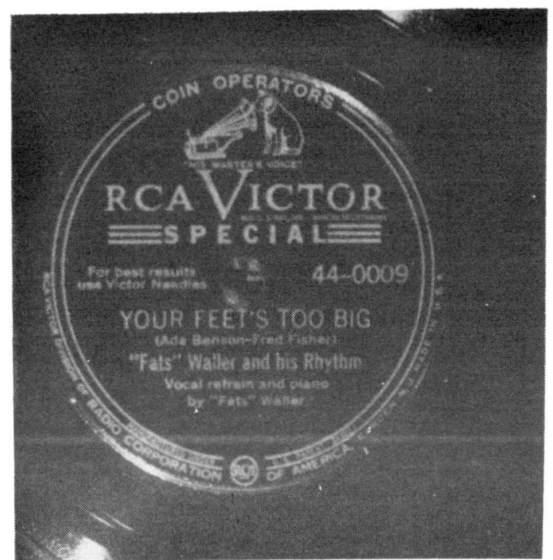

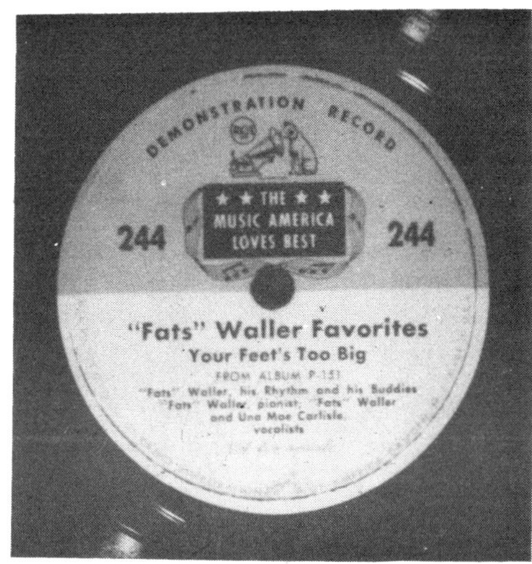

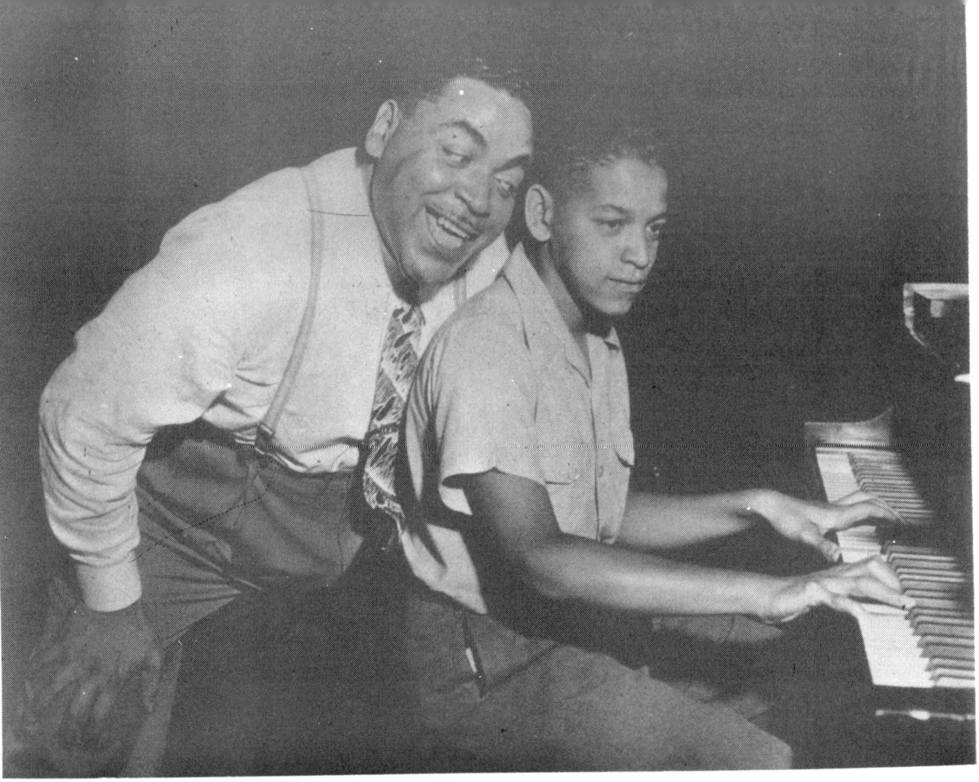

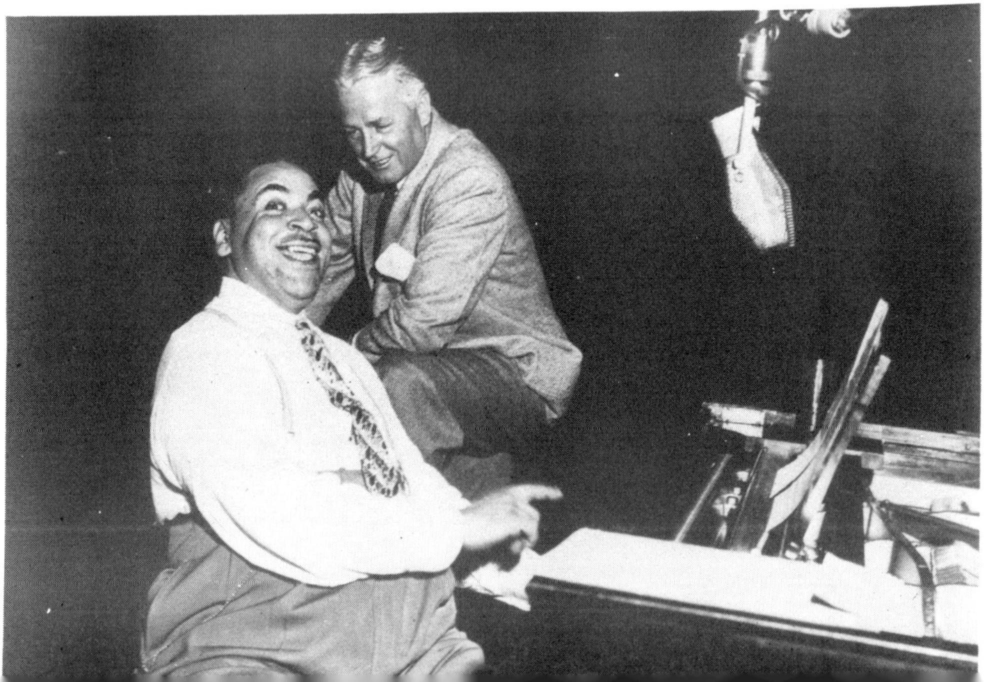

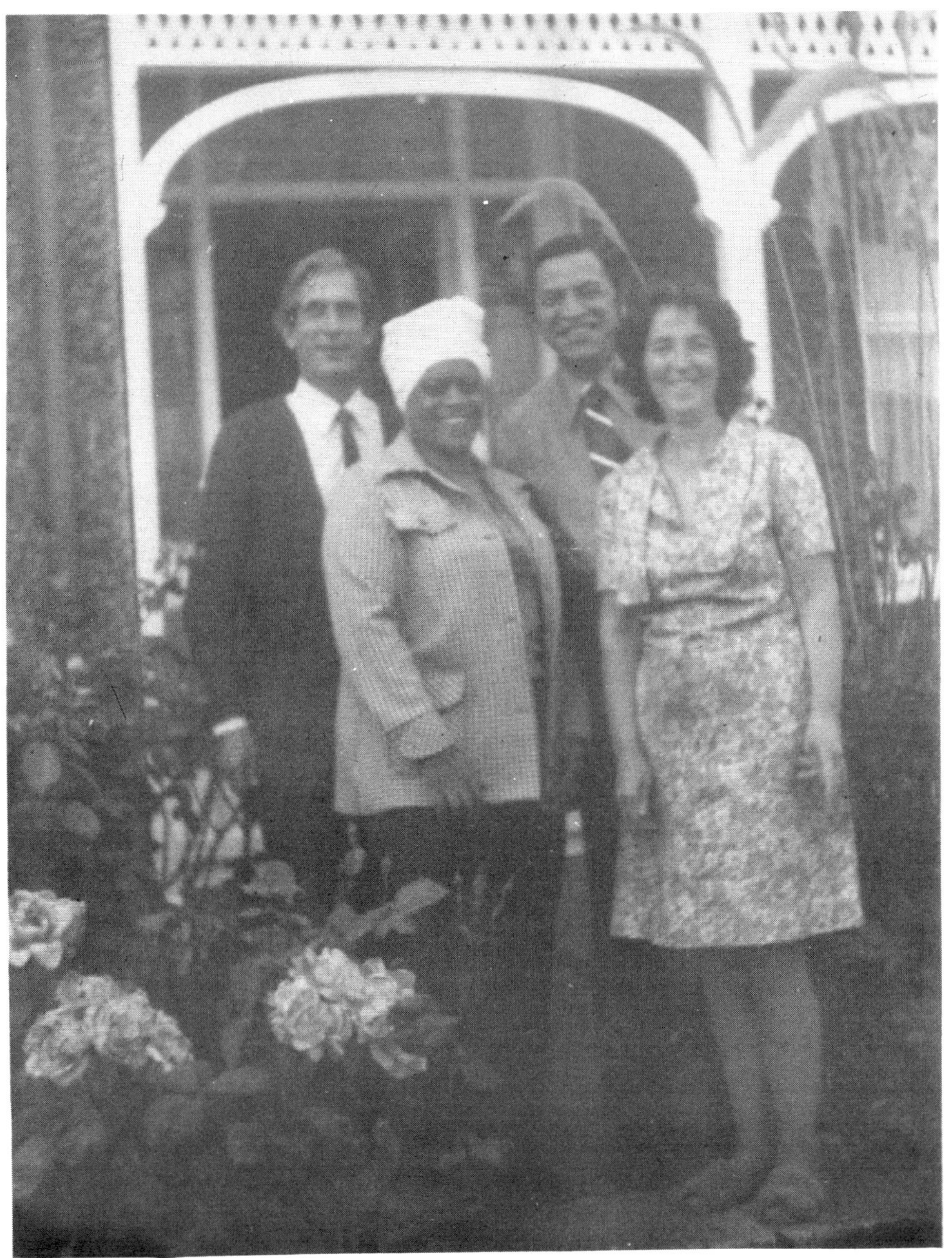

Above: Outside the author's home. L to R: Peter Carr, Mary and Maurice Waller, Peggy Wright.
Left: Two more shots from the final 'Rhythm' session. With his son Maurice and session director Leonard Joy.

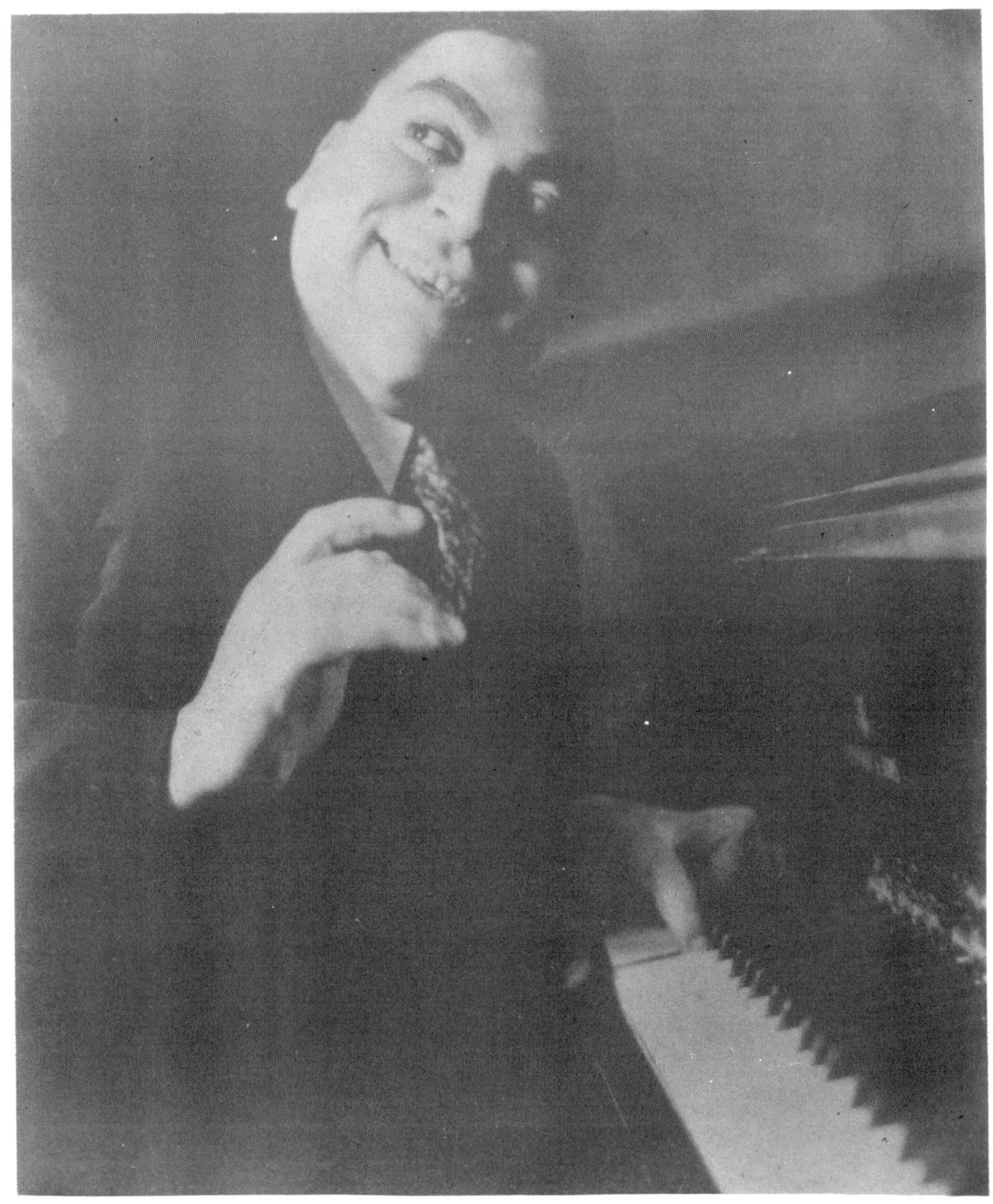

A Bluebird publicity photo and right, an action shot.

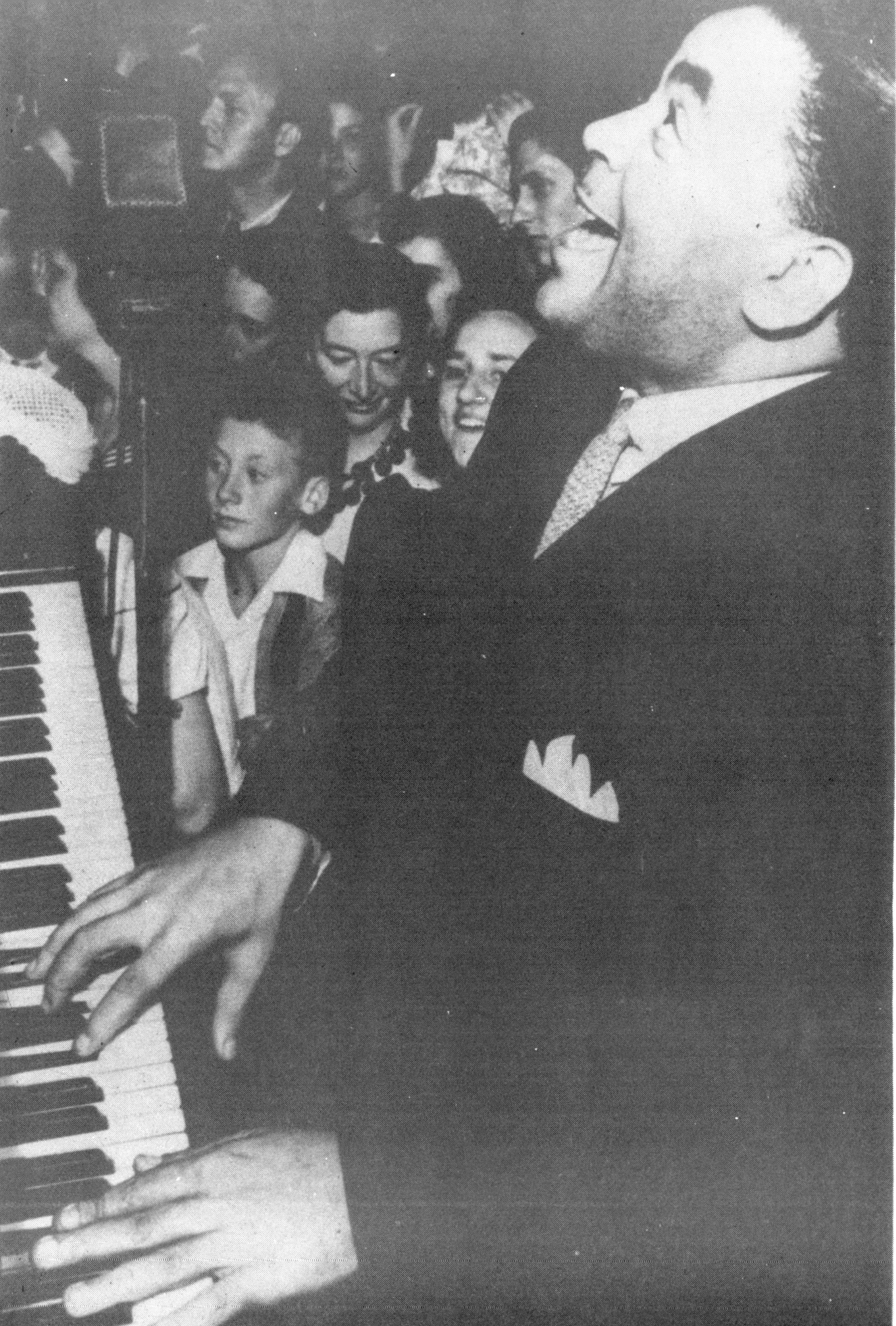

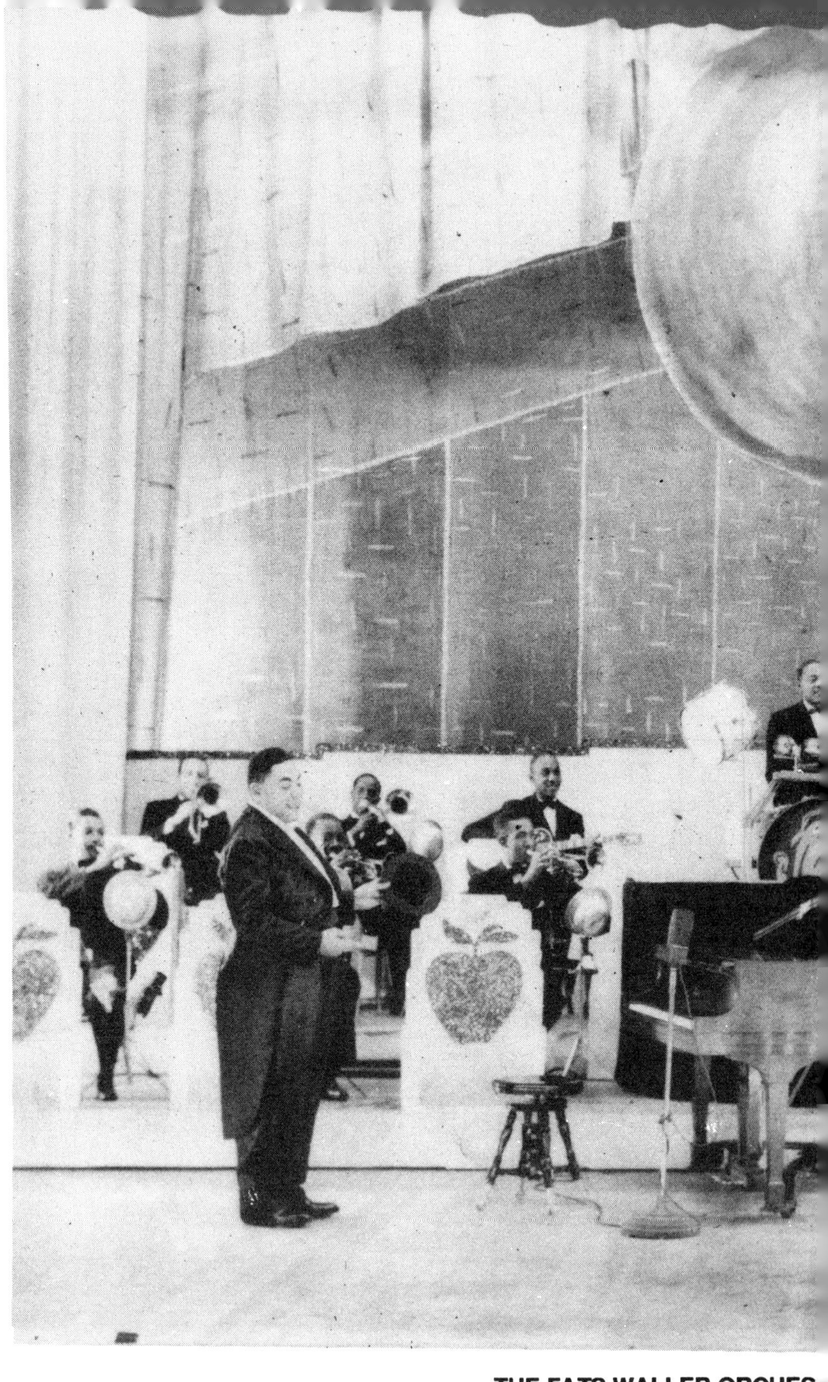

THE FATS WALLER ORCHES

L to R: John Hamilton, George Robinson, Fats, Herman Autrey, John Hau
Simmons, Jimmy Powell, D

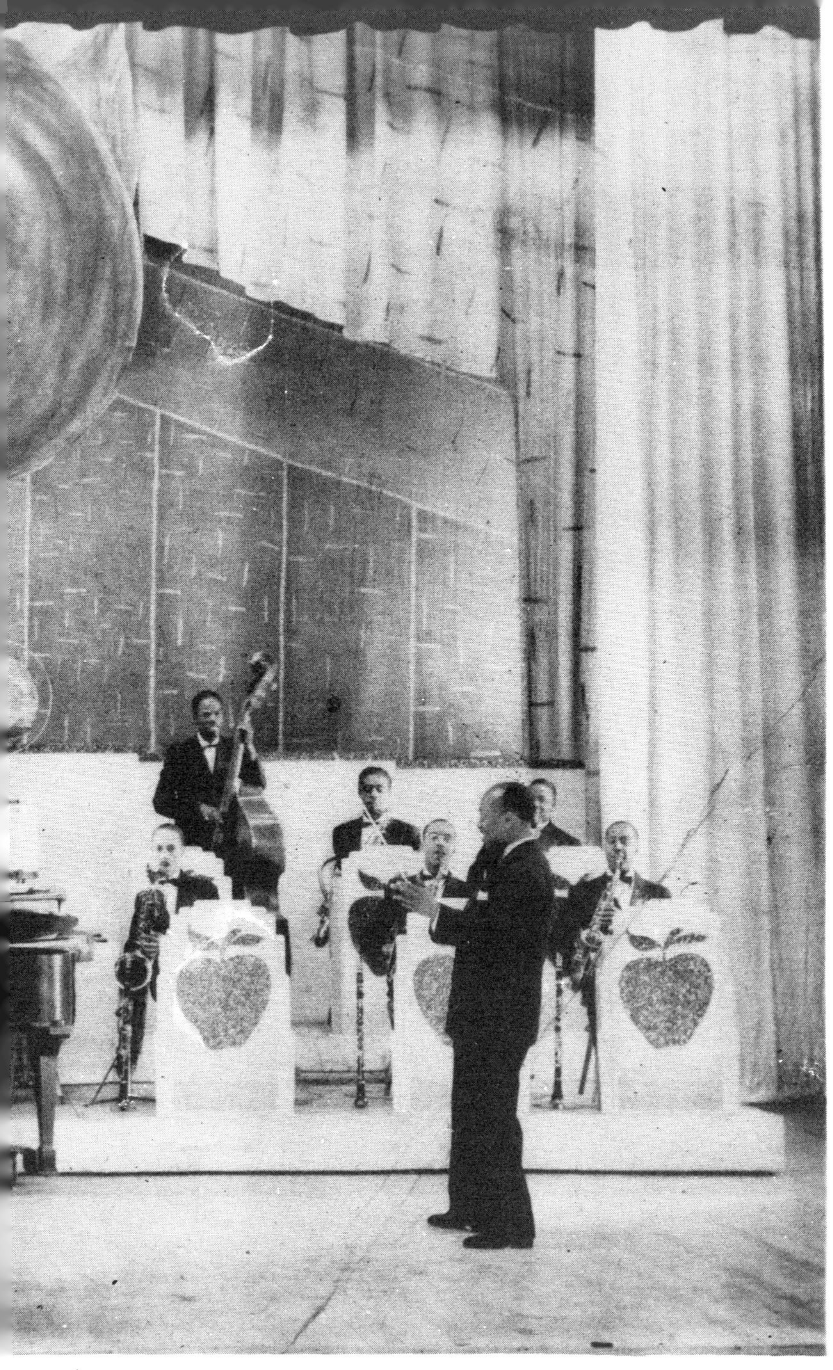

GE IN THE APOLLO THEATRE

ey Williams, Al Casey, Slick Jones, Freddie Skerritt, Cedric Wallace, Lonnie , Gene Sedric and Bill Alsop.

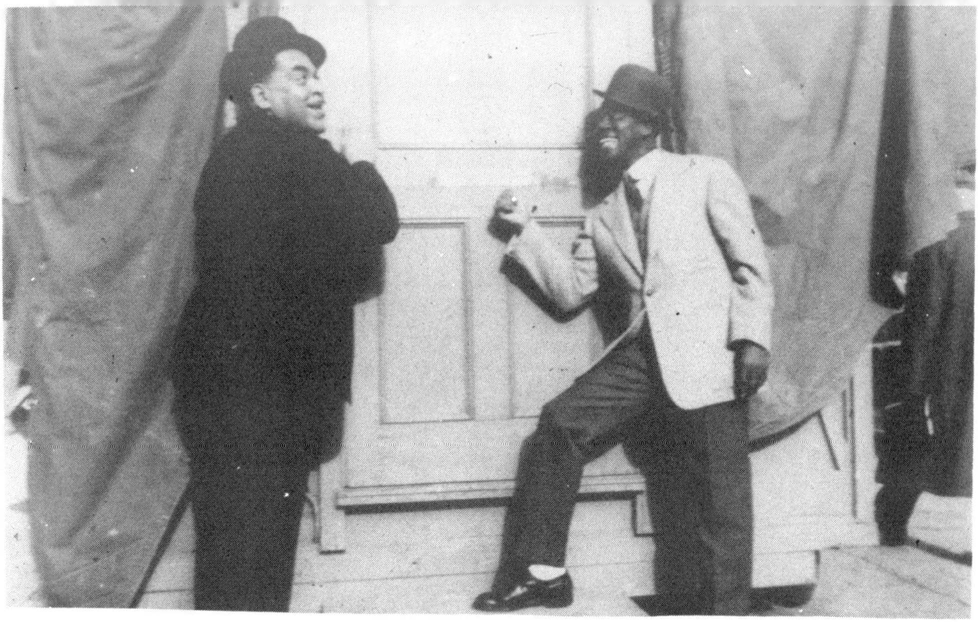

Publicity for *Stormy Weather:* Fats and Bojangles knocking on Lena Horne's dressing room door; Fats with Ada Brown and Lena Horne; at the piano; Ada Brown singing *That Ain't Right.*

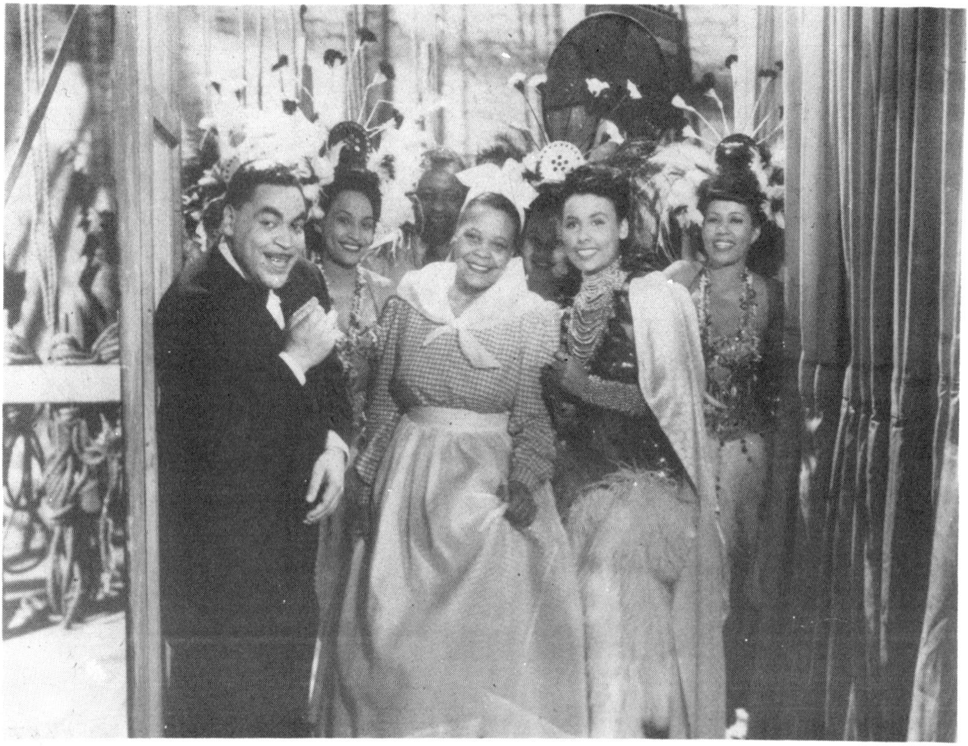

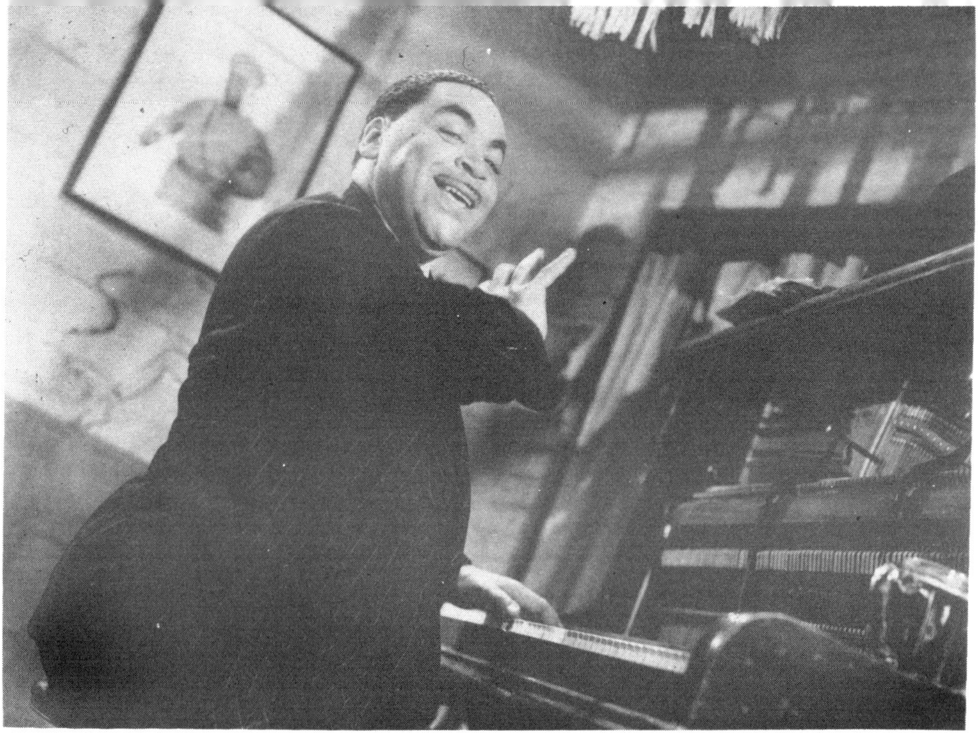

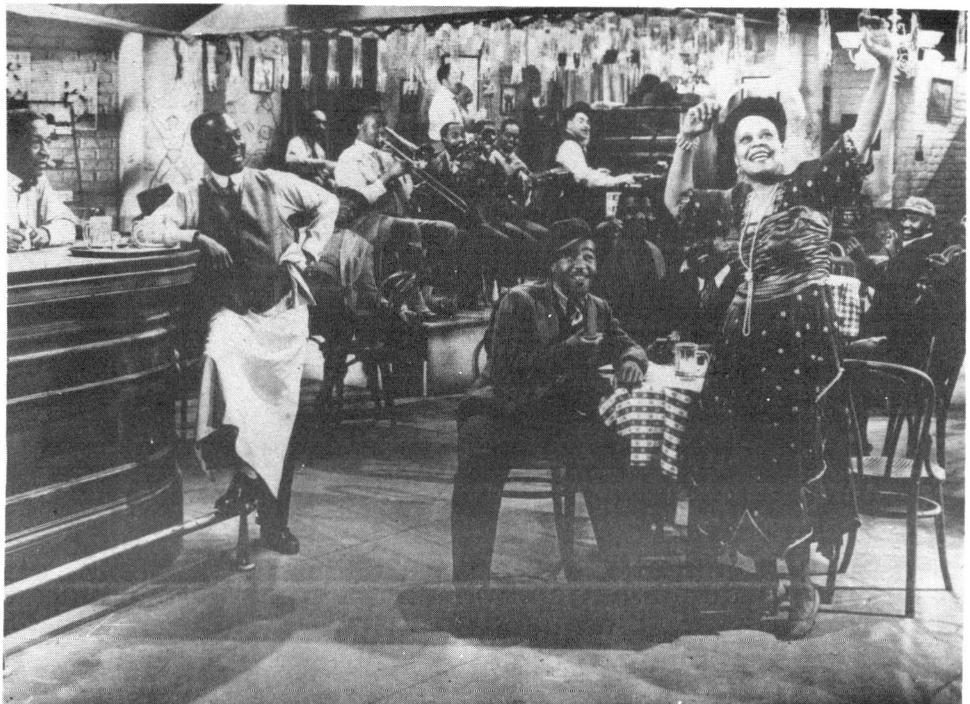

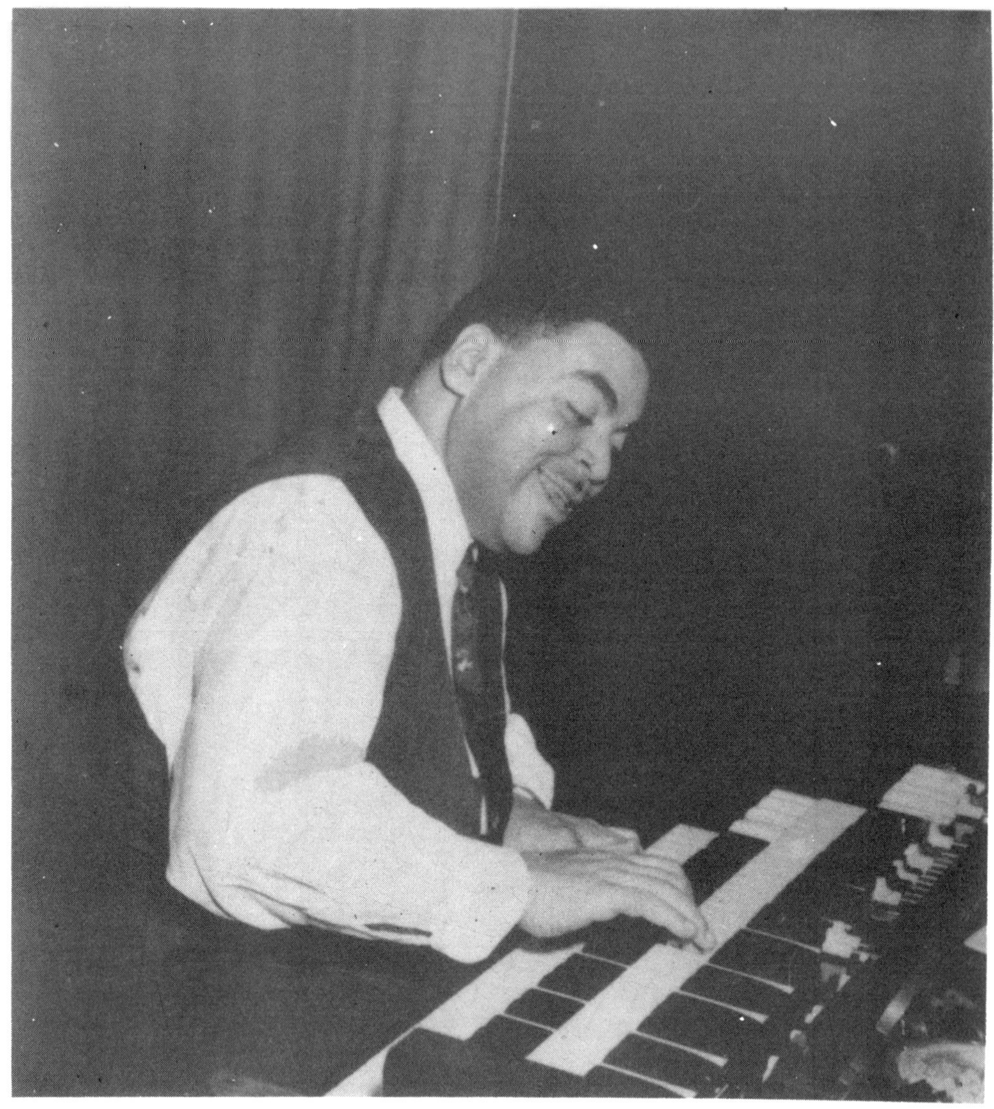

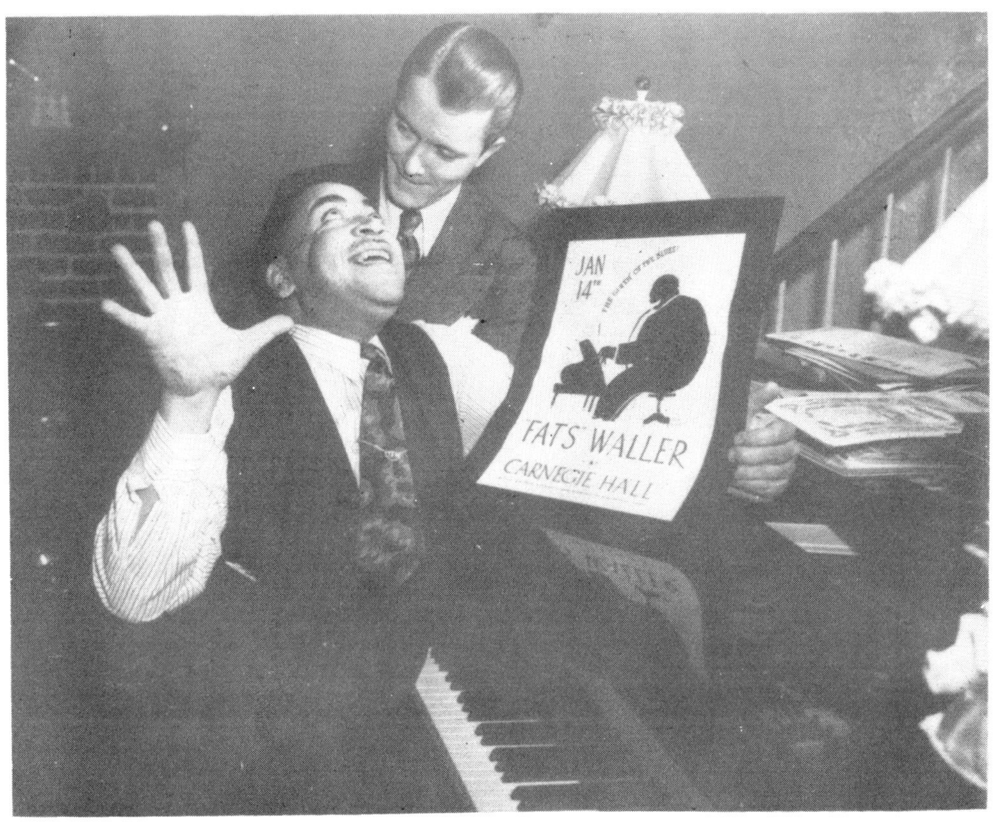

Above: A second pose with Eddie Condon and the Carnegie Concert Poster.
Left: Fats at his favourite instrument.

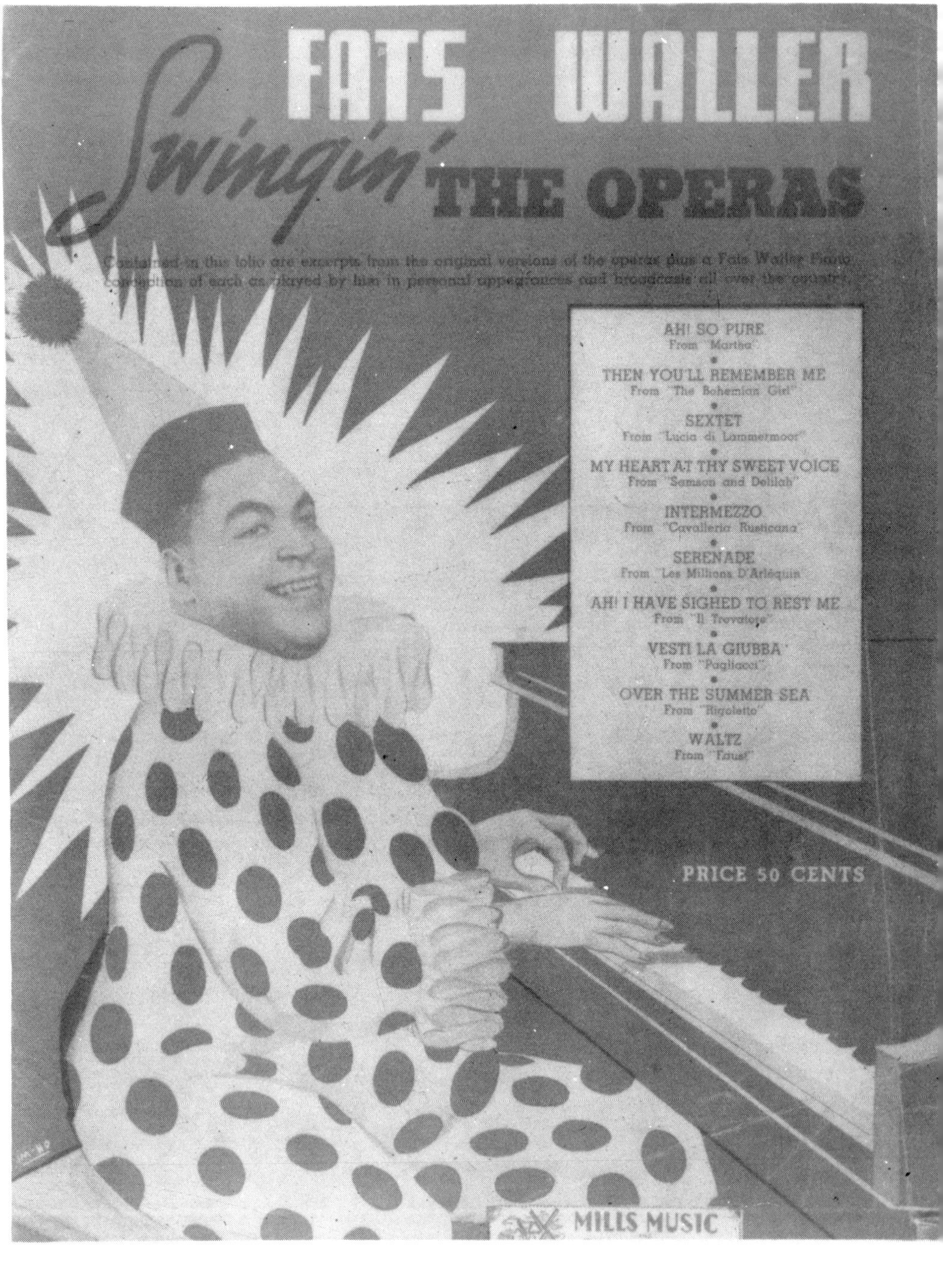

FATS WALLER

Swingin' THE OPERAS

Contained in this folio are excerpts from the original versions of the operas plus a Fats Waller Piano conception of each as played by him in personal appearances and broadcasts all over the country.

AH! SO PURE
From "Martha"

THEN YOU'LL REMEMBER ME
From "The Bohemian Girl"

SEXTET
From "Lucia di Lammermoor"

MY HEART AT THY SWEET VOICE
From "Samson and Delilah"

INTERMEZZO
From "Cavalleria Rusticana"

SERENADE
From "Les Millions D'Arlequin"

AH! I HAVE SIGHED TO REST ME
From "Il Trovatore"

VESTI LA GIUBBA
From "Pagliacci"

OVER THE SUMMER SEA
From "Rigoletto"

WALTZ
From "Faust"

PRICE 50 CENTS

MILLS MUSIC

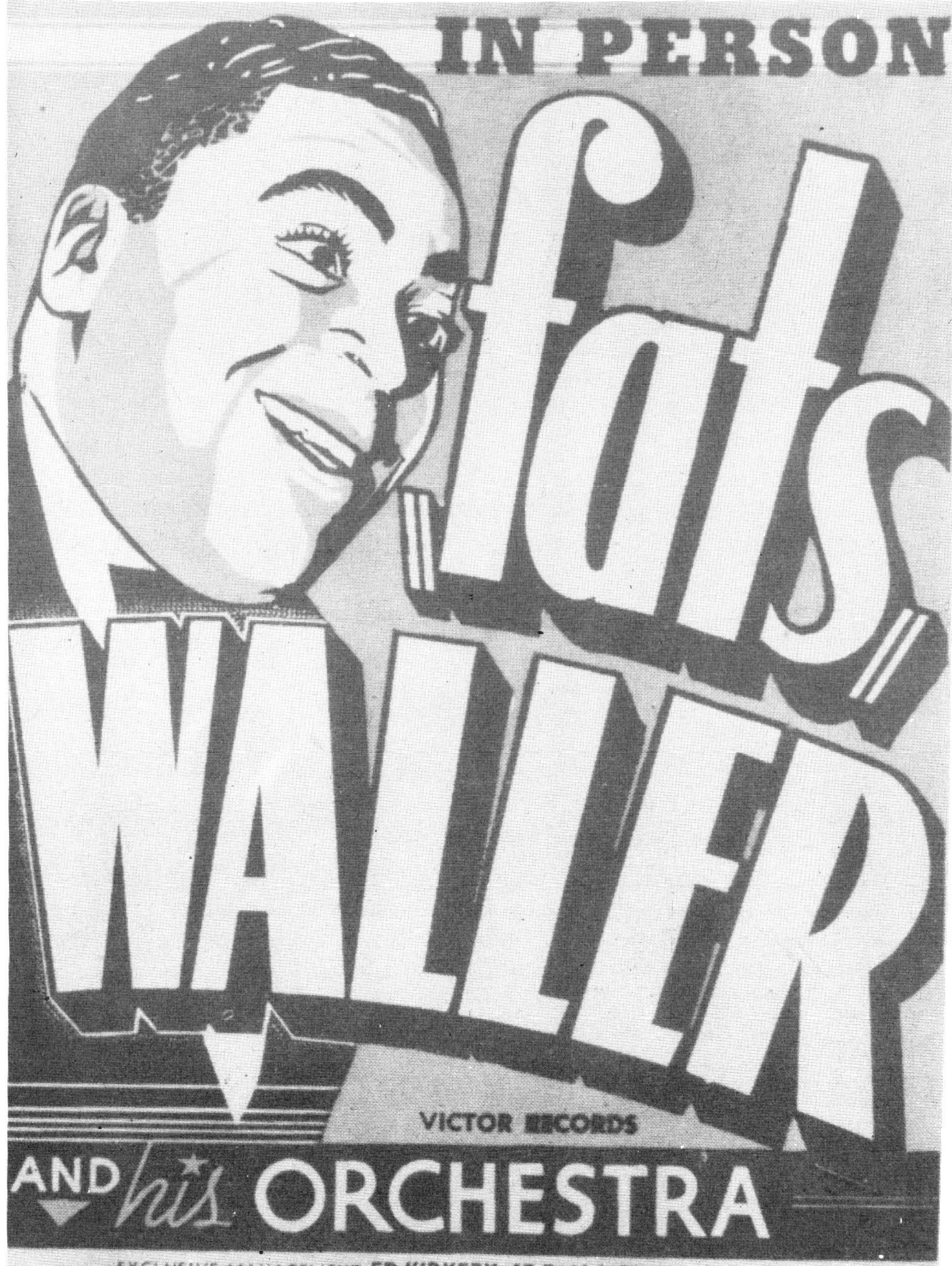

Left: A delightful folio cover from Mills Music. Above: A typical Waller advertising poster.

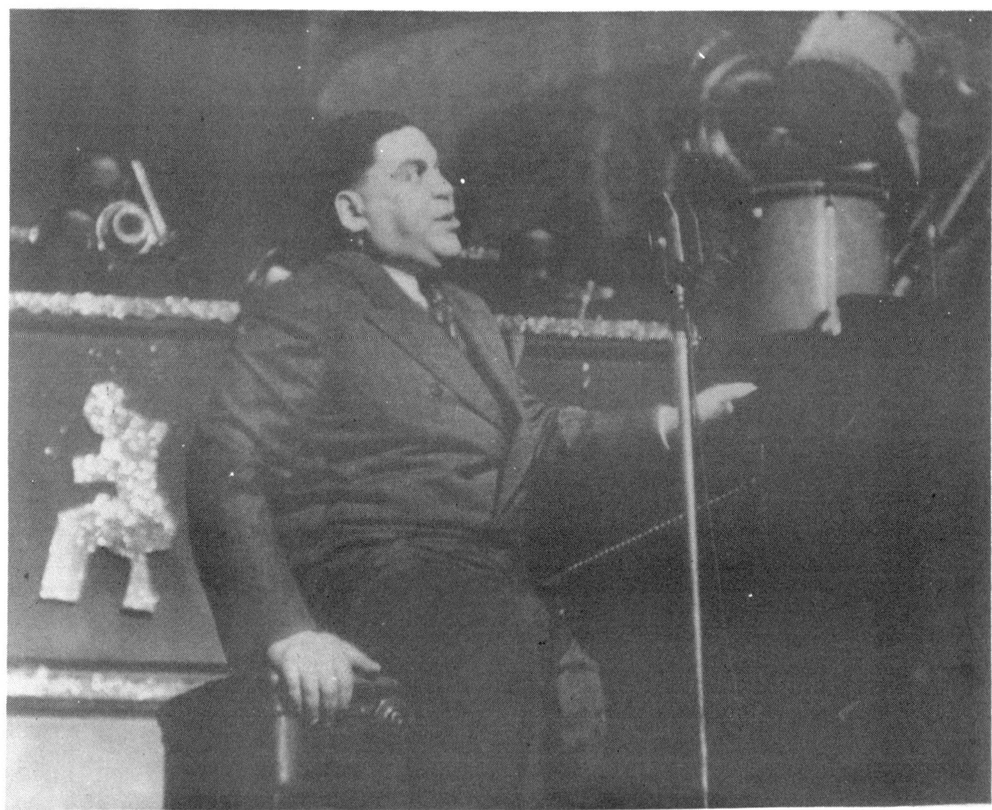

Above: Fats on stage with his orchestra at unknown date.
Top right: Two of Fats's musical collaborators; Andy Razaf and Alex Hill.
Bottom: The two sides of the Fats Waller medal issued by the American Negro Commemorative Society, struck in Sterling Silver. Actual size is 39mm.

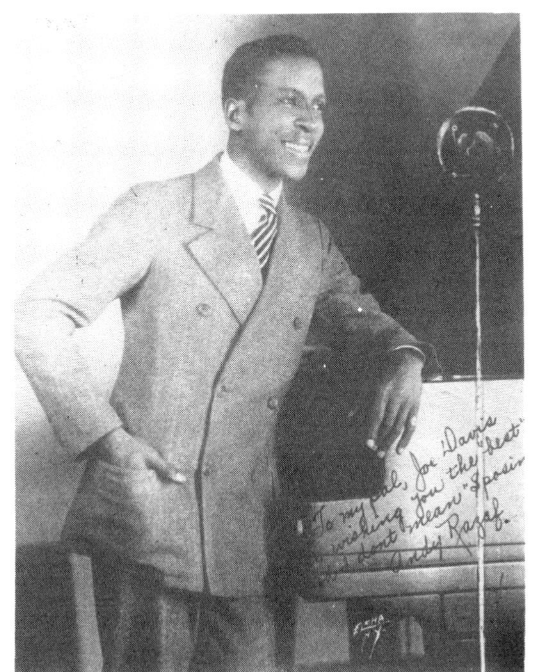
To my pal, Joe Davis
wishing you the "best"
Andy Razaf.

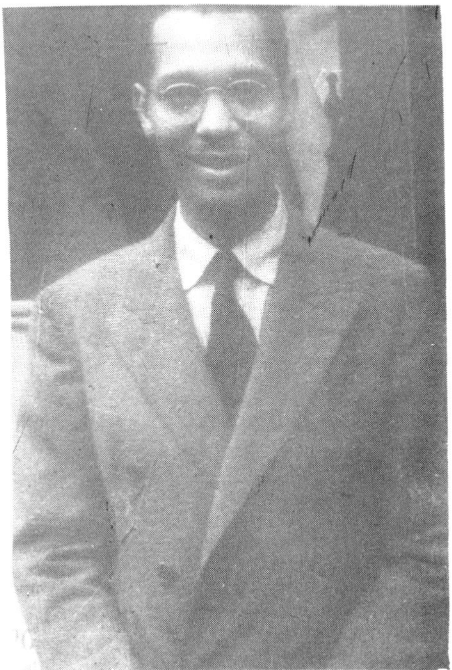

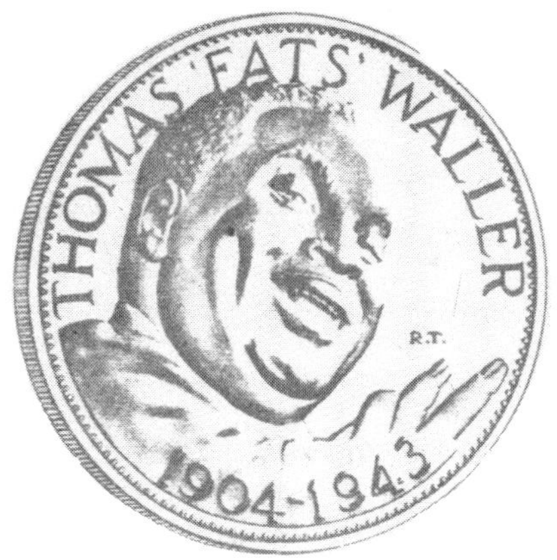
THOMAS 'FATS' WALLER
R.T.
1904-1943

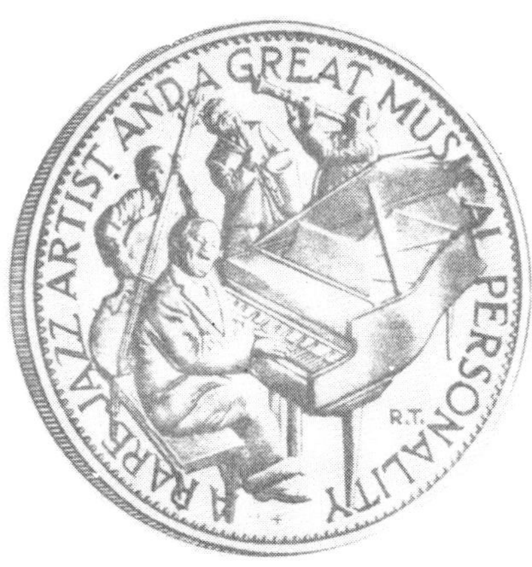
A RARE JAZZ ARTIST AND A GREAT MUSICAL PERSONALITY
R.T.

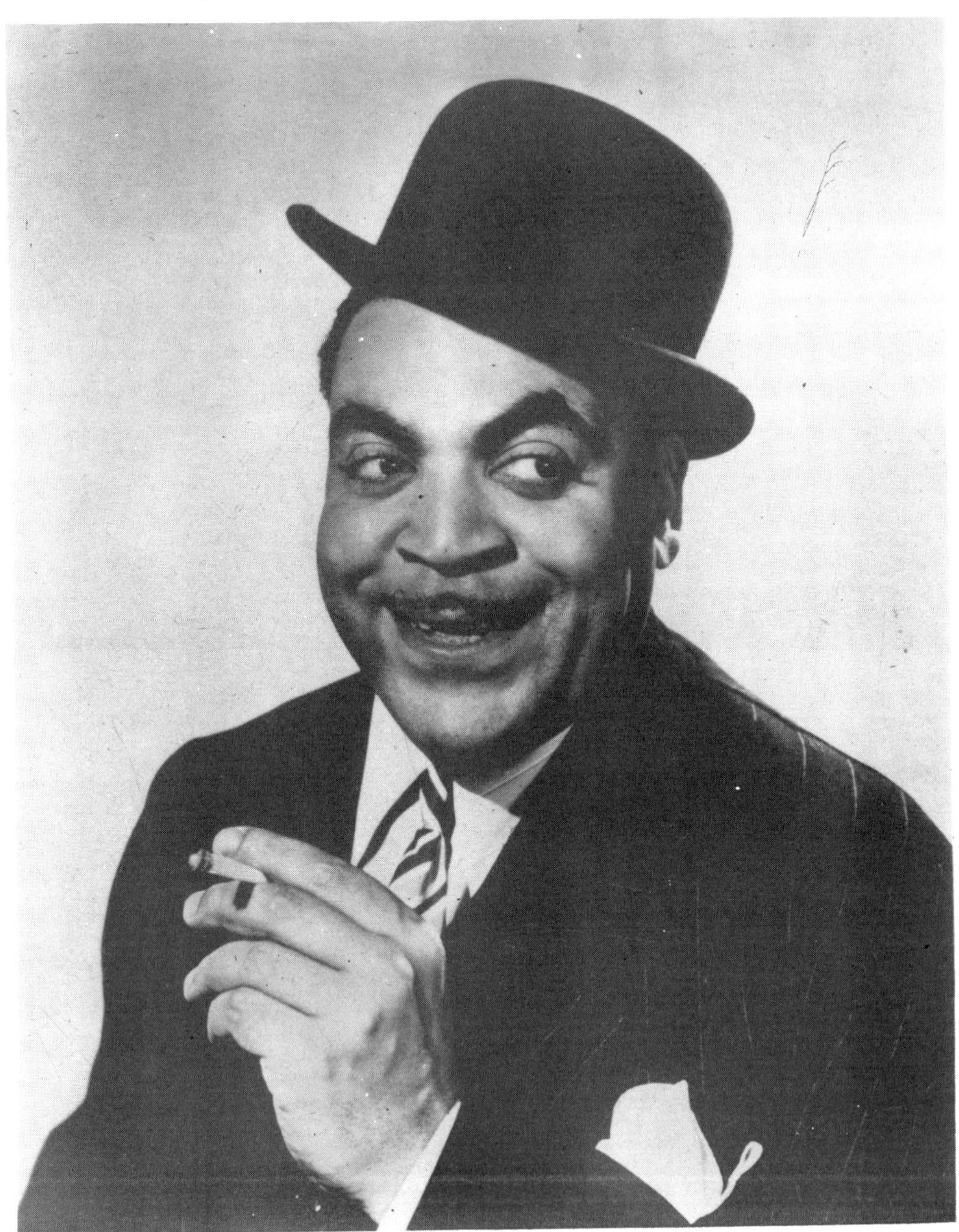

A final publicity still from *Stormy Weather*.

INDEX OF PEOPLE AND PLACES

This index includes all references to musicians, musical personalities and other people of interest, except for Waller himself and his latter-day manager, Ed Kirkeby and the names of artists on the reverses of Waller issues. Also included are musical shows and films (in an *italic face*) and theatres and other locations where Waller performed, plus recording formations which are not identified by the name of the leader. A page reference in bold type indicates an illustration.

INDEX OF TUNE TITLES

This index includes all references to tune titles except for piano rolls and non-Waller items on the reverse sides of Waller issues. A recording is indicated by the use of a **bold face** and where more than one version was made, the formation or instrument involved is noted.

INDEX OF RECORD CATALOGUE NUMBERS

This index lists the pages on which issues will be found, with the sides separated by an oblique stroke. Where the reverse is a non-Waller item this is indicated by a dash and further information will often be found at the foot of the session.

ILLUSTRATIONS

A number of people have contributed photographs and other material to add to my own resources. Special thanks are due to Roy Cooke who, early in this project turned over the files of the "Friends of Fats"; to Frank Driggs who was his usual helpful self and produced many snapshots which have not previously been published, and to Don Peterson, who combed the files of his father, the noted photographer Charles Peterson. Record label photographs are from the collections of Roy Cooke, Ken Crawford, Dave Gladen, Ron Jewson, Roy Rhodes and Laurie Wright.

v Gene Deitch
2 Roy Cooke
7 Laurie Wright
9 Laurie Wright
11 Frank Driggs
27 Laurie Wright
31 Laurie Wright
36 Laurie Wright
41 Laurie Wright
45 Bob Kumm
63 Laurie Wright
64 Laurie Wright
65 Roy Cooke
66 Roy Cooke
75 Frank Driggs
77 Frank Driggs
79 Top: Frank Driggs
Bottom: Duncan Schiedt via Ray Macnic
82 Frank Driggs
92 Harry Dial
108 Neva Peoples via Tom Stoddard
110 Frank Driggs
115 Laurie Wright
116 Laurie Wright
117 Frank Driggs
125 A Charles Peterson Photograph courtesy Don Peterson
133 Roy Cooke
137 A Charles Peterson Photograph courtesy Don Peterson
138 A Charles Peterson Photograph courtesy Don Peterson
141 Frank Driggs
147 Roy Cooke
156 Peter Stroud
157 Laurie Wright
158 Keith Evans
159 Laurie Wright
168 Morten Clausen
171 Royal Library, Copenhagen via Morten Clausen
172 Royal Libary, Copenhagen via Morten Clausen
174 Roy Cooke
176 Engstrøm and Sødring's Music House via Morten Clausen
179 Frank Driggs
183 Alf Lavér
186 Robert Pernet, Léon Dierckx and Georges Debroe
188 Roy Cooke
189 Laurie Wright
194 A Charles Peterson Photograph courtesy Don Peterson
203 Hazel Mundell
204 Hazel Mundell
205 Frank Driggs
206 Frank Driggs
213 Hazel Mundell
218 Frank Driggs
222 Frank Driggs
223 Frank Driggs
225 Frank Driggs

227 Frank Driggs
234 Freddie Skerritt via Frank Driggs
238 Laurie Wright (top)
Freddie Skerritt via Frank Driggs (bottom)
239 Freddie Skerritt via Frank Driggs
240 Freddie Skerritt via Frank Driggs (top)
Frank Driggs (bottom)
242 Frank Driggs
250 John R.T. Davies (top row)
Frank Driggs (remainder)
251 John R.T. Davies (all)
260 Ray Macnic
261 Charlie Peterson via John Heinz
263 Frank Driggs
267 Frank Driggs
268 Roy Cooke
269 Laurie Wright
271 Johnny Simmen
274 Frank Driggs
275 Roy Cooke
279 Frank Driggs (both)
281 Henry Parker
325 A Charles Peterson Photograph courtesy Don Peterson
345 Joey Bushkin via Ralph Sutton
351 Laurie Wright
352 Laurie Wright
363 A Charles Peterson Photograph courtesy Don Peterson
364 A Charles Peterson Photograph courtesy Don Peterson
377 Ernie Anderson (top),
Roy Cooke (bottom)
390 A Charles Peterson Photograph courtesy Don Peterson
392 A Charles Peterson Photograph courtesy Don Peterson
395 A Charles Peterson Photograph courtesy Don Peterson
403 Courtney Williams
475 Wally Fawkes
476 Frank Driggs
477 Frank Driggs
478 Frank Driggs
479 Frank Driggs
480 Laurie Wright
481 Laurie Wright
482 A Charles Peterson Photograph courtesy Don Peterson
483 Frank Driggs
484 Henry Parker (both)
485 Henry Parker
486 Laurie Wright
487 Frank Driggs
488 Roy Cooke (top),
Dave Gladen (bottom)
489 Frank Driggs (top),
Dave Gladen (bottom)
490 Freddie Skerritt via Frank Driggs (both)
491 Freddie Skerritt via Frank Driggs
492 Freddie Skerritt via Frank Driggs (both)
493 Freddie Skerritt via Frank Driggs
494 Andy Wittenborn (top),
Tomas Örnberg (rest)
495 Frank Driggs
496 Roy Cooke
497 A Charles Peterson Photograph courtesy Don Peterson
498 A Charles Peterson Photograph courtesy Don Peterson (both)
499 A Charles Peterson Photograph courtesy Don Peterson (both)
500 A Charles Peterson Photograph courtesy Don Peterson (both)
501 Frank Driggs (top), Roy Cooke (bottom)
502 Bill Andrews
503 Laurie Wright
504 Roy Cooke (top), Frank Driggs (bottom)

505 Laurie Wright
506 Bill Andrews
507 Laurie Wright
508/9 Frank Driggs
510 Frank Driggs (both)
511 Frank Driggs (top),
Roy Cooke (bottom)
512 Bill Andrews
513 Bill Andrews
514 Bill Andrews
515 Laurie Wright
516 Duncan Schiedt via Ray Macnic
517 Bruce Bastin (top L),
Frank Driggs (top R)
Henry Parker (bottom)
518 Frank Driggs

ADDITIONS AND CORRECTIONS

Inevitably in a book of this size and complexity errors will occur and new information will surface too late for inclusion. The following have been noted and additional new information will be given in the pages of *Storyville* magazine from time to time.

Acknowledgements: Please add Dave Dodd

25 Literally on the day this page was being prepared for printing, a cassette arrived from Steven Lasker marked "BVE-36773-2 St. Louis Blues Transferred from a vinyl test." It is somewhat shorter than the issued version (2' 41" compared to 2' 50"), and the fact that it is from a vinyl test indicates that the original metal was still intact in the 1950's.

42 The studio sheet for the Dunn session (courtesy of Steven Lasker) shows that it took place in Room 2 in the morning. The tunes are shown as 'Fox Trot' and 'Blues Fox-Trot' respectively and both bear the note 'Arrangements furnished by publisher' (Perry Bradford Music Co.). Seven men are shown to be present for a 3-hour session and there is an additional note '(Mr. Perry Bradford on date)' from which it might be assumed that he makes the number up to the seven mentioned, unless anyone can hear a banjo.

58 Add figures 1 and 2 to title of matrix 57702.

83 The Italian HMV issue against matrix 84422-1 should read HN727, not 707.

121 Matrix 102019-1 does not appear on HMVIn B.D.5354 (see p.143).

135 I asked Ernie Anderson if he knew of any Waller engagement at the Onyx Club on 52nd Street in 1936 and he replied, "Fats never worked at the Onyx at that time that I know of. Later, he was a fixture at the Yacht Club, one block further west. Stuff Smith & His Onyx Club Boys were the regular attraction. Jonah Jones was always in Stuff's band and you'd usually find Cozy Cole and maybe Buster Bailey. He had a proliferation of piano players before he settled on Clyde Hart. But Fats knew every piano on the Street, and there were a lot of them. Between sets on his own job he often wandered up the street to the Onyx, and if the piano stool happened to be unoccupied he took it over. It was a beatup upright, but the Onyx management kept it properly tuned and Fats liked its action. The barkeep would put a large measure of the best gin on top of the instrument. Then Fats would play for half an hour or so. After that he'd stroll back to the Yacht Club where Fritz Steinway had installed Fats's Steinway Concert Grand which was always in perfect tune. Steinway, whose premises were only five blocks north on 57th Street, invariably saw to this." Thus it would appear that Charlie Peterson had just caught Fats on a casual visit, unless the date on the photograph has been misread and should be 1936 (see page 324).

194 The photograph of Hugues Panassié and Fats in the Yacht Club was taken on 21

October 1938.

195 Howard Rye discovered an item in the December 1938 *International Musician* under the heading "Name Bands" which gives information on a hitherto unknown Waller charity engagement:

The list of bandleaders who contributed to the sell-out success of Local 802 A.F. of M. Medical Fund Benefit at the Manhattan Opera House on November 15 is long and complete. Among those present who played until 5:08 A.M. were: Paul Whiteman, Guy Lombardo, Benny Goodman, Tommy Dorsey, Fats Waller, Eddie DeLange, Jimmie Lunceford, Count Basie, Sammy Kaye, Kay Kyser, Eddy Duchin, Larry Clinton, Richard Himber, Russ Morgan, Ben Bernie, Cab Calloway, Vincent Lopez, Don Redman, Artie Shaw, Al Donahue, Phil Spitalny, Charles Barnet, Edgar Hayes, Merle Pitt, Lucky Millinder, George Hall, Ina Ray Hutton, Wood Herman (sic), *Enoch Light, Will Osborne, Noble Sissle and Les Brown.*

These 32 bands each gave a sample of their music on a stage built on tracks so that it could be shuttled back and forth on the stage proper. By alternately loading and dumping each end of the shuttle affair with bands, music was continuous until the early hours when the crowd of 5,000 fans had had their fill.

197 To further clarify the breakdown of the "This Is New York" broadcast, please add the numeral -4 to Studio Orchestra and add this numeral to the final three titles. There is also speech by Waller and Seldes after the *Introduction* and again after *Harlem* (a name given to a piece which lasts only a few bars, which may be something better known) in which Razaf also speaks.

233 Some of the conflicting reports on this page (and elsewhere in the book), may be the result of 'advance reporting' — in other words, of events which were scheduled, but which, for some reason, did not take place as expected, and were either truncated or cancelled.

Fats in Fact
9780902391147 2

7